This report contains the collective views of an international group of experts and does not necessarily represent the decisions or the stated policy of the International Commission of Non-Ionizing Radiation Protection, the International Labour Organization, or the World Health Organization.

Environmental Health Criteria 238

# EXTREMELY LOW FREQUENCY FIELDS

Published under the joint sponsorship of
the International Labour Organization,
the International Commission on
Non-Ionizing Radiation Protection, and
the World Health Organization.

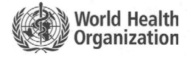

**World Health
Organization**

WHO Library Cataloguing-in-Publication Data

Extremely low frequency fields.

(Environmental health criteria ; 238)

1.Electromagnetic fields. 2.Radiation effects. 3.Risk assessment. 4.Environmental exposure. I.World Health Organization. II.Inter-Organization Programme for the Sound Management of Chemicals. III.Series.

ISBN 978 92 4 157238 5       (NLM classification: QT 34)

ISSN 0250-863X

© **World Health Organization 2007**

# Environmental Health Criteria

CONTENTS

# PREAMBLE

*The WHO Environmental Health Criteria Programme*

In 1973 the World Health Organization (WHO) Environmental Health Criteria Programme was initiated with the following objectives:

(i)     to assess information on the relationship between exposure to environmental pollutants and human health, and to provide guidelines for setting exposure limits;

(ii)    to identify new or potential pollutants;

(iii)   to identify gaps in knowledge concerning the health effects of pollutants;

(iv)    to promote the harmonization of toxicological and epidemiological methods in order to have internationally comparable results.

It should be noted in this context that WHO defines health as the state of complete physical, mental and social well being and not merely the absence of disease or infirmity (WHO, 1946).

The first Environmental Health Criteria (EHC) monograph, on mercury, was published in 1976 and since that time an ever-increasing number of assessments of chemical and of physical agents have been produced. In addition, many EHC monographs have been devoted to evaluating toxicological methodology, e.g. for genetic, neurotoxic, teratogenic and nephrotoxic agents. Other publications have been concerned with epidemiological guidelines, evaluation of short-term tests for carcinogens, biomarkers, effects on the elderly and so forth.

The original impetus for the Programme came from World Health Assembly resolutions and the recommendations of the 1972 UN Conference on the Human Environment. Subsequently the work became an integral part of the International Programme on Chemical Safety (IPCS), a cooperative programme of the United Nations Environment Programme (UNEP), the International Labour Office (ILO) and WHO. With the strong support of the new partners, the importance of occupational health and environmental effects was fully recognized. The EHC monographs have become widely established, used and recognized throughout the world.

*Electromagnetic Fields*

Three monographs on electromagnetic fields (EMF) address possible health effects from exposure to extremely low frequency (ELF) fields, static and ELF magnetic fields, and radiofrequency (RF) fields (WHO, 1984; WHO, 1987; WHO, 1993). They were produced in collaboration with UNEP, ILO and the International Non-Ionizing Radiation Committee (INIRC) of the International Radiation Protection Association (IRPA) and from 1992 the International Commission on Non-Ionizing Radiation Protection (ICNIRP).

xi

EHC monographs are usually revised if new data are available that would substantially change the evaluation, if there is public concern for health or environmental effects of the agent because of greater exposure, or if an appreciable time period has elapsed since the last evaluation. The EHCs on EMF are being revised and will be published as a set of three monographs spanning the relevant EMF frequency range (0–300 GHz); static fields (0 Hz), ELF fields (up to 100 kHz, this volume) and RF fields (100 kHz – 300 GHz).

WHO's assessment of any health risks produced by non-ionizing radiation emitting technologies (in the frequency range 0–300 GHz) falls within the responsibilities of the International EMF Project. This Project was established by WHO in 1996 in response to public concern over health effects of EMF exposure, and is managed by the Radiation and Environmental Health Unit (RAD) which is coordinating the preparation of the EHC Monographs on EMF.

The WHO health risk assessment exercise includes the development of an extensive database that comprises relevant scientific publications. Interpretation of these studies can be controversial, as there exists a spectrum of opinion within the scientific community and elsewhere. In order to achieve as wide a degree of consensus as possible, the health risk assessment also draws on, and in some cases includes sections of, reviews already completed by other national and international expert review bodies, with particular reference to:

- the International Agency for Research on Cancer (IARC) Monograph on static and extremely low frequency (ELF) fields ' IARC, 2002. In June 2001 IARC formally evaluated the evidence for carcinogenesis from exposure to static and ELF fields. The review concluded that ELF magnetic fields are possibly carcinogenic to humans.

- Reviews on physics/engineering, biology and epidemiology commissioned by WHO to the International Commission on Non-Ionizing Radiation Protection (ICNIRP), a non-governmental organization in formal relations with WHO (ICNIRP, 2003).

- Reviews by the Advisory Group on Non-Ionising Radiation (AGNIR) of the Health Protection Agency (HPA), United Kingdom (AGNIR, 2001a; 2001b; 2004; 2006).

*Scope*

The EHC monographs are intended to provide critical reviews on the effect on human health and the environment of chemicals, physical and biological agents. As such, they include and review studies that are of direct relevance for the evaluation. However, they do not describe *every* study carried out. Worldwide data are used and are quoted from original studies, not from abstracts or reviews. Both published and unpublished reports are considered but preference is always given to published data. Unpublished data are only used when relevant published data are absent or when they are pivotal to the risk assessment. A detailed policy statement is available that describes the procedures used for unpublished proprietary data so that this information can be used in the evaluation without compromising its confidential nature (WHO, 1990).

In the evaluation of human health risks, sound human data, whenever available, are generally more informative than animal data. Animal and in vitro studies provide support and are used mainly to supply evidence missing from human studies. It is mandatory that research on human subjects is conducted in full accord with ethical principles, including the provisions of the Helsinki Declaration (WMA, 2004).

All studies, with either positive or negative effects, need to be evaluated and judged on their own merit, and then all together in a weight of evidence approach. It is important to determine how much a set of evidence changes the probability that exposure causes an outcome. Generally, studies must be replicated or be in agreement with similar studies. The evidence for an effect is further strengthened if the results from different types of studies (epidemiology and laboratory) point to the same conclusion.

The EHC monographs are intended to assist national and international authorities in making risk assessments and subsequent risk management decisions. They represent an evaluation of risks as far as the data will allow and are not, in any sense, recommendations for regulation or standard setting. These latter are the exclusive purview of national and regional governments. However, the EMF EHCs do provide bodies such as ICNIRP with the scientific basis for reviewing their international exposure guidelines.

*Procedures*

The general procedures that result in the publication of this EHC monograph are discussed below.

A first draft, prepared by consultants or staff from a RAD Collaborating Centre, is based initially on data provided from reference databases such as Medline and PubMed and on IARC and ICNIRP reviews. The draft document, when received by RAD, may require an initial review by a small panel of experts to determine its scientific quality and objectivity. Once the document is acceptable as a first draft, it is distributed, in its unedited form, to well over 150 EHC contact points throughout the world who are asked to comment on its completeness and accuracy and, where necessary, provide additional material. The contact points, usually designated by governments, may be Collaborating Centres, or individual scientists known for their particular expertise. Generally some months are allowed before the comments are considered by the author(s). A second draft incorporating comments received and approved by the Coordinator (RAD), is then distributed to Task Group members, who carry out the peer review, at least six weeks before their meeting.

The Task Group members serve as individual scientists, not as representatives of their organization. Their function is to evaluate the accuracy, significance and relevance of the information in the document and to assess the health and environmental risks from exposure to the part of the electromagnetic spectrum being addressed. A summary and recommendations for further research and improved safety aspects are also required. The composition of the Task Group is dictated by the range of expertise required for the subject of the meeting (epidemiology, biological and physical sciences, medicine and public health) and by the need for a balance in the range of opinions on the science, gender and geographical distribution.

The membership of the WHO Task Groups is approved by the Assistant Director General of the Cluster on Sustainable Development and Health Environments. These Task Groups are the highest level committees within WHO for conducting health risk assessments.

Task Groups conduct a critical and thorough review of an advanced draft of the ELF EHC monograph and assess any risks to health from exposure to both electric and magnetic fields, reach agreements by consensus, and make final conclusions and recommendations that cannot be altered after the Task Group meeting.

The World Health Organization recognizes the important role played by non-governmental organizations (NGOs). Representatives from relevant national and international associations may be invited to join the Task Group as observers. While observers may provide a valuable contribution to the process, they can only speak at the invitation of the Chairperson. Observers do not participate in the final evaluation; this is the sole responsibility of the Task Group members. When the Task Group considers it to be appropriate, it may meet *in camera.*

All individuals who as authors, consultants or advisers participate in the preparation of the EHC monograph must, in addition to serving in their personal capacity as scientists, inform WHO if at any time a conflict of interest, whether actual or potential, could be perceived in their work. They are required to sign a conflict of interest statement. Such a procedure ensures the transparency and probity of the process.

When the Task Group has completed its review and the Coordinator (RAD) is satisfied as to the scientific consistency and completeness of the document, it then goes for language editing, reference checking, and preparation of camera-ready copy. After approval by the Director, Department of Protection of the Human Environment (PHE), the monograph is submitted to the WHO Office of Publications for printing. At this time a copy of the final draft is sent to the Chairperson and Rapporteur of the Task Group to check the proofs.

*Extremely Low Frequency Environmental Health Criteria*

This EHC addresses the possible health effects of exposure to extremely low frequency (>0 Hz – 100 kHz) electric and magnetic fields. By far the majority of studies concern the health effects resulting from exposure to power frequency (50–60 Hz) magnetic fields; a few studies address the effects of exposure to power frequency electric fields. In addition, a number of studies have addressed the effects of exposure to the very low frequency (VLF, 3–30 kHz) switched gradient magnetic fields used in Magnetic Resonance Imaging, and, more commonly, the weaker VLF fields emitted by visual display units (VDU's) and televisions.

The ELF EHC is organized by disease category; separate expert working groups met in order to develop drafts addressing neurodegenerative disorders (Chapter 7), cardiovascular disorders (Chapter 8), childhood leukaemia (section 11.2.1) and protective measures (Chapter 13). The membership of these expert working groups is given below. Drafts of the other chapters were prepared by consultants, staff from WHO collaborating centres and by RAD Unit staff. These included Prof. Paul Elliot, Imperial College of Science, Technology and Medicine, UK, Prof. Maria Stuchly, University of Victoria, Canada, and Prof. Bernard Veyret, ENSCPB, France, in addition to individuals who were also members of one of the expert working groups and/or the Task Group (see below). The draft chapters were individually reviewed by external referees prior to their collation as a draft document.

The draft EHC was subsequently distributed for external review. Editorial changes and minor scientific points were addressed by a WHO Editorial Group and the final draft was distributed to Task Group members prior to the Task Group meeting.

The Task Group met from October 3–7, 2005 at WHO headquarters in Geneva. The text of the EHC was subsequently edited for clarity and consistency by an Editorial Group consisting of Dr Emilie van Deventer and Dr Chiyoji Ohkubo, both from WHO, Geneva, Switzerland, Dr Rick Saunders, Health Protection Agency, Chilton, UK, Dr Eric van Rongen, Health Council of the Netherlands, Prof. Leeka Kheifets, UCLA School of Public Health, Los Angeles, CA, USA and Dr Chris Portier, NIEHS, Research Triangle Park, NC, USA. Following a final review by the Task Group and scientific and text editing, the EHC was published on the International EMF Projects website on 18 June 2007.

**Participants in the WHO Expert Working Groups**

## WHO Neurodegenerative Disorders Workshop, WHO HQ, Geneva. 12–13 December, 2002

Prof. Anders Ahlbom, Institute of Environmental Medicine, Karolinska Institute, Stockholm, Sweden

Prof. Laurel Beckett, School of Medicine UC Davis, Davis, CA, United States of America

Prof. Colin Blakemore, University of Oxford, Oxford, United Kingdom

Dr Zoreh Davanipour, Roswell Park Cancer Institute, Buffalo, NY, United States of America

Dr Michel Geffard, National Graduate School of Chemistry and Physics of Bordeaux (ENSCPB), Pessac, France

Dr Larry Goldstein, World Health Organization, Geneva, Switzerland

Dr Christoffer Johansen, Institute of Cancer Epidemiology, Copenhagen, Denmark

Dr Leeka Kheifets, World Health Organization, Geneva, Switzerland

Prof. Robert Olsen, Washington State University, Pullman, WA, United States of America

Dr Michael Repacholi, World Health Organization, Geneva, Switzerland

Prof. Eugene Sobel, Roswell Park Cancer Institute, Buffalo, NY, United States of America

## WHO Cardiovascular Disorders Workshop, Stockholm, Sweden, 27–28 May 2003

Prof. Anders Ahlbom, Institute of Environmental Medicine, Karolinska Institute, Stockholm, Sweden

Dr Christoffer Johansen, Institute of Cancer Epidemiology, Copenhagen, Denmark

Dr Leeka Kheifets, World Health Organization, Geneva, Switzerland

Dr Maria Feychting, Institute of Environmental Medicine, Karolinska Institute, Stockholm, Sweden

Dr Jack Sahl, Southern California Edison Co, Upland, CA, United States of America

## WHO Childhood Leukaemia Workshop, NIES, Japan, 16–18 September 2003

Prof. Abdelmonem Afifi, UCLA School of Public Health, Los Angeles, CA, United States of America

Prof. Anders Ahlbom, Institute of Environmental Medicine, Karolinska Institute, Stockholm, Sweden

Dr Emilie van Deventer, World Health Organization, Geneva, Switzerland

Dr Michinori Kabuto, National Institute for Environmental Studies, Tsukuba, Ibariki, Japan

Dr Bill Kaune, EMF Consultant, United States of America.

Prof. Leeka Kheifets, UCLA School of Public Health, Los Angeles, CA, United States of America.

Dr Gabor Mezei, Electric Power Research Institute, Palo Alto, CA, United States of America

Dr Chris Portier, National Institute of Environmental Health Sciences, Research Triangle Park, NC, United States of America

Dr Tomohiro Saito, National Centre for Child Health and Development, Japan

Dr John Swanson, National Grid Transco, London, United Kingdom

Dr Naoto Yamaguchi, Graduate School of Medicine, Tokyo Women's Medical University, Japan

## WHO Protective Measures for ELF EMFs Workshop, NIEHS, USA, 9–11 February, 2005

Dr Robert Bradley, Consumer and Clinical Radiation Protection Bureau, Ottawa, Canada

Mr Abiy Desta, Center for Devices and Radiological Health, Rockville, MD, United States of America

Mrs Shaiela Kandel, Soreq Nuclear Research Center, Yavne, Israel

Prof. Leeka Kheifets, UCLA School of Public Health, Los Angeles, CA, United States of America.

Dr Raymond Neutra, Division of Environmental and Occupational Disease Control, Californai Department of Health Services, Oakland, CA, United States of America

Dr Chris Portier, National Institute of Environmental Health Sciences, Research Triangle Park, NC, United States of America

Dr Michael Repacholi, World Health Organization, Geneva, Switzerland

Dr Jack Sahl, Southern California Edison Company, Upland, CA, United States of America

Dr John Swanson, National Grid Transco, London, United Kingdom

Dr Mary Wolfe, National Institute of Environmental Health Sciences, Research Triangle Park, NC, United States of America

## Task Group on ELF electric and magnetic fields, Geneva, 3–7 October, 2005

*Members*

Prof. Anders Ahlbom, Institute of Environmental Medicine, Karolinska Institute, Stockholm, Sweden

Dr Larry Anderson, Battelle Pacific Northwest National Laboratory, Richland, WA, United States of America

Dr Christoffer Johansen, Institute of Cancer Epidemiology, Copenhagen, Denmark

Dr Jukka Juutilainen, University of Kuopio, Kuopio, Finland

Dr Michinori Kabuto, National Institute for Environmental Studies, Tsukuba, Ibariki, Japan

Mrs Shaiela Kandel, Soreq Nuclear Research Center, Yavne, Israel

Prof. Leeka Kheifets, UCLA School of Public Health, Los Angeles, CA, United States of America

Dr Isabelle Lagroye, National Graduate School of Chemistry and Physics of Bordeaux (ENSCPB), Pessac, France

Dipl-Ing Rüdiger Matthes, Federal Office for Radiation Protection, Oberschleissheim, Germany

Prof. Jim Metcalfe, University of Cambridge, Cambridge, United Kingdom

Prof. Meike Mevissen, Institut für Tiergenetik, Bern, Switzerland

Prof. Junji Miyakoshi, Hirosaki University, Hirosaki, Japan

Dr Alastair McKinlay, Health Protection Agency, Chilton, United Kingdom

Dr Shengli Niu, International Labour Organization, Geneva, Switzerland

Dr Chris Portier, National Institute of Environmental Health Sciences, Research Triangle Park, NC, United States of America

Dr Eric van Rongen, Health Council of the Netherlands, The Hague, The Netherlands

Dr Nina Rubtsova, RAMS Institute of Occupational Health, Moscow, Russian Federation

Dr Paolo Vecchia, National Institute of Health, Rome, Italy

Prof. Barney de Villiers, University of Stellenbosch, Cape Town, South Africa

Prof. Andrew Wood, Swinburne University of Technology, Melbourne, Australia

Prof. Zhengping Xu, Zhejiang University School of Medicine, Hangzhou, China

*Observers*

Mr Kazuhiko Chikamoto, Japan NUS Co., Minato-Ku, Tokyo, Japan

Dr Robert Kavet, Electric Power Research Institute, Palo Alto, CA, United States of America

Prof. Hamilton Moss de Souza, CEPEL - Electrical Energy Research Center, Adrianópolis, Brazil

Dr Michel Plante, Hydro-Québec, Montreal, Canada

Dr Martine Souques, EDF Gaz de France, Paris, France

Dr John Swanson, National Grid Transco, London, United Kingdom

*WHO Secretariat*

Dr Houssain Abouzaid, World Health Organization – Regional Office for the Eastern Mediterranean (EMRO), Nasr City, Cairo, Egypt

Dr Emilie van Deventer, World Health Organization, Geneva, Switzerland

Dr Chiyoji Ohkubo, World Health Organization, Geneva , Switzerland

Dr Michael Repacholi, World Health Organization, Geneva, Switzerland

Dr Rick Saunders, c/o World Health Organization, Health Protection Agency, Chilton, United Kingdom

# ACKNOWLEDGEMENTS

This monograph represents the most thorough health risk assessment currently available on extremely low frequency electric and magnetic fields. WHO acknowledges and thanks all contributors to this important publication.

In particular, thanks go to the experts that drafted the initial version of the various chapters, including Prof. Paul Elliot, Prof. Maria Stuchly, and Prof. Bernard Veyret, the members of the Working Groups and the members of the Task Group.

Special thanks go to Dr Eric van Rongen, from the Health Council of the Netherlands, and Dr Rick Saunders, from the Health Protection Agency, United Kingdom, for their continuing work throughout the development of this monograph, and to Prof. Leeka Kheifets, who continued her involvement in the development of the document long after she left WHO.

WHO also acknowledges the generous support of the Health Council of the Netherlands for providing the scientific and language editing, and for performing the final layout of the document.


Dr. Emilie van Deventer
Acting Coordinator, Radiation and Environmental Health
World Health Organization
1 June 2007

# ABBREVIATIONS

| | |
|---|---|
| AC | alternating current |
| ACTH | adrenocorticotropic hormone |
| AD | Alzheimer's disease |
| AF | attributable fraction |
| AGNIR | Advisory Group on Non-Ionising Radiation |
| ALL | acute lymphocytic leukaemia |
| ALS | amyotrophic lateral sclerosis |
| AMI | acute myocardial infarction |
| AML | acute myeloid leukaemia |
| aMT6s | 6-sulphatoxymelatonin |
| AN | attributable number |
| BP | benzo(a)pyrene |
| CA | chromosomal aberrations |
| CAM | cell adhesion molecule |
| CBPI | cytokinesis-blocked proliferation index |
| CI | confidence interval |
| CNS | central nervous system |
| Con-A | concanavalin-A |
| Cx | connexin |
| DC | direct current |
| DENA | diethylnitrosamine |
| DMBA | 7,12-dimethylbenz(a)anthracene |
| DNA | desoxyribonucleic acid |
| EAS | electronic access and security system |
| EBCLIS | electric blanket cancer Long Island study |
| ECG | electrocardiogram |
| EEG | electroencephalograms |
| EHC | Environmental Health Criteria |
| ELF | extremely low frequency |
| EM | electromagnetic |
| EMF | electromagnetic fields |
| ENU | N-ethyl-N-nitrosourea |
| ER | estrogen receptor |
| ERP | evoked or event-related potentials |
| ES | embryonic stem cells |
| FDTD | finite-difference time-domain |
| FFT | fast Fourier transformation |
| FSH | follicle stimulating hormone |
| GABA | gamma-aminobutyric acid |
| GCS | ceramide glucosyltransferase |
| GH | growth hormone |
| GJIC | gap junction intercellular communication |
| H2O2 | hydrogenperoxyde |
| HIOMT | hydroxyindole-O-methyltransferase |
| HRV | heart rate variability |

| | |
|---|---|
| HSF | heat shock factor |
| hsp | heat shock protein |
| IARC | International Agency for Research on Cancer |
| ICNIRP | International Commission on Non-Ionizing Radiation Protection |
| IEEE | Institute of Electrical and Electronic Engineers |
| IEI | idiopathic environmental intolerance |
| IFN | interferon |
| Ig | immunoglobulin |
| IL | interleukin |
| JEM | job-exposure matrix |
| LAK | lymphokine activated killer |
| LH | luteinising hormone |
| LIBCSP | Long Island breast cancer study project |
| LPS | lipopolysaccharide |
| LTP | long-term potentiation |
| MBM | mouse bone marrow |
| MN | micronucleus |
| MRI | magnetic resonance imaging |
| mRNA | messenger ribonucleic acid |
| MS | multiple sclerosis |
| NA | noradrenaline |
| NADH | nicotinamide adenine dinucleotide |
| NADPH | nicotinamide adenine dinucleotide phosphate |
| NAT | N-acetyl-transferase enzyme |
| NDI | nuclear division index |
| NGF | nerve growth factor |
| NHL | non-Hodgkin lymphoma |
| NIEHS | National Institute for Environmental Health Sciences |
| NIOHS | National Institute for Occupational Safety and Health |
| NK | natural killer |
| NMDA | N-methyl-D-aspartate |
| NMU | N-methylnitrosurea |
| NO | nitric oxide |
| NRPB | National Radiological Protection Board |
| ODC | ornithine decarboxylase |
| OHCC | ordinary high current configuration |
| 8-OhdG | 8-hydroxydeoxyguanine |
| OLCC | ordinary low current configuration |
| OR | odds ratio |
| PAGE | poly-acrylamide gel electrophoresis |
| PARP | poly-ADP ribose polymerase |
| PBMC | peripheral blood mononuclear cells |
| PHA | phytohemagglutinin |
| PKC | protein kinase C |
| RAD | Radiation and Environmental Health Unit |
| RF | radiofrequency |
| RFID | radiofrequency identification |
| RNS | reactive nitrogen species |

| ROS | reactive oxygen species |
|---|---|
| RR | relative risk |
| SCE | sister chromatid exchange |
| SD | standard deviation |
| SES | socioeconomic status |
| SMR | standardized mortality ratio |
| SIR | standardized incidence ratio |
| SPFD | scalar potential finite difference |
| SRR | standardized relative mortality risk ratio |
| TGFR | transforming growth factor- receptor |
| TMS | transcranial magnetic stimulation |
| TNF | tumour necrosis factor |
| TNFR | tumour necrosis factor receptor |
| TPA | 12-0-tetradecanoylphorbol-13-acetate |
| TSH | thyroid-stimulating hormone |
| TWA | time-weighted average |
| UG | underground |
| UKCCSI | United Kingdom childhood cancer study investigators |
| ULF | ultra low frequency |
| UV | ultraviolet |
| VDU | visual display unit |
| VHCC | very high current configuration |
| VLCC | very low current configuration |
| VLF | very low frequency |
| WBC | white blood cell |
| WHO | World Health Organization |

## Units

| A | ampere |
|---|---|
| kA | kiloampere, $10^3$ ampere |
| eV | electronvolt |
| F | farad |
| $\mu$F | microfarad, $10^{-6}$ farad |
| Hz | hertz |
| kHz | kilohertz, $10^3$ hertz |
| MHz | megahertz, $10^9$ hertz |
| J | joule |
| kJ | kilojoule, $10^3$ joule |
| M | molar |
| nM | nanomolar, $10^{-9}$ molar |
| N | newton |
| pN | piconewton, $10^{-12}$ newton |
| V | volt |
| kV | kilovolt, $10^3$ volt |
| mV | millivolt, $10^{-3}$ volt |
| $\mu$V | microvolt, $10^{-6}$ volt |

| | |
|---|---|
| T | tesla |
| kT | kilotesla, $10^3$ tesla |
| mT | millitesla, $10^{-3}$ tesla |
| μT | microtesla, $10^{-6}$ tesla |
| nT | nanotesla, $10^{-9}$ tesla |
| W | watt |
| kW | kilowatt, $10^3$ watt |
| Ω | ohm |
| kΩ | kiloohm, $10^3$ ohm |

# 1 SUMMARY AND RECOMMENDATIONS FOR FURTHER STUDY

This Environmental Health Criteria (EHC) monograph addresses the possible health effects of exposure to extremely low frequency (ELF) electric and magnetic fields. It reviews the physical characteristics of ELF fields as well as the sources of exposure and measurement. However, its main objectives are to review the scientific literature on the biological effects of exposure to ELF fields in order to assess any health risks from exposure to these fields and to use this health risk assessment to make recommendations to national authorities on health protection programs.

The frequencies under consideration range from above 0 Hz to 100 khz. By far the majority of studies have been conducted on power-frequency (50 or 60 Hz) magnetic fields, with a few studies using power-frequency electric fields. In addition, there have been a number of studies concerning very low frequency (VLF, 3–30 kHz) fields, switched gradient magnetic fields used in magnetic resonance imaging, and the weaker VLF fields emitted by visual display units and televisions.

This chapter summarizes the main conclusions and recommendations from each section as well as the overall conclusions of the health risk assessment process. The terms used in this monograph to describe the strength of evidence for a given health outcome are as follows. Evidence is termed "limited" when it is restricted to a single study or when there are unresolved questions concerning the design, conduct or interpretation of a number of studies. "Inadequate" evidence is used when the studies cannot be interpreted as showing either the presence or absence of an effect because of major qualitative or quantitative limitations, or when no data are available.

Key gaps in knowledge were also identified and the research needed to fill these gaps has been summarized in the section entitled "Recommendations for research".

## 1.1 Summary

### 1.1.1 Sources, measurements and exposures

Electric and magnetic fields exist wherever electricity is generated, transmitted or distributed in power lines or cables, or used in electrical appliances. Since the use of electricity is an integral part of our modern lifestyle, these fields are ubiquitous in our environment.

The unit of electric field strength is volts per metre ($V\ m^{-1}$) or kilovolts per metre ($kV\ m^{-1}$) and for magnetic fields the flux density is measured in tesla (T), or more commonly in millitesla (mT) or microtesla ($\mu T$) is used.

Residential exposure to power-frequency magnetic fields does not vary dramatically across the world. The geometric-mean magnetic field in homes ranges between 0.025 and 0.07 $\mu T$ in Europe and 0.055 and 0.11 $\mu T$ in the USA. The mean values of the electric field in the home are in the range of several tens of volts per metre. In the vicinity of certain appliances, the instantaneous magnetic-field values can be as much as a few hundred microtesla. Near power lines, magnetic fields reach approximately 20 µT and electric fields up to several thousand volts per metre.

Few children have time-averaged exposures to residential 50 or 60 Hz magnetic fields in excess of the levels associated with an increased incidence of childhood leukaemia (see section 1.1.10). Approximately 1% to 4% have mean exposures above 0.3 µT and only 1% to 2% have median exposures in excess of 0.4 µT.

Occupational exposure, although predominantly to power-frequency fields, may also include contributions from other frequencies. The average magnetic field exposures in the workplace have been found to be higher in "electrical occupations" than in other occupations such as office work, ranging from 0.4–0.6 µT for electricians and electrical engineers to approximately 1.0 µT for power line workers, with the highest exposures for welders, railway engine drivers and sewing machine operators (above 3 µT). The maximum magnetic field exposures in the workplace can reach approximately 10 mT and this is invariably associated with the presence of conductors carrying high currents. In the electrical supply industry, workers may be exposed to electric fields up to 30 kV m$^{-1}$.

### 1.1.2    Electric and magnetic fields inside the body

Exposure to external electric and magnetic fields at extremely low frequencies induces electric fields and currents inside the body. Dosimetry describes the relationship between the external fields and the induced electric field and current density in the body, or other parameters associated with exposure to these fields. The locally induced electric field and current density are of particular interest because they relate to the stimulation of excitable tissue such as nerve and muscle.

The bodies of humans and animals significantly perturb the spatial distribution of an ELF electric field. At low frequencies the body is a good conductor and the perturbed field lines outside the body are nearly perpendicular to the body surface. Oscillating charges are induced on the surface of the exposed body and these induce currents inside the body. The key features of dosimetry for the exposure of humans to ELF electric fields are as follows:

•    The electric field inside the body is normally five to six orders of magnitude smaller than the external electric field.

•    When exposure is mostly to the vertical field, the predominant direction of the induced fields is also vertical.

•    For a given external electric field, the strongest induced fields are for the human body in perfect contact through the feet with ground (electrically grounded) and the weakest induced fields are for the body insulated from the ground (in "free space").

2

- The total current flowing in a body in perfect contact with ground is determined by the body size and shape (including posture), rather than tissue conductivity.

- The distribution of induced currents across the various organs and tissues is determined by the conductivity of those tissues

- The distribution of an induced electric field is also affected by the conductivities, but less so than the induced current.

- There is also a separate phenomenon in which the current in the body is produced by means of contact with a conductive object located in an electric field.

For magnetic fields, the permeability of tissue is the same as that of air, so the field in tissue is the same as the external field. The bodies of humans and animals do not significantly perturb the field. The main interaction of magnetic fields is the Faraday induction of electric fields and associated current densities in the conductive tissues. The key features of dosimetry for the exposure of humans to ELF magnetic fields are as follows:

- The induced electric field and current depend on the orientation of the external field. Induced fields in the body as a whole are greatest when the field is aligned from the front to the back of the body, but for some individual organs the highest values are for the field aligned from side to side.

- The weakest electric fields are induced by a magnetic field oriented along the vertical body axis.

- For a given magnetic field strength and orientation, higher electric fields are induced in larger bodies.

- The distribution of the induced electric field is affected by the conductivity of the various organs and tissues. These have a limited effect on the distribution of induced current density.

### 1.1.3   Biophysical mechanisms

Various proposed direct and indirect interaction mechanisms for ELF electric and magnetic fields are examined for plausibility, in particular whether a "signal" generated in a biological process by exposure to a field can be discriminated from inherent random noise and whether the mechanism challenges scientific principles and current scientific knowledge. Many mechanisms become plausible only at fields above a certain strength. Nevertheless, the lack of identified plausible mechanisms does not rule out the possibility of health effects even at very low field levels, provided basic scientific principles are adhered to.

Of the numerous proposed mechanisms for the direct interaction of fields with the human body, three stand out as potentially operating at lower field levels than the others: induced electric fields in neural networks, radical pairs and magnetite.

3

Electric fields induced in tissue by exposure to ELF electric or magnetic fields will directly stimulate single myelinated nerve fibres in a biophysically plausible manner when the internal field strength exceeds a few volts per metre. Much weaker fields can affect synaptic transmission in neural networks as opposed to single cells. Such signal processing by nervous systems is commonly used by multicellular organisms to detect weak environmental signals. A lower bound on neural network discrimination of 1 mV m$^{-1}$ has been suggested, but based on current evidence, threshold values around 10–100 mV m$^{-1}$ seem to be more likely.

The radical pair mechanism is an accepted way in which magnetic fields can affect specific types of chemical reactions, generally increasing concentrations of reactive free radicals in low fields and decreasing them in high fields. These increases have been seen in magnetic fields of less than 1 mT. There is some evidence linking this mechanism to navigation during bird migration. Both on theoretical grounds and because the changes produced by ELF and static magnetic fields are similar, it is suggested that power-frequency fields of much less than the geomagnetic field of around 50 $\mu$T are unlikely to be of much biological significance.

Magnetite crystals, small ferromagnetic crystals of various forms of iron oxide, are found in animal and human tissues, although in trace amounts. Like free radicals, they have been linked to orientation and navigation in migratory animals, although the presence of trace quantities of magnetite in the human brain does not confer an ability to detect the weak geomagnetic field. Calculations based on extreme assumptions suggest a lower bound for the effects on magnetite crystals of ELF fields of 5 $\mu$T.

Other direct biophysical interactions of fields, such as the breaking of chemical bonds, the forces on charged particles and the various narrow bandwidth "resonance" mechanisms, are not considered to provide plausible explanations for the interactions at field levels encountered in public and occupational environments.

With regard to indirect effects, the surface electric charge induced by electric fields can be perceived, and it can result in painful microshocks when touching a conductive object. Contact currents can occur when young children touch, for example, a tap in the bathtub in some homes. This produces small electric fields, possibly above background noise levels, in bone marrow. However, whether these present a risk to health is unknown.

High-voltage power lines produce clouds of electrically charged ions as a consequence of corona discharge. It is suggested that they could increase the deposition of airborne pollutants on the skin and on airways inside the body, possibly adversely affecting health. However, it seems unlikely that corona ions will have more than a small effect, if any, on long-term health risks, even in the individuals who are most exposed.

None of the three direct mechanisms considered above seem plausible causes of increased disease incidence at the exposure levels generally encountered by people. In fact they only become plausible at levels orders of

4

magnitude higher and indirect mechanisms have not yet been sufficiently investigated. This absence of an identified plausible mechanism does not rule out the possibility of adverse health effects, but it does create a need for stronger evidence from biology and epidemiology.

### 1.1.4 Neurobehaviour

Exposure to power-frequency electric fields causes well-defined biological responses, ranging from perception to annoyance, through surface electric charge effects. These responses depend on the field strength, the ambient environmental conditions and individual sensitivity. The thresholds for direct perception by 10% of volunteers varied between 2 and 20 kV m$^{-1}$, while 5% found 15–20 kV m$^{-1}$ annoying. The spark discharge from a person to ground is found to be painful by 7% of volunteers in a field of 5 kV m$^{-1}$. Thresholds for the discharge from a charged object through a grounded person depend on the size of the object and therefore require specific assessment.

High field strength, rapidly pulsed magnetic fields can stimulate peripheral or central nerve tissue; such effects can arise during magnetic resonance imaging (MRI) procedures, and are used in transcranial magnetic stimulation. Threshold induced electric field strengths for direct nerve stimulation could be as low as a few volts per metre. The threshold is likely to be constant over a frequency range between a few hertz and a few kilohertz. People suffering from or predisposed to epilepsy are likely to be more susceptible to induced ELF electric fields in the central nervous system (CNS). Furthermore, sensitivity to electrical stimulation of the CNS seems likely to be associated with a family history of seizure and the use of tricyclic antidepressants, neuroleptic agents and other drugs that lower the seizure threshold.

The function of the retina, which is a part of the CNS, can be affected by exposure to much weaker ELF magnetic fields than those that cause direct nerve stimulation. A flickering light sensation, called magnetic phosphenes or magnetophosphenes, results from the interaction of the induced electric field with electrically excitable cells in the retina. Threshold induced electric field strengths in the extracellular fluid of the retina have been estimated to lie between about 10 and 100 mV m$^{-1}$ at 20 Hz. There is, however, considerable uncertainty attached to these values.

The evidence for other neurobehavioural effects in volunteer studies, such as the effects on brain electrical activity, cognition, sleep, hypersensitivity and mood, is less clear. Generally, such studies have been carried out at exposure levels below those required to induce the effects described above, and have produced evidence only of subtle and transitory effects at best. The conditions necessary to elicit such responses are not well-defined at present. There is some evidence suggesting the existence of field-dependent effects on reaction time and on reduced accuracy in the performance of some cognitive tasks, which is supported by the results of studies on the gross electrical activity of the brain. Studies investigating whether magnetic fields affect sleep quality have reported inconsistent results. It is possible that these inconsistencies may be attributable in part to differences in the design of the studies.

Some people claim to be hypersensitive to EMFs in general. However, the evidence from double-blind provocation studies suggests that the reported symptoms are unrelated to EMF exposure.

There is only inconsistent and inconclusive evidence that exposure to ELF electric and magnetic fields causes depressive symptoms or suicide. Thus, the evidence is considered inadequate.

In animals, the possibility that exposure to ELF fields may affect neurobehavioural functions has been explored from a number of perspectives using a range of exposure conditions. Few robust effects have been established. There is convincing evidence that power-frequency electric fields can be detected by animals, most likely as a result of surface charge effects, and may elicit transient arousal or mild stress. In rats, the detection range is between 3 and 13 kV m$^{-1}$. Rodents have been shown to be aversive to field strengths greater than 50 kV m$^{-1}$. Other possible field-dependent changes are less well-defined; laboratory studies have only produced evidence of subtle and transitory effects. There is some evidence that exposure to magnetic fields may modulate the functions of the opioid and cholinergic neurotransmitter systems in the brain, and this is supported by the results of studies investigating the effects on analgesia and on the acquisition and performance of spatial memory tasks.

### 1.1.5    Neuroendocrine system

The results of volunteer studies as well as residential and occupational epidemiological studies suggest that the neuroendocrine system is not adversely affected by exposure to power-frequency electric or magnetic fields. This applies particularly to the circulating levels of specific hormones of the neuroendocrine system, including melatonin, released by the pineal gland, and to a number of hormones involved in the control of body metabolism and physiology, released by the pituitary gland. Subtle differences were sometimes observed in the timing of melatonin release associated with certain characteristics of exposure, but these results were not consistent. It is very difficult to eliminate possible confounding by a variety of environmental and lifestyle factors that might also affect hormone levels. Most laboratory studies of the effects of ELF exposure on night-time melatonin levels in volunteers found no effect when care was taken to control possible confounding.

From the large number of animal studies investigating the effects of power-frequency electric and magnetic fields on rat pineal and serum melatonin levels, some reported that exposure resulted in night-time suppression of melatonin. The changes in melatonin levels first observed in early studies of electric field exposures up to 100 kV m$^{-1}$ could not be replicated. The findings from a series of more recent studies, which showed that circularly-polarised magnetic fields suppressed night-time melatonin levels, were weakened by inappropriate comparisons between exposed animals and historical controls. The data from other experiments in rodents, covering intensity levels from a few microtesla to 5 mT, were equivocal, with some results showing depression of melatonin, but others showing no changes. In seasonally breeding animals, the evidence for an effect of exposure to power-frequency fields on melatonin levels and melatonin-dependent reproductive status is predominantly negative. No convincing effect on melatonin levels has been seen in a study of non-human primates chronically exposed to power-frequency fields, although a preliminary study using two animals reported melatonin suppression in response to an irregular and intermittent exposure.

The effects of exposure to ELF fields on melatonin production or release in isolated pineal glands were variable, although relatively few in vitro studies have been undertaken. The evidence that ELF exposure interferes with the action of melatonin on breast cancer cells in vitro is intriguing. However this system suffers from the disadvantage that the cell lines frequently show genotypic and phenotypic drift in culture that can hinder transferability between laboratories.

No consistent effects have been seen in the stress-related hormones of the pituitary-adrenal axis in a variety of mammalian species, with the possible exception of short-lived stress following the onset of ELF electric field exposure at levels high enough to be perceived. Similarly, while few studies have been carried out, mostly negative or inconsistent effects have been observed in the levels of growth hormone and of hormones involved in controlling metabolic activity or associated with the control of reproduction and sexual development.

Overall, these data do not indicate that ELF electric and/or magnetic fields affect the neuroendocrine system in a way that would have an adverse impact on human health and the evidence is thus considered inadequate.

### 1.1.6   Neurodegenerative disorders

It has been hypothesized that exposure to ELF fields is associated with several neurodegenerative diseases. For Parkinson disease and multiple sclerosis the number of studies has been small and there is no evidence for an association with these diseases. For Alzheimer disease and amyotrophic lateral sclerosis (ALS) more studies have been published. Some of these reports suggest that people employed in electrical occupations might have an increased risk of ALS. So far, no biological mechanism has been established which can explain this association, although it could have arisen because of confounders related to electrical occupations, such as electric shocks. Overall, the evidence for the association between ELF exposure and ALS is considered to be inadequate.

The few studies investigating the association between ELF exposure and Alzheimer disease are inconsistent. However, the higher quality studies that focused on Alzheimer morbidity rather than mortality do not indicate an association. Altogether, the evidence for an association between ELF exposure and Alzheimer disease is inadequate.

### 1.1.7 Cardiovascular disorders

Experimental studies of both short-term and long-term exposure indicate that while electric shock is an obvious health hazard, other hazardous cardiovascular effects associated with ELF fields are unlikely to occur at exposure levels commonly encountered environmentally or occupationally. Although various cardiovascular changes have been reported in the literature, the majority of effects are small and the results have not been consistent within and between studies. With one exception, none of the studies of cardiovascular disease morbidity and mortality has shown an association with exposure. Whether a specific association exists between exposure and altered autonomic control of the heart remains speculative. Overall, the evidence does not support an association between ELF exposure and cardiovascular disease.

### 1.1.8 Immunology and haematology

Evidence for the effects of ELF electric or magnetic fields on components of the immune system is generally inconsistent. Many of the cell populations and functional markers were unaffected by exposure. However, in some human studies with fields from 10 µT to 2 mT, changes were observed in natural killer cells, which showed both increased and decreased cell numbers, and in total white blood cell counts, which showed no change or decreased numbers. In animal studies, reduced natural killer cell activity was seen in female mice, but not in male mice or in rats of either sex. White blood cell counts also showed inconsistency, with decreases or no change reported in different studies. The animal exposures had an even broader range of 2 µT to 30 mT. The difficulty in interpreting the potential health impact of these data is due to the large variations in exposure and environmental conditions, the relatively small numbers of subjects tested and the broad range of endpoints.

There have been few studies carried out on the effects of ELF magnetic fields on the haematological system. In experiments evaluating differential white blood cell counts, exposures ranged from 2 µT to 2 mT. No consistent effects of acute exposure to ELF magnetic fields or to combined ELF electric and magnetic fields have been found in either human or animal studies.

Overall therefore, the evidence for effects of ELF electric or magnetic fields on the immune and haematological system is considered inadequate.

### 1.1.9 Reproduction and development

On the whole, epidemiological studies have not shown an association between adverse human reproductive outcomes and maternal or paternal exposure to ELF fields. There is some evidence for an increased risk of miscarriage associated with maternal magnetic field exposure, but this evidence is inadequate.

Exposures to ELF electric fields of up to 150 kV $m^{-1}$ have been evaluated in several mammalian species, including studies with large group sizes and exposure over several generations. The results consistently show no adverse developmental effects.

The exposure of mammals to ELF magnetic fields of up to 20 mT does not result in gross external, visceral or skeletal malformations. Some studies show an increase in minor skeletal anomalies, in both rats and mice. Skeletal variations are relatively common findings in teratological studies and are often considered biologically insignificant. However, subtle effects of magnetic fields on skeletal development cannot be ruled out. Very few studies have been published which address reproductive effects and no conclusions can be drawn from them.

Several studies on non-mammalian experimental models (chick embryos, fish, sea urchins and insects) have reported findings indicating that ELF magnetic fields at microtesla levels may disturb early development. However, the findings of non-mammalian experimental models carry less weight in the overall evaluation of developmental toxicity than those of corresponding mammalian studies.

Overall, the evidence for developmental and reproductive effects is inadequate.

### 1.1.10 Cancer

The IARC classification of ELF magnetic fields as "possibly carcinogenic to humans" (IARC, 2002) is based upon all of the available data prior to and including 2001. The review of literature in this EHC monograph focuses mainly on studies published after the IARC review.

*Epidemiology*

The IARC classification was heavily influenced by the associations observed in epidemiological studies on childhood leukaemia. The classification of this evidence as limited does not change with the addition of two childhood leukaemia studies published after 2002. Since the publication of the IARC monograph the evidence for other childhood cancers remains inadequate.

Subsequent to the IARC monograph a number of reports have been published concerning the risk of female breast cancer in adults associated with ELF magnetic field exposure. These studies are larger than the previous ones and less susceptible to bias, and overall are negative. With these studies, the evidence for an association between ELF magnetic field exposure and the risk of female breast cancer is weakened considerably and does not support an association of this kind.

In the case of adult brain cancer and leukaemia, the new studies published after the IARC monograph do not change the conclusion that the overall evidence for an association between ELF magnetic fields and the risk of these diseases remains inadequate.

For other diseases and all other cancers, the evidence remains inadequate.

*Laboratory animal studies*

There is currently no adequate animal model of the most common form of childhood leukaemia, acute lymphoblastic leukaemia. Three independent large-scale studies of rats provided no evidence of an effect of ELF magnetic fields on the incidence of spontaneous mammary tumours. Most studies report no effect of ELF magnetic fields on leukaemia or lymphoma in rodent models. Several large-scale long-term studies in rodents have not shown any consistent increase in any type of cancer, including haematopoietic, mammary, brain and skin tumours.

A substantial number of studies have examined the effects of ELF magnetic fields on chemically-induced mammary tumours in rats. Inconsistent results were obtained that may be due in whole or in part to differences in experimental protocols, such as the use of specific sub-strains. Most studies on the effects of ELF magnetic field exposure on chemically-induced or radiation-induced leukaemia/lymphoma models were negative. Studies of pre-neoplastic liver lesions, chemically-induced skin tumours and brain tumours reported predominantly negative results. One study reported an acceleration of UV-induced skin tumourigenesis upon exposure to ELF magnetic fields.

Two groups have reported increased levels of DNA strand breaks in brain tissue following in vivo exposure to ELF magnetic fields. However, other groups, using a variety of different rodent genotoxicity models, found no evidence of genotoxic effects. The results of studies investigating non-genotoxic effects relevant to cancer are inconclusive.

Overall there is no evidence that exposure to ELF magnetic fields alone causes tumours. The evidence that ELF magnetic field exposure can enhance tumour development in combination with carcinogens is inadequate.

*In vitro studies*

Generally, studies of the effects of ELF field exposure of cells have shown no induction of genotoxicity at fields below 50 mT. The notable exception is evidence from recent studies reporting DNA damage at field strengths as low as 35 $\mu$T; however, these studies are still being evaluated and our understanding of these findings is incomplete. There is also increasing evidence that ELF magnetic fields may interact with DNA-damaging agents.

There is no clear evidence of the activation by ELF magnetic fields of genes associated with the control of the cell cycle. However, systematic studies analysing the response of the whole genome have yet to be performed.

Many other cellular studies, for example on cell proliferation, apoptosis, calcium signalling and malignant transformation, have produced inconsistent or inconclusive results.

*Overall conclusion*

New human, animal and in vitro studies, published since the 2002 IARC monograph, do not change the overall classification of ELF magnetic fields as a possible human carcinogen.

### 1.1.11 Health risk assessment

According to the WHO Constitution, health is a state of complete physical, mental and social well-being and not merely the absence of disease or infirmity. A risk assessment is a conceptual framework for a structured review of information relevant to estimating health or environmental outcomes. The health risk assessment can be used as an input to risk management that encompasses all the activities needed to reach decisions on whether an exposure requires any specific action(s) and the undertaking of these actions.

In the evaluation of human health risks, sound human data, whenever available, are generally more informative than animal data. Animal and in vitro studies can support evidence from human studies, fill data gaps left in the evidence from human studies or be used to make a decision about risks when human studies are inadequate or absent.

All studies, with either positive or negative effects, need to be evaluated and judged on their own merit and then all together in a weight-of-evidence approach. It is important to determine to what extent a set of evidence changes the probability that exposure causes an outcome. The evidence for an effect is generally strengthened if the results from different types of studies (epidemiology and laboratory) point to the same conclusion and/or when multiple studies of the same type show the same result.

*Acute effects*

Acute biological effects have been established for exposure to ELF electric and magnetic fields in the frequency range up to 100 kHz that may have adverse consequences on health. Therefore, exposure limits are needed. International guidelines exist that have addressed this issue. Compliance with these guidelines provides adequate protection for acute effects.

*Chronic effects*

Scientific evidence suggesting that everyday, chronic low-intensity (above 0.3–0.4 µT) power-frequency magnetic field exposure poses a health

11

risk is based on epidemiological studies demonstrating a consistent pattern of increased risk for childhood leukaemia. Uncertainties in the hazard assessment include the role that control selection bias and exposure misclassification might have on the observed relationship between magnetic fields and childhood leukaemia. In addition, virtually all of the laboratory evidence and the mechanistic evidence fail to support a relationship between low-level ELF magnetic fields and changes in biological function or disease status. Thus, on balance, the evidence is not strong enough to be considered causal, but sufficiently strong to remain a concern.

Although a causal relationship between magnetic field exposure and childhood leukaemia has not been established, the possible public health impact has been calculated assuming causality in order to provide a potentially useful input into policy. However, these calculations are highly dependent on the exposure distributions and other assumptions, and are therefore very imprecise. Assuming that the association is causal, the number of cases of childhood leukaemia worldwide that might be attributable to exposure can be estimated to range from 100 to 2400 cases per year. However, this represents 0.2 to 4.9% of the total annual incidence of leukaemia cases, estimated to be 49 000 worldwide in 2000. Thus, in a global context, the impact on public health, if any, would be limited and uncertain.

A number of other diseases have been investigated for possible association with ELF magnetic field exposure. These include cancers in both children and adults, depression, suicide, reproductive dysfunction, developmental disorders, immunological modifications and neurological disease. The scientific evidence supporting a linkage between ELF magnetic fields and any of these diseases is much weaker than for childhood leukaemia and in some cases (for example, for cardiovascular disease or breast cancer) the evidence is sufficient to give confidence that magnetic fields do not cause the disease.

### 1.1.12 Protective measures

It is essential that exposure limits be implemented in order to protect against the established adverse effects of exposure to ELF electric and magnetic fields. These exposure limits should be based on a thorough examination of all the relevant scientific evidence.

Only the acute effects have been established and there are two international exposure limit guidelines (ICNIRP, 1998a; IEEE, 2002) designed to protect against these effects.

As well as these established acute effects, there are uncertainties about the existence of chronic effects, because of the limited evidence for a link between exposure to ELF magnetic fields and childhood leukaemia. Therefore the use of precautionary approaches is warranted. However, it is not recommended that the limit values in exposure guidelines be reduced to some arbitrary level in the name of precaution. Such practice undermines the scientific foundation on which the limits are based and is likely to be an expensive and not necessarily effective way of providing protection.

Implementing other suitable precautionary procedures to reduce exposure is reasonable and warranted. However, electric power brings obvious health, social and economic benefits, and precautionary approaches should not compromise these benefits. Furthermore, given both the weakness of the evidence for a link between exposure to ELF magnetic fields and childhood leukaemia, and the limited impact on public health if there is a link, the benefits of exposure reduction on health are unclear. Thus the costs of precautionary measures should be very low. The costs of implementing exposure reductions will vary from one country to another, making it very difficult to provide a general recommendation for balancing the costs against the potential risk from ELF fields.

In view of the above, the following recommendations are given.

- Policy-makers should establish guidelines for ELF field exposure for both the general public and workers. The best source of guidance for both exposure levels and the principles of scientific review are the international guidelines.

- Policy-makers should establish an ELF EMF protection programme that includes measurements of fields from all sources to ensure that the exposure limits are not exceeded either for the general public or workers.

- Provided that the health, social and economic benefits of electric power are not compromised, implementing very low-cost precautionary procedures to reduce exposure is reasonable and warranted.

- Policy-makers, community planners and manufacturers should implement very low-cost measures when constructing new facilities and designing new equipment including appliances.

- Changes to engineering practice to reduce ELF exposure from equipment or devices should be considered, provided that they yield other additional benefits, such as greater safety, or little or no cost.

- When changes to existing ELF sources are contemplated, ELF field reduction should be considered alongside safety, reliability and economic aspects.

- Local authorities should enforce wiring regulations to reduce unintentional ground currents when building new or rewiring existing facilities, while maintaining safety. Proactive measures to identify violations or existing problems in wiring would be expensive and unlikely to be justified.

- National authorities should implement an effective and open communication strategy to enable informed decision-making by all stakeholders; this should include information on how individuals can reduce their own exposure.

- Local authorities should improve planning of ELF EMF-emitting facilities, including better consultation between industry, local government, and citizens when siting major ELF EMF-emitting sources.

- Government and industry should promote research programmes to reduce the uncertainty of the scientific evidence on the health effects of ELF field exposure.

## 1.2 Recommendations for research

Identifying the gaps in the knowledge concerning the possible health effects of exposure to ELF fields is an essential part of this health risk assessment. This has resulted in the following recommendations for further research (summarized in Table 1).

As an overarching need, further research on intermediate frequencies (IF), usually taken as frequencies between 300 Hz and 100 kHz, is required, given the present lack of data in this area. Very little of the required knowledge base for a health risk assessment has been gathered and most existing studies have contributed inconsistent results, which need to be further substantiated. General requirements for constituting a sufficient IF database for health risk assessment include exposure assessment, epidemiological and human laboratory studies, and animal and cellular (in vitro) studies (ICNIRP, 2003; ICNIRP, 2004; Litvak, Foster & Repacholi, 2002).

For all volunteer studies, it is mandatory that research on human subjects is conducted in full accord with ethical principles, including the provisions of the Helsinki Declaration (WMA, 2004).

For laboratory studies, priority should be given to reported responses (i) for which there is at least some evidence of replication or confirmation, (ii) that are potentially relevant to carcinogenesis (for example, genotoxicity), (iii) that are strong enough to allow mechanistic analysis and (iv) that occur in mammalian or human systems.

### 1.2.1 Sources, measurements and exposures

The further characterization of homes with high ELF exposure in different countries to identify relative contributions of internal and external sources, the influence of wiring/grounding practices and other characteristics of the home could give insights into identifying a relevant exposure metric for epidemiological assessment. An important component of this is a better understanding of foetal and childhood exposure to ELF fields, especially from residential exposure to underfloor electrical heating and from transformers in apartment buildings.

It is suspected that in some cases of occupational exposure the present ELF guideline limits are exceeded. More information is needed on exposure (including to non-power frequencies) related to work on, for example, live-line maintenance, work within or near the bore of MRI magnets (and hence to gradient-switching ELF fields) and work on transportation systems. Similarly, additional knowledge is needed about general public exposure which could come close to guideline limits, including sources such as security systems, library degaussing systems, induction cooking and water heating appliances.

Exposure to contact currents has been proposed as a possible explanation for the association of ELF magnetic fields with childhood leukaemia. Research is needed in countries other than the USA to assess the capability of residential electrical grounding and plumbing practices to give rise to contact currents in the home. Such studies would have priority in countries with important epidemiological results with respect to ELF and childhood leukaemia.

### 1.2.2 Dosimetry

In the past, most laboratory research was based on induced electric currents in the body as a basic metric and thus dosimetry was focused on this quantity. Only recently has work begun on exploring the relationship between external exposure and induced electric fields. For a better understanding of biological effects, more data on internal electric fields for different exposure conditions are needed.

Computation should be carried out of internal electric fields due to the combined influence of external electric and magnetic fields in different configurations. The vectorial addition of out-of-phase and spatially varying contributions of electric and magnetic fields is necessary to assess basic restriction compliance issues.

Very little computation has been carried out on advanced models of the pregnant woman and the foetus with appropriate anatomical modelling. It is important to assess possible enhanced induction of electric fields in the foetus in relation to the childhood leukaemia issue. Both maternal occupational and residential exposures are relevant here.

There is a need to further refine micro-dosimetric models in order to take into account the cellular architecture of neural networks and other complex suborgan systems identified as being more sensitive to induced electric field effects. This modelling process also needs to consider influences in cell membrane electrical potentials and on the release of neurotransmitters.

### 1.2.3 Biophysical mechanisms

There are three main areas where there are obvious limits to the current understanding of mechanisms: the radical pair mechanism, magnetic particles in the body and signal-to-noise ratios in multicell systems, such as neuronal networks.

The radical pair mechanism is one of the more plausible low-level interaction mechanisms, but it has yet to be shown that it is able to mediate significant effects in cell metabolism and function. It is particularly important to understand the lower limit of exposure at which it acts, so as to judge whether this could or could not be a relevant mechanism for carcinogenesis. Given recent studies in which reactive oxygen species were increased in immune cells exposed to ELF fields, it is recommended that cells from the immune system that generate reactive oxygen species as part of their immune response be used as cellular models for investigating the potential of the radical pair mechanism.

Although the presence of magnetic particles (magnetite crystals) in the human brain does not, on present evidence, appear to confer a sensitivity to environmental ELF magnetic fields, further theoretical and experimental approaches should explore whether such sensitivity could exist under certain conditions. Moreover, any modification that the presence of magnetite might have on the radical pair mechanism discussed above should be pursued.

The extent to which multicell mechanisms operate in the brain so as to improve signal-to-noise ratios should be further investigated in order to develop a theoretical framework for quantifying this or for determining any limits on it. Further investigation of the threshold and frequency response of the neuronal networks in the hippocampus and other parts of the brain should be carried out using in vitro approaches.

### 1.2.4 Neurobehaviour

It is recommended that laboratory-based volunteer studies on the possible effects on sleep and on the performance of mentally demanding tasks be carried out using harmonized methodological procedures. There is a need to identify dose-response relationships at higher magnetic flux densities than used previously and a wide range of frequencies (i.e. in the kilohertz range).

Studies of adult volunteers and animals suggest that acute cognitive effects may occur with short-term exposures to intense electric or magnetic fields. The characterization of such effects is very important for the development of exposure guidance, but there is a lack of specific data concerning field-dependent effects in children. The implementation of laboratory-based studies of cognition and changes in electroencephalograms (EEGs) in people exposed to ELF fields is recommended, including adults regularly subjected to occupational exposure and children.

Behavioural studies on immature animals provide a useful indicator of the possible cognitive effects on children. The possible effects of pre- and postnatal exposure to ELF magnetic fields on the development of the nervous system and cognitive function should be studied. These studies could be usefully supplemented by investigations into the effects of exposure to ELF magnetic fields and induced electric fields on nerve cell growth using brain slices or cultured neurons.

There is a need to further investigate potential health consequences suggested by experimental data showing opioid and cholinergic responses in animals. Studies examining the modulation of opioid and cholinergic

16

responses in animals should be extended and the exposure parameters and the biological basis for these behavioural responses should be defined.

### 1.2.5 Neuroendocrine system

The existing database of neuroendocrine response does not indicate that ELF exposure would have adverse impacts on human health. Therefore no recommendations for additional research are given.

### 1.2.6 Neurodegenerative disorders

Several studies have observed an increased risk of amyotrophic lateral sclerosis in "electrical occupations". It is considered important to investigate this association further in order to discover whether ELF magnetic fields are involved in the causation of this rare neurodegenerative disease. This research requires large prospective cohort studies with information on ELF magnetic field exposure, electric shock exposure as well as exposure to other potential risk factors.

It remains questionable whether ELF magnetic fields constitute a risk factor for Alzheimer's disease. The data currently available are not sufficient and this association should be further investigated. Of particular importance is the use of morbidity rather than mortality data.

### 1.2.7 Cardiovascular disorders

Further research into the association between ELF magnetic fields and the risk of cardiovascular disease is not considered a priority.

### 1.2.8 Immunology and haematology

Changes observed in immune and haematological parameters in adults exposed to ELF magnetic fields showed inconsistencies, and there are essentially no research data available for children. Therefore, the recommendation is to conduct studies on the effects of ELF exposure on the development of the immune and haematopoietic systems in juvenile animals.

### 1.2.9 Reproduction and development

There is some evidence of an increased risk of miscarriage associated with ELF magnetic field exposure. Taking into account the potentially high public health impact of such an association, further epidemiological research is recommended.

### 1.2.10 Cancer

Resolving the conflict between epidemiological data (which show an association between ELF magnetic field exposure and an increased risk of childhood leukaemia) and experimental and mechanistic data (which do not support this association) is the highest research priority in this field. It is recommended that epidemiologists and experimental scientists collaborate on this. For new epidemiological studies to be informative they must focus on new aspects of exposure, potential interaction with other factors or on high exposure groups, or otherwise be innovative in this area of research. In addition, it is also recommended that the existing pooled analyses be updated, by adding data from recent studies and by applying new insights into the analysis.

Childhood brain cancer studies have shown inconsistent results. As with childhood leukaemia, a pooled analysis of childhood brain cancer studies should be very informative and is therefore recommended. A pooled analysis of this kind can inexpensively provide a greater and improved insight into the existing data, including the possibility of selection bias and, if the studies are sufficiently homogeneous, can offer the best estimate of risk.

For adult breast cancer more recent studies have convincingly shown no association with exposure to ELF magnetic fields. Therefore further research into this association should be given very low priority.

For adult leukaemia and brain cancer the recommendation is to update the existing large cohorts of occupationally exposed individuals. Occupational studies, pooled analyses and meta-analyses for leukaemia and brain cancer have been inconsistent and inconclusive. However, new data have subsequently been published and should be used to update these analyses.

The priority is to address the epidemiological evidence by establishing appropriate in vitro and animal models for responses to low-level ELF magnetic fields that are widely transferable between laboratories.

Transgenic rodent models for childhood leukaemia should be developed in order to provide appropriate experimental animal models to study the effect of ELF magnetic field exposure. Otherwise, for existing animal studies, the weight of evidence is that there are no carcinogenic effects of ELF magnetic fields alone. Therefore high priority should be given to in vitro and animal studies in which ELF magnetic fields are rigorously evaluated as a co-carcinogen.

With regard to other in vitro studies, experiments reporting the genotoxic effects of intermittent ELF magnetic field exposure should be replicated.

### 1.2.11 Protective measures

Research on the development of health protection policies and policy implementation in areas of scientific uncertainty is recommended, specifically on the use of precaution, the interpretation of precaution and the evaluation of the impact of precautionary measures for ELF magnetic fields and other agents classified as "possible human carcinogens". Where there are uncertainties about the potential health risk an agent poses for society, precautionary measures may be warranted in order to ensure the appropriate protection of the public and workers. Only limited research has been performed on this issue for ELF magnetic fields and because of its importance, more research is needed. This may help countries to integrate precaution into their health protection policies.

Further research on risk perception and communication which is specifically focused on electromagnetic fields is advised. Psychological and sociological factors that influence risk perception in general have been widely investigated. However, limited research has been carried out to analyse the relative importance of these factors in the case of electromagnetic fields or to identify other factors that are specific to electromagnetic fields. Recent studies have suggested that precautionary measures which convey implicit risk messages can modify risk perception by either increasing or reducing concerns. Deeper investigation in this area is therefore warranted.

Research on the development of a cost–benefit/cost-effectiveness analysis for the mitigation of ELF magnetic fields should be carried out. The use of cost–benefit and cost-effectiveness analyses for evaluating whether a policy option is beneficial to society has been researched in many areas of public policy. The development of a framework that will identify which parameters are necessary in order to perform this analysis for ELF magnetic fields is needed. Due to uncertainties in the evaluation, quantifiable and unquantifiable parameters will need to be incorporated.

**Table 1. Recommendations for further research**

| Sources, measurements and exposures | Priority |
|---|---|
| Further characterization of homes with high ELF magnetic field exposure in different countries | Medium |
| Identify gaps in knowledge about occupational ELF exposure, such as in MRI | High |
| Assess the ability of residential wiring outside the USA to induce contact currents in children | Medium |
| **Dosimetry** | |
| Further computational dosimetry relating external electric and magnetic fields to internal electric fields, particularly concerning exposure to combined electric and magnetic fields in different orientations | Medium |
| Calculation of induced electric fields and currents in pregnant women and in the foetus | Medium |
| Further refinement of microdosimetric models taking into account the cellular architecture of neural networks and other complex suborgan systems | Medium |
| **Biophysical mechanisms** | |
| Further study of radical pair mechanisms in immune cells that generate reactive oxygen species as part of their phenotypic function | Medium |
| Further theoretical and experimental study of the possible role of magnetite in ELF magnetic field sensitivity | Low |
| Determination of threshold responses to internal electric fields induced by ELFs on multicell systems, such as neural networks, using theoretical and in vitro approaches | High |

Table 1. Continued

## Neurobehaviour

| | |
|---|---|
| Cognitive, sleep and EEG studies in volunteers, including children and occupationally exposed subjects, using a wide range of ELF frequencies at high flux densities | Medium |
| Studies of pre- and post-natal exposure on subsequent cognitive function in animals | Medium |
| Further study of opioid and cholinergic responses in animals | Low |

## Neurodegenerative disorders

| | |
|---|---|
| Further studies of the risk of amyotrophic lateral sclerosis in "electric" occupations and in relation to ELF magnetic field exposure and of Alzheimer's disease in relation to ELF magnetic field exposure | High |

## Immunology and haematology

| | |
|---|---|
| Studies of the consequences of ELF magnetic field exposure on immune and haematopoietic system development in juvenile animals. | Low |

## Reproduction and development

| | |
|---|---|
| Further study of the possible link between miscarriage and ELF magnetic field exposure | Low |

## Cancer

| | |
|---|---|
| Update existing pooled analyses of childhood leukaemia with new information | High |
| Pooled analyses of existing studies of childhood brain tumour studies | High |
| Update existing pooled and meta-analyses of adult leukaemia and brain tumour studies and of cohorts of occupationally exposed individuals | Medium |
| Development of transgenic rodent models of childhood leukaemia for use in ELF studies | High |
| Evaluation of co-carcinogenic effects using in vitro and animal studies | High |
| Attempted replication of in vitro genotoxicity studies | Medium |

## Protective measures

| | |
|---|---|
| Research on the development of health protection policies and policy implementation in areas of scientific uncertainty | Medium |
| Further research on risk perception and communication focused on electromagnetic fields | Medium |
| Development of a cost–benefit/cost-effectiveness analysis for the mitigation of ELF fields | Medium |

## 2      SOURCES, MEASUREMENTS AND EXPOSURES

### 2.1      Electric and magnetic fields

This chapter describes the nature of electric and magnetic fields, provides information on sources and exposures, and discusses the implications for exposure assessment for epidemiology. Generation and measurement of fields in experimental laboratory settings is outside the scope of this chapter.

#### 2.1.1      *The field concept*

The field concept is very general in physics and describes for each point in a region of space the specific state of a physical quantity. Although a field can be defined for almost any physical quantity, it is in common use only for those which are capable of exerting a force. The gravitational field, for example, describes the force exerted on a unit mass at each point in space. Accordingly, the electric field describes the force exerted on a unit electric charge, and the magnetic field is defined in terms of the force exerted on a moving unit charge.

Electric fields are produced by electric charges, irrespective of their state of motion. A single charge at a point produces an electric field in all directions in a pattern with spherical symmetry and infinite dimension. A line of charges (e.g. a power line) produces an electric field around the line in a pattern with cylindrical symmetry. In practice, it is not possible to have a single isolated charge or a single isolated charged object, and instead of indefinitely long field lines, they will terminate on another charge (which could be another charge already present in a conductor or could be a charge induced by the field itself in a conducting object). The overall shape of the pattern of electric field experienced at any point thus depends on the distribution of charges and of objects in the vicinity. In technical systems, electric charges are related to voltages, and not to currents or power.

Magnetic fields are produced by moving charges and thus are proportional to electric currents in a system, irrespective of the voltage used. A current flowing in any conductor, no matter how complicated the shape of the conductor, can be broken down into a series of infinitesimally small segments, joined end-to-end. The magnetic field produced by a short element of current is given by the Biot-Savart law:

$$\frac{|dH|}{dl} = \frac{i}{4\pi r^2} \sin(\varphi)$$

where $dH$ is the element of magnetic field produced by the current element $i$ in the conductor element $dl$ at a position $r$ in space, and $\varphi$ is the angle between $dl$ and $r$.

As long as charges and currents are static, electricity and magnetism are distinct phenomena. Time varying charge distributions however result in a coupling of electric and magnetic fields that become stronger with increasing frequency. The characteristics and interactions of electric and magnetic fields are completely described by Maxwell's equations.

In addition to the "quasi static fields" from resting and moving charges, accelerating charges produce a radiation component. At extremely low frequencies the radiating field of a source is negligible. In practical exposure situations, radiation is absolutely negligible in the ELF range. Radiation only becomes dominant at distances that are large compared to the wavelength.

The wavelength is the distance between two successive cycles of the wave. In free space it is related to the frequency by the formula wavelength = speed of light / frequency. At 50 Hz, the wavelength is very long, 6000 km (60 Hz: 5000 km). In comparison, a radio wave with a frequency of 100 kHz has a wavelength of 3 km.

### 2.1.2 Quantities and units

For magnetic fields, there are two different quantities: the magnetic flux density, usually designated $B$, and the magnetic field strength, usually designated $H$. The distinction between $B$ and $H$ becomes important for the description of magnetic fields in matter, especially for materials which have certain magnetic (ferromagnetic) properties, such as iron. Biological tissue generally has no such properties and for practical purposes, either $B$ or $H$ can be used to describe magnetic fields outside and inside biological tissues.

Similarly, for the description of electric fields there are also different quantities: the electric field strength $E$ and the dielectric displacement $D$. $D$ is not useful for the description of electric fields in biological tissue. All these parameters are vectors; vectors are denoted in italics in this Monograph (see also paragraph 3.1).

The SI unit of magnetic flux density ($B$) is the tesla (T), and of magnetic field strength ($H$) is the ampere per metre (A m$^{-1}$). In the absence of magnetic material, 1 $\mu$T = $4\pi\times10^{-7}$ A m$^{-1}$. Either $B$ or $H$ can be used to describe fields, but $B$ (i.e. tesla) is more common and is used here. Older literature, especially American, often uses the Gauss (G): 1 $\mu$T = $10^4$ G (1 $\mu$T= 10 mG).

The SI unit of the electric field strength ($E$) is volt per metre (V m$^{-1}$).

### 2.1.3 Polarization

Electric and magnetic fields are vector quantities; they are characterized by an intensity (field strength) and a direction. In static (direct current, DC) fields, direction and intensity are constant over time. A time varying (alternating current, AC) field usually has a constant direction but a variable intensity. The field oscillates in a defined direction. This is often referred to as linear polarization.

22

In complex exposure scenarios, fields with different vector quantities may overlap. The resultant field is the addition of the two or more field vectors. In DC fields the result is a field with a different intensity and in most cases a different orientation. In AC fields, the situation becomes more complex because the vector addition may result in a time varying orientation of the resulting field. The field vector rotates in space; with the varying intensity of AC fields, the tip of the vector traces out an ellipse in a plane. This is often referred to as elliptical or circular polarization. This situation needs to be considered with respect to field measurement.

### 2.1.4   Time variation, harmonics and transients

The basic AC field can be described as a sine wave over time. The peak field strength is called the amplitude and the number of wave cycles within a second is called the frequency. The most common frequencies used in the electricity system of many countries are 50 Hz and 60 Hz. When fields of more than one frequency are combined, the resultant field is no longer a sine wave when plotted against time. Depending on the parameters of the combined fields (amplitude, frequency) any time course of the resultant field can be achieved, for example a square wave or a triangular wave. Conversely, any shape waveform can be split into a number of sinusoidal components at different frequencies. The process of splitting a waveform into its component frequencies is known as Fourier analysis, and the components are called the Fourier components.

In many electrical systems, sinusoidal signals are distorted by a non-linear behaviour of the loads. This happens when the electrical properties of the system depend on the signal strength. Such distortions introduce Fourier components in addition to the fundamental frequency of the signal, which are called harmonics. Harmonics are a precise multiple of the fundamental frequency. Given a 50 Hz fundamental frequency, 100 Hz is the second harmonic, 150 Hz is the third harmonic, and so forth.

Note that the terminology used in electrical engineering is different to musical terminology: a frequency of twice the fundamental is the second harmonic to the engineer but only the first harmonic to the musician. In electrical engineering, "fundamental" and "first harmonic" are equivalent terms.

The term "harmonic" is generally used only for those components of the current or voltage with a frequency which is an integral multiple of the power frequency (and is locked into that frequency) and that are produced as part of the operation of the electricity system. These will produce harmonic frequencies in the magnetic or electric fields produced. If there are currents or voltages at other frequencies, which are not tied to the power frequency, these frequencies will also appear in the magnetic or electric fields produced.

There is a number of possible sources of such currents and voltages, particularly at frequencies rather higher than the power frequencies. With regard to exposure of the public, the main sources are the 16 2/3(20 or sometimes 15) Hz used by some electric transport systems, 400 Hz used by most aeroplanes, the screen-refresh frequencies of video display units (VDUs) (which have varied over the years with advances in computer design but is typically 50–160 Hz), and the variable frequencies increasingly used by variable-speed traction drives for trains and trams. It can be seen that these are all specific to particular situations, and, with the exception of the VDU, it would not be expected to find fields at these frequencies in normal domestic settings. In a normal domestic setting, any non-harmonic frequencies are generally negligible. There are many other sources in occupational settings related to specific industrial processes.

All the frequency components of the field so far considered are periodic: that is, although the amplitude of the field varies over time, the pattern of the variation repeats itself at fixed intervals (e.g. at 20 ms intervals for signals with a fundamental frequency of 50 Hz).

Natural and man made field sources often produce signals which are not repeated periodically but rather occur only once. The resulting time variation of the field is called transient. Over the course of a period of time, say a day, there may be a number of transients, but there is no regularity or periodicity to them, and they are sufficiently far apart to be treated as separate isolated events.

Transients accompany virtually all switching operations and are characterized by a high rate of change of the field. In fact there is a wide range of events which fit the basic definition of a transient as a non-periodic event. The characteristics of transients are numerous, which makes measurement complex.

### 2.1.5 Perturbations to fields, shielding

Magnetic fields are perturbed by materials that have a very high relative permeability. This effectively means they are perturbed only by ferromagnetic materials, and the most common example is iron and its compounds or alloys. An object made of such material will produce a region of enhanced field where the field enters and leaves the object, with a corresponding reduction in the field to the sides.

Shielding of ELF magnetic fields with such material is in practice only an option to protect small areas, for example VDU's from magnetic interference. Another option with only little practical relevance for field reduction purposes is the compensation of the magnetic field with a specially designed field source.

Electric fields, in contrast to magnetic fields, are readily perturbed by materials with a high relative permittivity (dielectrics) and even more significantly by conducting objects. A conducting enclosure eliminates the electric field within it. A conducting object also perturbs the field outside it, increasing it in line with the field and reducing it to the sides. At power frequencies, a metal box is effectively a perfect screen, and buildings are sufficiently conducting to reduce the electric field within them from an external source by factors of 10–100 or more.

Electric fields are particularly affected by earthed conducting objects including not just the ground, but also trees, hedges, fences, many buildings, and human beings. Any conducting object has a charge induced on it by the electric field. This induced charge itself then becomes part of the set of charges which constitutes the field. The consequence is that to determine the electric field produced by, say, a transmission line it is necessary to consider not just the positions of the conductors of the line but the position of the ground relative to them and the positions of any other conducting objects. In terms of human exposure to power lines, the main effect is that close to a vertical object that is tall compared to a person – e.g. a tree or a house – field exposure on the ground is reduced.

## 2.2 Sources of alternating fields

### 2.2.1 Electric fields

#### 2.2.1.1 Naturally occurring fields

The natural electric field encountered above the surface of the Earth varies greatly with time and location. The primary cause of the field is the charge separation that occurs between the Earth and the ionosphere, which acts as a perfect conductor separated by air of negligible conductivity (König et al., 1981). The field near the surface in fair weather has a typical strength of about 130 V m$^{-1}$ (Dolezalek, 1979). The strength generally depends on height, local temperature, humidity profile and the presence of ions in the atmosphere. Deviations of up to 200% from fair-weather levels have been recorded in the presence of fog or rain. Daily changes are attributed to meteorological phenomena, such as thunderstorms, which affect the rate of charge transfer between the ground and the upper atmosphere.

Variations of up to 40 kV m$^{-1}$ occur near thunderstorms, although even in the absence of local lightning, fields can reach up to 3 kV m$^{-1}$. Because the dominant component usually changes very slowly, the phenomenon is often described as "electrostatic". However a variety of processes in the atmosphere and magnetosphere produce a wide range of signals with frequencies reaching up to several megahertz. Atmospheric inversion layer phenomena produce electric fields at the lower end of the ELF range (König et al., 1981). Atmospheric fields related to lightning discharges have spectral components below 1 Hz but the largest amplitude components have frequencies between 1 and 30 kHz. Generally the range of frequencies and field strengths vary widely with geographical location, time of day and season. Characteristics of the Earth's electric field in the ELF range are summarized in Table 2. The intensity of time-varying fields related to atmospherics such as lightning between 5 Hz and 1 kHz are typically less than 0.5 V m$^{-1}$ and amplitudes generally decrease with increasing frequency. The natural electric field strength at the power frequencies of 50 or 60 Hz is about $10^{-4}$ V m$^{-1}$ (EC, 1996).

**Table 2. Characteristics of the Earth's electric field in the ELF range**

| Frequency range (Hz) | Electric field strength (V m$^{-1}$) | Comment |
|---|---|---|
| 0.001–5 | 0.2–10$^3$ | Short duration pulses of magnetohydrodynamic origin |
| 7.5–8.4 and 26–27 | 0.15–0.6×10$^{-6}$ | Quasi-sinusoidal pulses of underdetermined origin |
| 5–1000 | 10$^{-4}$–0.5 | Related to atmospheric changes (atmospherics) |

The Earth-atmosphere system approximates electromagnetically to a three conductive layer radial shell, denoted as the Earth-ionosphere cavity, in which electromagnetic radiation is trapped. In this cavity broadband electromagnetic impulses, like those from lightning flashes, create globally the so-called Schumann resonances at frequencies 5–50 Hz (Bliokh, Nickolaenko & Filippov, 1980; Schumann, 1952; Sentman, 1987). Electric fields of up to a few tenths of a millivolt per metre can be attributed to the Schumann resonances (König et al., 1981).

### 2.2.1.2 Artificial fields

The dominant sources of ELF electric fields are invariably the result of human activity, in particular, the operation of power systems or the operation of mains appliances within a home.

#### 2.2.1.2.1 Overhead power lines

The electric field at a point near a power line depends on the voltage of the line, its distance, and how close together the various charged conductors making up the line are. The radius of the conductors is also relevant. Other factors being equal, thicker conductors result in larger electric fields at ground level. In addition, electric fields are affected by conducting objects.

Electric fields are lower and fall more rapidly with distance for point symmetric systems than for others. Electric fields are lowest when the three phases are balanced and rise with the unbalance. At ground level, electric fields are highest towards the middle of a span where the sag of the conductors brings them nearest the ground and reduce towards the end of the span.

The highest electric field strength at ground level from overhead lines is typically around 10 kV m$^{-1}$ (AGNIR, 2001b; NIEHS, 1995).

#### 2.2.1.2.2 House wiring and appliances

The electric field produced by any source outside the home will be attenuated considerably by the structure of the home. All common building

26

materials are sufficiently conducting to screen fields, and the ratio of the field outside to the field inside typically ranges from 10 to 100 or more (AGNIR, 2001b).

Within homes, however, there are sources of electric field just as there are sources of magnetic field. House wiring can produce electric fields, which are clearly strongest close to the wiring but which can be significant over the volume of a house as well. The electric field produced by wiring depends partly on how it is installed; wiring installed in metal trunking or conduit produces very small external fields, and the fields produced by wiring installed within walls is attenuated by an amount depending on the building materials (AGNIR, 2001b).

The other main source of electric fields within a home is mains appliances. Any mains appliance produces power-frequency electric fields whenever it is connected to the mains (in contrast to magnetic fields, which are produced only when current is being drawn), and appliances are often left plugged in even when not operating. The size of the electric field depends on the wiring of the appliance, and on how much of the wiring is enclosed by metal which will screen the electric field. The electric field from an appliance falls rapidly with distance from the appliance, just as the magnetic field does. The magnetic field from an appliance typically merges into the background magnetic field within a metre or two. With electric fields, except in those few homes very close to a source of high electric field, there is no background field from sources outside the home. Therefore the electric field from an appliance is still appreciable, albeit rather small, at greater distances from the appliance than is the case for magnetic fields.

Because electric fields are so easily perturbed by conducting objects, fields within the volume of a room are rarely uniform or smoothly varying. Many objects, in particular metal objects, perturb the field and can create local areas of high electric field strength.

### 2.2.1.2.3 Underground cables and substations

When a cable is buried underground, it still produces a magnetic field above the ground (see section 2.2.2.2.2). By contrast, a buried cable produces no electric field above ground, partly because of the screening effect of the ground itself, but mainly because underground cables practically always include a metal sheath which screens the electric field.

Substations also rarely produce significant electric fields outside their perimeter. In the case of a ground-mounted final distribution substation, this is because all the busbars and other equipment are contained either in metal cabinets and pillars or in a building, both of which screen electric fields. Higher-voltage substations are not so rigorously enclosed, but are usually surrounded by a security fence, which because it is metal again screens the electric field.

#### 2.2.1.2.4 Electric power industry

Bracken and colleagues have characterized the electric field environment within towers of transmission lines rated between 230 and 765 kV. During various operations that include climbing the towers, electric fields may reach anywhere from 10 to 30 kV m$^{-1}$. These fields would not typically be oriented parallel to the body (Bracken, Senior & Dudman, 2005; Bracken, Senior & Tuominen, 2004). In some operations, such as bare hand live line work, linemen wear a conductive suit, which shields the individual from the electric field.

### 2.2.2 Magnetic fields

#### 2.2.2.1 Naturally occurring fields

The Earth's magnetic field changes continually at periods ranging from a few milliseconds up to $10^{12}$ seconds. The broad spectrum of variation is summarized in Table 3. The main feature of the geomagnetic field is its close resemblance to a dipole field aligned approximately with the spin axis of the Earth. The dipole field is explained by electrical currents that flow in the core. The vertical component of the field reaches a maximum of about 70 µT at the magnetic poles, and approaches zero at the magnetic equator; conversely the horizontal component is close to zero at the poles and has a maximum just over 30 µT at the magnetic equator. Changes of the dipole field with periods of the order of 100 years or so constitute the secular variation, and are explained by eddy currents located near the core boundary (Bullard, 1948).

**Table 3. The broad spectrum of variation in the Earth's magnetic field**

| Type | Period (seconds) | Typical amplitudes | Origin | Comment |
|---|---|---|---|---|
| Reversals | ~$10^{12}$ | 100 µT | Internal | Current systems in the earth |
| Secular change | $10^9$–$10^{10}$ | 10 µT | | |
| Magnetic storms | $10^8$–$10^9$ | hundreds nT | External | 11 year period of maximum |
| Sunspot activity | $10^6$ | | | |
| Storm repetition | | | | 27 day period |
| Diurnal | $10^5$ | tens nT | | 24 hour period |
| Lunar | $10^5$ | | | 25 hour period |
| Pulsations | $10^{-1}$–$10^2$ | 0.02–100 nT | | Solar-terrestrial interaction |
| Cavity resonances | $10^{-2}$–$10^{-1}$ | $10^{-2}$ nT | | Solar-terrestrial interaction |
| Atmospherics | $10^{-6}$–$10^0$ | $10^{-2}$ nT (ELF) | | Lightning discharges |

**Table 4. Characteristics of the Earth's magnetic field across the ELF part of the spectrum**

| Nature and origin | Amplitude changes (µT) | Typical frequency (Hz) | Comment |
|---|---|---|---|
| Regular solar and lunar variations | 0.03–0.05 (solar) 0.005–0.006 (lunar) | $10^{-5}$ $10^{-5}$ | Increases in energy during summer and towards the equator. Also increases at a period of 11 years due to sunspot activity. |
| Irregular disturbances, such as magnetic storms related to sunspot activity | 0.8–2.4 | Wide range of frequencies | Repetition after 27 day period corresponding to the sun's rotation time on its axis. |
| Geomagnetic pulsations (micropulsations) related to changes in the magnetosphere | $2\times10^{-5}$–$8\times10^{-2}$ | 0.002–5 Hz | Amplitudes quoted for moderate activity at mid-latitudes. |
| Cavity resonances | $2\times10^{-5}$–$5\times10^{-5}$ | 5–50 Hz | Schumann resonance oscillations excited by broadband lightning discharges |
| Atmospherics related to lightning discharges | $5\times10^{-5}$ | < 1–2 kHz | Energy peak at 100–200 Hz. Some spectral components < 1 Hz and VLF components in the range 1–30 kHz. |

The main characteristics of the Earth's magnetic field across the ELF and VLF part of the spectrum are summarized in Table 4. All of the spectrum of time variations of period shorter than the most rapid secular change have their primary cause outside the Earth, associated with processes in the ionosphere and magnetosphere (Garland, 1979). These include the regular solar and lunar daily variations upon which more irregular disturbances are superimposed. The typical solar diurnal cycle shows variations of no more than a few tens of nanoteslas depending on magnetic latitude. Large magnetic disturbances known as storms show typical variations of 0.5 µT over 72 hours and are closely related to sunspot activity and the sun's rotation time. Geomagnetic pulsations arise from effects in the magnetosphere and typically cover the frequency range from 1 MHz to 1 Hz. At mid-latitudes during periods of moderate activity up to several tens of nanotesla can be attributed to pulsations (Allan & Pouler, 1992; Anderson, 1990).

The ELF variations arise mainly from the effects of solar activity in the ionosphere and atmospheric effects such as lightning discharges which cause resonance oscillations in the Earth-ionosphere cavity. Changes in ELF signals over 11-year and 27-day periods and circadian variations reflect the solar influences (EC, 1996). The electromagnetic fields that arise from lightning discharges, commonly known as atmospherics, have a very broad frequency range with spectral components from below 1 Hz up to a few megahertz. In the ELF range the peak intensity from lightning discharges occurs typically at 100–200 Hz. The Schumann resonances are a source of ELF magnetic fields of the order of $10^{-2}$ nT at frequencies of up to a few tens of hertz (König et al., 1981). The measurement of signals with frequencies below 100 Hz is extremely difficult because of the interference from man-made signals. At 50 Hz or 60 Hz the natural magnetic field is typically of the order of $10^{-6}$ µT (Polk, 1974).

### 2.2.2.2 Artificial fields

### 2.2.2.2.1 Transmission lines

*Factors affecting fields*

The magnetic field produced by a transmission line depends on several factors.

- The number of currents carried by the line (usually three for a single-circuit line, 6 for a two-circuit line, etc.).

- The arrangement of those currents in space, including:
  o *The separation of the currents.* This is usually determined by the need to avoid sparkover between adjacent conductors, including an allowance for displacement of conductors caused by wind. The separation therefore usually increases as the voltage of the line increases.
  o *The relative phasing of multiple circuits.* Suppose the three phases of one circuit are arranged in the order a-b-c from top to bottom. If the second circuit is similarly arranged a-b-c, the two circuits produce magnetic fields which are aligned with each other and reinforce each other. But if the second circuit is arranged in the opposite order, c-b-a, its magnetic field will be in the opposite direction and the two fields will partially cancel each other. The resultant field falls more nearly as the reciprocal of distance cubed instead of squared. This is variously known as transposed, reversed, or rotated phasing. Other arrangements of the relative phasing are clearly possible and generally produce higher fields at ground level.

- The currents carried by the line, which include:
  o the load current;
  o any out of balance currents.

- Any currents carried by the earth conductor or in the ground itself.

- The height of the currents above ground: the minimum clearance allowed for a given voltage line is usually determined by the need to avoid sparkover to objects on the ground.

Higher voltage lines usually carry higher currents and have larger spacing between conductors. They therefore usually produce higher magnetic fields, even though the magnetic field itself does not depend on the voltage.

Currents in power lines vary over the course of a day, seasonally and from year to year as electricity demand varies. This affects the magnetic field both directly and also because the load carried affects the conductor temperature and hence sag and ground clearance. Lines usually operate at significantly less load than their rating, and therefore average magnetic fields encountered are usually significantly less than the theoretical maximum field a line is capable of producing.

*Harmonics and transients*

The nature of the electricity system and the use of electricity means that some harmonics are more prevalent than others. In particular, the third harmonic, 150 (180) Hz, is usually the strongest, and even harmonics (2nd, 4th, 6th etc.) are usually smaller than odd harmonics (3rd, 5th, 7th etc.). In many situations, harmonics are very small, perhaps a few percent or less of the fundamental. In some situations, however, particularly in buildings with certain types of apparatus, or near certain industrial users of electricity, the harmonic content can increase, and on occasion the third harmonic can be comparable in magnitude to the fundamental. In general, harmonics above the third or fifth are very small, but there are certain processes which lead to harmonics as high as the 23rd and 25th. Some harmonics occur as a result of the operation of the electricity system itself – for instance, small amounts of 11th, 13th, 23rd and 25th harmonics are produced by common types of AC-to-DC conversion equipment – but most occur as a result of the loads consumers connect to the electricity system. A particular example is dimmer switches used in lighting applications. Harmonics are regarded as undesirable on an efficiently operated electricity system. Harmonics tend to be lower in the transmission system, higher in the distribution system, and highest in final-distribution circuits and homes.

Transients also occur in electrical systems. Transients in the voltage (and hence in the electric field) are produced by the following causes.

- *Lightning strikes to an overhead power line.* Most lightning strikes hit the earth conductor (where one is present). If the lightning hits a phase conductor instead, or jumps across to the phase conductor having initially hit something else, a very high voltage can be applied to that phase conductor. This voltage rapidly dissipates, not least over the spark gaps which are installed partly for this very purpose.

- *Switching events*. When a switch in a circuit carrying a current is opened and the current is interrupted, a voltage is generated in that circuit. The voltage dissipates over a period of time determined by the electrical characteristics of the circuit. Switching surges occur whenever circuits are interrupted, so also occur in distribution systems and in homes.

- *Short circuits*. These can occur either between two phase conductors or from a phase conductor to earth or to an earthed conductor. Examples of how short circuits occur with overhead lines include when two phase conductor, both oscillating in the wind, clash, or when an object such as a tree or a hot-air balloon bridges the gap between a phase conductor and another conductor or the earth. With underground circuits and circuits in homes, short circuits can occur when a drill cuts the cable, or as a result of corroded insulation. Short circuits should usually result in the circuit concerned being rapidly disconnected (by the operation of a circuit breaker or by the blowing of a fuse). For the duration of the short circuit, which could be as short as 40 ms on parts of the transmission system or as long as a second on parts of the distribution system, the voltage of the circuit concerned is forced by the fault to a different value from normal.

Transients in the current (and in the resulting magnetic field) result from the following causes.

- *Short circuits*. For the duration of the short circuit (until either the short circuit is removed, or more usually, until the circuit is disconnected by the fuse or circuit breaker) abnormally high currents will be flowing. On the UK transmission system, the highest "fault current" that is allowed to flow is 63 kA. At lower voltages, the "fault level" (the amount of current that can flow in the event of a short circuit) is lower, but can still be many times the normal current in the circuit.

- *Switching events*. Transient currents can be produced when a circuit is first switched on (such currents are often called "inrush" currents which describes their nature quite well).

Some transients affect only the circuit they are generated on. More usually, they affect neighbouring circuits as well, but to a lesser extent. For instance, at high voltages, a lightning strike to a transmission circuit may cause a sufficiently large transient voltage on that circuit to cause the protection circuits to operate the circuit breaker and to disconnect the circuit. On other nearby circuits, it may cause a large transient voltage, but not large enough to cause the protection to operate. On circuits further away, the transient may still be present but may be much smaller and for practical purposes negligible. At low voltages, switching an appliance in one home may produce a transient that affects adjoining homes as well. Thus it is only transient voltages or currents which are generated close to a given point which are likely to produce significant transient electric or magnetic fields at that point.

*Field levels*

Transmission lines can produce maximum magnetic flux densities of up to a few tens of microteslas during peak demand, however mean levels are usually no more than a few microteslas. The magnetic flux density reduces typically to a few hundred nanotesla at distances of several tens of metres from a transmission line. The magnetic flux density decreases in lower voltage systems, mainly due to progressively smaller currents and conductor separations used.

Overhead transmission lines operate at various voltages up to 1150 kV. In the UK, the largest power lines in use operate at 400 kV with ratings up to 4 kA per circuit and a minimum ground clearance of 7.6 m. This theoretically produces up to 100 μT directly beneath the conductors. In practice, because the load is rarely the maximum and the clearance rarely the minimum, the typical field at ground level directly beneath the conductors is 5 μT. Table 5 gives more detail on the average magnetic field at various distances from a typical National Grid line. These figures were calculated from one year's recorded load data and are the average for a representative sample of 43 different lines.

**Table 5. Average magnetic field at various distances from National Grid line [a]**

| Distance (m) | Average field (μT) |
|---|---|
| 0 | 4.005 |
| 50 | 0.520 |
| 100 | 0.136 |
| 200 | 0.034 |
| 300 | 0.015 |

[a] Source: National Grid, 2007b.

**Table 6. Typical magnetic field levels in μT for power transmission lines [a]**

| Type of line | Usage | Maximum on right-of-way | Distance from lines | | | |
|---|---|---|---|---|---|---|
| | | | 15 m | 30 m | 61 m | 91 m |
| 115 kV | Average | 3 | 0.7 | 0.2 | 0.04 | 0.02 |
| | Peak | 6.3 | 1.4 | 0.4 | 0.09 | 0.04 |
| 230 kV | Average | 5.8 | 2.0 | 0.7 | 0.18 | 0.08 |
| | Peak | 11.8 | 4.0 | 1.5 | 0.36 | 0.16 |
| 500 kV | Average | 8.7 | 2.9 | 1.3 | 0.32 | 0.14 |
| | Peak | 18.3 | 6.2 | 2.7 | 0.67 | 0.30 |

[a] Source: NIEHS, 1995.

tances from a typical National Grid line. These figures were calculated from one year's recorded load data and are the average for a representative sample of 43 different lines. Typical values for the US at various distances, voltages, and power usage are summarized in Table 6.

### 2.2.2.2.2  Underground cables

When a high-voltage line is placed underground, the individual conductors are insulated and can be placed closer together than with an overhead line. This tends to reduce the magnetic field produced. However, the conductors may only be 1 m below ground instead of 10 m above ground, so can be approached more closely. The net result is that to the sides of the underground cable the magnetic field is usually significantly lower than for the equivalent overhead line, but on the line of the route itself the field can be higher. Examples of fields for UK underground cables are given in Table 7.

**Table 7. Examples of fields for underground cables calculated at 1 m above ground level** [a]

| Voltage | Specifics | Location | Load | Magnetic field in μT at distance from centreline | | | |
|---|---|---|---|---|---|---|---|
| | | | | 0 m | 5 m | 10 m | 20 m |
| 400 kV and | trough | 0.13 m spacing 0.3 m depth | maximum typical | 83.30 20.83 | 7.01 1.75 | 1.82 0.46 | 0.46 0.12 |
| 275 kV | direct buried | 0.5 m spacing 0.9 m depth | maximum typical | 96.17 24.06 | 13.05 3.26 | 3.58 0.90 | 0.92 0.23 |
| 132 kV | separate cores | 0.3 m spacing 1 m depth | typical | 9.62 | 1.31 | 0.36 | 0.09 |
| | single cable | 1 m depth | typical | 5.01 | 1.78 | 0.94 | 0.47 |
| 33 kV | single cable | 0.5 m depth | typical | 1.00 | 0.29 | 0.15 | 0.07 |
| 11 kV | single cable | 0.5 m depth | typical | 0.75 | 0.22 | 0.11 | 0.06 |
| 400 V | single cable | 0.5 m depth | typical | 0.50 | 0.14 | 0.07 | 0.04 |

[a] Source: National Grid, 2007a.

Depending on the voltage of the line, the various conductors can be contained within an outer sheath to form a single cable. Not only is in that case the separation of the conductors further reduced, but they are usually wound helically, which produces a further significant reduction in the magnetic field produced.

## 2.2.2.2.3   Distribution lines

In power system engineering, it is common to distinguish between transmission lines and distribution lines. Transmission lines are high voltage (more than a few tens of kV), usually carried on lattice steel towers or substantial metal or concrete structures, capable of carrying large currents (hundreds or sometimes thousands of amps), and used for long-distance bulk transmission of power. Distribution lines are usually lower voltage (less than a few tens of kV), more often carried on wood poles or simpler structures, designed to carry lower currents, and used for more local distribution of power, including the final distribution of power to individual homes. Distribution lines may also have a neutral conductor whereas transmission lines rarely do.

Viewed from the standpoint of production of electric and magnetic fields, the difference between transmission lines and distribution lines is one of degree rather than kind. As the voltage of a circuit reduces, generally so does the spacing of the conductors and the load. All of these factors tend to mean that as the voltage decreases, so do both the electric and magnetic fields. Thus, conceptually, a distribution line without grounding currents is no different to a transmission line, it simply produces lower fields. In practice, the main difference between transmission and distribution lines is often that distribution lines do carry grounding currents but transmission lines do not.

The situation described for transmission lines also applies for a distribution circuit where the neutral is isolated from ground for most of its length. The neutral is often connected to the earth once at or near the transformer or substation which supplies the line, but that is the only earth connection. However, it was realised in various countries that by connecting the earth to the neutral at further points along their length other than just at the transformer/substation, extra security and safety could be obtained. When this is done, the neutral is usually connected to the mass of earth itself at various points, and in some configurations, there is a combined neutral-and-earth conductor rather than separate neutral and earth conductors.

This is the basis of much distribution wiring round the world. Practical systems are more complicated than this simple description, and there are usually numerous regulations and practices associated with them. However, for the present purposes, it is sufficient to note that much distribution wiring results in the neutral conductor being earthed at various points along its length. The situation in different countries is summarized in Table 8.

Each time the neutral conductor is earthed, there is the possibility that neutral current can divert out of the line into the earth itself (or more likely, into a convenient conducting earthed utility such as a water pipe) and return to the transformer/substation by a different route altogether. As soon as any neutral current diverts out of the lines, the currents left in the line are no longer exactly balanced. This can be expressed in various ways, for instance by saying that the neutral current is no longer equal and opposite to

**Table 8. Wiring practices in different countries**

| Country | What is known about distribution earthing practices | Source of information |
|---|---|---|
| Australia | Neutral is earthed at entrance to each house | Rauch et al., 1992 |
| France | Multiple earthing should not occur | |
| Germany | Cities: neutral multiply earthed (optional but common). Rural: neutral not normally earthed. | Rauch et al., 1992 |
| Japan | Multiple earthing not normal but can occur with certain motors and telecommunications equipment | Rauch et al., 1992 |
| Norway | Multiple earthing should not occur | Vistnes et al., 1997b |
| UK | Multiple earthing becoming more common. Over 64% of circuits with multiple earthing. | Swanson, 1996 |
| USA | Multiple earthing of neutral universal | Rauch et al., 1992 |

the zero-sequence current. The commonest and most useful way of describing the situation is to say that the line now has a net current, that is, a non-zero vector sum of all the currents flowing within the line.

Grounding currents – diverted neutral currents – flow on various conducting services, such as water pipes, and these may pass through a home. Where this happens there can be a region of elevated field within the home.

The net current clearly has a return path (all currents must flow in complete circuits). However, the return path, comprising water pipes, the ground, and maybe other distribution circuits or the same circuit further along its length, are likely to be rather distant from the line with the net current. So at any given point, for instance in a home supplied by the line, there is likely to be rather poor cancellation between the magnetic fields produced by the net current in the line and its return path. Often, it is accurate enough to calculate the magnetic field in a home based just on the net current in the distribution line supplying it, ignoring the return current altogether.

Net currents tend to be low — typically varying from a fraction of an amp to a few amps — and so these magnetic fields produced by net currents are also rather low compared to the magnetic fields produced directly underneath transmission lines. However, in homes which are distant from transmission lines (which is in fact the majority of homes in most countries), and from heavily loaded 3 phase distribution lines, there are no other significant sources of magnetic field outside the home, so it is the field produced by the net current which constitutes the dominant source of field, usually referred to as the "background field". If the return path is distant and we are regarding the field as produced by a single net current, it falls as one over the

36

distance from the source, so varies comparatively little over the volume of a typical home.

Note that, although the concept of a net current was introduced by reference to deliberate multiple earthing of a neutral conductor, there are two other ways net currents can arise. These are, firstly, where two adjacent distribution circuits meet and their neutral conductors are connected; and secondly, where faulty house wiring or a faulty appliance results in an unintended earth connection to the neutral (this probably occurs in 20% or more of homes in the UK and is also common in the USA). Both have the effect of allowing neutral current to divert out of the line, and thus of creating a net current. In practical situations, a net current could be created by any of these three mechanisms, or more likely by a combination of two or all three of them, and the magnetic field it produces is unaffected by which of the mechanisms produced it (Maslanyj et al., 2007).

With overhead distribution, the phase conductors are sometimes close together in a single cable. Often, however, they are not as close together as they are with underground distribution, and significant fields may arise from load currents as well as net currents. Net currents still exist, and the magnetic field is produced by both net current and the currents in the phase conductors.

The size of a net current depends on the size of the neutral current, which in turn depends on the size of the currents in the phase conductors. These vary over time, as loads are switched on and off. In fact, electricity use shows characteristic variations both diurnally and annually. Because net currents do not depend directly on loads, they do not vary over time in exactly the same way, but net currents (and hence the background magnetic fields in homes produced by them) do usually show characteristic variations over time.

Supplies to houses in the USA have two phases each at 110 V. Appliances connected at 220 V between the two phases do not contribute neutral current and therefore do not contribute to net currents. Appliances connected between one or other phase and earth do contribute to neutral current. The neutral current, and hence the net current and magnetic field, depends on the difference between the loads connected to the two phases rather than to the total load.

Another wiring source of magnetic field within homes is two-way switching of lights. If wired in orthodox fashion, no net currents are produced by two-way switched lights. However, the layout of the lighting circuits, switches and lights in a home often makes it tempting to wire the light in a way which effectively creates a loop of net current connecting the light and the two switches and enclosing part of the rest of the volume of the home. This loop of net current constitutes a source of magnetic field. Again, this source only operates when the relevant light is switched on.

*Spatial distribution*

EMF strength from any source diminishes as the distance from the source increases. Quite often, fields decrease with a power of the distance, depending on the configuration of the source (Kaune & Zafanella, 1992).

The field strength at any distance r is proportional to $1/r$, $1/r^2$, or $1/r^3$. The higher the power of r, the steeper the decrease of the field. When the field strength is proportional to one over the distance cubed ($1/r^3$), the field is reduced to an eighth with every doubling of the distance. Although good approximations, in practice, fields rarely follow these power laws exactly, departing from them particularly at very small distances or very large distances.

Within homes, the background field – the general level of field over the volume of the home – varies relatively little, as it usually comes from sources outside the home, and the inverse distance or inverse distance square relationship with distance does not produce great variation over a limited volume. However, superimposed on that background variation, there are local areas of higher fields, from appliances, or house wiring. The fields from such devices tend to decay at $1/r^3$.

*Temporal variation*

Because magnetic fields stem from currents, they vary over time as electricity demand varies over time. The relationship is not precise, as magnetic fields usually depend on net currents, which may not be precisely proportional to loads. Nonetheless, magnetic fields do show daily, weekly and annual variations. The magnetic field in a home in the UK can vary typically by a factor of 2 during the day above and below the daily average and by 25% during the year above and below the annual average.

Direct measurements of fields in the same property are available only up to about 5 years apart. Dovan et al. (Dovan, Kaune & Savitz, 1993) conducted measurements in a sample of homes from the childhood cancer study of Savitz et al. (1988) five years after they were first measured and reported a correlation of 0.7 between the spot measurements for the two periods. For longer periods, changes in fields have to be estimated from models, taking account of changes in loads, numbers of consumers, lengths of circuits, etc. Kaune et al. (1998) examined the correlation of loads over time for over one hundred transmission circuits in Sweden. The correlation decayed substantially over time (after about ten years) and thus, contemporaneous measurements are not reliable for retrospective estimation of ambient residential fields. Simple models look just at some measure of per capita consumption. Swanson (1996) developed a more sophisticated model which looks at changes in electricity systems and wiring practices as well. Even so, there are some changes which such models cannot easily take into account, so the results should be interpreted with caution. The models all suggest that average fields have increased over time, for example by a factor of 4.2 in the UK from 1949 to 1989.

Several authors (e.g. Kaune et al., 1994; Kaune & Zaffanella, 1994; Merchant, Renew & Swanson, 1994a; Merchant, Renew & Swanson, 1994c; Perry et al., 1981; Silva et al., 1989; UKCCSI, 2000) have found that the distribution of fields in domestic settings was approximately lognormal, and other published data also appear to exhibit this structure. It is therefore assumed here that all distributions are approximately lognormal and, thus, are better characterised by their geometric mean (GM) and geometric standard deviation (GSD) than by their arithmetic mean (AM) and standard deviation (SD). For a log-normal distribution, GM and GSD can be calculated from AM and SD using the following formulae (Swanson & Kaune, 1999):

$$GM = \frac{AM^2}{\sqrt{AM^2 + SD^2}}$$

$$GSD = e^{\sqrt{\ln\left[1 + \left(\frac{SD}{AM}\right)^2\right]}}$$

Data from various countries show, that the geometric mean of spot measurements in homes do not vary dramatically. Geometric means of the data provided range between 48 nT and 107 nT in Canada (Donnelly & Agnew, 1991; Mader et al., 1990; McBride, 1998), 60 nT in Finland (Juuti-lainen, 1989), 26 nT to 29 nT in Germany (Michaelis et al., 1997; Schüz et al., 2000), 29 nT in New Zealand (Dockerty et al., 1998; 1999), 37 nT to 48 nT in Sweden (Eriksson et al., 1987; Tomenius, 1986), 29 nT to 64 nT in the UK (Coghill, Steward & Philips, 1996; Merchant, Renew & Swanson, 1994c; Preece et al., 1996; UKCCSI, 1999), and 47 nT to 99 nT in the USA (Banks et al., 2002; Bracken et al., 1994; Davis, Mirick & Stevens, 2002; Kaune et al., 1987; Kaune et al., 1994; Kaune & Zaffanella, 1994; Kavet, Silva & Thornton, 1992; Linet et al., 1997; London et al., 1991; Zaffanella, 1993; Zaffanella & Kalton, 1998). There is a tendency of higher fields in countries with lower distribution voltage. These data should, however, be interpreted with care, given great differences in the evaluation conditions (e.g. number of homes included).

### 2.2.2.2.4   Electrical equipment, appliances, and devices

The commonest source of magnetic field within a home is not the fixed wiring of the home but mains appliances. Every mains appliance produces a magnetic field when it is drawing current (and with some appliances, the mains transformer is still connected and drawing current whenever the appliance is plugged in, regardless of whether it is switched on or not). In a typical home the magnetic field consists of the background field with "peaks" of field surrounding each appliance. Exposure to magnetic fields from home appliances can sometimes usefully be considered separately from exposure to fields due to power lines. Power lines produce relatively low-intensity, small-gradient fields that are always present throughout the home, whereas fields produced by appliances are invariably more intense, have much steeper spatial gradients, and are, for the most part, experienced only sporadically. The appropriate way of combining the two field types into a single measure of exposure depends critically on the exposure metric considered.

Magnetic fields from appliances are produced by electric current used by the devices. Currents in an appliance can often be approximated as small closed loops. Appliances of that type usually produce a comparatively small field, because any current within the appliance is balanced by a return current a comparatively short distance away. It is usually only in some appliances such as kettles, convection fires, electric blankets, that the current flows in the heating element round a reasonably large loop.

However, many appliances contain an electric motor, a transformer, or a choke or inductor. These all depend on magnetic fields for their operation: that is, they deliberately create a magnetic field inside the appliance. The magnetic field around those appliances (stray field) depends strongly on the design, which aims to keep stray fields as low as possible. If the design priorities are not efficiency but low cost, small size or low weight, the result will be an appliance that produces higher magnetic fields.

Thus higher fields are often produced by small and cheap transformers (e.g. mains adaptors, transistor radios) and small, cheap and compact motors (e.g. mains razors, electric can openers). A survey of 57 mains appliances conducted for National Grid in 1992 (Swanson, 1996) found that the field produced by an appliance was, on average, independent of the power consumed by the appliance.

Whether it is produced directly by the currents or indirectly by leakage field from a transformer or motor, the magnetic field produced by an appliance usually falls as one over the distance cubed. In consequence, magnetic fields from appliances tend to be significant only close to the appliance itself. More than a metre or two away, they have usually become so small that they have effectively merged into the background field. Very close to an appliance, the fields can rise to quite high levels; hundreds of microteslas on the surface of many mains radios, and over a millitesla on the surface of some mains razors. Exactly how high the field rises depends not just on the size of the field produced by the source (motor or transformer) inside the appliance, but also on how close the source can be approached. This depends on where within the volume of the appliance the source is located.

Examples of the field levels likely to be encountered at short distances from various appliances are presented in Table 9.

**Table 9. Examples of magnetic flux densities from 50 and 60 Hz domestic electrical appliances** [a]

| | Source | Magnetic flux densities (µT) | | | |
|---|---|---|---|---|---|
| | | 60 Hz at 30 cm [b] | | 50 Hz at 50 cm [c] | |
| | | Median | Range [d] | Computed field | SD |
| Bathroom | Hair dryers | 1 | bg***–7 | 0.12 | 0.1 |
| | Electric shavers | 2 | bg–10 | 0.84 | |
| | Electric showers | | | 0.44 | 0.75 |
| | Shaver socket | | | 1.24 | 0.27 |
| Kitchen | Blenders | 1 | 0.5–2 | 0.97 | 1.05 |
| | Can openers | 15 | 4–30 | 1.33 | 1.33 |
| | Coffee makers | bg | bg–0.1 | 0.06 | 0.07 |
| | Dishwashers | 1 | 0.6–3 | 0.8 | 0.46 |
| | Food processors | 0.6 | 0.5–2 | 0.23 | 0.23 |
| | Microwave ovens | 0.4 | 0.1–20 | 1.66 | 0.63 |
| | Mixers | 1 | 0.5–10 | 0.69 | 0.69 |
| | Electric ovens | 0.4 | 0.1–0.5 | 0.39 | 0.23 |
| | Refrigerators | 0.2 | bg–2 | 0.05 | 0.03 |
| | Freezers | | | 0.04 | 0.02 |
| | Toasters | 0.3 | bg–0.7 | 0.09 | 0.08 |
| | Electric knives | | | 0.12 | 0.05 |
| | Liquidisers | | | 0.29 | 0.35 |
| | Kettle | | | 0.26 | 0.11 |
| | Extractor fan | | | 0.5 | 0.93 |
| | Cooker hood | | | 0.26 | 0.10 |
| | Hobs | | | 0.08 | 0.05 |
| Laundry/Utility | Clothes dryers | 0.2 | bg–0.3 | 0.34 | 0.42 |
| | Washing machines | 0.7 | 0.1–3 | 0.96 | 0.56 |
| | Irons | 0.1 | 0.1–0.3 | 0.03 | 0.02 |
| | Portable heaters | 2 | 0.1–4 | 0.22 | 0.18 |
| | Vacuum cleaners | 6 | 2–20 | 0.78 | 0.74 |
| | Central heating boiler | | | 0.27 | 0.26 |
| | Central heating timer | | | 0.14 | 0.17 |
| Living room | TVs | 0.7 | bg–2 | 0.26 | 0.11 |
| | VCRs | | | 0.06 | 0.05 |
| | Fish tank pumps | | | 0.32 | 0.09 |
| | Tuners/tape players | bg | bg–0.1 | 0.24 | |

| | | | | | |
|---|---|---|---|---|---|
| Table 9. Continued. | | | | | |
| | Audio systems | | | 0.08 | 0.14 |
| | Radios | | | 0.06 | 0.04 |
| | Bedroom | | | | |
| | Clock alarm | 0-50 | | 0.05 | 0.05 |
| Office | Air cleaners | 3.5 | 2–5 | | |
| | Copy machines | 2 | 0.2–4 | | |
| | Fax machines | bg | bg–0.2 | | |
| | Fluorescent lights | 0.6 | bg–3 | | |
| | VDUs | 0.5 | 0.2–0.6 | 0.14 | 0.07 |
| Tools | Battery chargers | 0.3 | 0.2-0.4 | | |
| | Drills | 3 | 2-4 | | |
| | Power saws | 4 | 0.9-30 | | |
| Miscellaneous | Central heating pump | | | 0.51 | 0.47 |
| | Burglar alarm | | | 0.18 | 0.11 |

[a] Source: ICNIRP, 2003.
[b] Source: EPA, 1992.
[c] Source: Preece et al., 1997.
[d] bg: background.

Preece et al. (1997) assessed broadband magnetic fields at various distances from domestic appliances in use in the United Kingdom. The magnetic fields were calculated from a mathematical model fitted to actual measurements made on the numbers of appliances. They reported that few appliances generated fields in excess of 0.2 µT at 1 meter distance: microwave cookers $0.37 \pm 0.14$ µT; washing machines $0.27 \pm 0.14$ µT; dishwashers $0.23 \pm 0.13$ µT; some electric showers $0.11 \pm 0.25$ µT and can openers $0.20 \pm 0.21$ µT.

Gauger (1984) and Zaffanella & Kalton (1998) reported narrow band and broadband data, respectively, for the USA. In Gauger's analysis of hand held hair dryers, at 3 cm from their surfaces, magnetic felds of about 6, 15, and 22 µT were produced for three types of hair dryers. Zaffanella (1993) found that at a distance of 27 cm from digital and analog clocks/clock radios, the median fields were 0.13 µT and 1.5 µT for digital and analog clocks, respectively. Preece et al. (1997) also measured the magnetic fields produced by hair dryers and electric clocks. At distances of 5 and 50 cm from hair dryers field measurements were 17 and 0.12 µT, respectively, and from electric clocks 5.0 and 0.04 µT, respectively.

Florig & Hoburg (1990) characterized fields from electric blankets, using a three-dimensional computer model; maximum, minimum, and volume-average fields within human forms were presented as a function of blanket type and geometric factors such as body size, body-blanket separation, and lateral body position. They reported that when blankets are heating, typical flux densities range from a few tenths of microtesla on the side of the body farthest from the blanket to a few tens of microtesla on the side closest to the blanket. Wilson et al. (1996) used spot measurements made in the home and in the laboratory. They reported that the average magnetic fields from electric blankets to which the whole body is exposed are between 1 and 3T. More recently, from eight-hour measurements, Lee et al. (2000) estimated that the time-weighted average magnetic field exposures from overnight use of electric blankets ranged between 0.1 and 2 $\mu$T.

It should be noted that many appliances produce a wide range of harmonics. The interpretation of results from broad band measurements can be misleading, if the spectral content of the fields is not known. Another problem with the interpretation of field measurements from appliances may result from the huge spatial and temporal variability of the fields.

### 2.2.2.2.5  Distribution substations and transformers

Overhead lines and underground cables at whatever voltage usually terminate at substations. All substations usually contain apparatus to perform similar functions: transforming, switching metering and monitoring. Substations range from large complexes several hundred metres in extent at one end of the scale to simple pole-mounted transformers at the other end of the scale. One feature they all have in common is that members of the general public are excluded from most of the functional regions of the substation, either by a perimeter fence or enclosure (for ground-based substations) or by the height of the pole (for pole-mounted substations).

Although substations vary in their complexity and size, the principles which determine the magnetic fields they produce are common. Firstly, in all substations, there are a number of components which produce a negligible magnetic field outside the confines of the substation. These include the transformers, virtually all switches and circuit breakers, and virtually all metering and monitoring equipment. Secondly, in many cases the largest fields in publicly accessible regions are produced by the overhead lines and underground cables running in and out of the substation. Thirdly, all substations contain a system of conductors (often referred to as 'busbars') which connect the various components within it, and these busbars usually constitute the main source of magnetic field within the substation producing appreciable field outside.

The size of the currents and the separation of the busbars are both larger in higher-voltage substations than in lower-voltage ones. However, the perimeter fence also tends to be further away from the busbars in higher-voltage substations. Therefore, the resulting field to which the public can be exposed can be somewhat greater at higher-voltage substations than at lower-voltage ones. In both cases, the magnetic field falls very rapidly with distance from the substation.

43

Typical values in the United Kingdom for substations of 275 and 400 kV at the perimeter fence is 10 µT, and 1.6 µT for an 11 kV substation. Renew, Male & Maddock found the mean field at the substation boundary, measured at about 0.5 m above ground level, to be 1.6 µT (range: 0.3–10.4 µT) (Renew, Male & Maddock, 1990). They also found (for the 19 substations where the background field was low enough to enable this measurement to be made) the mean distance at which the field at the substation boundary was halved to be 1.4 m (range: 0.6–2.0 m). NRPB has performed similar measurements on 27 substations in the UK with similar findings (Maslanyj, 1996). The mean field at the substation boundary was 1.1 µT, with a field of 0.2 µT at between 0–1.5 m from the boundary and a field of 0.05 µT at between 1–5 m.

### 2.2.2.2.6 Transport

Dietrich & Jacobs (1999) have reported magnetic fields associated with various transportation systems across a range of frequencies. AC currents of several hundred amperes are commonly used in electric railway systems, and magnetic fields are highly variable with time, the maxima often occurring during braking and acceleration. Up to a few millitesla can be generated near motor equipment, and up to a few tens of microteslas elsewhere on the trains (Table 10). Elevated ELF exposure levels also occur in the areas adjacent to electrified rail lines. Peak magnetic flux densities up to a few tens of microteslas have been recorded on the platform of a local city railway line (EC, 1996). Magnetic flux densities of a few microteslas were measured at 5 m from the line reducing to a microtesla or so at 10 m. In France, measurements inside a high-speed train and at a distance of 10 m outside the train showed peak values around 6 to 7 µT during high-speed drive (Gourdon, 1993). In a Swedish study (Anger, Berglund & Hansson Mild, 1997) field values in the driver cabinet range from a few to over 100 µT with mean values for a working day between a few to up to tens of microteslas depending on the engine. Some UK results are summarized in Table 10.

The magnetic fields encountered in electrified rail systems vary considerably because of the large variety of possible arrangements of power supply and traction. Many of the conventional rail systems use DC traction motors and AC power supplies with frequencies of 16 2/3 Hz or 50 Hz AC power in Europe and 25 Hz or 60 Hz in North America. Such systems often rely on pulse rectification either carried out on board or prior to supply and this gives rise to a significant alternating component in the static or quasi–static magnetic fields from the traction components of the trains (Chadwick & Lowes, 1998). Major sources of static and alternating magnetic fields are the smoothing and line filter inductors and not the motors themselves, which are designed to minimise flux leakage. Alternatively where DC supplies are used, voltage choppers are used to control the power by switching the power supply on and off regularly. Recently AC motors have become more common with the advances in high capacity solid-state technologies. When the required frequency differs from that of the supply frequency, converters are used to supply the correct frequency, or inverters are used when the power supply is DC (Muc, 2001).

**Table 10. Alternating magnetic fields from UK electrified rail systems** [a]

| System and Source | AC magnetic flux density | Frequency | Comments |
|---|---|---|---|
| London underground | Up to 20 µT | 100 Hz | In the driver's cab; arising from traction components and on board smoothing inductors |
| Suburban trains | | | |
| 750 DC Electric | Up to 1 mT | 100 Hz | Floor level |
| Motor Units | 16–64 µT | 100 Hz | In passenger car at table height |
| | 16-48 µT | 100 Hz | Outside train on platform |
| Mainline trains | | | |
| Electric Motor Units | Up to 15 mT | 100 Hz | Floor level above inductor |
| Mainline trains | | | |
| Locomotives | Up to 2.5 mT | 100 Hz | 0.5 m above floor in equipment car |
| | 5–50 µT | 50 Hz | In passenger coaches |

[a] Source: Allen et al., 1994; Chadwick & Lowes, 1998.

Train drivers and railway workers incur higher exposures than passengers because they often work closer to important sources. Nordenson et al. (2001) reported that engine drivers were exposed to 16 2/3 Hz magnetic fields ranging from a few to more than 100 µT. Hamalainen et al. (1999) reported magnetic fields ranging in frequency from 10 Hz to 2 kHz measured in local and long distance electrified trains in Finland where roughly more than half of the rail network is electrified with 50 Hz. Average levels to which workers and passengers were exposed varied by a factor of 1000 (0.3–290 µT for passengers and 10–6000 µT for workers). On Swedish trains, Nordenson et al. (2001) found values ranging from 25 to 120 µT for power-frequency fields in the driver's cabin, depending on the type (age and model) of locomotive. Typical daily average exposures were in the range of 2–15 µT.

Wenzl (1997) reported measurements on a 25 Hz AC electrified portion of the Northeast Rail Corridor in Maryland and Pennsylvania. Averages for workers were found to range between 0.3 and 1.8 µT , although 60 Hz and 100 Hz fields were also present from transmission lines suspended above the railway catenaries and from the railway safety communications and signalling system respectively. Chadwick & Lowes (1998) reported flux densities of up to 15 mT modulated at 100 Hz at floor level on British Electric Motor Units and 100 Hz fields of up to 2.5 mT in mainline locomotives (Table 10).

Other forms of transport, such as aeroplanes and electrified road vehicles are also expected to increase exposure, but have not been investigated extensively. Other possible ELF exposures associated with transport are discussed in 2.2.2.2.8.

### 2.2.2.2.7 Heating

The magnetic fields associated with underfloor heating systems depend on the configuration and depth of the cables, and the current flowing in them (Allen et al., 1994). Typically magnetic flux densities of up to a few microtesla can occur at floor level falling to a few tenths of a microtesla at 1 m above the floor. Systems operating at commercial premises can give up to a few hundred microtesla at floor level falling to a few tens of microtesla at 1 m above the floor. Many systems only draw current overnight, relying on off-peak electricity, and the heat capacity of the floor to provide warmth during the day.

### 2.2.2.2.8 Miscellaneous sources of ELF fields (other than power frequencies)

ELF magnetic fields are also generated in the home by petrol engine-powered devices such as lawnmowers, strimmers and chainsaws. Personal localised exposures of up to a few hundred microteslas can result when using such equipment (EC, 1996).

The pulsating battery current in the mobile phone generates a low-frequency nonsinusoidal magnetic field in the vicinity of the phone (Jokela, Puranen & Sihvonen, 2004). The time course is approximately a square wave with a pulse cycle similar to the radiation pattern of the phone (pulse width 0.7 to 1 ms with a repetition period of 4.6 ms). As the current drawn by the phones investigated (seven different types) was up to 3 A and the devices are used very close to the brain (approximately 10 mm), the field may exceed 50 $\mu$T.

Occupational exposure to ELF electric and magnetic fields from video display units (VDUs) has recently received attention. VDUs produce both power-frequency fields and higher-frequency fields ranging from about 50 Hz up to 50 kHz (NIEHS, 1998). Sandström et al. (1993) measured magnetic fields from VDUs in 150 offices and found that rms values measured at 50 cm from the screen ranged up to 1.2 $\mu$T (mean: 0.21 $\mu$T) in the ELF range (0–3 kHz) and up to 142 nT (mean: 23 nT) in the VLF range (3–30 kHz).

Cars are another source of ELF magnetic field exposure. Vedholm (1996) measured the field in 7 different cars (two of them with the battery underneath the back seat or in the trunk), engines running idle. In the left front seat the magnetic field, at various ELF frequencies ranged from 0.05 to 3.9 $\mu$T and in the left back seat from 0.02 to 3.8 $\mu$T. The highest values where parts of the body are likely to be were found at the left ankle at the left front seat, 0.24–13 $\mu$T. The higher values were found in cars with the battery located underneath the back seat or in the trunk.

Another source of ELF magnetic fields result from the steel belts in car tires that are permanently magnetized. Depending on the speed of the car,

46

this may cause magnetic fields in the frequency range below 20 Hz. The field has a fundamental frequency determined by the speed (rotation rate of the tire) and a high harmonic content. At the tread fields can exceed 500 μT and on the seats the maximum is approximately 2 μT (Milham, Hatfield & Tell, 1999).

### 2.2.2.2.9 Occupational exposure in the electric power industry

Strong magnetic fields are encountered mainly in close proximity to high currents (Maddock, 1992). In the electric power industry, high currents are found in overhead lines and underground cables, and in busbars in power stations and substations. The busbars close to generators in power stations can carry currents up to 20 times higher than those typically carried by the 400-kV transmission system (Merchant, Renew & Swanson, 1994b).

Exposure to the strong fields produced by these currents can occur either as a direct result of the job, e.g. a lineman or cable splicer, or as a result of work location, e.g. when office workers are located on a power station or substation site. It should be noted that job categories may include workers with very different exposures, e.g. linemen working on live or dead circuits. Therefore, although reporting magnetic-field exposure by job category is useful, a complete understanding of exposure requires a knowledge of the activities or tasks and the location as well as measurements made by personal exposure meters.

The average magnetic fields to which workers are exposed for various jobs in the electric power industry have been reported as follows: 0.18–1.72 μT for workers in power stations, 0.8–1.4 μT for workers in substations, 0.03–4.57μT for workers on lines and cables and 0.2–18.48 μT for electricians (AGNIR, 2001b; NIEHS, 1998).

### 2.2.2.2.10 Other occupational sources

Exposure to magnetic fields varies greatly across occupations. The use of personal dosimeters has enabled exposure to be measured for particular types of job.

Measurements by the National Institute for Occupational Safety and Health (NIOSH) in various industries are summarized in Table 11 (NIOSH, 1996).

In some cases the variability is large. This indicates that there are instances in which workers in these categories are exposed to far stronger fields than the means listed here.

Floderus et al. (1993) investigated sets of measurements made at 1015 different workplaces. This study covered 169 different job categories, and participants wore the dosimeters for a mean duration of 6.8 h. The most common measurement was 0.05 μT and measurements above 1 μT were rare.

**Table 11. Magnetic flux densities from equipment in various industries** [a]

| Industry | Source | ELF magnetic flux density (µT) | Comments | Other frequencies |
|---|---|---|---|---|
| Manufacturing | Electrical resistance heater | 600–1400 | Tool exposures measured at operator's chest | VLF |
| | Induction heater | 1–46 | | |
| | Hand-held grinder | 300 | | |
| | Grinder | 11 | | |
| | Lathe, drill press etc | 0.1–0.4 | | |
| Electrogalvanizing | Rectification | 200–460 | Rectified DC current (with an ELF ripple) galvanized metal parts | Static fields |
| | Outdoor electric line and substation | 10–170 | | |
| Aluminum refining | Aluminum pot rooms | 0.34–3 | Highly-rectified DC current (with an ELF ripple) refines aluminum | Static field |
| | Rectification room | 30–330 | | Static field |
| Steel foundry | Ladle refinery, electrodes active | 17–130 | Highest ELF field was at the chair of control room operator | ULF from ladle's magnetic stirrer |
| | Electrodes inactive | 0.06–0.37 | | |
| | Electrogalvanizing unit | 0.2–110 | | VLF |
| Television broadcasting | Video cameras (studio and minocam) | 0.72–2.4 | Measured at 30 cm | VLF |
| | Video tape degaussers | 16–330 | | |
| | Light control centres | 0.1–30 | | |
| | Studios and newsrooms | 0.2–0.5 | Walk-through surveys | |

**Table 11. Continued.**

| Telecommuni cations | Relay switching racks | 0.15–3.2 | Measured 5-7 cm from relays | Static fields and ULF-ELF tran-sients |
|---|---|---|---|---|
| | Switching rooms (relay and elec-tronic switches) | 0.01–130 | Walk-through sur-vey | Static fields and ULF-ELF tran-sients |
| | Underground phone vault | 0.3–0.5 | Walk-through sur-vey | Static fields and ULF-ELF tran-sients |
| Hospitals | Intensive care unit | 0.01–22 | Measured at nurse's chest position | VLF |
| | Post anaesthe-sia care unit | 0.01–2.4 | | VLF |
| | Magnetic reso-nance imaging | 0.05–28 | Measured at technician's work locations | Static, VLF and RF |
| Government offices | Desk work loca-tions | 0.01–0.7 | Peaks due to laser printers | |
| | Desks near power centre | 1.8-5 | | |
| | Power cables in floor | 1.5–17 | | |
| | Computer centre | 0.04–0.66 | | |
| | Desktop cooling fan | 100 | Appliances mea-sured at 15 cm | |
| | Other office appliances | 1–20 | | |
| | Building power supplies | 2.5–180 | | |

[a] Source: (NIOSH, 1996).

### 2.2.2.2.11  Arc and spot welding

In arc welding, metal parts are fused together by the energy of a plasma arc struck between two electrodes or between one electrode and the metal to be welded. A power-frequency current usually produces the arc but higher frequencies may be used in addition to strike or to maintain the arc. A feature of arc welding is that the insulated welding cable, which can carry currents of hundreds of amperes, can touch the body of the operator. Mag-netic flux densities in excess of 1 mT have been measured at the surface of a welding cable and 100 μT close to the power supply (Allen et al., 1994).

Stuchly & Lecuyer (1989) surveyed the exposure of arc welders to magnetic fields and determined the exposure at 10 cm from the head, chest, waist, gonads, hands and legs. Whilst it is possible for the hand to be exposed to fields in excess of 1 mT, the trunk is typically exposed to several hundred microtesla. Once the arc has been struck, these welders work with comparatively low voltages and this is reflected in the electric field strengths measured; i.e. up to a few tens of volts per metre (AGNIR, 2001b).

Bowman et al. (1988) measured exposure for a tungsten-inert gas welder of up to 90 µT. Similar measurements reported by the National Radiological Protection Board indicate magnetic flux densities of up to 100 µT close to the power supply, 1 mT at the surface of the welding cable and at the surface of the power supply and 100–200 µT at the operator position (AGNIR, 2001b). London et al. (1994) reported the average workday exposure of 22 welders and flame cutters to be much lower (1.95 µT).

### 2.2.2.2.12 Induction furnaces

Electrically conducting materials such as metals and crystals can be heated as a consequence of eddy current losses induced by alternating magnetic fields. Typical applications include drying, bonding, zone refining, melting, surface hardening, annealing, tempering, brazing and welding. The main sources of electromagnetic fields in induction heaters are the power supply, the high frequency transformer and the induction heater coil, and the product being processed. The latter is positioned within a coil, which acts like a primary winding of a transformer. This coil generates magnetic fields that transfer power to the load, which behaves like a single turn short-circuited secondary winding.

The frequency determines the penetration of the field, a lower frequency being used for volume heating and a higher frequency for surface heating. For example frequencies of a few tens of hertz are used for heating copper billets prior to forging, whereas frequencies of a few megahertz are used for sealing bottle tops. The heating coils range in size depending on the application. Small single turn devices of a few centimetres diameter are used for localised heating of a product, and large multi-turn systems of 1 or 2 m diameter are used in furnaces capable of melting several tons of iron. Power requirements also depend on the application, and range from about 1 kW for small items to several megawatt for induction furnaces (Allen et al., 1994).

Studies of magnetic flux densities in the vicinity of induction furnaces and equipment heaters have shown that operators may have some of the highest maximum exposure levels found in industry (Table 12). Typical maximum flux densities for induction heaters operating at frequencies up to 10 kHz are presented in Table 13. Somewhat higher levels of 1–60 mT have been reported in Sweden (Lövsund, Öberg & Nilsson, 1982), at distances of 0.1–1 m.

**Table 12. Maximum exposures to power frequency magnetic flux densities in the workplace** [a]

| Workplace | Occupation / source | Magnetic flux density (µT) |
|---|---|---|
| Industry | Induction workers | $10^4$ |
|  | Railway workers | $10^3$ |
|  | Power industry | $10^3$ |
|  | Arc welders | $10^2$ |
| Office | Tape erasers | $10^2$ |
|  | VDUs | 1 |
| General | Underfloor heating | 10 |
|  | Electric motors | 10 |

[a] Source: Allen et al., 1994.

**Table 13. Examples of magnetic fields produced by induction heaters operating up to 10 kHz** [a]

| Machine | Input power | Frequency | Position | Maximum magnetic flux density (µT) |
|---|---|---|---|---|
| Copper billet heater | Up to 6 MW | 50 Hz | 1 m from coil line | 540 |
| Steel billet heater | ~ 800 kW | 1.1 kHz | 1 m from coil | 125 |
| Axle induction hardener | 140 kW | 1.65 kHz | Operator position | 29 |
| Copper tube annealer | 600 kW | 2.9 kHz | 0.5 m from coil | 375 |
| Chain normalisers | 20 kW | 8.7–10 kHz | 0.5 m from coils | 25 |

[a] Source: Allen et al., 1994.

Electric field strengths in the vicinity of induction heaters that operate in the frequency range of interest are usually no more than several volts per metre.

### 2.2.2.2.13 Induction cooking equipment

Originally induction cooking equipment was restricted largely to commercial catering environments where three phase power supplies were available; however, single phase domestic varieties are now common (IEC, 2000). Induction cooking hobs normally operate at frequencies of a few tens of kilohertz. In domestic environments a frequency of over 20 kHz is necessary to avoid pan noise and below 50 kHz to have a maximum efficiency and comply with electromagnetic compatibility product standards. Powers normally range between 1–3 kW used for domestic appliances and 5–10 kW for commercial equipment. Under worst-case exposure conditions, corresponding to poor coupling between the coil and pan, maximum magnetic flux densities are usually less than a few microtesla at a few tens of centimetres from the front edge of the hobs. Electric field strengths are usually no more than a few tens of volt per metre because the appliances do not use high voltage electricity. Usually the fundamental frequency induction dominates the magnetic field; however, some models produce harmonic components comparable in magnitude to that of the fundamental (Allen et al., 1994).

### 2.2.2.2.14  Security and access control systems

A number of devices generate electromagnetic fields for security purposes and for controlling personal access. These include metal detectors, radiofrequency identification (RFID) equipment and electronic article surveillance (EAS) systems, also known as anti-theft systems. RFID and EAS equipment use a broad range of frequencies, ranging from sub-kilohertz frequencies to microwave frequencies.

*Metal detectors*

Metal detectors are used for security, e.g. at airports. The two main types are the free-standing walk-through systems and the hand-held detectors. Walk-through detectors usually consist of two columns, one which houses the transmitter unit and uses conducting coils to produce a pulsed magnetic field, and the other which contains a receiver which employs a set of coils to detect the electric currents induced in metallic objects by the pulsed field. The magnetic field waveforms from both detectors consist of a train of bipolar pulses and fast Fourier transforms (FFTs) of the pulses exhibit broad spectral content with an amplitude peak in the region of 1 kHz. Peak magnetic fields are usually a few tens of microtesla (Cooper, 2002).

Hand-held detectors normally contain a coil, which carries an alternating current, at frequencies of a few tens of kilohertz. If electrically conducting material is brought within the detection range of the device, eddy currents are produced in the material that disturb the configuration of the magnetic field. The corresponding change in the behaviour of the coil, which may be resonant, can then be detected by the instrument.

The magnetic fields from hand-held metal detectors tend to be weaker and more localised than those from walk-through devices. The maximum magnetic flux density encountered near the casing is typically a few microtesla (Cooper, 2002).

*Electronic access and security systems (EAS)*

EAS systems use electromagnetic fields to prevent unauthorised removal of items from shops, libraries and supermarkets and are even used in hospitals to stop abduction of babies. The detection panels are the most significant source of electromagnetic fields. The tags or labels serve only to cause a slight perturbation of the fields in the detection systems and are usually passive in the sense that they do not contain any power source, although they may contain a small number of electronic components such as diodes.

The third component of EAS systems is known as "deactivators". These are used to "switch off" disposable tags or to remove re-usable tags. The deactivator fields are usually higher in absolute amplitude than the main detection fields, though they are confined to a small region.

There are two main types of EAS system that operate within the ELF-VLF range. Both use inductive fields, so the field is almost completely magnetic in nature, and the field propagation is negligible (ICNIRP, 2002; IEC, 2000).

The electromagnetic (EM) type operates at frequencies of 20 Hz–20 kHz and detects harmonics in the detection field that are set up during the non-linear magnetisation of the magnetically soft tag. The magnetic flux density at the point midway through panels normally placed 1–3 m apart is from a few tens of microtesla up to about 100 μT. Typical field strengths fall as the operating frequency rises and some systems use more than one frequency simultaneously.

The resonant acousto-magnetic (AM) type operates at typical frequencies around 60 kHz, and detects the ringing of the tag's magnetic field caused by an element that resonates in the presence of a specific frequency pulsed magnetic field that occurs in the detection zone.

Some examples of maximum magnetic flux densities inside EAS gates are reported in Table 14.

Table 14. Examples of peak magnetic flux densities within magnetic type EAS gates

| Type | Frequency (waveform [a]) | Magnetic flux density (μT) | Distance from transmitter (cm) |
|---|---|---|---|
| Electromagnetic (EM) | 73 Hz (SCW) | 146 | 31.5 |
| | 219 Hz (SCW) | 122 | 36 |
| | 230 Hz (SCW) | 93 | 42 |
| | 535.7 Hz (SCW) | 72 | 36 |
| | 6.25 kHz (SCW) | 39 | 45 |
| | 5 kHz / 7.5 kHz (CW) | 43 | 48.5 |
| | 1 kHz (PMS) | 100 | 41 |
| | 6.25 kHz (CW) | 58 | 25.7 |
| Acoustomagnetic (AM) | 58 kHz (PMS) | 65 | 36 |
| | 58 kHz (PMS) | 17.4 | 62.5 |
| | 58 kHz (CW) | 52 | 37.2 |

[a] CW – Continuous Wave, SCW – Sinusoidal Continuous Wave, PMS = Pulsed Modulated Sinusoid.

Members of the public receive transient exposure to the main detection field because of the method of use of EAS systems; workers receive longer-term whole body exposure to lower amplitude fields outside the detection system and transient localised exposures from the deactivators.

### 2.2.2.2.15 Sewing machines

Hansen et al. (2000) reported higher-than-background magnetic fields near industrial sewing machines, because of proximity to motors, with field strengths ranging from 0.32–11.1 μT at a position corresponding approximately to the sternum of the operator. The average exposure for six workers working a full work-shift in the garment industry ranged from 0.21–3.20 μT. A more extensive study of the personal exposures of 34 workers using sewing machines reported exposures (Kelsh et al., 2003) at the waist, where the mean 60-Hz magnetic field was 0.9 μT with a range between 0.07–3.7 μT.

## 2.3     Assessment of exposure

### 2.3.1     General considerations

Electric and magnetic fields are complex and can be characterized by many different physical parameters. Some of these parameters are discussed more fully in section 2.1. In general, they include transients, harmonic content, peak values and time above thresholds, as well as average levels. It is not known which of these parameters or what combination of parameters, if any, are relevant for the induction of health effects. If there were a known biophysical mechanism of interaction for e.g. carcinogenesis, it would be possible to identify the critical parameters of exposure, including relevant timing of exposure. However, in the absence of a generally accepted mechanism, most exposure assessments in epidemiological studies are based on a time-weighted average of the field, a measure that is also related to some, but not all field characteristics (Zaffanella & Kalton, 1998).

The physical characteristics of electric and magnetic fields have been described in detail in section 2.1. Some of the characteristics of exposure to electric and magnetic fields which make exposure assessment for the purposes of epidemiological studies particularly difficult are listed below.

- *Prevalence of exposure.* Everyone in the population is exposed to some degree to ELF electric and magnetic fields and therefore exposure assessment can only separate the more from the less exposed individuals, as opposed to separating individuals who are exposed from those who are not.

- *Inability of subjects to identify exposure.* Exposure to electric and magnetic fields, whilst ubiquitous, is usually not detectable by the exposed person nor memorable, and hence epidemiological studies cannot rely solely on questionnaire data to characterize past exposures adequately.

- *Lack of clear contrast between "high" and "low" exposure.* The difference between the average field strengths to which "highly exposed" and "less highly exposed" individuals in a population are subjected is not great. The typical average magnetic fields in homes appear to be about 0.05–0.1 µT. Pooled analyses of childhood leukaemia and magnetic fields, such as that by Ahlbom et al. (2000), have used 0.4 µT as a high-exposure category. Therefore, an exposure assessment method has to separate reliably exposures which may differ by factors of only 2 or 4. Even in most of the occupational settings considered to entail "high exposures" the average fields measured are only one order of magnitude higher than those measured in residential settings (Kheifets et al., 1995).

- *Variability of exposure over time: short-term.* Fields (particularly magnetic fields) vary over time-scales of seconds or longer. Assessing a person's exposure over any period involves using a single summary figure for a highly variable quantity.

- *Variability of exposure over time: long-term.* Fields are also likely to vary over time-scales of seasons and years. With the exception of historical data on loads carried by high-voltage power lines, data on such variation are rare. Therefore, when a person's exposure at some period in the past is assessed from data collected later, an assumption has to be made. The usual assumption is that the exposure has not changed. Some authors (e.g. Jackson, 1992; Petridou et al., 1993; Swanson, 1996) have estimated the variations of exposure over time from available data, for example, on electricity consumption. These apply to population averages and are unlikely to be accurate for individuals.

- *Variability of exposure over space.* Magnetic fields vary over the volume of, for example, a building so that, as people move around, they may experience fields of varying intensity. Personal exposure monitoring captures this, but other assessment methods generally do not.

People are exposed to fields in different settings, such as at home, at school, at work, while travelling and outdoors. Current understanding of the contributions to exposure from different sources and in different settings is limited. Most studies make exposure assessments within a single environment, typically at home for residential studies and at work for occupational studies. Some recent studies have included measures of exposure from more than one setting (e.g. Feychting, Forssen & Floderus, 1997; Forssén et al., 2000; UKCCSI, 1999).

In epidemiological studies, the distribution of exposures in a population has consequences for the statistical power of the study. Most populations are characterized by an approximately log-normal distribution with a heavy preponderance of low-level exposure and much less high-level exposure. Pilot studies of exposure distribution are important for developing effective study designs.

Since most epidemiological studies have investigated magnetic rather than electric fields, the next six sections will deal with aspects of magnetic field exposure and section 2.3.7 with electric field exposure.

### 2.3.2 Assessing residential exposure to magnetic fields: methods not involving measurement

#### 2.3.2.1 Distance

The simplest possible way of assessing exposure is to record proximity to a facility (such as a power line or a substation) which is likely to be a source of field. This does provide a very crude measure of exposure to both electric and magnetic fields from that source, but takes no account of other sources or of how the fields vary with distance from the source (which is different for different sources). Distances reported by study subjects rather than measured by the investigators tend to be unreliable. Recently over half of the time-averaged magnetic field exposures above 0.4 µT in the UKCCS were attributable to sources other than high-voltage power lines (Maslanyj et al., 2007).

#### 2.3.2.2 Wire code

Wire coding is a non-intrusive method of classifying dwellings on the basis of their distance from visible electrical installations and the characteristics of these installations. This method does not take account of exposure from sources within the home. Wertheimer & Leeper (1979) devised a simple set of rules to classify residences with respect to their potential for having a higher-than-usual exposure to magnetic fields. Their assumptions were simple:

- the field strength decreases with distance from the source;

- current flowing in power lines decreases at every pole from which "service drop" wires deliver power to houses;

- if both thick and thin conductors are used for lines carrying power at a given voltage, and more than one conductor is present, it is reasonable to assume that more and thicker conductors are required to carry greater currents; and

- when lines are buried in a conduit or a trench, their contribution to exposure can be neglected. This is because buried cables are placed close together and the fields produced by currents flowing from and back to the source cancel each other much more effectively than when they are spaced apart on a cross beam on a pole (see section 2.2.2.2.2).

Wertheimer & Leeper (1979) used these four criteria to define two and later four (Wertheimer & Leeper, 1982), then five (Savitz et al., 1988) classes of home: VHCC (very high current configuration), OHCC (ordinary high current configuration), OLCC (ordinary low current configuration), VLCC (very low current configuration) and UG (underground, i.e. buried). The houses with the higher classifications were assumed to have stronger background fields than those with lower classifications. According to this classification scheme, residences more than 40 m from power lines were considered to be not exposed to magnetic fields.

Wire coding, in the original form developed by Wertheimer and Leeper, has been used in a number of studies. The ranges of measurements by wire code category for five substantial data sets – the control groups from the Savitz et al. (1988) and London et al. (1991) studies, the HVTRC survey (Zaffanella, 1993), the EMDEX Residential Project (Bracken et al., 1994) and the NCI study (Tarone et al., 1998) – indicate a positive relationship between the mean of the distributions and the wire code (i.e. higher averages are seen for higher wire code categories), but there is a large overlap among the various categories.

Kheifets, Kavet & Sussman (1997) evaluated relationships between wire codes and measured fields in the data sets available to them (EMDEX; HVTRC and London). The relationships were quite similar across data sets; thus only selected examples are presented below. Log-transformed spot mea-surement data for all 782 single and duplex residences and for all wire codes, except VLCC, from the HVTRC survey, were distributed log-normally. The data indicate a 10th-to-90th percentile interval of about an order of magni-tude for all the wire codes, considerable overlap in the field range across wire codes (as mentioned above), equivalent fields for UG and VLCC (which are sometimes grouped as referent categories), and a trend of increasing field with wire code. For this data, wire code explains 14.5% of the total variance in the log of the spot-measured fields (Kheifets, Kavet & Sussman, 1997).

There are many reasons for a discordance between wire codes and measurement classifications (for simplicity, a dichotomous classification scheme is used). For example, while number and thickness of wires reflect the total current carrying capacity of a system of wires, this does not take into account differences in geometry, phasing schemes in multi-circuit systems that enhance field cancellation, and actual loading patterns. Thus high wire code homes may actually have relatively low fields. Similarly, low wire code homes may exhibit high readings due to high field levels from non-power line sources, or from very heavily loaded external sources. Data available to date shows that the "high wire code–low measurement" situation is far more prevalent than the "low wire code–high measurement" circumstance.

While wire codes explain little of the variance of measured residen-tial magnetic fields, they are useful in identifying homes with potentially high magnetic fields. In particular, the majority of homes with high interior measurements fell into the VHCC category. And although most of the mis-classification occurs from homes in high wire code categories having low measurements, the VHCC category still performs reasonably well in exclud-ing homes with low measurements (Kheifets, Kavet & Sussman, 1997).

The concept of wire coding has been shown to be a usable crude surrogate even when tailored to local wiring practices. For example, the correlation between wiring code and measured magnetic fields in homes in the Savitz et al. (1988) study accounted for only 16% of the variance in the measured field values. Rankin et al. (2002) report that wire code predicts < 21% of the variance in magnetic field measurements. The wire code is overall an imperfect surrogate for magnetic field exposure in a variety of environments. In general, wire codes have been used only in North American studies, as their applicability is limited in other countries, where power drops to homes are mostly underground.

### 2.3.2.3 Calculated historical fields

Feychting & Ahlbom (1993) carried out a case–control study nested in a cohort of residents living in homes within 300 m of power lines in Sweden. The geometry of the conductors on the power line, the distance of the houses from the power lines and historical records of currents, were all available. This special situation allowed the investigators to calculate the fields to which the subjects' homes were exposed at various times (e.g. prior to diagnosis) (Kheifets et al., 1997).

The common elements between wire coding and the calculation model used by Feychting & Ahlbom (1993) are the reliance on the basic physical principles that the field increases with the current and decreases with the distance from the power line, and the fact that both neglect magnetic-field sources other than visible power lines. There is, however, one important difference: in the Wertheimer and Leeper code, the line type and thickness are a measure of the potential current carrying capacity of the line. In the Feychting & Ahlbom (1993) study, the approximate yearly average current was obtained from utility records; thus the question of temporal stability of the estimated fields did not even arise: assessment carried out for different times, using different load figures, yielded different estimates.

The approach of Feychting & Ahlbom (1993) has been used in various Nordic countries and elsewhere, although the likely accuracy of the calculations has varied depending in part on the completeness and precision of the available information on historical load. The necessary assumption that other sources of field are negligible is reasonable only for subjects relatively close to high-voltage power lines. The validity of the assumption also depends on details such as the definition of the population chosen for the study and the size of average fields from other sources to which the relevant population is exposed.

There is some evidence from Feychting & Ahlbom (1993) that their approach may work better for single-family homes than for apartments. When Feychting & Ahlbom (1993) validated their method by comparing calculations of present-day fields with present-day measurements, they found that virtually all homes with a measured field < 0.2 µT, whether single-family or apartments, were correctly classified by their calculations. However, for homes with a measured field > 0.2 μT, the calculations were able to classify correctly 85% of single-family homes, but only half of the apartments.

The difference between historical calculations and contemporary measurements was also evaluated by Feychting & Ahlbom (1993) who found that calculations using contemporary current loads resulted in a 45% increase in the fraction of single-family homes estimated to have a field > 0.2 μT, compared with calculations based on historical data. If these calculations of historical fields do accurately reflect exposure, this implies that present-day spot measurements overestimate the number of exposed homes in the past.

When fields are calculated from transmission lines and then used as an estimate of the exposure of a person, the assumption is made that fields from other sources are negligible. Close to the transmission line where the field from the line is high, it would be rare for other (principally distribution) sources to produce as high a field, and this is a valid assumption. As the distance from the power line is increased (or equivalently as the threshold between exposed and non-exposed is lowered), the assumption becomes less valid, and misclassification will result. An example of this can be seen in the Feychting & Ahlbom (1993) study where it has been observed that there is substantial calculation error by comparing their contemporary calculations and measurements (Jaffa, Kim & Aldrich, 2000). This error was more pronounced in the lower exposure categories (Feychting & Ahlbom, 2000). These calculation errors in the lower exposure categories are likely the result of not including the field contribution from local sources, which make a greater contribution to exposures at larger distances from transmission lines. This error can negate the value of estimating historical exposures such that contemporary measurements can be a more reliable metric for effect estimates (Jaffa, 2001; Maslanyj et al., 2007; Mezei & Kheifets, 2001).

### 2.3.3 Assessing residential exposure to magnetic fields using measurements

Following the publication of the Wertheimer & Leeper (1979; 1982) studies, doubt was cast on the reported association between cancer and electrical wiring configurations on the grounds that exposure had not been measured. Consequently, many of the later studies included measurements of various types.

All measurements have the advantage that they capture exposure from whatever sources are present, and do not depend on prior identification of sources, as wire codes and calculated fields do. Furthermore, because measurements can classify fields on a continuous scale rather than in a limited number of categories, they provide greater scope for investigating different thresholds and exposure–response relationships.

#### 2.3.3.1 Spot measurements in the home

The simplest form of measurement is a reading made at a point in time at one place in a home. To capture spatial variations of field, some studies have made multiple spot measurements at different places in or around the home. In an attempt to differentiate between fields arising from sources inside and outside the home, some studies have made spot measurements under "low-power" (all appliances turned off) and "high-power" (all appliances turned on) conditions. Neither of these alternatives truly represents the usual exposure conditions in a home, although the low-power conditions are closer to the typical conditions.

The major drawback of spot measurements is their inability to capture temporal variations. As with all measurements, spot measurements can assess only contemporary exposure, and can yield no information about historical exposure, which is an intrinsic requirement for retrospective studies of cancer risk. An additional problem of spot measurements is that they give only an approximation even for the contemporary field, because of short-term temporal variation of fields, and unless repeated throughout the year do not reflect seasonal variations.

A number of authors have compared the time-stability of spot measurements over periods of up to five years (reviewed in Kheifets et al., 1997; UKCCSI, 2000). The correlation coefficients reported were from 0.7–0.9, but even correlation coefficients this high may result in significant misclassification (Neutra & Del Pizzo, 1996).

### 2.3.3.2 Longer-term measurements in homes

Because spot measurements capture short-term temporal variability poorly, many studies have measured fields at one or more locations for longer periods, usually 24–48h, most commonly in a child's bedroom, which is an improvement on spot measurements. Comparisons of measurements have found only a poor-to-fair agreement between long-term and short-term measurements. This was mainly because short-term increases in fields caused by appliances or indoor wiring do not affect the average field measured over many hours (Schüz et al., 2000).

Measurements over 24–48 h cannot account for longer-term temporal variations. One study (UKCCSI, 1999) attempted to adjust for longer-term variation by making 48-h measurements, and then, for subjects close to high-voltage power lines, modifying the measurements by calculating the fields using historical load data. In a study in Germany, Schüz et al. (2001) identified the source of elevated fields by multiple measurements, and attempted to classify these sources as to the likelihood of their being stable over time. Before beginning the largest study in the USA (Linet et al., 1997), a pilot study was conducted (Friedman et al., 1996) to establish the proportion of their time children of various ages spent in different parts of the home. These estimates were used to weight the individual room measurements in the main study (Linet et al., 1997) for the time-weighted average measure. In addition, the pilot study documented that magnetic fields in dwellings rather than schools accounted for most of the variability in children's exposure to magnetic fields.

**Table 15. Exposure distribution of the arithmetic mean based on exposure of controls in a case-control study or all respondents in an exposure survey**

| Country | Authors | Study type | Measure-ment | Magnetic field category (µT) | | | | N |
|---|---|---|---|---|---|---|---|---|
| | | | | ≤ 0.1 | > 0.1–≤ 0.2 | > 0.2–≤ 0.3 | > 0.3 | |
| Belgium | Decat, Van den Heuvel & Mulpas, 2005 | Exposure survey | 24-hr personal | 81.9% | 11.5% | 1.6% | 5.1% | 251 |
| Canada | McBride et al., 1999[a] | Case-control | 48-hr personal | 59.0% | 29.2% | 8.5% | 3.3% | 329 |
| Germany | Michaelis et al., 1998 | Case-control | 24-hr bedroom | 89.9% | 7.0% | 1.7% | 1.4% | 414 |
| | Brix et al., 2001 | Exposure survey | 24-hr personal | 73.6% | 17.8% | 4.1% | 4.5% | 1952 |
| | Schüz et al., 2001[b] | Case-control | 24-hr bedroom | 93.0% | 5.6% | 0.9% | 0.5% | 1301 |
| Japan | Kabuto et al.,2006[b] | Case-control | 7-day home | 89.9% | 6.0% | 2.5% | 1.6% | 603 |
| Korea | Yang, Ju & Myung, 2004 | Exposure survey | 24-hr personal | 64.0% | 24.2% | 4.0% | 7.8% | 409 |
| UK | UKCCSI, 1999[b] | Case-control | 48-hr home | 92.3% | 5.8% | 1.2% | 0.8% | 2226 |
| USA | London et al., 1991[a] | Case-control | 24-hr bedroom | 69.2% | 19.6% | 4.2% | 7.0% | 143 |
| | Linet et al., 1997 | Case-control | 24-hr bedroom | 65.7% | 23.2% | 6.6% | 4.5% | 620 |
| | Zaffanella & Kalton, 1998 | Exposure survey | 24-hr personal | 64.2% | 21.1% | 7.8% | 4.2% | 995 |
| | Zaffanella, 1993 | Exposure survey | 24-hr home | 72.3% | 17.5% | 5.6% | 4.6% | 987 |

[a] Based on the distribution for pooled analysis reported by Greenland et al., 2000.

[b] Given exposure categories: < 0.1, 0.1–< 0.2, 0.2–< 0.4, > 0.4 µT; approximated categories in the table by applying the ratios of exposures in the high categories of the EMF Rapid Survey (Zaffanella & Kalton, 1998).

Five extensive exposure surveys have been conducted to evaluate ELF exposures of the general population (Brix et al., 2001; Decat, Van den Heuvel & Mulpas, 2005; Yang, Ju & Myung, 2004; Zaffanella, 1993; Zaffanella & Kalton, 1998). As indicated in Tables 15 and 16, these surveys generally estimate that approximately 4–5% had mean exposures above 0.3 µT, with the exception of Korea where 7.8% had mean exposures above 0.3 µT (Kheifets, Afifi & Shimkhada, 2006). Only 1–2% have median exposures in excess of 0.4 µT.

Estimating exposures using the control-exposures from case-control studies allows a look at a broader spectrum of countries and results in a range of 0.5–7.0 % having mean exposures greater than 0.3? µT and 0.4–3.3% having median exposures above 0.4 µT. Two countries, the USA and Germany, had both exposure surveys and case-control studies. In the USA, the mean exposures were virtually equal from the two methods but for the case-control median eight estimates were less than the survey median estimates. In Germany, the case-control mean exposure estimates were substantially smaller than the survey estimates (median estimates were not available for the case-control study), which could be due to regional differences and the inclusion of occupational exposures in the survey estimates. In some studies, the exposure distribution for 0.2–0.3 µT and 0.3–0.4 µT had to be estimated since only data for the 0.2–0.4 µT intervals were given; the ratio from the EMF Rapid Survey from the USA was used to calculate these estimates.

Table 16. Exposure distribution of the geometric mean based on exposure of controls in a case-control study or all respondents in an exposure survey

| Country | Authors | Study type | Measurement | Magnetic field category (µT) | | | | N |
|---|---|---|---|---|---|---|---|---|
| | | | | ≤ 0.1 | > 0.1– ≤ 0.2 | > 0.2– ≤ 0.4 | > 0.4 | |
| Belgium | Decat, Van den Heuvel & Mulpas, 2005 | Exposure survey | 24-hr personal | 91.9% | 4.1% | 2.8% | 1.2% | 251 |
| Canada | McBride et al., 1999[a] | Case-control | 48-hr personal | 70.7% | 17.4% | 8.6% | 3.3% | 304 |
| Germany | Michaelis et al., 1998[a] | Case-control | 24-hr bedroom | 92.9% | 5.1% | 1.5% | 0.5% | 409 |
| UK | UKCCSI, 1999[a] | Case-control | 48-hr home | 94.4% | 4.1% | 1.2% | 0.4% | 2224 |
| USA | Zaffanella & Kalton, 1998 | Exposure survey | 24-hr personal | 72.6% | 17.6% | 7.5% | 2.3% | 995 |
| | Linet et al., 1997[a] | Case-control | 24-hr bedroom | 72.8% | 17.9% | 8.3% | 0.9% | 530 |

[a] Based on the distribution for pooled analysis reported by Ahlbom et al., 2000.

### 2.3.3.3 Personal exposure monitoring

Monitoring the personal exposure of a subject by a meter worn on the body is attractive because it captures exposure to fields from all sources and at all places the individual encounters. Because all sources are included, the average fields measured tend to be higher than those derived from spot or long-term measurements in homes. However, the use of personal exposure monitoring in case–control studies could be problematic, due to age- or disease-related changes in behaviour. The latter could introduce differential misclassification in exposure estimates. However, personal exposure monitoring can be used to validate other types of measurements or estimates.

Table 17 summarizes results from studies which have measured the personal exposure of representative samples of people in different countries. Geometric mean and geometric standard deviation are given on the assumption of log-normal distributions.

**Table 17. Summary of measurements of residential personal exposure [a]**

| Authors | Area | Sample type | Measurement type | Time of year | Sample size | Type of statistics [b] | Geometric mean (nT) | Geometric standard deviation |
|---|---|---|---|---|---|---|---|---|
| Donnelly & Agnew, 1991 | Toronto, Canada | Utility employees, contacts, and general public, chosen for variety of exposure environments | Roughly 48 h, single axis | June–October | 31 | Children at home (D) | 117 | 2.98 |
| | | | | | | Adults at home (D) | 133 | 2.80 |
| Skotte, 1994 | Denmark | From industry. Homes near power lines excluded for this analysis. | Personal exposure, 24 h | | 298 (includes some duplication) | "Non-work" (P) | 50 | 2.08 |
| Brix et al., 2001 | Bavaria, Germany | Volunteers recruited for exposure assessment | Personal exposure, 24 h | | 1952 | (U) | 6.4 | 2.41 |
| Vistnes et al., 1997a | Suburb of Oslo, Norway | Children from two schools. This analysis only of homes > 275 m from power line | Personal exposure, 24 h | | 6 | At home (P,A) | 15 | 2.40 |

**Table 17. Continued**

| Reference | Location | Population | Duration | Season | N | Measurement location | Value | GM |
|---|---|---|---|---|---|---|---|---|
| Merchant, Renew & Swanson, 1994a | England and Wales, UK | Volunteers from electricity industry. HV lines excluded for this analysis | 3–7 days | Spread over year | 204 | At home (P,F) | 54 | 2.05 |
| Preece et al., 1996 | Avon, UK | Random selection from mothers with surviving children | 24 h | Dec–May | 44 | (A) | 42 | 2.65 |
| Kavet, Silva & Thornton, 1992 | Maine, USA | Random-digit dialing; adults | 24 h | June/August | 15 | At home (D) | 134 | 1.80 |
| Zaffanella & Kalton, 1998 | USA | Random-digit dialling | 24 h personal measurement (bedroom & home) | | 994 | (D) | 92 | 1.36 |
| Bracken et al., 1994 | USA | Employees of EPRI member utilities, weighted to random samples of wire codes | 24 h | | 396 | At home, not in bed (F) | 111 | 1.88 |
| Kaune et al., 1994 | Washington DC, USA | Children of volunteers from NCI and private daycare facility, overhead wiring | 24 h | Spring | 29 | Residential (P) | 96 | 2.38 |
| Kaune & Zaffanella, 1994 | California and Mass., USA | Children from volunteers from industry, chosen for variety of distribution arrangements | 24 h | | 31 | (P) | 96 | 2.45 |

[a] Source: Swanson & Kaune, 1999.

[b] P = geometric statistics are given in Swanson & Kaune, 1999; A = calculated from arithmetic statistics given in Swanson & Kaune, 1999 using the equations given in Section 2.2.2.2.3 Distribution lines, subsection Data on fields in different countries; D =calculated from data given in Swanson & Kaune, 1999; F = fitted to statistics given in Swanson & Kaune, 1999 using least-squares procedure; U = calculated from unpublished data.

**Table 18. Comparisons of personal exposure and background fields**

| Country | Authors | Subjects | Sample size | Personal exposures: geometric mean (nT) | Long-term background field: geometric mean (nT) | Ratio personal exposure / background |
|---------|---------|----------|-------------|------------------|----------------|------------------|
| USA | Kavet, Silva & Thornton, 1992 | Adults, at home | 15 | 134 | 58 | 2.3 |
| | Bracken et al., 1994 | Adults, at home, not in bed | 396 | 111 | 74 | 1.5 |
| | Kaune et al., 1994 | Children, residential | 29 | 96 | 99 | 1.0 |
| | Kaune & Zaffanella, 1994 | Children | 31 | 96 | 67 | 1.4 |
| Canada | Donnelly & Agnew, 1991 | Children, at home | 31 | 117 | 107 | 1.1 |
| | | Adults, at home | 31 | 133 | | 1.2 |
| UK | Merchant, Renew & Swanson, 1994a | Adults, at home | 204 | 54 | 37 | 1.5 |
| | Preece et al., 1996 | Adults | 44 | 42 | 29 | 1.5 |

In general, personal-exposure measurements are higher than fields measured away from appliances, largely because of the extra contributions of appliances and any other sources within the home. Seven studies that include both personal exposure measurements and long-term measurements of fields away from appliances in the homes of the subjects are compared in Table 18. The ratio of average personal exposure to average field away from appliances varies from 1.0 to 2.3, with an average of 1.44. This shows the relative magnitude of short-term exposure to appliances emitting relatively high magnetic fields compared with background exposure. There may be a tendency for the ratio to be smaller for children than for adults, but it would be unwise to draw firm conclusions from these limited data.

### 2.3.4 Assessing exposure to magnetic fields from appliances

Only little is known about the magnitude and distribution of EMF exposures from appliances. The contribution to overall exposure by appliances depends, among other things, on the type of appliance, its age, its distance from the person using it, and the pattern and duration of use. The assessment of appliance use in epidemiological studies has generally relied on questionnaires, sometimes answered by proxies such as other household members (Mills et al., 2000). These questionnaires ascertain some (but not usually all) of these facts, and are subject to recall bias. It is not known how well data from even the best questionnaire approximate to the actual exposure. Mezei et al. (2001) reported that questionnaire-based information on appliance use, even when focused on use within the last year, has limited value in estimating personal exposure to magnetic fields. Limited attempts have been made (e.g. UKCCSI, 1999) to include some measurements as well as questionnaire data.

According to Mader & Peralta (1992), appliances are not a significant source of whole-body exposure, but they may be the dominant source of exposure of extremities. Delpizzo (1990) suggested that common domestic electrical appliances were responsible for an exposure comparable to that from power lines. Recently, Mezei et al. (2001) showed that computers contributed appreciablyto overall exposure while other appliances each contributed less than 2%. Most of the time, a low contribution was the result of infrequent and short duration of appliance use. When limited to only those subjects who actually used certain appliances, the analysis showed that computers (16%) and cellular phones (21%) could contribute appreciablyto total daily exposure.

Because exposure to magnetic fields from appliances tends to be short-term and intermittent, the appropriate method for combining assessments of exposure from different appliances and chronic exposure from other sources would be particularly dependent on assumptions made about exposure metrics. Such methods have yet to be developed.

### 2.3.5 *Assessing exposure at schools*

Exposure to ELF electric and magnetic fields while at school seldom represents a major fraction of a child's total exposure.

A study involving 79 schools in Canada took a total of 43009 measurements of 60-Hz magnetic fields (141–1543 per school) (Sun et al., 1995). Only 7.8% of all the fields measured were above 0.2 µT. For individual schools, the average magnetic field was 0.08 µT (SD: 0.06 µT). In the analysis by use of room, only typing rooms had magnetic fields that were above 0.2 µT. Hallways and corridors were above 0.1 µT and all other room types were below 0.1 µT. The percentage of classrooms above 0.2 µT was not reported. Magnetic fields above 0.2 µT were mostly associated with wires in the floor or ceiling, proximity to a room containing electrical appliances or movable sources of magnetic fields such as electric typewriters, computers and overhead projectors. Eight of the 79 schools were situated near high-voltage power lines. The survey showed no clear difference in overall magnetic field strength between the schools and domestic environments.

Kaune et al. (1994) measured power-frequency magnetic fields in homes and in the schools and daycare centres of 29 children. Ten public shools, six private schools and one daycare centre were included in the study. In general, the magnetic field strengths measured in schools and daycare centres were smaller and less variable than those measured in residential settings.

The UKCCSI (1999) carried out an epidemiological study of children in which measurements were made in schools as well as homes. Only three of 4452 children aged 0–14 years who spent 15 or more hours per week at school during the winter, had an average exposure during the year above 0.2 µT as a result of exposure at school.

### 2.3.6 Assessing non-occupational exposure to magnetic fields: discussion

One crucial question in case-control studies in general, and of magnetic fields and childhood cancer in particular, is how to span time. By definition, all exposures of interest in these studies are historical. Thus, measurements, wire codes, and historic models are only surrogates for the critical exposure, which occurred at some unknown time in the past. The question is then, what is a better surrogate for historic exposure: wire codes, area measurements or personal exposure? Each method has distinct advantages. Wire codes are relatively simple categorical scales that are thought to be stable over time. This method allows magnetic fields to be estimated without resident participation, thus reducing potential bias due to non-participation and maximizing study size. Measured fields, on the other hand, are more appealing because they can account for all sources within the residence and entail fewer implicit assumptions. However, one would expect measurements taken soon after diagnosis to be better surrogates than measurements taken long after diagnosis. Although it is generally considered that such long term measurements are the best available estimate of average magnetic field exposure, wire codes may be better indicators of high historical exposure because they may be less biased, and may produce less misclassification and measurement error. This might be especially true when one has to estimate exposure that has occurred several years to decades in the past. Epidemiological studies with personal measurements are yet to be completed. However, in case-control settings personal measurements could be problematic due to age or disease-related changes in behavior and thus, exposure.

Epidemiological studies that estimated the historical exposures of subjects to magnetic fields from power lines by calculations did not usually report using documented computer programs or publish the details of the computation algorithms, e.g. Olsen, Nielsen & Schulgen (1993), Verkasalo et al. (1993; 1996), Feychting & Ahlbom (1994), Tynes & Haldorsen (1997), though others, e.g. UKCCSI (2000), did. However, for exposure assessment in these studies, it is important to consider how accurate the calculations are in a specific study when interpreting results. For example in the seminal Feychting & Ahlbom study (1993), the calculation error (contemporary calculations vs. contemporary measurements) is greater than any advantage that might have been gained by estimating exposure at the time of diagnosis with historical calculations. As a result, contemporary spot measurements appear to provide better estimates of historical exposures in this study (Jaffa, Kim & Aldrich, 2000).

### 2.3.7 Assessing occupational exposure to magnetic fields

Following Wertheimer and Leeper's report of an association between residential magnetic fields and childhood leukaemia, Milham (1982; 1985a; 1985b) noted an association between cancer and some occupations (often subsequently called the "electrical occupations") intuitively expected to involve proximity to sources of electric and magnetic fields. However, classification based on job title is a very coarse surrogate. Critics (Guenel et al., 1993; Loomis & Savitz, 1990; Theriault et al., 1994) have pointed out that, for example, many electrical engineers are basically office workers and that many electricians work on disconnected wiring.

Much less is known about exposures in non-electrical occupations. Little data, if any, is available for many jobs and industrial environments. Of note in the few surveys conducted are high exposures among railway engine drivers (about 4 µT) and seamstresses (about 3 µT). The best information on work exposures is available in a survey conducted by Zaffannela (Zaffanella & Kalton, 1998). The survey included 525 workers employed in a variety of occupations (Table 19).

Table 19. Parameters of the distributions of average magnetic field during work for different types of occupations [a]

| Description | Sample size | Mean (µT) | Standard deviation (µT) | Geometric mean (µT) | Geometric standard deviation |
|---|---|---|---|---|---|
| Managerial and professional speciality occupations | 204 | 0.164 | 0.282 | 0.099 | 2.47 |
| Technical, sales, and administrative supports occupation | 166 | 0.158 | 0.167 | 0.109 | 2.03 |
| (Protective, food, health, cleaning, and personal) service occupations | 71 | 0.274 | 0.442 | 0.159 | 2.55 |
| Farming, forestry, and fishing occupations | 19 | 0.091 | 0.141 | 0.045 | 2.97 |
| Precision production, craft, and repair occupations, and operators, fabricators, and laborers | 128 | 0.173 | 0.415 | 0.089 | 2.80 |
| Electrical occupations [b] | 16 | 0.215 | 0.162 | 0.161 | 2.25 |

[a] Source: Zaffanella & Kalton, 1998.

[b] As classified by Milham (1982; 1985a; 1985b): electronic technicians, radio and telegraph operators, electricians, linemen (power and telephone), television and radio repairmen, power station operators, aluminium workers, welders and flame cutters, motion picture projectionists, electrical enigineers and subway motormen.

The largest geometric mean (0.161 μT) for magnetic field exposure during work occurred in electrical occupations. Service occupations followed at 0.159 μT. Technical, sales, and administrative support positions had a geometric mean of 0.109 μT; managerial and professional specialty occupations, 0.099 μT; and precision production, craft and repair work, operation, fabrication, and labor, 0.089 μT. At 0.045 μT, farming, forestry, and fishing occupations had the lowest geometric mean. Work exposures were often significantly higher and more variable than other exposures: people spent significantly more time, for example, in fields exceeding 1.6 μT at work than at home. Nevertheless, average work exposures for the general population are low, with only 4% exposed to magnetic fields above 0.5 μT.

Intuitive classification of occupations by investigators can be improved upon by taking account of judgements made by appropriate experts (e.g. Loomis et al., 1994), and by making measurements in occupational groups (e.g. Bowman et al., 1988).

A study by Forssén et al. (2004) provides a first attempt to comprehensively evaluate occupational magnetic field exposure assessment among women. The results for the work-site environments are presented in Table 20. "Large scale kitchens" and "Shops and stores" are both environments with high exposure.

Table 20. Exposures to extremely low frequency magnetic fields by occupational environment [a]

| Environment | Sample size | Arithmetic/geometric means (arithmetic standard deviations) (μT) | | Proportion of time spent at exposure level (n) | | | |
|---|---|---|---|---|---|---|---|
| | | Time-weighted average | Maximum | < 0.1 μT | 0.1– 0.2 μT | 0.2– 0.3 μT | ≥ 0.3 μT |
| Health care | 67 | 0.11 / 0.10 (0.07) | 2.62 / 2.10 (1.90) | 66% (29) | 20% (18) | 8% (10) | 7% (10) |
| Hospitals | 27 | 0.09 / 0.08 (0.05) | 3.01 / 2.37 (2.26) | 77% (21) | 13% (14) | 6% (8) | 4% (6) |
| Elsewhere | 40 | 0.13 / 0.11 (0.08) | 2.35 / 1.94 (1.58) | 59% (31) | 24% (20) | 9% (11) | 9% (12) |
| Schools and childcare | 55 | 0.15 / 0.12 (0.10) | 5.41 / 2.12 (16.49) | 62% (27) | 20% (16) | 8% (8) | 10% (12) |
| Large scale kitchens | 34 | 0.38 / 0.28 (0.43) | 5.97 / 4.67 (4.55) | 30% (27) | 20% (11) | 15% (12) | 36% (27) |
| Offices | 127 | 0.16 / 0.12 (0.13) | 2.41 / 1.73 (2.32) | 55% (38) | 25% (26) | 9% (14) | 12% (22) |
| Shops and stores | 33 | 0.31 / 0.26 (0.17) | 5.84 / 2.55 (18.21) | 26% (29) | 17% (13) | 17% (13) | 40% (30) |

[a] Source: Forssén et al., 2004.

A further improvement is a systematic measurement programme to characterize exposure in a range of jobs corresponding as closely as possible to those of the subjects in a study, thus creating a "job-exposure matrix", which links measurement data to job titles.

Forssén et al. (2004) constructed a job-exposure matrix for women. Analysis of the exposure distribution in the female working population showed that about 16% of the women are highly exposed (0.20 μT). However, only 5% would be classified as such if the job-exposure matrix for men (Floderus, Persson & Stenlund, 1996) was used (Table 21). Furthermore, only 20% of the women with high exposure would be correctly classified as highly exposed by the job-exposure matrix for men. Using the job-exposure matrix for men in an epidemiological study that involves women would hence cause not only loss of power but could also dilute any effects through misclassification of the exposure.

Table 21. Distribution of exposure in the population of women gainfully employed in Stockholm County 1980 by using job-exposure matrices (JEM)

| Geometric mean of time-weighted average (μT) | Pecentage of women exposed | |
| --- | --- | --- |
| | JEM for women [a] | JEM for men [b] |
| ≤ 0.10 | 21.4 | 7.2 |
| 0.11–0.20 | 48.3 | 47.4 |
| 0.21–0.30 | 13.7 | 4.4 |
| > 0.30 | 3.0 | 1.0 |
| Missing | 13.6 | 40.0 |

[a] Source: Forssén et al., 2004.
[b] Source: Floderus, Persson & Stenlund, 1996.

Despite the improvements in exposure assessment, the ability to explain exposure variability in complex occupational environments remains poor. Job titles alone explain only a small proportion of exposure variability. A consideration of the work environment and of the tasks undertaken by workers in a specific occupation leads to a more precise estimate (Kelsh, Kheifets & Smith, 2000). Harrington et al. (2001) have taken this approach one stage further by combining job information with historical information not only on the environment in general but on specific power stations and substations. The within-worker and between-worker variability which account for most of the variation are not captured using these assessments.

In addition to the need for correct classification of jobs, the quality of occupational exposure assessment depends on the details of work history available to the investigators. The crudest assessments are based on a single job (e.g. as mentioned on a death certificate). This assessment can be improved by identifying the job held for the longest period, or even better, by obtaining a complete job history which would allow for the calculation of the

70

subject's cumulative exposure over his professional career, often expressed in µT–years.

### 2.3.8    Assessing exposure to electric fields

Assessment of exposure to electric fields is generally more difficult and less well developed than the assessment of exposure to magnetic' fields. All of the difficulties encountered in assessment of exposure to magnetic fields discussed above also apply to electric fields. In addition, electric fields are easily perturbed by any conducting object, including the human body.Although most studies that have assessed electric fields have attempted to assess the unperturbed field, the very presence of subjects in an environment means that they are not being exposed to an "unperturbed field".

Because electric fields are perturbed by the body, the concept of personal exposure is difficult to define, and readings taken with a meter attached to the body are likely to be dominated by local perturbations affected by the precise location of the meter on the body.

A number of electric and magnetic field exposure studies have included measurements of electric fields within homes. Some of these consisted of wearing personal exposure meters for periods of 24 or 48 hours, while others consisted of spot measurements within specific rooms. The majority of studies were epidemiological studies, although one compared homes near to a power line to homes at a considerable distance from any power lines.

In each of the studies data are presented for controls as well as for the cases. A comparison has been made between the measurements for the controls in different studies. Green et al. (1999a) performed continuous monitoring and reported that the average electric field exposure at home for controls was below 16 V m$^{-1}$ for 90% of the group. London et al. (1991) and Savitz et al. (1988) performed spot measurements in the centre of the controls' sitting rooms. London et al. reported a mean of 7.98 V m$^{-1}$ and Savitz et al. reported a median below 9 V m$^{-1}$. A number of other studies involved monitoring of electric fields over a 24 or 48 hour period. McBride et al. (1999) carried out 48-h personal exposure monitoring, reporting a median exposure for controls of 12.2 V m$^{-1}$. However no distinction was made between exposure at home and away from home. Studies by Dockerty et al. (1998) and Kaune et al. (1987) performed 24-h monitoring within specific rooms of the home. Both monitored electric field within the sitting room, while the Dockerty et al. study also monitored electric field levels within the bedroom. The study by Dockerty et al. reported arithmetic means less than 10.75 V m$^{-1}$ in at least 60% of the homes, regardless of the room, while Kaune et al. reported a mean value of 33 V m$^{-1}$ across the homes investigated. Kaune et al. reported higher levels that other studies reported to date. Levallois et al. (1995) carried out 24-h monitoring of the electric fields in homes both near to a 735 kV line, and distant to any overhead lines. For those homes distant to power lines, a geometric mean electric field of 14 V m$^{-1}$ was reported. Finally, Skinner et al. (2002) made measurements in several locations in the home with geometric means around 10 V m$^{-1}$.

### 2.3.9 *Exposure assessment: conclusions*

Electric and magnetic fields exist wherever electricity is generated, transmitted or distributed in power lines or cables, or used in electrical appliances. Since the use of electricity is an integral part of our modern lifestyle, these fields are ubiquitous in our environment.

Residential exposure to power frequency magnetic fields does not vary dramatically across the world. The geometric mean magnetic field in homes ranges between 0.025 and 0.07 μT in Europe and 0.055 and 0.11 μT in the USA. The mean values of electric field in the home are in the range of several tens of volts per metre. In the vicinity of certain appliances, the instantaneous magnetic-field values can be as much as a few hundred microtesla. Near power lines, magnetic fields reach approximately 20 μT and electric fields up to several thousand volts per metre.

Few children have time-averaged exposures to residential 50 or 60 Hz magnetic fields in excess of the levels associated with an increased incidence of childhood leukaemia. Approximately 1% to 4 % have mean exposures above 0.3 μT and only 1% to 2% have median exposures in excess of 0.4 μT.

Occupational exposure, although predominantly to power-frequency fields, may also include contributions from other frequencies. The average magnetic field exposures in the workplace have been found to be higher in "electrical occupations" than in other occupations such as office work, ranging from 0.4–0.6 μT for electricians and electrical engineers to approximately 1.0 μT for power line workers, with the highest exposures for welders, railway engine drivers and sewing machine operators (above 3 μT). The maximum magnetic field exposures in the workplace can reach up to approximately 10 mT and this is invariably associated with the presence of conductors carrying high currents. In the electrical supply industry, workers may be exposed to electric fields up to 30 kV m$^{-1}$.

# 3    ELECTRIC AND MAGNETIC FIELDS INSIDE THE BODY

## 3.1    Introduction

Chapter 2 describes the fields to which people are exposed. Exposure to these fields in turn induces fields and currents inside the body. This chapter describes and quantifies the relationship between external fields and contact currents with 'the current density and electric fields induced within the body. Only the induced electric field and resultant current density in tissues and cells are considered, as the internal magnetic field in tissues and cells is the same as the external field. The chapter first considers calculations on a macroscopic scale referring to dimensions much greater than those of cells or cell assemblies, and then on a microscopic scale when dimensions considered are comparable to, or smaller than a cell.

At extremely low frequencies, exposure is characterized by the electric field strength ($E$) or the electric flux density (also called the displacement) vector ($D$), and the magnetic field strength ($H$) or the magnetic flux density (also called the magnetic induction) ($B$). All these parameters are vectors; vectors are denoted in italics in this Monograph (see also paragraph 2.1.1). The flux densities are related to the field strengths by the properties of the medium in a given location $r$ as:

$$D(r) = \hat{\varepsilon}\, E(r)$$
$$B(r) = \hat{\mu}\, H(r)$$

where $\hat{\varepsilon}$ is the complex permittivity and $\hat{\mu}$ is the permeability. For biological media. $\hat{\mu} \cong \mu_0$ where $\mu_0$ is the permeability of free space (air). The electric and magnetic fields are effectively decoupled, since quasi-static conditions can be assumed (Olsen, 1994). To determine exposure in a given location, both the electric and magnetic field have to be computed or measured separately. Similarly, the internal induced fields are also evaluated separately. For simultaneous exposure to electric and magnetic fields, the internal measures can be obtained by superposition. Exposures to either electric or magnetic fields result in the induction of electric fields and associated current density in conductive tissue. The magnitudes and spatial patterns of these fields depend on the type of the exposure field (electric vs. magnetic), their characteristics (frequency, magnitude, orientation, etc.), and the size, shape, and electrical properties of the exposed body (human, animal). A biological body significantly perturbs an external electric field, and the exposure also results in an electric charge on the body surface. The external electric field is also strongly perturbed by metallic or other conductive objects.

The primary dosimetric measure is the local induced electric field. This measure is selected because thresholds of the excitable tissue stimulation are defined by the electric field and its spatial variation. However, current density is used in some exposure guidelines (ICNIRP, 1998a). Among the measurements often reported are the average, root mean square (rms) and maximum induced electric field and current density values (Stuchly & Dawson, 2000). Additional measurements more recently introduced are the 50th, 95th, and 99th percentiles, which indicate values not exceeded in the given volume of tissue, e.g. the 99th percentile shows the dosimetric measure exceeded in 1% of a given tissue volume (Kavet et al., 2001). Some exposure guidelines (ICNIRP, 1998a) specify dosimetry limit values as current density averaged over 1 cm$^2$ of tissue. The electric field in tissue is typically expressed in V m$^{-1}$ or mV m$^{-1}$ and the current density in A m$^{-2}$ or mA m$^{-2}$.

The internal (induced) electric field ($E$) and conduction current density ($J$) are related through Ohm's law:

$$J = \sigma E$$

where $\sigma$ is the bulk tissue conductivity, and may be a tensor in anisotropic tissues (e.g. muscle).

Early dosimetry modeled a human body as homogeneous ellipsoids or other overly simplified shapes. In addition, limited measurements of currents through the whole body and body parts have been performed. During the last few years, a few research laboratories have performed extensive computations of the induced electric field and current density in heterogeneous models of the human body in uniform and non-uniform electric or magnetic fields at 50 or 60 Hz. There is convergence of the results obtained by various groups and agreement with earlier measurements, where such measurements are available (Caputa et al., 2002; Stuchly & Gandhi, 2000). Microscopic dosimetry data remain very limited.

### 3.2    Models of human and animal bodies

Currently, a number of laboratories have developed heterogeneous models of the human body with realistic anatomy and numerous tissues identified. Most of these models have been developed by computer segmentation of data from magnetic resonance imaging (MRI) and allocation of proper tissue type (Dawson, 1997; Dawson, Moerloose & Stuchly, 1996; Dimbylow, 1997; Dimbylow, 2005; Gandhi, 1995; Gandhi & Chen, 1992; Zubal, 1994). Special care has been taken to make these models anatomically realistic. Table 22 summarizes essential characteristics of some of these models.

Typically, over 30 distinct organs and tissues are identified and represented by cubic cells (voxels) of 1 to 10 mm on a side. Voxels are assigned a conductivity value based on measured values for various organs and tissues (Gabriel, Gabriel & Corthout, 1996). A human body model constructed from several geometrical bodies of revolution has also been used (Baraton, Cahouet & Hutzler, 1993; Hutzler et al., 1994). The model is symmetric and is divided into about 100000 tetrahedral elements, which represent only the major organs. This can be contrasted with over eight million of tissue voxels used in the hybrid method with resolution of 3.6 mm (Dawson, Caputa & Stuchly, 1998). In the hybrid method, the FDTD part of the modeling requires that the body model is enclosed in a parallelpiped. To illustrate the quality of such models Figure 1 shows the external view, the skeleton and skin, and the main internal organs.

Table 22. Main characteristics of the MRI-derived models of the human body

| Model | NRPB [a] | University of Utah [b] | University of Victoria [c] |
|---|---|---|---|
| Height and mass | 1.76 m, 73 kg | 1.76 m, 64 kg scaled to 71 kg | 1.77 m, 76 kg |
| Original voxels | 2.077 x 2.077 x 2.021 mm | 2 x 2 x 3 mm | 3.6 x 3.6 x 3.6 mm |
| Posture | upright, hands at sides | upright, hands at sides | upright, hands in front |

[a] Source: Dimbylow, 1997.
[b] Source: Gandhi & Chen, 1992.
[c] Source: Dawson, 1997.

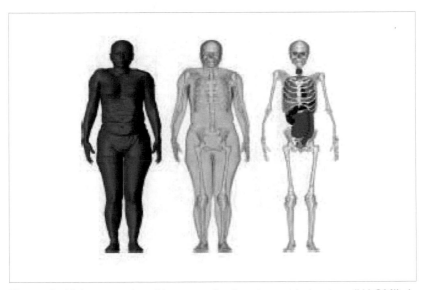

**Figure 1.** Volume rendered images of a female voxel phantom (NAOMI). In the image on the left the opacity of the skin has been hardened and the image is illuminated to display the outside surface. In the middle image the opacity of the skin has been reduced to enable the internal skeleton to be seen. The image on the right shows the skeleton and internal organs. The skin, fat, muscle and breasts have been removed. (Dimbylow, 2005)

A few animal models, namely rats, mice and monkeys have also been developed. The quality of the models varies.

## 3.3 Electric field dosimetry

### 3.3.1 Basic interaction mechanisms

As mentioned earlier the human (or animal) body significantly perturbs a low-frequency electric field. In most practical cases of human exposure, the field is vertical (with respect to the ground). At low frequencies, the body is a good conductor, and the electric field is nearly normal to its surface. The electric field inside the body is many orders of magnitude smaller than the external field. Non-uniform charges are induced on the surface of the body and the current direction inside the body is mostly vertical. Figure 2 illustrates the electric fields in air around the human body and body surface charge density for the model in free space and on perfect ground.

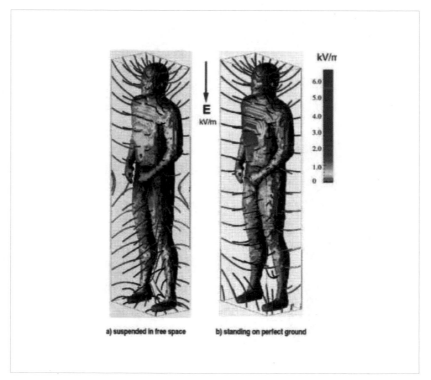

**Figure 2.** Human body in a uniform electric field of 1 kV m$^{-1}$ at 60 Hz showing the external electric field and surface charge density on the body surface: (a) in free space, and (b) in contact with perfect ground (Stuchly & Dawson, 2000).

The electric field in the body strongly depends also on the contact between the body and the electric ground, where the highest fields are found when the body is in perfect contact with ground through both feet (Deno & Zaffanella, 1982). The further away from the ground the body is located, the lower the electric fields in tissues. For the same field, the maximum ratio of internal fields for grounded to free space models is about two.

### 3.3.2    Measurements

Kaune & Forsythe (1985) performed measurements of currents in models consisting of manikins standing in a vertical electric field with both feet grounded. The model was filled with saline solution whose conductivity is equal to that of the average human tissues. The results of the measurements are shown in Figure 3.

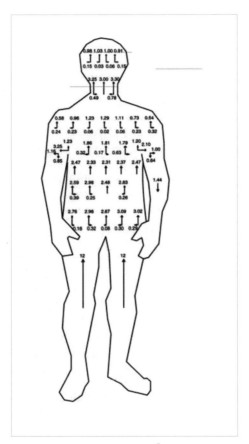

**Figure 3.** Measured current density (mA m$^{-2}$) in a saline filled homogeneous phantom grounded through both feet. The electric field strength is 10 kV m$^{-1}$, the field vector is directed along the long axis of the body, and the frequency is 60 Hz (Kaune & Forsythe, 1985).

### 3.3.3    Computations

Early dosimetry computations represented the human (or animal) body as a homogeneous body of revolution with a single conductivity value.

Examples of analytic solutions in homogeneous geometric shapes for electric field exposure are available in Shiau & Valentino (1981), Kaune and McCreary (1985), Tenforde & Kaune (1987), Spiegel (1977), Foster and Schwan (1989) and Hart (1992). Measurements of currents within the body have also been performed (Deno & Zaffanella, 1982; Kaune & Forsythe, 1985; Kaune, Kistler & Miller, 1987). As an intermediate development, highly simplified body-like shapes have been evaluated by numerical methods (Chen, Chuang & Lin, 1986; Chiba et al., 1984; Dimbylow, 1987; Spiegel, 1981).

Various computational methods have been used to evaluate induced electric fields in high-resolution models. Computations of exposure to electric fields are generally more difficult than for the magnetic field exposure, since the human body significantly perturbs the exposure field. Suitable numerical methods are limited by the highly heterogeneous electrical properties of the human body and equally complex external and organ shapes. The methods that have been successfully used so far for high-resolution dosimetry are the finite difference (FD) method in frequency domain and time domain (FDTD) and the finite element method (FEM). Each method and its implementation offer some advantages and have limitations, as reviewed by Stuchly and Dawson (2000). Some of the methods and computer codes have undergone extensive verification by comparison with analytic solutions (Dawson & Stuchly, 1996; Stuchly et al., 1998). An extensive valuation of accuracy of various dosimetric measures is also available (Dawson, Potter & Stuchly, 2001).

Several numerical computations of the electric field and current density induced in various organs and tissues have been performed (Dawson, Caputa & Stuchly, 1998; Dimbylow, 2000; Furse & Gandhi, 1998; Hirata et al., 2001). In a more recent publication (Dimbylow, 2000), the maximum current density is averaged over 1 cm$^2$ for excitable tissues. The latter computation is clearly aimed at compliance with the most recent ICNIRP guideline (ICNIRP, 1998a and a later published clarification on tissue-related applicability of the limit (ICNRIP, 1998b).

Effects of two sets of conductivity have been examined in high-resolution models (Dawson, Caputa & Stuchly, 1998). The difference between calculation with either set is negligible on short-circuit current and very small on the average and maximum electric field and current density values in horizontal slices of the body. This conclusion is in agreement with the basic physical laws as explained by Dawson, Caputa & Stuchly (1998). The average and maximum electric fields vary, but less than the induced current density values for the same organ for the two different sets of conductivity. It is also apparent that not only the conductivity of a given organ determines its current density, but also the conductivity of other tissues. In general, lower induced electric fields (higher current density) are associated with higher conductivity of tissue. The exceptions are locations in the body associated with the concave curvature, e.g. tissue surrounding the armpits, where the electric field is enhanced. For the whole-body the averages are within 2%.

The maximum values of the electric field differ by up to 20% for the two sets of conductivity.

Model resolution influences how accurately the induced quantities are evaluated in various organs. Organs small in any dimension are poorly represented by large voxels. The maximum induced quantities are consistently higher as the voxel dimension decreases. The differences are typically of the order of 30–50% for voxels of 3.6 compared with 7.2 mm (Dawson, Caputa & Stuchly, 1998).

The main features of dosimetry for exposures to the ELF electric field can be summarized as follows.

- Magnitudes of the induced electric fields are typically $10^{-4}$ to $10^{-7}$ of the magnitude of external unperturbed field.

- Since the exposure is mostly to the vertical field, the predominant direction of the induced fields is also vertical.

- In the same exposure field, the strongest induced fields are for the human body in contact through the feet with a perfectly conducting ground plane, and the weakest induced fields are for the body in free space, i.e. infinitely far from the ground plane.

- The global dosimetric measure of short-circuit current for a body in contact with perfect ground is determined by the body size and shape (including posture) rather than tissue conductivity.

- The induced electric field values are to a lesser degree influenced by the conductivity of various organs and tissues than are the values of the induced current density.

Figure 4 shows vertical current computed in models of an adult and a child exposed to the vertical electric field in free space and in contact with perfect ground.

Table 23 gives various dosimetric measures for the human body model in a vertical field of 1 kV/m at 60 Hz (Dawson, Caputa & Stuchly, 1998; Kavet et al., 2001). Equivalent data for 50 Hz is shown in Table 24 (Dimbylow, 2005). In these calculations the body is in contact with perfectly conducting ground through both feet, the body height is 1.76 m for NORMAN and 1.63 m for NAOMI and weight is 73 kg for NORMAN and 60 kg for NAOMI. Table 25 gives dosimetric measures for a simplified model of a 5-year old child of 1.10 m and 18.7 kg (Hirata et al., 2001). The voxel maximum values in these models are significantly overestimated, thus 99th percentiles are more representative (Dawson, Potter & Stuchly, 2001).

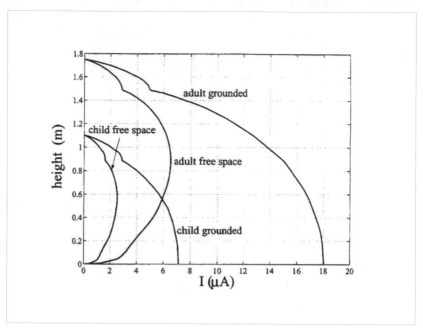

**Figure 4.** Current in body cross-sections for a human body model in contact with perfect ground at 1 kV m$^{-1}$ and 60 Hz (Hirata et al., 2001).

**Table 23. Induced electric fields (mV m$^{-1}$) of a grounded human body model in a vertical uniform electric field of 1 kV m$^{-1}$ and 60 Hz$^a$ or 50 Hz$^b$**

| Tissue/Organ | Mean | | 99th percentile | | Maximum | |
|---|---|---|---|---|---|---|
| | 50 Hz | 60 Hz | 50 Hz | 60 Hz | 50 Hz | 60 Hz |
| Bone | 5.72 | 3.55 | 49.4 | 34.4 | 88.8 | 40.8 |
| Tendon | 9.03 | | 37.9 | | 55.1 | |
| Skin | 2.74 | | 33.1 | | 67.3 | |
| Fat | 2.31 | | 25.2 | | 84.4 | |
| Trabecular bone | 2.80 | 3.55 | 15.1 | 34.4 | 56.5 | 40.8 |
| Muscle | 1.65 | 1.57 | 8.14 | 10.1 | 24.1 | 32.1 |
| Bladder | 1.86 | | 6.49 | | 8.58 | |
| Prostate | | 1.68 | | 2.81 | | 3.05 |
| Heart muscle | 1.29 | 1.42 | 3.98 | 2.83 | 5.83 | 3.63 |
| Spinal cord | 1.16 | | 2.92 | | 4.88 | |
| Liver | 1.63 | | 2.88 | | 5.05 | |
| Pancreas | 1.09 | | 2.76 | | 6.03 | |
| Lung | 1.09 | 1.38 | 2.54 | 2.42 | 5.69 | 3.57 |

**Table 23. Continued.**

| | | | | | | |
|---|---|---|---|---|---|---|
| Spleen | 1.33 | 1.79 | 2.49 | 2.61 | 5.07 | 3.22 |
| Vagina | 1.46 | | 2.34 | | 3.23 | |
| Uterus | 1.14 | | 2.13 | | 3.01 | |
| Thyroid | 1.16 | | 2.03 | | 3.29 | |
| White matter | 0.781 | 0.86 | 2.02 | 1.95 | 6.13 | 3.70 |
| Kidney | 1.29 | 1.44 | 1.86 | 3.12 | 4.10 | 4.47 |
| Stomach | 0.739 | | 1.86 | | 3.29 | |
| Adrenals | 1.35 | | 1.83 | | 2.32 | |
| Ovaries | 0.802 | | 1.69 | | 2.03 | |
| Blood | 0.690 | 1.43 | 1.66 | 8.91 | 3.06 | 23.8 |
| Grey matter | 0.474 | 0.86 | 1.62 | 1.95 | 4.85 | 3.70 |
| Oesophagus | 0.995 | | 1.61 | | 4.16 | |
| Duodenum | 0.765 | | 1.60 | | 2.92 | |
| Lower LI | 0.897 | | 1.53 | | 3.79 | |
| Breast | 0.705 | | 1.46 | | 2.68 | |
| Gall bladder | 0.439 | | 1.36 | | 2.03 | |
| Small intestine | 0.709 | | 1.20 | | 4.29 | |
| CSF | 0.271 | 0.35 | 1.15 | 1.02 | 2.38 | 1.58 |
| Thymus | 0.719 | | 1.09 | | 1.70 | |
| Cartilage nose | 0.598 | | 1.03 | | 1.40 | |
| Upper LI | 0.557 | | 0.989 | | 3.57 | |
| Testes | | 0.48 | | 1.19 | | 1.63 |
| Bile | 0.352 | | 0.805 | | 1.26 | |
| Urine | 0.295 | | 0.700 | | 1.29 | |
| Lunch | 0.370 | | 0.621 | | 1.14 | |
| Sclera | 0.292 | | 0.567 | | 0.623 | |
| Retina | 0.314 | | 0.552 | | 0.582 | |
| Humour | 0.188 | | 0.276 | | 0.321 | |
| Lens | 0.211 | | 0.268 | | 0.268 | |

[a] Source: Dawson, Caputa & Stuchly, 1998; Kavet et al., 2001.
[b] Source: Dimbylow, 2005.

Table 24. Induced electric field for 99th percentile voxel value at 50 Hz for an applied electric field in a female phantom (NAOMI) and a male phantom (NORMAN). The external field is that required to produce a maximum induced electric field in the brain, spinal cord (sc) or retina of 100 mV m$^{-1}$ [a]

| Geometry | Electric field mV m$^{-1}$ per kV m$^{-1}$ for 99th percentile | | | | |
| | Brain | Spinal cord | Retina | Largest | External field (kV m$^{-1}$) |
| --- | --- | --- | --- | --- | --- |
| NAOMI, GRO [b] | 2.02 | 2.92 | 0.552 | 2.92 sc | 34.2 |
| NORMAN, GRO | 1.62 | 3.42 | 0.514 | 3.42 sc | 29.2 |
| NAOMI, ISO | 1.22 | 1.40 | 0.336 | 1.40 sc | 71.4 |
| NORMAN, ISO | 0.811 | 1.63 | 0.262 | 1.63 sc | 61.3 |

[a] Source: Dimbylow, 2005.

[b] GRO: grounded; ISO: isolated.

Table 25. Induced electric fields (mV m$^{-1}$) of a grounded child body model in a vertical uniform electric field of 60 Hz, 1 kV m$^{-1}$ [a]

| Tissue/Organ | Mean | 99th percentile | Maximum |
| --- | --- | --- | --- |
| Blood | 1.52 | 9.18 | 18.06 |
| Bone marrow | 3.70 | 32.85 | 41.87 |
| Brain | 0.70 | 1.58 | 3.07 |
| CSF | 0.28 | 0.87 | 1.37 |
| Heart | 1.60 | 3.07 | 3.69 |
| Lungs | 1.55 | 2.63 | 3.69 |
| Muscle | 1.65 | 9.97 | 30.56 |

[a] Source: Hirata et al., 2001.

The current density averaged over 1 cm$^2$, which is the basic exposure unit in the ICNIRP guidelines (ICNIRP, 1998a), is illustrated in Figure 5.

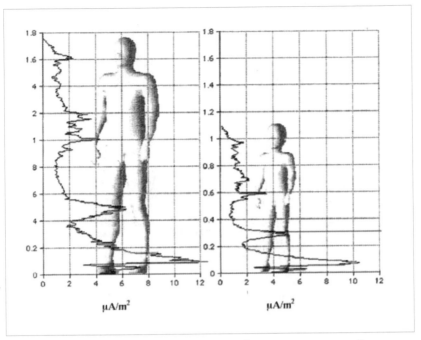

**Figure 5.** Maximum current density in μA m$^{-2}$ averaged over 1 cm$^2$ in vertical body layers for grounded models exposed to a vertical electric field of 1 kV m$^{-1}$ and 60 Hz (Hirata et al., 2001).

With certain exposures in occupational situations, e.g. in a substation, when the human body is close to a conductor at high potential, higher electric fields are induced in some organs (e.g. the brain) than calculated using the measured field 1.5 m above ground (Potter, Okoniewski & Stuchly, 2000). This is to be expected, as the external field increases above the ground.

### 3.3.4 Comparison of computations with measurements

Computed (Gandhi & Chen, 1992) and measured (Deno, 1977) current distributions for ungrounded and grounded human of 1.77 m height standing in a vertical homogeneous electric field are illustrated in Figure 6.

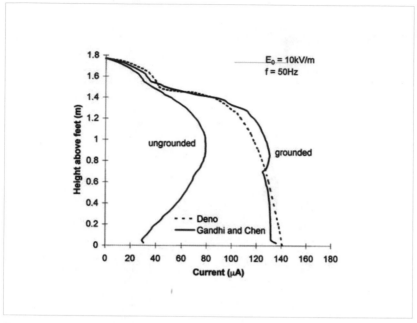

**Figure 6.** Computed (Gandhi & Chen, 1992) and measured (Deno, 1977) current distribution for an ungrounded and grounded human of 1.77 m in height standing in a vertical homogeneous electric field of 10 kV m$^{-1}$ at 50 Hz.

Table 26 shows a comparison of the computed (Dawson, Caputa & Stuchly, 1998) vertical current across a few cross-sections of the human body with the measurements (Tenforde & Kaune, 1987). Given the modelling differences among the laboratories, the agreement can be considered very acceptable.

**Table 26. Induced vertical current (μA) in a human body model in a vertical uniform electric field of 60 Hz and 1 kV m$^{-1}$**

| Body position | Grounded | | Elevated above ground | | Free space | |
|---|---|---|---|---|---|---|
| | Computed[a] | Measured[b] | Computed[a] | Measured[b] | Computed[a] | Measured[b] |
| Neck | 4.9 | 5.4 | 3.7 | 4.0 | 2.9 | 3.1 |
| Chest | 9.8 | 13.5 | 7.0 | 8.7 | 5.3 | 5.4 |
| Abdomen | 13.8 | 14.6 | 9.1 | 9.3 | 6.6 | 5.7 |
| Thigh | 16.6 | 15.6 | 9.7 | 9.4 | 6.1 | 5.6 |
| Ankle | 17.6 | 17.0 | 7.3 | 8.0 | 3.0 | 3.0 |

[a] Source: Dawson, Caputa & Stuchly, 1998.
[b] Source: Tenforde & Kaune, 1987.

## 3.4    Magnetic field dosimetry

### 3.4.1    Basic interaction mechanisms

Human and animal bodies do not perturb the magnetic field, and the field in tissue is the same as the external field, since the magnetic permeability of tissues is the same as that of air. The quantities of magnetic material that are present in some tissues are so minute that they can be neglected in macroscopic dosimetry. The main interaction of a magnetic field with the body is the Faraday induction of an electric field and associated current in conductive tissue. In a homogeneous tissue the lines of electric flux (and current density) are solenoidal. In the case of heterogeneous tissues, consisting of regions of different conductivities, currents are flowing also at the interfaces between the regions. In the simplest model of an equivalent circular loop corresponding to a given body contour the induced electric field is

$$E = \pi \, f \, r \, B$$

and the current density is

$$J - \pi f \sigma r B$$

where f is the frequency, r is the loop radius and $B$ is the magnetic flux density vector normal to the current loop. Similarly, ellipsoidal loops can be considered to better fit into the body shape.

Electric fields and currents induced in the human body cannot be measured easily. Measurements in animals have been performed, but data are limited, and the accuracy of measurements is relatively poor.

### 3.4.2    Computations – uniform field

Heterogeneous models of the human body similar to those used for electric field exposures have been numerically analyzed using the impedance method (IM) (Gandhi et al., 2001; Gandhi & Chen, 1992; Gandhi & DeFord, 1988), and the scalar potential finite difference (SPFD) technique (Dawson & Stuchly, 1996; Dimbylow, 1998). Even more extensive data than for the electric field are available for the magnetic field. The influence on the induced quantities of the model resolution, tissue properties in general and muscle anisotropy specifically, field orientation with respect to the body, and to a certain extent body anatomy have been investigated (Dawson, Caputa & Stuchly, 1997b; Dawson & Stuchly, 1998; Dimbylow, 1998; Stuchly & Dawson, 2000). In the past, the maximum current density in a body part has often been calculated using the largest loop of current that can be incorporated in it. Dawson, Caputa & Stuchly (1999b) have shown that induced parameters should be calculated for organs in situ instead of for isolated ones, since there is a significant influence of surrounding structures.

The main features of dosimetry for exposures to the uniform ELF magnetic field can be summarized as follows.

- The electric fields induced in the body depend on the orientation of the magnetic field with respect to the body.

- For most organs and tissues, as expected, the magnetic field orientation normal to the torso (front-to-back) gives maximum induced quantities.

- In the brain, cerebrospinal fluid, blood, heart, bladder, eyes and spinal cord, the highest quantities are induced by the magnetic field oriented side-to-side.

- Consistently lowest induced fields are for the magnetic field oriented along the vertical body axis.

- For a given field strength and orientation, greater electric fields are induced in a body of a larger size.

- The induced electric field values are to the lesser degree influenced by the conductivity of various organs and tissues than the values of the induced current density.

Table 27 presents electric field induced in several organs and tissues at 60 Hz, 1 µT magnetic field oriented front-to-back (Dawson, Caputa & Stuchly, 1997b; Dawson & Stuchly, 1998; Kavet et al., 2001). Comparable data at 50 Hz and normalized to 1 mT are shown in Table 28 (Dimbylow, 2005). An example of the current distribution in the body compared to the body anatomy is illustrated in Figure 7. The layer averaged electric field and current density for two sets of tissue conductivity are shown in Figure 8.

Table 27. Induced electric fields (mV m⁻¹) in the human body model in a uniform magnetic field of 1 mT and 60 Hz or 50 Hz oriented front-to-back [a]

| Tissue/organ | Mean | | 99th percentile | | Maximum | |
|---|---|---|---|---|---|---|
| | 50 Hz | 60 Hz | 50 Hz | 60 Hz | 50 Hz | 60 Hz |
| Bone | 11.6 | 16 | 50.9 | 23 | 166 | 83 |
| Tendon | 2.81 | | 9.35 | | 14.9 | |
| Skin | 13.5 | | 36.0 | | 65.6 | |
| Fat | 13.7 | | 33.5 | | 129 | |
| Trabecular bone | 6.40 | 16 | 24.3 | 23 | 48.5 | 83 |
| Muscle | 8.44 | 15 | 23.0 | 51 | 67.6 | 147 |
| Bladder | 11.8 | | 45.8 | | 64.7 | |
| Heart muscle | 9.62 | 14 | 28.0 | 38 | 42.0 | 49 |
| Spinal | 8.90 | | 27.0 | | 53.0 | |
| Liver | 13.2 | | 38.2 | | 73.1 | |
| Pancreas | 3.52 | | 13.6 | | 24.9 | |
| Lung | 8.22 | 21 | 24.4 | 49 | 93.3 | 86 |
| Spleen | 8.16 | 41 | 18.4 | 72 | 27.2 | 92 |
| Vagina | 3.76 | | 12.0 | | 19.4 | |

**Table 27. Continued.**

| | | | | | |
|---|---|---|---|---|---|
| Uterus | 3.81 | | 9.44 | | 17.0 | |
| Prostate | | 17 | | 36 | | 52 |
| Thyroid | 12.6 | | 21.8 | | 37.9 | |
| White matter | 10.1 | 11 | 31.4 | 31 | 82.5 | 74 |
| Kidney | 10.8 | 25 | 22.5 | 53 | 39.2 | 71 |
| Stomach | 4.52 | | 15.0 | | 26.8 | |
| Adrenals | 9.91 | | 19.2 | | 24.5 | |
| Ovaries | 2.40 | | 5.30 | | 7.87 | |
| Blood | 5.99 | 6.9 | 17.5 | 23 | 30.9 | 83 |
| Grey matter | 8.04 | 11 | 30.2 | 31 | 74.8 | 74 |
| Oesophagus | 4.86 | | 10.0 | | 14.1 | |
| Duodenum | 5.22 | | 14.1 | | 22.1 | |
| Lower LI | 4.30 | | 12.2 | | 27.4 | |
| Testes | | 15 | | 41 | | 73 |
| Breast | 18.1 | | 31.0 | | 51.6 | |
| Gall bladder | 3.41 | | 9.64 | | 14.8 | |
| Small intestine | 3.98 | | 10.4 | | 24.8 | |
| CSF | 5.25 | 5.2 | 14.8 | 17 | 33.3 | 25 |
| Thymus | 12.2 | | 19.6 | | 30.7 | |
| Cartilage nose | 13.4 | | 31.5 | | 38.3 | |
| Upper LI | 5.85 | | 12.7 | | 21.1 | |
| Bile | 2.56 | | 6.63 | | 9.56 | |
| Urine | 2.16 | | 4.71 | | 7.55 | |
| Lunch | 2.31 | | 6.47 | | 7.58 | |
| Sclera | 7.78 | | 16.3 | | 18.2 | |
| Retina | 6.69 | | 13.5 | | 15.1 | |
| Humour | 4.51 | | 7.41 | | 9.20 | |
| Lens | 5.22 | | 6.70 | | 6.70 | |

[a] Sources: Dawson & Stuchly, 1998 (60 Hz), Dimbylow, 2005 (50 Hz).

**Table 28.** Induced electric field for 99th percentile voxel value at 50 Hz for an applied magnetic field in a female phantom (NAOMI) and a male phantom (NORMAN). The external field (in terms of magnetic flux density) is that required to produce a maximum induced electric field in the brain (br), spinal cord (sc) or retina of 100 mV m$^{-1}$ [a]

| Geometry | Induced electric field mV m$^{-1}$ per mT for 99th percentile | | | | |
|---|---|---|---|---|---|
| | Brain | Spinal cord | Retina | Largest | External field (mT) |
| NAOMI, AP [b] | 25.7 | 17.7 | 6.98 | 25.7 br | 3.89 |
| NORMAN, AP | 30.7 | 29.7 | 7.05 | 30.7 br | 3.26 |
| NAOMI, LAT | 31.4 | 27.0 | 13.5 | 31.4 br | 3.18 |
| NORMAN, LAT | 33.0 | 48.6 | 14.6 | 48.6 sc | 2.06 |
| NAOMI, TOP | 25.1 | 8.60 | 6.90 | 25.1 br | 3.98 |
| NORMAN, TOP | 22.1 | 23.0 | 10.2 | 23.0 sc | 4.35 |

[a] Source: Dimbylow, 2005.

[b] AP: front-to-back; LAT: side-to-side; TOP: head-to-feet.

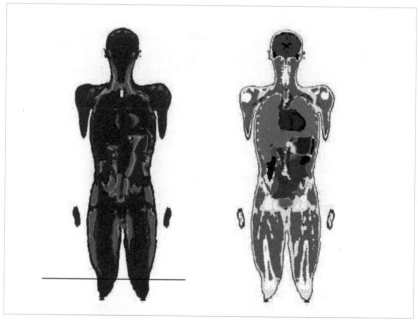

**Figure 7.** Distribution of the current density (left) induced by a uniform magnetic field of 50 Hz perpendicular to the frontal plane, calculated for an anatomically shaped heterogeneous model of the human body (right) (Dimbylow, 1998). The colour map of the current density (left) is a spectrum, the highest values in red and the lowest values in violet, and is only intended to give a general view of current density patterns.

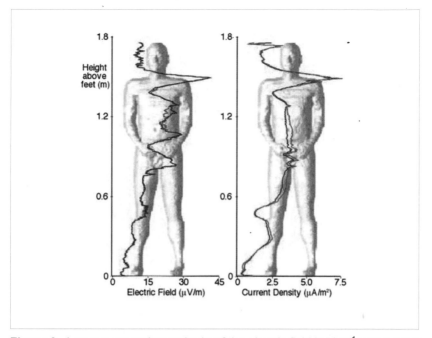

**Figure 8.** Layer-averaged magnitude of the electric field in V m$^{-1}$ and current density in A m$^{-2}$ for exposure to a uniform magnetic flux density of 1 µT and 60 Hz oriented front-to-back. The two curves on each graph correspond to two sets of conductivity (Dawson & Stuchly, 1998).

### 3.4.3   Computations – non-uniform fields

Human exposure to relatively high magnetic flux density values most often occurs in occupational settings. Numerical modeling has been considered mostly for workers exposed to high-voltage transmission lines (Baraton & Hutzler, 1995; Dawson, Caputa & Stuchly, 1999a; Dawson, Caputa & Stuchly, 1999c; Stuchly & Zhao, 1996). In those cases, current-carrying conductors can be represented as infinite straight-line sources. However, some of the exposures occur in more complex scenarios, two of which have been analyzed, a more-realistic representation of the source conductors based on finite line segments has been used (Dawson, Caputa & Stuchly, 1999d). Table 29 gives dosimetry for two representative exposure scenarios illustrated in Figure 9 (Dawson, Caputa & Stuchly, 1999c). Current in each conductor is 250 A for a total of 1000 A in a four-conductor bundle.

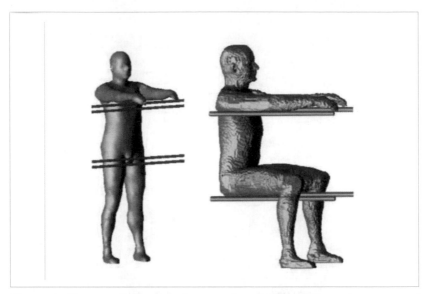

**Figure 9.** Two exposure scenarios used in calculations for workers exposed to high-voltage transmission lines (Dawson, Caputa & Stuchly, 1999c).

Table 29. Calculated electric fields (mV m$^{-1}$) induced in a model of an adult human for the occupational exposure scenarios shown in Figure 9 (total current in conductors: 1000 A; 60 Hz) [a]

| Tissue/organ | Scenario A | | Scenario B | |
|---|---|---|---|---|
| | $E_{max}$ | $E_{rms}$ | $E_{max}$ | $E_{rms}$ |
| Blood | 20 | 3.7 | 15 | 2.4 |
| Bone | 90 | 11 | 58 | 7.2 |
| Brain | 22 | 4.6 | 28 | 5.9 |
| Cerebrospinal fluid | 9.2 | 2.3 | 14 | 3.7 |
| Heart | 27 | 11 | 9.0 | 3.2 |
| Kidneys | 22 | 7.9 | 2.8 | 0.9 |
| Lungs | 31 | 10 | 9.9 | 2.9 |
| Muscle | 59 | 6.9 | 33 | 5.5 |
| Prostate | 5.5 | 1.9 | 2.6 | 1.2 |
| Testes | 18 | 5.5 | 2.7 | 1.2 |

[a] Source: Stuchly & Dawson, 2000.

### 3.4.4 Computations – inter-laboratory comparison and model effects

To assess the reliability of data obtained by using anatomy based body models and numerical methods, an interlaboratory comparison was performed (Caputa et al., 2002). Two groups in the UK and Canada used the 3.6 mm and 2 mm resolution models of average size. Each group applied its own, independently developed, field solver based on the Scalar Potential Finite Difference (SPFD) method. For a great majority of tissues, the difference in calculated parameters between the two groups was 1% or less. Only in a few cases it reaches 2–3 %. Differences of the order of 1–2 % are typically expected on the basis of the accuracy analysis (Dawson, Potter & Stuchly, 2001).

In addition, a larger size model was used to investigate effects of body size and anatomy (Caputa et al., 2002). The size of the body model and its shape (including anatomy and resolution) influenced the average ($E_{avg}$), voxel maximum and 99 percentile values of the induced electric field ($E_{99}$). The large size model mass was about 40% greater than that of the two average size models. Correspondingly, the whole-body-average electric fields were also about 40% greater, while 99 percentile electric fields were 41% and 34% greater. Such simple mass-based scaling did not apply even approximately to specific organs and tissues. The actual anatomy of persons represented by the models, as well as the accuracy of the models, both influenced differences in the two dosimetric measures for organs that are computed accurately, namely $E_{avg}$ and $E_{99}$. The two models of similar size showed typically differences by about 10% or less in the average and 99 percentile values, e.g. $E_{avg}$ in blood, brain, heart, kidney, muscle, and $E_{99}$ in blood, brain, muscle, for the same model resolution. Relatively small organs, such as the testes, or thin organs, such as the spinal cord, indicated larger differences in induced electric field strengths that could be directly ascribed to the differences in the shape and size of these organs in the models.

## 3.5   Contact current

Contact currents produce electric fields in tissue that are similar to and often much greater than those induced by external electric and magnetic fields. Contact currents occur when a person touches conductive surfaces at different potentials and completes a path for current flow through the body. Typically, the current pathway is hand-to-hand and/or from a hand to one or both feet. Contact current sources may include the appliance chassis that, because of typical residential wiring practices (in North America), carry a small potential above a home ground. Also, large conductive objects situated in an electric field, such as a vehicle parked under a transmission line, serve as a source of contact current. The possible role of contact currents as a factor responsible for the reported association of magnetic fields with childhood leukaemia was first introduced by Kavet et al. (2000) in a scenario that involved contact with appliances. In subsequent papers, a more plausible exposure scenario has been developed that entails contact currents to children with low contact resistance while bathing and touching the water fixtures (Kavet et al., 2004; Kavet, 2005; Kavet & Zaffanella, 2002).

Recently, electric fields have been computed in an adult and a child model with electrodes on hands and feet simulating contact current (Dawson et al., 2001). Three scenarios are considered based on the combinations of electrodes. In all scenarios contact is through one hand. In scenario A the opposite hand and both feet are grounded. In scenario B only the opposite hand is grounded. This scenario represents touching a charged object with one hand and grounded object with another hand. Scenario C has both feet grounded. This is perhaps the most common and represents touching an ungrounded object while both feet are grounded. Dosimetric measures can be scaled linearly for other contact current values. These in turn can be obtained for a given contact resistance (or impedance) for a known open-circuit voltage. Table 30 gives representative measures for the electric field in bone marrow, which do not vary significantly, for the three scenarios. The measures in the bone marrow are of interest in view of the reports by Kavet and colleagues cited above. It should be noted that the electric fields in the brain are negligibly small in the case of contact currents.

**Table 30. Calculated electric field (mV m$^{-1}$) induced by a contact current of 60 Hz, 1 µA in voxels of bone marrow of a child** [a]

| Body part | $E_{avg}$ | $E_{99}$ |
|---|---|---|
| Lower arm | 5.1 | 14.9 |
| Upper arm | 0.9 | 1.4 |
| Whole body | 0.4 | 3.3 |

[a] Source: Dawson et al., 2001.

Examination of data in Table 30 indicates that, averaged across the body, electric fields of the order of 1 mV m$^{-1}$ are produced in bone marrow of children from a contact current of 1 µA. However, much higher values occur in the marrow of the lower contacting arm: 5 mV m$^{-1}$ per µA averaged across this anatomical site and an upper 5th percentile of 13 mV m$^{-1}$ per µA in this tissue. As discussed in section 4.6.2, 50 µA may result from the upper 4% of contact voltages measured between the water fixture and the drain (the site of exposure) in one US measurement study (Kavet et al., 2004); such a voltage would produce bone marrow doses of about 650 mV m$^{-1}$ (see section 4.6.2). In contrast, current resulting from contact with an appliance would be very limited owing to the resistance of structural materials, shoes, and dry skin (Kavet et al., 2000). Contact with vehicle-sized objects in an electric field would produce currents in excess of roughly 5 µA per kV m$^{-1}$ (Dawson et al., 2001), and would depend on the grounding of the vehicle relative to the contacting person's grounding.

## 3.6    Comparison of various exposures

It is interesting to compare different electric and magnetic field exposures that produce equivalent internal electric fields in different organs. Such comparisons are given in Table 31 based on published data (Dawson, Caputa & Stuchly, 1997a; Dimbylow, 2005; Stuchly & Dawson, 2002).

Table 31. Electric (grounded model) or magnetic field (front-to-back) source levels at 50 or 60 Hz needed to induce mean and maximum electric field of 1 mV m⁻¹, calculated from data of tables 23 and 27

| Organ | Electric field ($kV\ m^{-1}$) | | | |
|---|---|---|---|---|
| | Mean | | 99th percentile | |
| | 50 Hz | 60 Hz | 50 Hz | 60 Hz |
| Blood | 1.45 | 0.70 | 0.60 | 0.11 |
| Bone | 0.17 | 0.28 | 0.020 | 0.029 |
| Brain | 1.28 | 1.16 | 0.50 | 0.51 |
| CSF | 3.69 | 2.86 | 0.87 | 0.98 |
| Heart | 0.78 | 0.70 | 0.25 | 0.35 |
| Kidneys | 0.78 | 0.69 | 0.54 | 0.32 |
| Liver | 0.61 | | 0.35 | |
| Lungs | 0.92 | 0.72 | 0.39 | 0.41 |
| Muscle | 0.61 | 0.64 | 0.12 | 0.000 |
| Prostate | | 0.60 | | 0.36 |
| Testes | | 2.08 | | 0.84 |

| Organ | Magnetic field (µT) | | | |
|---|---|---|---|---|
| | Mean | | 99th percentile | |
| | 50 Hz | 60 Hz | 50 Hz | 60 Hz |
| Blood | 166.9 | 144.9 | 57.1 | 43.5 |
| Bone | 86.2 | 62.5 | 19.6 | 43.5 |
| Brain | 99.0 | 90.9 | 31.8 | 32.3 |
| CSF | 190.5 | 192.3 | 67.6 | 58.8 |
| Heart | 104.0 | 71.5 | 35.7 | 26.3 |
| Kidneys | 92.6 | 40.0 | 44.4 | 18.9 |
| Liver | 75.8 | | 26.2 | |
| Lungs | 121.7 | 47.6 | 41.0 | 20.4 |
| Muscle | 118.5 | 66.7 | 43.5 | 19.6 |
| Prostate | | 58.8 | | 27.8 |
| Testes | | 66.7 | | 24.4 |

## 3.7 Microscopic dosimetry

Macroscopic dosimetry that gives induced electric fields in various organs and tissues can be extended to more spatially refined models of subcellular structures to quantitatively predict and understand biophysical interactions. The simplest subcellular modeling that considers linear systems requires evaluation of induced fields in various parts of a cell. Such models, for instance, have been developed to understand neural stimulation (Abdeen & Stuchly, 1994; Basser & Roth, 1991; Malmivuo & Plonsey, 1995; Plonsey

& Barr, 1988; Reilly, 1992). Also, in the past, simplified models of cells consisting of a membrane, cytoplasm and nucleus, and suspended in conductive medium have been considered (Foster & Schwan, 1989). The membrane potential has been computed for spherical (Foster & Schwan, 1996), ellipsoidal (Bernhardt & Pauly, 1973) and spheroidal cells (Jerry, Popel & Brownell, 1996) suspended in a lossy medium. Computations are available as a function of the applied electric field and its frequency. Because cell membranes have high resistivity and capacitance (nearly constant for all mammalian cells and equal to 1 F cm$^{-2}$), at sufficiently low frequencies high fields are produced at the two faces of the membrane. The field is nearly zero inside the cell, as long as the frequency of the applied field is below the membrane relaxation frequency. This specific relaxation frequency depends on the total membrane resistance and capacitance. The larger the cell, the higher the induced membrane potential for the same applied field. However, the larger the cell, the lower the membrane relaxation frequency.

Gap junctions connect most cells. A gap junction is an aqueous pore or channel through which neighboring cell membranes are connected. Thus, cells can exchange ions, for example, providing local intercellular communication (Holder, Elmore & Barrett, 1993). Certain cancer promoters inhibit gap communication and allow the cells to multiply uncontrollably. It has been hypothesized with support from some suggestive experimental results, that low-frequency electric and magnetic fields may affect intercellular communication. Gap-connected cells have previously been modeled as long cables (Cooper, 1984). Also, very simplified models have been used, in which gap-connected cells are represented by large cells of the size of the gap-connected cell-assemblies (Polk, 1992). With such models relatively large induced membrane potentials have been estimated, even for moderate applied fields.

A numerical analysis has been performed to compute membrane potentials in more realistic models (Fear & Stuchly, 1998a; 1998b; 1998c). Various assemblies of cells connected by gap-junctions have been modeled with cell and gap-junction dimensions and conductivity values representative of mammalian cells. These simulations have indicated that simplified models can only be used for some specific situations. However, even in those cases, equivalent cells have to be constructed in which cytoplasm properties are modified to account for the properties of gap-junctions. These models predict reasonably well the results for very small assemblies of cells of certain shapes and at very low frequencies (Fear & Stuchly, 1998b). On the other hand, numerical analysis can predict correctly the induced membrane potential as well as the relaxation frequency (Fear & Stuchly, 1998a; 1998c). It has been shown that, as the size of the cell-assembly increases, the membrane potential even at DC does not increase linearly with dimensions, as it does for very short elongated assemblies. There is a characteristic length for elongated assemblies beyond which the membrane potential does not increase significantly. There is also a limit of increase for the membrane potential for assemblies of other shapes. Even more importantly, as the assembly size (volume) increases, the relaxation frequency decreases (at the relaxation frequency the induced membrane potential is half of that at DC).

From this linear model of gap-connected cells, it is concluded that at 50 or 60 Hz the induced membrane potential in any organ of the human body exposed to a uniform magnetic flux density of up to 1 mT or to an electric field of approximately 10 kV m$^{-1}$ or less, does not exceed 0.1 mV. This is small in comparison to the endogenous resting membrane potential in the range 20-100 mV.

## 3.8    Conclusions

Exposure to external electric and magnetic fields at extremely low frequencies induces electric fields and currents inside the body. Dosimetry describes the relationship between the external fields and the induced electric field and current density in the body, or other parameters associated with exposure to these fields. The local induced electric field and current density are of particular interest because they relate to the stimulation of excitable tissue such as nerve and muscle.

The bodies of humans and animals significantly perturb the spatial distribution of an ELF electric field. At low frequencies the body is a good conductor and the perturbed field lines outside the the body are nearly normal to the body surface. Oscillating charges are induced on the surface of the exposed body and these induce currents inside the body. The key features of dosimetry for the exposure of humans to ELF electric fields are as follows:

• The electric field inside the body is normally five to six orders of magnitude smaller than the external electric field.

• When exposure is mostly to the vertical field, the predominant direction of the induced fields is also vertical.

• For a given external electric field, the strongest induced fields are for the human body in perfect contact through the feet with the ground (electrically grounded) and the weakest induced fields are for the body insulated from the ground (in "free space").

• The total current flowing in a body in perfect contact with ground is determined by the body size and shape (including posture) rather than tissue conductivity.

• The distribution of induced currents across the various organs and tissues is determined by the conductivity of those tissues.

• The distribution of an induced electric field is also influenced by the conductivities, but less so than the induced current.

• There is also a separate phenomenon in which the current in the body is produced by means of contact with a conductive object located in an electric field.

For magnetic fields, the permeability of tissues is the same as that of air, so the field in tissue is the same as the external field. The bodies of humans and animals do not significantly perturb the field. The main interaction of magnetic fields with the body is the Faraday induction of electric fields and associated current densities in the conductive tissues. The key features of dosimetry for the exposure to ELF magnetic fields are as follows:

- The induced electric field and current depend on the orientation of the external field. Induced fields in the body as a whole are greatest when the fields are aligned from the front or back of the body, but for some individual organs the highest values are induced for the field aligned from side-to-side.

- The consistently lowest induced electric fields are found when the external magnetic field is oriented along the vertical body axis.

- For a given magnetic field strength and orientation, higher electric fields are induced in a body of a larger size.

- The distribution of the induced electric field values is affected by the conductivity of various organs and tissues. These have a limited effect on the distribution of the induced current density.

# 4 BIOPHYSICAL MECHANISMS

## 4.1 Introduction

This chapter considers the biophysical plausibility of various proposed interaction mechanisms for ELF electric and magnetic fields; in particular whether a "signal" generated in a biological process by exposure to ELF fields can be discriminated from inherent random noise. It covers both direct mechanisms (the field interacts directly with sites in the body) and indirect mechanisms (the field affects or is related to another environmental factor, which in turn affects the body).

For exposure to ELF electric and magnetic fields to cause adverse health effects, the following sequence of events must occur. First, the field must interact with a fundamental component of the matter from which the person is made up – an atom or molecule or a characteristic of atoms or molecules such as a dipole moment. This interaction must then produce an effect at the cellular level that ultimately produces biological changes in the person that are regarded as detrimental to health.

Note that if it can be demonstrated that electric or magnetic field exposure, even at very low levels, can adversely affect health, then it follows that a mechanism of interaction must exist, even if this appears biophysically implausible. [An analogy comes from particle physics, where parity conservation was regarded as a fundamental law. However, when a convincing experimental demonstration of parity violation was made (Wu et al., 1957), it was recognised that this "law" was no longer tenable.] The converse, that if a plausible interaction mechanism cannot exist then there can be no health effects from such exposure, cannot be proven. Nevertheless, repeated failure to identify a plausible interaction mechanism might suggest, in the absence of contrary information, that such health effects are unlikely.

This chapter considers the first of the events outlined above, the biophysical interaction mechanism. It first considers the principles on which to assess whether a proposed biophysical interaction mechanism is physically plausible or not. It then surveys the various mechanisms that have been suggested and assesses their plausibility according to the criteria established.

## 4.2 The concept of plausibility

In the context of this document, the degree of plausibility of a mechanism relates to the extent to which it challenges scientific principles and current scientific knowledge. The degree of plausibility for a mechanism to play a role is strongly linked to the exposure level under consideration. Nevertheless, even the lack of identified plausible mechanisms would not exclude the possibility of a health effect existing even at very low field levels.

For any given mechanism of direct interaction, the magnitude of the response at a molecular level can be calculated from the physical laws involved. However, in order for the mechanism of interaction to count as biophysically plausible, it will have to produce a significant change to some biological parameter (e.g. the transmembrane voltage) that conveys information about the external field through some signalling mechanism, such as an intracellular or neural signalling pathway. However, the parameter in question will itself be subject to random variation that conveys nothing of biological significance. For example, any voltage has a noise level caused by thermal agitation. The effect produced by the field can be of biological significance only if it can be distinguished from random fluctuations.

A convenient way of expressing this concept is in terms of a signal-to-noise ratio. In this context, the "signal" is the effect on a given parameter produced by the field, and the "noise" is the level of random fluctuations that occur in that parameter. If the signal-to-noise ratio is less than one, there will be no "detectable" change in the parameter that can be attributed to the field and no possibility of subsequent biological effects that are similarly attributable. If the signal-to-noise ratio is one or greater, then there could be a change in the parameter that is attributable to the field, and there is a possibility of subsequent events producing an effect in the organism.

Random fluctuations in biological systems typically extend across a wide range of frequencies. If the biological "transducer", the cellular component that responds to an external signal such as an applied ELF field, is itself sensitive to a wide range of frequencies, then the comparison should be made with the amplitude of the noise over its whole frequency range. However, if the transducer concerned is sensitive only to a narrow range of frequencies, then the applied signal should be compared only to that component of the noise over the frequency range of sensitivity. Vision and hearing are two such phenomena where sensitivity is highly frequency-dependent.

Other factors that could increase the signal-to-noise ratio are amplification mechanisms for the signal. They include enhancement of the signal due to cell geometry or signal processing by large electrically coupled cell aggregates. Those mechanisms are discussed in detail in the following sections.

With indirect effects the principle still applies that the agent (for example chemicals, ions etc.) influenced by or occurring in concert with the fields must be sufficiently large to produce a detectable change in the biological system.

In summary therefore, a proposed biophysical mechanism can only constitute a plausible mechanism for fields to interact with living tissue as to be potentially capable of causing disease if it causes a variation in some parameter that is larger than the background noise. The mechanism will be more plausible if this variation is either substantially larger than the random noise, or if the organism has developed frequency-specific sensitivity.

## 4.3    Stochastic effects, thresholds and dose-response relationships

The nature of the various possible interaction mechanisms discussed below affects the way in which health effects might be induced. At a fundamental level, stochastic interactions, such as random genotoxic damage to DNA by, for example, reactive oxygen species, increase the probability of inducing a mutation and hence the risk of initiating cancer. Deterministic effects, on the other hand, occur when some threshold is passed, for example when applied electric fields cause sufficient sodium ion channels in a nerve membrane to have opened so that nerve excitation becomes self-sustaining. Such thresholds usually show a distribution of sensitivity within populations (of cells and of people), and so the induction of an effect will vary over this range within the population.

The way in which a subsequent health effect might vary with exposure can be estimated from the biophysical nature of the interaction alone, although this will tend to neglect the contribution made by the intervening chain of biological responses at the cellular and whole organism level, and so can only be suggestive. For example, the ability to reverse acute physiological changes such as ion fluxes, and to repair for example potentially long term effects like oxidative damage, will affect the overall health outcome.

With regard to alternating fields, if the effect of an interaction depends on the size of the field and not its spatial direction, then the magnitude of the effect depends simply on the size of the field. However, any effect that depends on the direction of the field as well as its size will, to a first order, average to zero over time; as one half cycle increases an effect, the other decreases it by the same amount.

Non-linearities in the interaction mechanism mean that these effects do not average out exactly to zero. (It is worth noting here that any subsequent biological responses are almost certain to be non-linear.) The effect produced, which is the difference between two first-order or linear effects, is a second-order effect, proportional to the field squared (or to an even higher power) rather then the field. Subsequent stages in the mechanism may modify this further, but are unlikely to restore any component proportional to the field itself.

Mathematically, the effect of the field can be expressed as a Taylor expansion. For any effect proportional to the field $B$, the first order term of the Taylor expansion averages to zero and the lowest order non-zero term is the second power of field (Adair, 1994). However, for an effect proportional to the modulus of $B$, the first order term can be non-zero as well.

The practical consequence of this is that if the mechanism is proportional to the square of the field or a higher power, the effects will be produced more by short exposures to high fields than by long exposures to low fields. In particular, high fields are experienced predominantly from domestic appliances, so a mechanism proportional to a higher power of field would be expected to show effects related to appliance use more clearly than effects related to background fields in homes. However, this might depend to some extent on the way in which the initial interaction was subsequently modified by biological processes.

## 4.4    Induced currents and fields

### 4.4.1    Currents induced by fields

Power-frequency fields, both electric and magnetic, induce electric fields and hence currents in the body. An external electric field is attenuated greatly inside the body, but the internal field then drives a current in the body. A magnetic field induces an electric field, which will in turn drive a current in the conducting body. This is discussed in detail in Chapter 3, where results from numerical modelling are presented.

### 4.4.2    Comparison with noise

The observation of several cellular and membrane responses to weak ELF fields has raised the question of how the magnitudes of these signals compare with the intrinsic electrical noise present in cell membranes. The three major sources of electrical noise in biological membranes are (Leuchtag, 1990): (1) Johnson-Nyquist thermally-generated electrical noise, which produces a 3-$\mu$V transmembrane voltage shift at physiological temperatures; (2) "shot" noise, which results from the discrete nature of ionic charge carriers and can be a major source of membrane electrical noise; and (3) 1/f noise associated with ion current flows through membrane channels, which typically produces a 10-$\mu$V transmembrane voltage shift.

Any material (including but not confined to biological material) has fluctuating electric fields and corresponding currents within it, due to the random movement of the charged components of matter. From basic physical consideration, an expression can be derived for a lower limit to the thermal noise voltage or field that appears between two points across any element of material. This thermal noise field depends on the resistance of the element (and hence for a given material its size), the temperature (which for the present purposes can always be taken as the body temperature), and the frequency range. (Strictly speaking, it is the noise in a given frequency band that depends on the resistance; the total noise across all frequencies is independent of the resistance and depends instead on the capacitance.)

There are other sources of noise as well, which in some instances may be much larger than the thermal noise, but the thermal noise always constitutes a lower limit on the noise. One particular other source of noise, shot noise, is considered separately in the next section.

In regard to shot noise, when a process depends on discrete particles, and some property produced by the process depends on the average number of particles fulfilling some condition, there will be a random variation in the number of particles involved, which can be regarded as a noise level superimposed on the average number. This is known as "shot" noise. This can be applied to passage of ions or molecules through a voltage-gated channel in a cell membrane. The number of ions passing through such a channel in the absence of a field depends on the maximum possible flux of ions, a property of the cell membrane, and how often the gates or channels are open, a function of the transmembrane potential, the noise energy density, the cell gating charge, and the exposure time. The signal-to-noise ratio will be maximised by considering either a long cell parallel to the in situ electric field with the channels confined to the ends (so as to minimise the number of channels which are not affected by the applied field), or by a large spherical cell (so as to maximise the cell's area). For a cylindrical cell 1 mm long and radius 25 μm, or for a spherical cell radius 100 μm, and for typical values of the other parameters, the value of the in situ electric field for a signal-to-noise ratio of one is around 100 mV·m$^{-1}$ (Weaver & Vaughan, 1998). By optimising the noise level and the transmembrane potential, the threshold field can be improved, to around 10 mV m$^{-1}$, corresponding to external fields of 5 kV m$^{-1}$ and 300 μT.

The shot noise considered above is mostly in relation to the spontaneous opening and closing of voltage-gated channels. The arrival of neurotransmitters (synaptic events) also causes voltage fluctuations in nerve and muscle cells. In an experimental study by Jacobson et al. (2005) it was shown that voltage noise in neurons fluctuated with a standard deviation up to 0.5 mV, and that these fluctuations were dominated by synaptic events in the 5–100 Hz range. Shot noise associated with these neurotransmitter events may thus be much more relevant in estimating excitation thresholds in the retinae (Jacobson et al., 2005).

Despite the presence of thermal and shot noise, it appears that 1/f noise is the dominant source of noise on the membrane and represents a reasonable baseline for signal-to-noise considerations, and for the estimation of equivalent external field values. External field values required to produce a signal discernable from noise depend on the specific characteristics of the biological system in question. However, at least for small isolated cells in the human body, the range of external fields would be of the order of 10 mT and 100 kV m$^{-1}$.

### 4.4.3    Myelinated nerve fibre stimulation thresholds

The electrical excitability of neurons (nerve cells) results from the presence of voltage-gated ion channels, principally sodium, potassium, calcium and chloride, in the cell membrane (e.g. McCormick, 1998). Sodium, calcium and chloride ions exist in higher concentrations on the outside of each neuron, and potassium and membrane-impermeant anions are concentrated on the inside. The net result is that the interior of the cell is negatively charged compared to the exterior; generally, inactive mammalian neurons exhibit a "resting" membrane potential of –60 to –75 mV. An externally applied electric field will stimulate the peripheral nerve cell axon resulting in one or more action potentials if the induced membrane depolarisation is above a threshold value sufficient for the opening of the voltage gated sodium channels to become self-sustaining. For many nerve axons, the action potential threshold is around –50 mV to –55 mV, some 10–15 mV above the "resting" potential.

Electrical stimulation of myelinated nerve fibres can be modelled using electrical cable theory applied to the membrane conductance changes originally described by Hodgkin and Huxley (1952) and Frankenhaeuser and Huxley (1964). Reilly, Freeman & Larkin (1985) proposed a spatially extended nonlinear nodal (SENN) model for myelinated nerve fibres that has been used to derive thresholds for various applied electrical fields and currents. Minimum, orientation-dependent stimulus thresholds for large diameter myelinated nerve axons were estimated to lie around 6 V m$^{-1}$ (Reilly, 1998b), which equates to a current density of about 1.2 A m$^{-2}$ assuming a tissue conductivity of 0.2 S m$^{-1}$. Electric field thresholds were estimated to be larger for smaller diameter neurons. Note however that passive cable theory does not apply to neuronal dendrites in the CNS (e.g. Takagi, 2000).

### 4.4.4    Neural networks and signal detection

The previous section described estimates of thresholds for stimulating individual nerve fibres. The nervous system itself, however, comprises a network of interacting nerve cells, communicating with each other principally via chemical "junctions" or synapses in which neurotransmitter released by the pre-synaptic terminal binds to specific receptor molecules on the post-synaptic cell, usually in a one-way process. The activation of receptors by the neurotransmitter may then cause a variety of post-synaptic responses, many of which result in an alteration of the probability that a particular type of ion channel will open. Such neural networks are thought to have complex non-linear dynamics that can be very sensitive to small voltages applied diffusely across the elements of the network (e.g. Saunders, 2003). The sensitivity of N interacting neuronal units increases theoretically in proportion to $\sqrt{N}$ (Barnes, 1992). Essentially, the signal-to-noise ratio improves if the noise is added randomly, but the signals are added coherently.

The theoretical basis for neural network sensitivity has been explored by Adair, Astumian & Weaver (1998) and Adair (2001), considering the detection of weak electric fields by sharks, and other elasmobranchs. These fish are known to be able to respond behaviorally to electric fields in seawater as low as 0.5 μV m$^{-1}$ that generate small electrical potentials, of the order of 200 nV, in the "detector" cells of the ampullae of Lorenzini. Adair (2001) suggests that such a weak signal would generate a signal-to-noise ratio greater than 1 within 100 ms with the convergence of approximately 5000 sensory detector cells onto a secondary neuron that exhibits coincidence detection, a property of certain types of neurotransmitter receptor (Hille, 2001).

Such convergence is a common property of sensory systems; evolutionary pressure exists to maximise the sensitivity with which environmental stimuli can be detected. In the peripherey of the mammalian retina, for example, up to 1000 rods converge on one ganglion (retinal output) cell (Taylor & Smith, 2004). In addition, brain function depends on the collective activity of very large numbers of interacting neurons. EMF effects on nervous system function and behaviour are described in Chapter 5. However, a lower limit on neural network sensitivity in humans has been estimated to lie around 1 mV m$^{-1}$ (Adair, Astumian & Weaver, 1998); a similar value of a lower limit was agreed at an ICNIRP/WHO workshop on weak electric field sensitivity held in 2003 (McKinlay & Repacholi, 2003). Modelling of the human phosphene response and neurphysiological studies of brain tissue function suggest such thresholds are more likely to lie in the 10–100 mV m$^{-1}$ region (see section 5.2.3).

### 4.4.5 Transients

The current induced by both electric and magnetic fields is directly proportional to the frequency. Thus, a higher frequency could result in an improved signal-to-noise ratio. Induced current effects are plausible from continuous high-frequency signals. Fields produced by power systems have no significant continuous higher frequency component. They can, however, contain transients, that is, short-lasting components of higher frequency. Because they are short-lasting rather than continuous, different considerations apply. Adair (1991) analysed the effect of short-term pulses from a consideration of momentum transfer to various entities. The external pulse is modelled as the sum of exponential rise and fall terms and this is used to calculate the frequency and amplitude components of the corresponding internal pulse. The momentum transferred by the pulse is compared with the thermal momentum for representative ions, molecules, and cells. For an external electric-field pulse of 100 kV m$^{-1}$ the effect of the pulse is small compared to thermal motion.

### 4.4.6 Heating effects of induced currents

The current induced by an electric or magnetic field produces heating in the tissues through which it passes. From a knowledge of the resistivities of the various components of tissue and of cells it is possible to calculate the heat produced. Combined with knowledge of tissue thermal conductivities and of the effect of circulation, it is then possible to calculate the temperature rise.

Kotnik & Miklavcic (2000) calculated power dissipation in various portions of cells, including the membrane. They do not calculate corresponding temperature rises, which are expected to be small.

### 4.4.7 Summary on induced currents

Comparisons have been made between the signal produced by external fields and various noise levels or levels of established effects, as shown in Table 32.

Essentially, the effects of weak fields on synapses can only be detected as a biologically meaningful signal through some sort of neural network showing convergence. This characterizes sensory systems like the ampullae of Lorenzini of the sharks, and the periphery of the retina, which have evolved to detect weak signals.

Complex neural circuits exist within the rest of the brain (see Shepherd & Koch, 1998 for a review); the extent to which these might show sensitivity to electric fields induced by EMF exposure is discussed in Chapter 5.

Table 32. Comparison between the signal produced by external fields and various of in situ electric field noise levels or nervous system effect thresholds

| Comparison | | In situ electric field (mV m⁻¹) | Corresponding external electric field (V m⁻¹) [a] | Corresponding external magnetic field [b] |
|---|---|---|---|---|
| Thermal noise | Volume of cell | 20 | $10^4$ | 600 µT |
| | Complete membrane | 200 | $10^5$ | 5 mT |
| | Element of membrane | 1000 | $10^9$ | 40 T |
| Shot noise | Typical cell | 100 | $5\times10^4$ | 3 mT |
| | Optimised cell | 10 | 5000 | 300 µT |
| 1/f noise | | | $1\times10^5$ | 10 mT |
| Myelinated nerve stimulation threshold (SENN) | | 5000 | | |
| Phosphene threshold (dosimetric calculation) | | 10–100 | | |
| Estimated lower limit for neural network threshold | | 1 | | |

[a] Source: Dimbylow, 2000.
[b] Source: Dimbylow, 1998.

Essentially, the effects of weak fields on synapses can only be detected as a biologically meaningful signal through some sort of neural network showing convergence. This characterizes sensory systems like the ampullae of Lorenzini of the sharks, and the periphery of the retina, which have evolved to detect weak signals.

Complex neural circuits exist within the rest of the brain (see Shepherd & Koch, 1998 for a review); the extent to which these might show sensitivity to electric fields induced by EMF exposure is discussed in Chapter 5.

## 4.5    Other direct effects of fields

### 4.5.1    Ionization and breaking of bonds

The bonds that hold molecules together can be broken by delivering sufficient energy to them. Electromagnetic radiation is quantised, and the energy of each quantum is given by Plank's constant, h, multiplied by the frequency. The energy required to break various bonds that are found in biological systems has been quantified, e.g. by Valberg, Kavet & Rafferty (1997). Typical covalent bonds require 1–10 electronvolt (eV), and typical hydrogen bonds require 0.1 eV. The quantum energy of 50 Hz radiation is

$10^{-12}$ eV. Thus a single quantum of 50 or 60-Hz radiation clearly does not have adequate energy to break bonds. The quantum energy becomes comparable to the energy of covalent bonds at around the frequencies of visible light.

Vistnes & Gjotterud (2001) have pointed out that the wavelength at 50 Hz, 6000 km, is so much larger than the distance scales of the interactions being considered in the body that it is inappropriate to consider single-quantum events. They calculate that in the human body in a 10 kV m$^{-1}$ field, far from a situation of single photons, there are in fact of order $10^{34}$ "overlapping" photons present within the volume that a single photon can be said to occupy. It is still correct to say that chemical bonds cannot be broken by absorption of a single photon, but it would not be correct to use that to rule out any other possible effects of EMFs.

As an alternative to transfer of energy to a bond by quantum energy, fields might transfer sufficient energy to break a bond by accelerating a charged particle and thereby imparting energy to it. The "noise" here is the thermal kinetic energy of the particle, determined from fundamental thermodynamics, and is about 0.04 eV for room or body temperature. If the maximum distance over which a particle can be accelerated is assumed to be limited to 20 μm, the dimension of a typical cell, the fields required to impart equal energy to this thermal energy are of order $10^9$ V m$^{-1}$ and 1 μT. In practice the maximum distance would be even shorter and hence the required field even higher.

### 4.5.2 *Forces on charged particles*

Both electric and magnetic fields exert forces on charged particles. The force exerted by an electric field on a charge q is $F=qE$, directed in the same direction as the field. The force exerted by a magnetic field appears only on a moving charge and is $F=vqB$, directed perpendicularly to both velocity v and field $B$.

These forces can be compared to those required to produce various effects in biological systems (Valberg, Kavet & Rafferty, 1997). These range (to the nearest order of magnitude) from 1 picoNewton (pN) to activate a single hair cell in the inner ear, through 10 pN to open a mechanoreceptor transmembrane ion channel, to 100 pN which equals the force binding a ligand molecule to a protein receptor.

To produce 1 pN would require an external electric field (in air) in the order of $10^{10}$ V m$^{-1}$ (assuming a molecule with 10 charges located in a cell membrane); or a field of 10 μT (the Lorentz force acting on the same molecule moving with average thermal velocity is less than the force due to the induced electric field).

### 4.5.3 *Forces on magnetic particles*

A magnetic field will exert a turning force (a moment or torque) on any entity that has a magnetic moment. If ferromagnetic crystals existed in the body, they could have a magnetic moment, and hence the field could exert an oscillating moment on them and cause them to vibrate.

The size of the turning force is determined by the size of the field and the size of the magnetic moment. One magnetic material which is known to exist in some biological systems is magnetite. If it is assumed that a particle of magnetite exists where all its individual magnetic domains are aligned, the magnetic moment of the particle is the saturation magnetization of magnetite multiplied by the volume. Thus the maximum turning force exerted on the particle is proportional to its volume. If the magnetic field were a static field, the particle would rotate until either restoring forces equalled the turning force, or it was aligned with the field. With an alternating field, however, the amplitude of oscillation is determined by the viscosity of the surrounding medium as well.

In this instance, the "signal" produced by the field, an amplitude of oscillation at the power frequency, has to be compared to the "noise", the amplitude of oscillation of the same particle produced randomly by thermal noise (i.e. Brownian motion). Adair (1994) has calculated that, for a single-domain magnetite particle of diameter 0.2 $\mu$m, and a viscosity of the surrounding medium of seven times water, both of which are regarded as extreme assumptions, the "signal" becomes equal to the "noise" for a field of 5 $\mu$T. If alternative assumptions are made, equivalent field values can be calculated, given that the effect is proportional to the diameter of the particle cubed and to the field squared. More plausible choices of the particle size and viscosity lead to an equivalence between noise and signal levels at higher fields.

It is known that some animals use magnetite to detect small changes in the earth's static magnetic field, for navigation purposes (ICNIRP, 2003). For example, certain bee species have been shown to detect a change in static field of 26 nT (Kirschvink & Kirschvink, 1991; Walker & Bitterman, 1985). This appears to be achieved by means of magnetite particles, in air, attached to large numbers of sensory hairs. Signal discrimination by the nervous system dramatically improves the signal-to-noise ratio, and such sensitivity is plausible without requiring a signal-to-noise ratio more than one.

Kirschvink et al. (1992) describe the existence of trace levels of magnetite in the human brain and other tissues, and postulate that such crystals might act as transducers, opening mechanically sensitive transmembrane ion channels in hypothesised "receptor" neurons within the central nervous system. Such a "detector" would be subject to the constraints described above. However, attempts to confirm that humans can use the geomagnetic field for orientation and direction-finding have so far failed (ICNIRP, 2003). These authors concluded that the presence of magnetite crystals in the human brain does not confer an ability to detect the weak geomagnetic field, although some mechanisms of magnetic sensitivity remain to be explored (Kirschvink, 1997). Interestingly, Scaiano, Monahan & Renaud (2006) note that magnetite particles can dramatically effect the way in which external magnetic fields affect radical pair interactions.

### 4.5.4    Free radicals

The radical pair mechanism is the only generally accepted way in which static and ELF magnetic fields can affect the chemistry of individual molecules (e.g. see Brocklehurst & McLauchlan, 1996; Eveson et al., 2000; Grissom, 1995; Hore, 2005; McLauchlan, 1992; Steiner & Ulrich, 1989). This involves a specific type of chemical reaction: the recombination of a pair of short-lived, reactive free radicals generated either from a single molecule or from two molecules by intermolecular electron or hydrogen atom transfer. The effect of an applied magnetic field depends upon its interaction with the spin of unpaired electrons of the radicals. Importantly, this effect may constitute a mechanism for the biological effects of very weak fields (Adair, 1999; Timmel et al., 1998). Field-sensitivity occurs over the period of radical pair formation and recombination, typically tens of nanoseconds in normal solutions, but possibly extended to a few microseconds in micelles (Eveson et al., 2000) or other biological structures. Power frequency magnetic fields are essentially static over these short time intervals, an equivalence that was confirmed experimentally by Scaiano et al. (1994) and that may extend up to frequencies of a few MHz (Adair, 1999).

Free radicals are a chemical species formed during many metabolic processes and thought to contribute to various disease states such as neurodegenerative disease (see Chapter 7). During normal metabolism, for example, oxygen is reduced to $H_2O$ in mitochondria during energy production by oxidative phosphorylation. This involves the sequential addition of four electrons, producing intermediate reactive oxygen species such as the superoxide anion radical ($O_2^{-}$), hydrogen peroxide ($H_2O_2$) and the hydroxyl radical ($OH\cdot$). Most cells contain a variety of radical scavengers such as glutathione peroxidase that provide anti-oxidant defence mechanisms. If these are depleted, for example from exposure to an agent such as long wavelength ultraviolet radiation (UVA) that generates excess reactive oxygen species, tissue damage may ensue (AGNIR, 2002).

Free radicals can also be formed by the homolytic scission of a covalent bond. Most biological molecules exist in a low energy, singlet state in which the angular momentum of a molecule containing pairs of electrons is zero because the spins of electron pairs are antiparallel (reviewed by e.g. Brocklehurst & McLauchlan, 1996; Eveson et al., 2000; McLauchlan, 1992; Timmel et al., 1998). The scission of a covalent bond in such a molecule can result in the formation of two geminate radicals, each bearing an unpaired electron with a spin anti-parallel to the other. The energy released by the reaction causes the free radicals to separate rapidly so that relatively little instantaneous reaction ensues. Subsequently, the magnetic interactions (hyperfine couplings) of the electron spins with the nuclei of nearby hydrogen and nitrogen atoms modify the spin state of the radical pair, giving it some triplet character (Zeeman effect). For applied magnetic fields typically greater than 1–2 mT, the probability of reaction during a re-encounter of the radicals is increased, with a concomitant decrease in the number of free radicals that escape recombination and diffuse into the surrounding medium.

Conversely, in magnetic fields of less than ~1 mT, the free radical concentration is increased with possibly harmful effects. Experimental evidence for such effects in biochemical systems has been recently reported by Hore, McLauchlan and colleagues (e.g. Eveson et al., 2000; Liu et al., 2005). In contrast, effects on the recombination of randomly diffusing radicals with uncorrelated spins that encounter by chance are thought to be negligible (Brocklehurst & McLauchlan, 1996).

Hore (2005) notes that more than 60 enzymes use radicals or other paramagnetic molecules as reaction intermediates, although most do not involve radical pairs with correlated electron spins. The maximum size of an effect of a field of less than ~1 mT on a wide variety of geminate radical pairs has been calculated by Timmel et al. (1998). It was found that a weak field, even one comparable to the geomagnetic field, could alter the yield of any free radical recombination by 15–30%. This depended however, on the radical pair existing in close proximity for a sufficiently long time for the applied field to have an effect. Durations of the order of 100–1000 ns have been suggested as necessary (e.g. Brocklehurst & McLauchlan, 1996; Timmel et al., 1998) but these might only exist where some form of physical constraint applied, such as within a membrane for example, or bound to an enzyme. In addition, theoretical calculation and experimental investigation indicate that variation of the magnitude of these effects with magnetic field intensity is highly non-linear (Brocklehurst & McLauchlan, 1996; Grissom, 1995; Hore, 2005; Timmel et al., 1998).

The biological significance of these types of effects is not clear at present. They have been suggested (Cintolesi et al., 2003; Ritz, Adem & Schulten, 2000; Schulten, 1982) as a mechanism by which animals, particularly birds, may use the Earth's magnetic field as a source of navigational information during migration and there is some experimental support for this view (Ritz et al., 2004). The Earth's magnetic field is ~50 µT, varying from about 30 µT near the equator to about 60 µT at the poles. Apart from this rather specialised instance however, since static and ELF magnetic fields are equivalent in their interactions, Scaiano et al. (1994) and Adair (1999) suggest that power frequency fields of much less than around 50 µT are unlikely to be of much biological significance. Several specific requirements have to be fulfilled for small, but significant modifications to the recombination rate at 50 µT and these conditions are sufficiently special to be considered unlikely (Adair, 1999). Liu et al. (2005) note that, given the efficiency of homeostatic buffering processes such as the radical scavenging mechanisms described above, there does not appear to be a strong likelihood of physiologically significant changes in cellular functions or of long term mutagenic effects resulting from low magnetic field-induced variations in free radical concentrations or fluxes. In addition, processes such as modulation of anisotropic magnetic interactions by radical tumbling may set a lower bound on the detection of this low field effect.

### 4.5.5  Effects with narrow bandwidths

When comparing the signal to the noise, the comparison must be with the noise over the correct frequency range. If a postulated mechanism is sensitive only to a narrow range of frequencies, the noise must be assessed over that same range, which will in general be less than over a wider range of frequencies. A number of mechanisms have been proposed which achieve this narrow bandwidth, usually by some form of resonance condition involving the static field.

#### 4.5.5.1  Cyclotron resonance

A moving charged particle in a magnetic field will perform circular orbits (if left undisturbed for sufficiently long) with a frequency determined by the charge q, the field $B$ and the mass m, the frequency being $Bq/m$. An AC field at the same frequency could then interact in a resonant fashion. However, to produce cyclotron resonance of a biologically relevant particle such as a calcium ion at power frequencies requires unconstrained orbits of order 1 m diameter lasting several cycles, whereas molecular collisions (i.e. damping) occur which would destroy the orbit and the resonance on timescales of $10^{-12}$ s.

#### 4.5.5.2  Larmor precession

A charged particle vibrating in a magnetic field will have its direction of vibration rotated about the field at the Larmor frequency, which is half the cyclotron frequency. If the field itself is modulated at this frequency, the particle will vibrate for longer in certain directions than others, with the potential for altering reaction probabilities (Edmonds, 1993). This mechanism again requires the vibration to continue unperturbed by other factors for an implausible length of time.

#### 4.5.5.3  Quantum mechanical resonance phenomena

A number of quantum mechanical phenomena have been suggested to explain biological observations involving low levels of exposure. Among these, one particular phenomenon has been investigated in some detail, ion parametric resonance, whereby the DC field creates various sublevels of a vibrating ion, and the AC field then causes transitions between them. It predicts effects at the cyclotron resonance frequency and integral fractions of it (Blanchard & Blackman, 1994; Lednev, 1991; Lednev, 1993; Lednev, 1994).

The mechanism has been extensively investigated, with the conclusion that it is not plausible. It requires unfeasibly narrow vibrational energy levels, a fixed phase relationship between the vibrational states and the externally applied field, and implausible symmetry of the binding of the ion (Adair, 1992; 1998).

### 4.5.6    Stochastic resonance

Stochastic resonance is the phenomenon whereby random noise, added to an oscillating, non-linear system, can produce responses which are not seen in the absence of the noise. Under some circumstances it is possible for the addition of noise to a system to produce a dramatic change in the response. However, this applies primarily to the addition of small amounts of noise to a larger signal. It is relevant, for example, when considering the exact threshold for shot noise, and is included in those calculations; but it cannot explain a response to small signals in the presence of a larger noise (Adair, 1996; Weaver & Vaughan, 1998).

## 4.6    Indirect effects of fields

### 4.6.1    Surface charge and microshocks

In a power-frequency electric field, a charge is induced on the surface of a body. If the field is large enough (see section 5.2.1) this can be perceived through the vibration of hairs.

In an electric field, different objects acquire different potentials, depending on whether they are grounded or not. A person touching a conducting object, where one is grounded and the other is not, experiences a microshock or small spark discharge (see section 5.2.1). This can be painful and can lead to burns to the skin in extreme circumstances.

### 4.6.2    Contact currents

When a person simultaneously contacts two conductive objects that are at different electrical potential, that person will conduct a contact current whose magnitude is inversely proportional to the electrical resistance between those two points. A fraction of the pathway's resistance is that which exists between the object's points of contact and the subdermal layers. This fraction is high for a dry fingertip contact and much lower for a wet full-handed grip (large surface area shorted by the moisture across the outer dermal layer). Body resistance exclusive of the skin contact points is much less variable, but depends on body dimensions, fat-to-muscle content, etc.

Kavet and colleagues have identified a child in a bathtub as the most likely scenario for exposure to contact current and have suggested that the electric field induced in the bone marrow of children so exposed might offer a plausible interaction mechanism underlying the increased risk of childhood leukaemia (see section 11.4.2) associated with magnetic field exposure (Kavet et al., 2004; Kavet, 2005; Kavet & Zaffanella, 2002). When bathing, young children frequently engage in exploratory behaviours that include contact with the faucet handle, the spout, or the water stream itself. In residential electrical systems in which a home's water line is connected to the electrical service neutral, a small voltage (usually less than a volt) can appear between the water line, and thus the water fixtures, and earth. If the tub's drain is conductive and sunk into the earth, a child can complete the circuit by touching the water fixtures or water stream. Because both ends of the contact are wet, body resistance is minimised (to perhaps 1–2 kiloohm [k$\Omega$]).

The voltage on the water line may arise from either return current in the grounding system producing an ohmic voltage difference between the water line and earth, or as a result of Faraday induction on the neutral/grounding system, or from both. Measurement studies in the USA indicated that the closed circuit voltage (i.e., with a 1 kΩ resistor replacing a person) from the water line to the drain may exceed 100 mV in a small percentage of homes (~ 4%) (Kavet et al., 2004). Under such conditions roughly 50 µA could enter a child's hand. Dosimetric modelling by Dawson, Potter & Stuchly (2001) estimated that a 50 µA exposure would produce about 650 mV m$^{-1}$ or more in 5% of the marrow in the lower arm of an 18 kg child (normal weight for a 4-year old). Smaller (i.e. younger) children would experience larger internal fields. Chiu & Stuchly (2005) computed that a local field of 1 V m$^{-1}$ could produce 0.2 mV across the gap junctional apparatus connecting two bone marrow stromal cells; these are the cells that orchestrate hematopoiesis that includes lymphocyte precursor cellular proliferation (LeBien, 2000). For the scenario described above, Chiu & Stuchly's (2005) values would scale to 0.13 mV across the gap junction. Bulk tissue fields and transmembrane potentials of these magnitudes constitute signals that exceed competing noise.

There is at present, however, no biological evidence indicating that such fields and currents within bone marrow are either carcinogenic or stimulate the proliferation of initiated cells. Nor is there any epidemiological evidence linking contact current in children to the risk of childhood leukaemia. However, measurement studies (Kavet et al., 2004; Kavet & Zaffanella, 2002) together with computer modelling of typical US neighborhoods (Kavet, 2005) indicate that, across a geographic region characteristic of a population-based epidemiology study, residential magnetic fields are very likely to be positively associated with the source voltage for contact current exposure. These results offer support to this proposed hypothesis.

To date engineering research concerning contact currents has focused largely on electrical systems characteristic of the USA. Some countries in which ELF epidemiology has been conducted have electrical systems with multiple ground points (e.g. the UK; see Rauch et al., 1992) that include the water supply. Others without explicit connections may very well have inadvertent water-line-to-earth voltages, primarily via the water heater connection.

### 4.6.3    Deflection of cosmic rays

Cosmic rays are produced by the sun, in space, and in the atmosphere, and are known to be able to cause harm to humans through energy deposition in biological tissue. Hopwood (1992) suggested that both electric and magnetic fields from power lines could deflect cosmic rays which pass close to the power lines in such a way as to produce a focussing effect close to the power line. Hopwood reported measuring a doubling of sky particle count a few metres to the side of a power line, though subsequent more sophisticated measurements have failed to show any increase (Burgess & Clark, 1994). Simple analytical calculations suggest the deflections are likely to be of the order of only centimetres, and then only for those particles which pass very close to the conductors. Skedsmo & Vistnes (2000) have performed sophisticated numerical modelling, and showed that even for low energy electrons (the particles most susceptible to deflection) the difference in particle flux density under and to the sides of the line is less than 0.15%, and for all particles combined it is less than 0.01%. Such differences are too small to be relevant for health effects.

### 4.6.4 Effects on airborne pollutants

A category of mechanisms has been suggested (Fews et al., 1999b; Fews et al., 1999a; Fews et al., 2002; Henshaw et al., 1996a; Henshaw et al., 1996b) where the electric fields produced by overhead power lines interact with airborne pollutant particles in such a way as to increase the harmful effects of these particles on the body.

Airborne particles having the greatest effects on health include tobacco smoke, radon decay products, chemical pollutants, spores, bacteria and viruses (AGNIR, 2004). If inhaled, some become deposited in the airways of the respiratory system. Others can be deposited on the skin. Since charged particles are more likely than uncharged particles to be deposited when close to the walls of the respiratory airways or to the skin, an increase in the proportion of particles that are charged could lead to an increase in adverse health effects. Fews et al. (1999b) suggested that such an increase could arise from the generation of corona ions by power lines. These positive or negative ions arise when electrical potentials of a few thousand volts or greater cause electrical breakdown of the air by corona discharges. A further increase in the deposition of charged particles could arise due to an increase in the probability of their impact with surfaces of the skin and respiratory airways in the presence of electric fields (Henshaw et al., 1996b).

#### 4.6.4.1 Production of corona ions

As a consequence of corona discharges, high voltage AC power lines may produce clouds of negative or positive ions that are readily blown downwind (AGNIR, 2004). Negative ions are more often produced, especially in fog or misty conditions. Although high voltage AC transmission lines are designed to operate without generating corona discharges, small local intensifications of the conductor surface electric field can occur at dust and dirt accumulations, or at water drops, sometimes causing corona discharges to occur. In addition, some high voltage lines are operated above their original design voltage and can be more prone to corona discharge in adverse weather conditions. An increase of charge density downwind of power lines can often be observed at distances up to several kilometres (Fews et al., 1999a; Fews et al., 2002; Swanson & Jeffers, 1999; Swanson & Jeffers, personal communication in AGNIR, 2004). However, recently, Bracken Senior & Bailey (2005) have reported measurements carried out over two years of DC electric fields and ion concentrations upwind and downwind of 230-kV and 345-kV transmission lines at two sites. They found some evidence of an excess downwind, but the downwind values only exceeded the range of upwind (ambient) values for a small percentage of the time under most conditions.

The ion clouds charge particles that pass through them. These particles will already carry some charge because of the naturally occurring ions that exist in the atmosphere, but it seems likely that in some regions this will be increased even at ground level as a result of corona discharge. Calculating this increase as a function of particle size is possible but only if a number of simplifying assumptions are made. The effects indoors, where the majority of people spend most of their time, are likely to be less than outdoors, for example because of deposition of corona ions on the surfaces of small apertures through which some air enters buildings.

### 4.6.4.2 Inhalation of pollutant particles

People may be exposed to these more highly charged pollutant particles and the possibility that electrostatic charge could increase their respiratory tract deposition has been recognised for some time (AGNIR, 2004). In principle, the effect could be significant and AGNIR (2004) estimated that in the size range of about 0.1–1 μm, where lung deposition is normally low (about 10%) there is potential to increase lung deposition by up to a theoretical maximum factor of about 3–10, depending on particle size. The actual increase will depend on the number of charges and particle size, though neither experimental results nor theory currently allow reliable predictions. Nevertheless, experimental and theoretical studies indicate that increased deposition should be very small for particles larger than about 0.3 μm because of the high charge per particle needed to produce a significant effect. For smaller particles, the effect of charge on deposition of a pollutant within the lungs will be appreciably less than the theoretical maximum for various reasons. Indeed, for the smallest (less than about 10 nm diameter) particles, charge may even decrease the probability of deposition in the lungs since a higher proportion will be deposited in the upper airways.

The effect of exposure on individuals will be lower still because of their "occupancy" factor: the fraction of the time to which they are exposed to particles charged by corona ions. One estimate, Henshaw and Fews (personal communication in AGNIR, 2004), is that people downwind of power lines in corona might have 20–60% more particles deposited in their lungs than those upwind. This estimate is for people exposed out of doors to pollutant particles which originate out of doors. When outdoor air enters houses, many of the pollutant particles will be carried with it (Liu & Nazaroff, 2003), so a similar but smaller effect would be expected indoors due to the deposition of some of the pollutant particles on the surfaces of small apertures. The effects of corona ions on lung deposition of particles which originate indoors will be substantially less. There are substantial difficulties in the way of modelling such effects, making all such estimates very uncertain. Furthermore, since wind directions vary, the excess for any one group of people would be lower, but more groups will be affected, than if the wind direction was constant.

### 4.6.4.3 Deposition under power lines

Particles which are electrically charged oscillate with a frequency of 50 Hz along the electric fields produced by the power lines. The distance over which a particle oscillates depends on its charge and inertia, and the strength of the field which is usually greatest immediately underneath the line. However field directions and strengths can be altered by objects in the field and are, for example, normally perpendicular to a conducting object such as a human body. Field strengths are particularly high around pointed conductors. If the oscillation of a particle makes it hit a surface, it will generally stick.

The oscillation of particles in the electric field causes people underneath or near power lines in the open air to have increased numbers of such particles deposited on their clothing and skin compared with the numbers deposited away from the line. Because buildings and other objects screen out the electric field, power lines do not cause increased deposition indoors. Henshaw et al. (1996a; 1996b) considered whether such electric fields could cause increased deposition within the respiratory tract. They calculated that the field is a factor of $10^4$ lower inside the body than outside, but nevertheless suggested that this might have an effect on unattached radon decay products. Stather et al. (1996) pointed out that the unattached decay products mainly deposit in the upper airways, so any increase in internal deposition would probably reduce lung deposition.

With regard to deposition of airborne particles on the skin, AGNIR (2004) concluded that it is likely that there will be a small increase downwind of power lines caused by corona discharge. The increase will be mainly of small particles and so any adverse health effects are likely to come from increased surface activity from radon decay products rather than surface effects from chemical pollutants. The change in surface deposition of radon decay products on skin is also very sensitive to the electrostatic charge on the skin and the wind speed over it. It seems likely that even downwind of power lines, these last two variations will be much larger than the increases from corona ions.

There is experimental evidence supported by theoretical analysis (Fews et al., 1999a) that the deposition of particles of sizes associated both with radon decay products and chemical pollutants are somewhat larger directly underneath power lines. The reported increase is ~ 2.4 for radon decay products and ~ 1.2 for chemical pollutants. The increased deposition is attributable to the increase in impact rate and therefore deposition rate of the naturally charged particles in the oscillating electric fields. The oscillation amplitude decreases rapidly with the mass of the particle. Since the mass of chemical pollutants is mostly associated with larger particles, the increased deposition of these would be insignificant in still air. Fews et al. (Fews et al., 1999a) calculate, however, that this is not the case when the air flow is turbulent.

Swanson & Jeffers (personal communication in AGNIR, 2004) agreed that increased deposition of radon decay products will occur under power lines. However they attribute the increased deposition observed of larger particles, and therefore the likely increased deposition of chemical pollutants, to the design of the experiments. They also attribute the theoretically predicted increased deposition of larger particles to the specific parametric values and analytical expressions used by Fews et al. (1999a).

The extent of skin deposition under power lines cannot be determined without further experimental measurements. It is possible that the differences in the theoretical analysis might be reduced by further work. However the physical situation is very complicated and it seems unlikely that it can be modelled with sufficient accuracy to provide reliable information in the foreseeable future.

### 4.6.4.4  Implications for health

The main health hazards of airborne particulate pollutants are cardio-respiratory disease and lung cancer (AGNIR, 2004). There is strong evidence that the risk of cardio-respiratory disease is increased by inhalation of particles generated outdoors, mainly from motor vehicle exhaust, and of environmental tobacco smoke produced within buildings. The risk of lung cancer is increased by particulate pollution in outdoor air, and by radon decay products and environmental tobacco smoke in buildings. Any health risks from the deposition of environmental particulate air pollutants on the skin appear to be negligible.

In their recent review, AGNIR (2004) conclude that the potential impact of corona ions on health will depend on the extent to which they increase the dose of relevant pollutants to target tissues in the body. It was not possible to estimate the impact precisely, because of uncertainties about: a) the extent to which corona effects increase the charge on particles of different sizes, particularly within buildings; b) the exact impact of this charging on the deposition of particles in the lungs and other parts of the respiratory tract; and c) the dose-response relation for adverse health outcomes in relation to different size fractions of particle. However, it seemed unlikely that corona ions would have more than a small effect on the long-term health risks associated with particulate air pollutants, even in the individuals who are most affected. In public health terms, AGNIR conclude that the proportionate impact will be even lower because only a small fraction of the general population live or work close to sources of corona ions.

## 4.7    Conclusions

Various proposed direct and indirect interaction mechanisms for ELF electric and magnetic fields are examined for plausibility, in particular whether a "signal" generated in a biological process by exposure to electric or magnetic fields can be discriminated from inherent random noise and whether the mechanism challenges scientific principles and current scientific knowledge. Many mechanisms become plausible only at fields above a certain strength. Nevertheless, the lack of identified plausible mechanisms does not rule out the possibility of health effects existing even at very low field levels providing the basic scientific principles are adhered to.

Of the numerous suggested mechanisms proposed for the direct interaction of fields with the human body, three stand out as potentially operating at lower field levels than the others: induced electric fields in neural networks, radical pairs, and magnetite.

Electric fields induced in tissue by exposure to ELF electric and magnetic fields will directly stimulate myelinated nerve fibres in a biophysically plausible manner when the internal electric field strength exceeds a few volts per metre. Much weaker fields can affect synaptic transmission in neural networks as opposed to single cells. Such signal processing by nervous systems is commonly used by multicellular organisms to discriminate weak environmental signals. A lower bound of 1 mV m$^{-1}$ on neural network discrimination was suggested, but based on current evidence threshold values around 10-100 mV m$^{-1}$ seem more likely.

The radical pair mechanism is an accepted way in which magnetic fields can affect specific types of chemical reactions, generally increasing reactive free radical concentration in low fields and decreasing them in high fields. These increases have been seen at less than 1 mT. There is some evidence linking this mechanism to navigation during bird migration. Both on theoretical grounds, and because the changes produced by ELF and static magnetic fields are similar, it is suggested that power frequency fields of much less than the geomagnetic field of around 50 μT are unlikely to be of much biological significance.

Magnetite crystals, small ferromagnetic crystals of various forms of iron oxide are found in animal and human tissues, although in trace amounts. Like free radicals, they have been linked to orientation and navigation in migratory animals, although the presence of trace quantities of magnetite in the human brain does not confer an ability to detect the weak geomagnetic field. Calculations based on extreme assumptions suggest a lower bound for the effects on magnetite crystals of ELF fields of 5 μT.

Other direct biophysical interactions of fields, such as the breaking of chemical bonds, forces on charged particles and the various narrow bandwidth "resonance" mechanisms, are not considered to provide plausible explanations for the interactions at field levels encountered in public and occupational environments.

With regard to indirect effects, the surface electric charge induced by exposure to ELF electric fields can be perceived and it can result in painful microshocks when touching a conductive object. Contact currents can occur when young children touch, for example, a tap in a bathtub in some homes. This produces small electric fields, possibly above background noise levels, in bone marrow. However, whether these present a risk to health is unknown.

High voltage power lines produce clouds of electrically charged ions as a consequence of corona discharge. It is suggested that they could increase the deposition of airborne pollutants on the skin and on airways inside the body, possibly adversely affecting health. However, it seems unlikely that corona ions will have more than a small effect, if any, on long-term health risks, even in the individuals who are most exposed.

None of the three direct mechanisms considered above seem plausible causes of increased disease incidence at the exposure levels generally encountered by people. In fact they only become plausible at levels orders of magnitude higher and indirect mechanisms have not yet been sufficiently investigated. This absence of an identified plausible mechanism does not rule out the possibility of adverse health effects, but it does increase the need for stronger evidence from biology and epidemiology.

# 5       NEUROBEHAVIOUR

Neurobehavioural studies encompass the effects of exposure to ELF electromagnetic fields on the nervous system and its responses at different levels of organization. These include the direct stimulation of peripheral and central nerve tissue, perceptual effects resulting from sensory stimulation, and effects on central nervous system function. Effects on the latter can be assessed both electrophysiologically by recording the electrical activity of the brain, and by tests of cognition, assessment of mood, and other studies.

The nervous system also has a central role in the control of other body systems, particularly the cardiovascular system, through direct nervous control, and the endocrine system, through neural input into the pineal and pituitary glands. These glands in turn influence reproduction and development, and in a more general way, physiology and well-being.

The brain and nervous systems function by using electrical signals, and may therefore be considered particularly vulnerable to low frequency EMFs and the resultant induced electric fields and currents. Substantial numbers of laboratory experiments with volunteers and animals have investigated the possible consequences of exposure to weak EMFs on various aspects of nervous system function, including cognitive, behavioural and neuroendocrine responses. In addition, epidemiological studies have been carried out on the relationship between EMF exposure and both suicide and depression.

These studies have been reviewed by NRC (1997), NIEHS (1998), IARC (2002), ICNIRP (2003) and McKinlay et al. (2004). In particular, ICNIRP (2003) reviewed in detail some of the evidence summarized here.

In general, there are few effects for which the evidence is strong, and even the more robust field-induced responses seen in the laboratory studies tend to be small in magnitude, subtle and transitory in nature (Crasson et al., 1999; Sienkiewicz et al., 1993).

## 5.1       Electrophysiological considerations

An examination of the electrophysiological properties of the nervous system, particularly the central nervous system (CNS: brain and spinal cord) gives an indication of its likely susceptibility to the electric fields induced in the body by EMF exposure. Ion channels in cell membranes allow passage of particular ionic species across the cell membrane in response to the opening of a "gate" which is sensitive to the transmembrane voltage (Catterall, 1995; Hille & Anderson, 2001; Mathie, Kennard & Veale, 2003). It is well established that electric fields induced in the body either by direct contact with external electrodes, or by exposure to low frequency magnetic fields, will, if of sufficient magnitude, excite nerve tissue through their interaction with these voltage-gated ion channels. Sensitivity is therefore primarily to the transmembrane electric field and varies widely between different ion channels (Hille & Anderson, 2001; Mathie, Kennard & Veale, 2003; Saunders & Jefferys, 2002). Many voltage-gated ion channels are associated with electrical excitability and electrical signalling. Such electrically excit-

118

able cells not only comprise neurons, glial and muscle cells, but also endocrine cells of the anterior pituitary, adrenal medulla and pancreas, gametes and, with reservations, endothelial cells (Hille & Anderson, 2001).

All these cells generally express voltage-gated sodium and calcium channels. Both of these ion channels are involved in electrical signaling and calcium ions activate a number of crucial cellular processes including neurotransmitter release, excitation-contraction coupling in muscle cells and gene expression (Catterall, 2000; Hille & Anderson, 2001). Some ion channels, for example voltage-gated potassium and chloride ion channels, also exist in other, non-excitable tissues such as those in the kidney and liver and show slow electric potential changes but their voltage sensitivity is likely to be lower (Begenisich & Melvin, 1998; Cahalan, Wulff & Chandy, 2001; Catterall, 2000; Jan & Jan, 1989; Nilius & Droogmans, 2001). Since voltage-gated ion channels in excitable cells are steeply sensitive to the transmembrane electric potential, electric field strength in tissue is a more relevant parameter to relate to electrically excitable cell thresholds than current density (Bailey et al., 1997; Blakemore & Trombley, 2003; Reilly, 2005; Sheppard, Kavet & Renew, 2002). In fact, the relevant parameter in determining the transmembrane current and hence the excitability is the linear gradient in electric field (Tranchina & Nicholson, 1986), which in turn relates to geometric parameters of the neuron, including the degree of bending of the axon.

Peripheral nerves comprise neurons whose cell bodies are located within the CNS with extended processes (axons) that lie outside the CNS. They conduct action potentials (impulses) towards (sensory nerves) or from (motor nerves) the spinal cord and nerve stimulation shows an all-or-nothing threshold behaviour. Excitation results from a membrane depolarisation of between 10–20 mV, corresponding to an electric field in tissue of 5–25 V m$^{-1}$ (McKinlay et al., 2004). Pulsed magnetic fields, where the rate of change of field induces large localised electric fields, can directly stimulate peripheral nerves and nerve fibres located within the brain (see below).

Cells of the central nervous system are considered to be sensitive to electric fields induced in the body by exposure to ELF magnetic fields at levels that are below threshold for impulse initiation in nerve axons (Jefferys, 1995; Jefferys et al., 2003; Saunders, 2003; Saunders & Jefferys, 2002). Such weak electric field interactions have been shown in experimental studies mostly using isolated animal brain tissue to have physiological relevance. These interactions result from the extracellular voltage gradients generated by the synchronous activity of a number of neurons, or from those generated by applying pulsed or alternating currents directly through electrodes placed on either side of the tissue. Jefferys and colleagues (Jefferys, 1995; Jefferys et al., 2003) identified in vitro electric field thresholds of around 4–5 V m$^{-1}$. Essentially, the extracellular gradient alters the potential difference across the neuronal membrane with opposite polarities at either end of the neuron; a time-constant of a few tens (15–60) of milliseconds results from the capacitance of the neuronal membrane (Jefferys et al., 2003) and indicates a limited frequency response. Similar arguments concerning the limited frequency response of weak electric field effects due to the long time-constants (25 ms) arising from cell membrane capacitance have been given by Reilly (2002) regarding phosphene data.

The CNS in vivo is likely to be more sensitive to induced low frequency electric fields and currents than are in vitro preparations (Saunders & Jefferys, 2002). Spontaneous activity is higher, and interacting groups or networks of nerve cells exposed to weak electrical signals would be expected, on theoretical grounds, to show increased sensitivity through improved signal-to-noise ratios compared with the response of individual cells (Adair, 2001; Stering, 1998; Valberg, Kavet & Rafferty, 1997). Much of normal cognitive function of the brain depends on the collective activity of very large numbers of neurons; neural networks are thought to have complex non-linear dynamics that can be very sensitive to small voltages applied diffusely across the elements of the network (Adair, 2001; ICNIRP, 2003; Jefferys et al., 2003). Gluckman et al. (2001) placed the detection limit for network modulation in hippocampal slices by electric fields at around 100 mV m$^{-1}$. Recent experimental work by Francis, Gluckman & Schiff (2003) confirms a neural network threshold of around 140 mV m$^{-1}$, which the authors found was lower than single neuron thresholds, based on a limited number of measurements. A lower limit on neural network sensitivity to physiologically weak induced electric fields has elsewhere been considered on theoretical grounds to be around 1 mV m$^{-1}$ (Adair, Astumian & Weaver, 1998; Veyret, 2003). The time-course of the opening of the fastest voltage-gated ion channels can be less than 1 ms (Hille & Anderson, 2001), suggesting that effects at frequencies up to a few kilohertz should not be ruled out. Accommodation to a slowly changing stimulus resulting from slow inactivation of the sodium channels will raise thresholds at frequencies less than around 10 Hz.

Other electrically excitable tissues with the potential to show network behaviour include glial cells located within the CNS (e.g. Parpura et al., 1994), and the autonomic and enteric nervous systems (see Sukkar, El-Munshid & Ardawi, 2000), which comprise interconnected non-myelinated nerve cells and are distributed throughout the body and gut, respectively. These systems are involved in regulating the visceral or "housekeeping" functions of the body; for example, the autonomic nervous system is involved in the maintenance of blood pressure. Muscle cells also show electrical excitability; only cardiac muscle tissue has electrically interconnected cells. However, Cooper, Garny & Kohl et al. (2003), in a review of cardiac ion channel activity, conclude that weak internal electric fields much below the excitation threshold are unlikely to have any significant effect on cardiac physiology. EMF effects on the heart could theoretically result from indirect effects mediated via the autonomic nervous system and CNS (Sienkiewicz, 2003). Effects on the endocrine system could potentially also be mediated this way, although the evidence from volunteer experiments indicates that acute ELF magnetic field exposure up to 20 µT does not influence the circadian variation in circulating levels of the hormone melatonin (Warman et al., 2003b), nor other plasma hormone levels (ICNIRP, 2003).

## 5.2 Volunteer studies

An electric charge is induced on the surface of a human (or other living organism) exposed to a low frequency electric field that alternates in amplitude with the frequency of the applied field. The alternation of the surface charge with time induces an electric field and therefore current flow within the body; in addition, exposure to a low frequency magnetic field induces circulating eddy currents and associated electric fields. If of sufficient magnitude, these induced electric fields and currents can interact with electrically excitable nerve and muscle tissue. Generally, however, the surface charge effects of exposure to low frequency electric fields become prohibitive long before the internal electric fields become large enough to elicit a response in the tissue.

### 5.2.1 Surface electric charge

The surface electric charge can be perceived directly through the induced vibration of body hair and tingling sensations in areas of the body, particularly the arms, in contact with clothing, and indirectly through spark discharges between a person and a conducting object within the field. In several studies carried out in the 1970's and 1980's (summarized by Reilly, 1998a; 1999), the threshold for direct perception has shown wide individual variation; 10% of the exposed subjects had detection thresholds of around 2–5 kV m$^{-1}$ at 60 Hz, whereas 50% could detect fields of 7–20 kV m$^{-1}$. These effects were considered annoying by 5% of the test subjects exposed under laboratory conditions above electric field strengths of about 15–20 kV m$^{-1}$. In addition to showing a wide variation in individual sensitivity, these responses also vary with environmental conditions, particularly humidity; the studies referred to above, however, included both wet and dry exposure conditions.

It has been estimated that spark discharges would be painful to 7% of subjects who are well-insulated and who touch a grounded object within a 5 kV m$^{-1}$ field (Reilly, 1998a; Reilly, 1999) whereas they would be painful to about 50% in a 10 kV m$^{-1}$ field. Unpleasant spark discharges can also occur when a grounded person touches a large conductive object such as a large vehicle that is "well-insulated" from ground and is situated within a strong electric field. Here, the threshold field strength required to induce such an effect varies inversely with the size of the conductive object. In both cases, the presence in the well-insulated person or object of a conductive pathway to ground would tend to mitigate the intensity of any effect (Reilly, 1998a; Reilly, 1999), as would the impedance to earth of the grounded object or person.

People can perceive electric currents directly applied to the body through touching, for example, a conductive loop in which current is induced by exposure to environmental electromagnetic fields. Thresholds for directly applied currents have also been characterised. At 50 to 60 Hz, the male median threshold for perception was between 0.36 mA (finger contact) and 1.1 mA (grip contact), while pain occurred at 1.8 mA (finger contact).

Median thresholds for women were generally found to be two thirds of the male thresholds, while children were assumed to have median thresholds half of male threshold values (WHO, 1993). There is also a wide variety in the individual's ability to detect currents, there is, for example, about one order of magnitude difference in the perception threshold at the 0.5 percentile and the 99.5 percentile at 50/60 Hz (Kornberg & Sagan, 1979). Generally, the ability to detect fields or currents decreases with increasing frequency. This has been characterised for the perception of currents; the threshold is increasing by about two orders of magnitude at higher frequencies: 0.36 mA at 50/60 Hz, 4 mA at 10 kHz and 40 mA at 100 kHz (WHO, 1993).

A series of extensive studies on 50 Hz population thresholds in more than 1000 people from all ages have recently been carried out by Leitgeb and colleagues. Leitgeb & Schröttner (2002) examined perception thresholds in 700 people aged between 16 and 60 years, approximately half of them women. This study was recently extended to include 240 children aged 9–16 years, and about 20 people aged 61 years or more (Leitgeb, Schroettner & Cech, 2005). In both studies, electric current was applied to the forearm using pre-gelled electrodes, and considerable care was taken to rule out subjective bias.

A summary of the studies on perception of electric currents directly applied to the body is given in Table 33.

Table 33. 50 Hz electric current perception values ($I_w$) for different perception probabilities (p) for men, women and the general population [a]

|  | $I_w$ (µA) | | | |
| --- | --- | --- | --- | --- |
| p (%) | Men | Women | Children | Population |
| 90 | 602 | 506 | 453 | 553 |
| 50 | 313 | 242 | 252 | 268 |
| 10 | 137 | 93 | 112 | 111 |
| 5 | 106 | 68 | 78 | 78 |
| 0.5 | 53 | 24 | 35 | 32 |

[a] Source: Leitgeb & Schroettner, 2002; Leitgeb, Schroettner & Cech, 2005.

Leitgeb, Schroettner & Cech (2005) note that the median perception threshold for the population is 268 µA, almost 50% lower than the present limit of 500 µA recommended by the IEC (1994). They also note that whilst the median threshold for women is approximately two thirds of the male threshold values, children aged between 9 and 16 do not exhibit as a high a sensitivity as had been assumed.

An issue with perception levels is that they really depend on the site of application of the current (cheek and inner forearm being very sensitive) and the area of application of the current (i.e. current density). The latter makes the comparison of current values difficult (Reilly, 1998a).

## 5.2.2    Nerve stimulation

Large, rapidly changing, pulsed magnetic fields used in various specialised medical applications such as magnetic resonance imaging (MRI) and transcranial magnetic stimulation (TMS) can induce electric fields large enough to stimulate nervous tissue in humans. Minimum, orientation-dependent stimulus thresholds for large diameter (20 µm) myelinated nerve axons have been estimated to be approximately 6 V m$^{-1}$ at frequencies up to about 1–3 kHz (Reilly, 1998a; Reilly, 1999). In addition, accommodation to a slowly changing stimulus resulting from slow inactivation of sodium channels will raise thresholds at low frequencies. In MRI, nerve stimulation is an unwanted side effect of a procedure used to derive cross-sectional images of the body for clinical diagnosis (see Shellock, 2001). Threshold rates of change of the switched gradient magnetic fields used in MRI for perception, discomfort and pain resulting from peripheral nerve stimulation are extensively reviewed by Nyenhuis et al. (2001). Generally, median, minimum threshold rates of change of magnetic field (during periods of < 1 ms) for perception were 15–25 µT s$^{-1}$ depending on orientation and showed considerable individual variation (Bourland, Nyenhuis & Schaefer, 1999). These values were somewhat lower than previously estimated by Reilly (1998a; 1999), possibly due to the constriction of eddy current flow by high impedance tissue such as bone (Nyenhuis et al., 2001). Thresholds rose as the pulse width of the current induced by the switched gradient field decreased; the median pulse width (the chronaxie) corresponding to a doubling of the minimum threshold (the rheobase) ranged between 360 and 380 µs but again showing considerable individual variation (Bourland, Nyenhuis & Schaefer, 1999). Numerical calculations of the electric field induced by pulses in the 84 subjects tested by Nyenhuis et al. (2001) have been used to estimate the median threshold for peripheral nerve stimulation at 60 Hz as 48 mT (Bailey & Nyenhuis, 2005). Furthermore, Nyenhuis et al. (2001) using data from measurements on human volunteers estimated a rheobase electric field of 2.2 V m$^{-1}$ in tissue.

In TMS, parts of the brain are deliberately stimulated in order to produce a transient, functional impairment for use in the study of cognitive processes (see Reilly, 1998a; Ueno, 1999; Walsh, Ashbridge & Cowey, 1998). Furthermore, in TMS, brief, localised, suprathreshold stimuli are given, typically by discharging a capacitor through a coil situated over the surface of the head, in order to stimulate neurons in a small volume (a few cubic centimetres) of underlying cortical tissue (Reilly, 1998a). The induced current causes the neurons within that volume to depolarise synchronously, followed by a period of inhibition (Fitzpatrick & Rothman, 2000). When the pulsed field is applied to a part of the brain thought to be necessary for the performance of a cognitive task, the resulting depolarisation interferes with the ability to perform the task. In principle then, TMS provides cognitive neuroscientists with the capability to induce highly specific, temporally and spatially precise interruptions in cognitive processing – sometimes known as "virtual lesions". Reilly (1998a) noted induced electric field thresholds to be of the order of 20 V $m^{-1}$. However, Walsh & Cowey (1998) cited typical rates of change of magnetic field of 30 kT $s^{-1}$ over a 100 µs period transiently inducing an electric field of 500 V $m^{-1}$ in brain tissue.

People are likely to show variations in sensitivity to induced electric fields. In particular, epileptic syndromes are characterised by increased neuronal excitability and synchronicity (Engelborghs, D'Hooge & De Deyn, 2000); seizures arise from an excessively synchronous and sustained discharge of a group of neurons (Engelborghs, D'Hooge & De Deyn, 2000; Jefferys, 1994). TMS is widely used, apparently without adverse effects. However, repetitive TMS has been observed to trigger epileptic seizure in some susceptible subjects (Fitzpatrick & Rothman, 2000; Wassermann, 1998). These authors also reported short- to medium-term memory impairments and noted the possibility of long-term cognitive effects from altered synaptic activity or neurotransmitter balance. Contraindications for TMS use agreed at an international workshop on repetitive TMS safety (Wassermann, 1998) include epilepsy, a family history of seizure, the use of tricyclic antidepressants, neuroleptic agents and other drugs that lower seizure threshold. Serious heart disease and increased intracranial pressure have also been suggested as contraindications due to the potential complications that would be introduced by seizure.

### 5.2.3    Retinal function

The effects of exposure to weak low frequency magnetic fields on human retinal function are well established. Exposure of the head to magnetic flux densities above about 5 mT at 20 Hz, rising to about 15 mT at 50 Hz, will reliably induce faint flickering visual sensations called magnetic phosphenes (Attwell, 2003; Sienkiewicz, Saunders & Kowalczuk, 1991; Taki, Suzuki & Wake, 2003). It is generally agreed that these phosphenes result from the interaction of the induced electric current with electrically sensitive cells in the retina. Several lines of evidence suggest the production of phosphenes by a weak induced electric field does not involve the initial transduction of light into an electrical signal. Firstly, the amplification of the initial signal generated by the absorption of light takes place primarily through an intracellular "second-messenger cascade" of metabolic reactions prior to any change in ion channel conductivity (Hille & Anderson, 2001). Secondly, the phosphene threshold appears unaffected by "dark" adaptation to low light levels (Carpenter, 1972). In addition, phosphenes have been induced in a patient with retinitis pigmentosa, a degenerative illness primarily affecting the pigment epithelium and photoreceptors (Lövsund et al., 1980).

There is good reason to view retinal circuitry as an appropriate model for induced electric field effects on CNS neuronal circuitry in general (Attwell, 2003). Firstly, the retina displays all the processes present in other CNS areas, such as graded voltage signalling and action potentials, and has a similar biochemistry. Secondly, in contrast to more subtle cognitive effects, phosphenes represent a direct and reproducible perception of field interaction. A clear distinction can be made in this context between the detection of a normal visual stimulus and the abnormal induction of a visual signal by non-visual means (Saunders, 2003); the latter suggests the possibility of direct effects on cognitive processes elsewhere in the CNS.

Thresholds for electrically induced phosphenes have been estimated to be about 10–14 mA m$^{-2}$ at 20 Hz (Adrian, 1977; Carstensen, 1985). A similar value (10 mA m$^{-2}$ at 20 Hz), based on studies of magnetically induced phosphenes, has been derived by Wake et al. (1998). The equivalent electric field threshold can be estimated as around 100–140 mV m$^{-1}$ using a tissue conductivity for brain tissue of about 0.1 S m$^{-1}$ (Gabriel, Gabriel & Corthout, 1996). More recently, Reilly (2002) has calculated an approximate 20 Hz electric field threshold in the retina of 53 mV m$^{-1}$ for phosphene production. A similar value (60 mV m$^{-1}$) has been reported elsewhere (see Saunders, 2003). Subsequently, however, Taki et al. (2003) indicated that calculations of phosphene thresholds suggested that electrophosphene thresholds were around 100 mV m$^{-1}$, whereas magnetophosphene thresholds were around 10 mV m$^{-1}$ at 20 Hz.

More detailed calculation by Attwell (2003) based on neuroanatomical and physiological considerations, suggests that the phosphene electric field threshold in the extracellular fluid of the retina is in the range 10–60 mV m$^{-1}$ at 20 Hz. There is however, considerable uncertainty attached to these values. In addition, the extrapolation of values in the extracellular fluid to those appropriate for whole tissue, as used in most dosimetric models, is complex, depending critically on the extracellular volume and other factors. With regard to the frequency response, Reilly (2002) suggests that the narrow frequency response is the result of relatively long membrane time constants of around 25 ms. However, at present, the exact mechanism underlying phosphene induction is unknown. It is not clear whether the narrow frequency response is due to intrinsic physiological properties of the retinal neurons, as suggested by Reilly (2002) above and by Attwell (2003) considering active amplification process in the retinal neuron synaptic terminals, or is the result of central processing of the visual signal (Saunders, 2003; Saunders & Jefferys, 2002). This issue can only be resolved through further investigation.

### 5.2.4 Brain electrical activity

Since the first suggestion that occupational exposure to EMFs resulted in clinical changes in the electroencephalogram (EEG) was published in 1966 (Asanova & Rakov, 1966; 1972), various studies have investigated if exposure to magnetic fields can affect the electrical activity of the brain. Such methods can provide useful diagnostic information regarding the functional state of the brain, not only from recordings of the spontaneous activity at rest but also from recording the sensory functions and subsequent cognitive processes evoked in response to specific stimuli (evoked or event-related potentials, ERPs). Nevertheless, neurophysiological studies using magnetic fields need to be performed with much care and attention since they can be prone to many potential sources of error and artefact (NIEHS, 1998). Changes in arousal and attention of volunteers, in particular, can substantially affect the outcome of these studies.

Various studies have investigated the effects of magnetic fields on brain activity by analysing the spectral power of the main frequency bands of the EEG (Bell et al., 1992; Bell et al., 1991; Bell, Marino & Chesson, 1994a; Bell, Marino & Chesson, 1994b; Gamberale et al., 1989; Heusser, Tellschaft & Thoss, 1997; Lyskov et al., 1993b; Lyskov et al., 1993a; Marino, Bell & Chesson, 1996; Schienle et al., 1996; Silny, 1986). These studies have used a wide variety of experimental designs and exposure conditions, as well as healthy volunteers and patients with neurological conditions, and thus are difficult to compare and evaluate. Despite some scattered field-dependent changes, most notably in the alpha frequency band, and with intermittent exposure perhaps more effective than continuous exposure, these studies have produced inconsistent and sometimes contradictory results.

A difficulty with interpretation of the EEG in individuals at rest is that the intra-individual variability is very high. The variability of ERPs is much lower, resulting in better reproducibility, and other studies have investigated the effects of magnetic fields and combined electric and magnetic fields on these potentials within the EEG waveform. There are some differences between studies, but generally, the early components of the evoked response corresponding to sensory function do not appear affected by exposure (Graham & Cook, 1999; Lyskov et al., 1993b). In contrast, large and sustained changes on a later component of the waveform representing stimulus detection may be engendered by exposure at 60 mT (Silny, 1984; 1985; 1986), with lesser effects occurring using fields of 1.26 mT (Lyskov et al., 1993b), and nothing below 30 µT (Graham & Cook, 1999). Finally, exposure during the performance of some discrimination and attention tasks may affect the late major components of the EEG which are believed to reflect cognitive processes involved with stimulus evaluation and decision making (Cook et al., 1992; Crasson et al., 1999; Graham et al., 1994), although Crasson and Legros (2005) were unable to replicate the effects they reported previously. There also is some evidence that task difficulty and field intermittency may be important experimental variables. However, all these subtle effects are not well defined, and some inconsistencies between studies require additional investigation and explanation.

A summary of studies on changes in brain electrical activity while awake is given in Table 34.

**Table 34. Brain electrical activity**

| Test [a] | Exposure | Response | Comments | Authors |
|---|---|---|---|---|
| **During exposure to magnetic fields up to 10 Hz** | | | | |
| Standard EEG: $C_{3,4}$; $P_{3,4}$; $O_{1,2}$; FFT at 10 Hz, no records during exposure 6 female and 4 male volunteers | 10 Hz 100 µT 10 min | Immediately after exposure the spectral power of the brain activity was lower than before exposure and 10 min afterwards, but only at the occipital electrodes was this difference significant. | Data for individual volunteers are not presented, and there is no information concerning the rate of responders. | Bell, Marino & Chesson, 1994b |
| Standard EEG: $C_{3,4}$; $P_{3,4}$; $O_{1,2}$; FFT at 1.5 Hz or 10 Hz band 13 healthy subjects and 6 patients | 5 or 10 Hz 20, 40 µT 2 s on, 5 s off | In each person, the magnetic field altered the brain activity at the frequency of stimulation, but no systematic changes of brain activity. | The strength of the effect was proportional neither to frequency nor to field strength. | Bell, Marino & Chesson, 1994a |
| Standard EEG: $C_{3,4}$; $P_{3,4}$; $O_{1,2}$; frequency spectrum analysis except for < 2.5 Hz and 9-11 Hz. 13 volunteers, 6 patients | 1.5 or 10 Hz 80 µT 2 s on, 5 s off | ICOS (intra-subject comparison of stimulus and non-stimulus state) was altered by ELF exposure in 58% of the subjects. | | Marino, Bell & Chesson, 1996 |
| Standard EEG, $O_{1,2}$ spectral analysis of theta (3.5-7.5 Hz), alpha (7.5-12.5 Hz) and beta bands (12.5-25 Hz) 25 female and 36 male volunteers | 3 Hz 100 µT$_{pp}$ 20 min one exposure and one control session | Significant changes in theta and beta frequency bands after exposure relative to controls, interpreted as slightly pronounced reduct on of alertness during exposure. | Exposure and control sessions on different days, the two session days were not treated as a double blind study. | Heusser, Tellschaft & Thoss, 1997 |
| **During exposure to magnetic fields between 45 and 60 Hz** | | | | |
| Standard EEG 26 experienced power utility linemen | 50 Hz exposure during workday average exposure 23 µT one day live, one day sham | No changes in alpha EEG, nor evidence of EEG abnormalities. | Intervention study, not laboratory. | Gamberale et al., 1989 |

127

**Table 34. Continued**

| | | | |
|---|---|---|---|
| Standard EEG (10-20 system): $C_{3,4}$; $P_{3,4}$; $O_{1,2}$; FFT at 1-18.5 Hz in 0.5 Hz steps 3 female, 11 male volunteers | 60 Hz 25 or 50 µT 2 s on, 8 s off, first 2 s used as control | No systematic effects for frequency bands and activity-power intensities. In 50 % of volunteers diminished EEG power was observed as a response to the field. | Bell et al., 1991 |
| Standard EEG: $C_{3,4}$; $P_{3,4}$; $O_{1,2}$; FFT at 1-18.5 Hz in 0.5 Hz steps 10 healthy volunteers and 10 neurological patients | 60 Hz $B_{DC}$: 78 µT, $B_{AC}$: 78 µT, single and combined 2 s on, 5 s off, first 2 s used as control | 19 out of 20 persons responded to the fields: overall 35% to $B_{DC}$; 70% of the patients and 80% of the volunteers to $B_{AC}$, response to $B_{AC}$ was not different from the responses to the combination $B_{AC}$+ $B_{DC}$. Field-induced increase and decrease of brain activity, no systematic changes were observed for the hemispheres or activity loci. EEG changes were lower in patients than in healthy subjects. | Bell et al., 1992 |
| Standard EEG spectral analysis 6 female and 8 male volunteers | 45 Hz 1.26 mT 1s on, 1s off cycle over 15 min, one exposure and one control session | Significant increase of the power values of alpha and beta bands after exposure, no changes in delta- and theta-bands. | Lyskov et al., 1993a |
| Standard EEG spectral analysis. before and after exposure 11 female and 9 male volunteers | 45 Hz 1.26 mT 10 persons: 1 h continuous field, 10 persons: 1s on/off intermittent field for 1 h One exposure and one control session | Several statistically significant changes; increase of alpha activity during intermittent exposure and decrease of delta activity. Increase of beta waves in frontal but not in occipital derivations. | Inhomogeneous results, consistent with increased relaxation. Double blind study. Lyskov et al., 1993b |

**Table 34. Continued**

### During exposure to magnetic fields at higher frequencies

| | | | |
|---|---|---|---|
| Standard EEG, $F_{3,4}$, $P_{3,4}$, $O_{1,2}$, traditional frequency bands 0.1 - 30 Hz, psychological parameters and questionnaires<br>26 female and 26 male volunteers | Spherics simulation:<br>10 kHz<br>500 µs duration, random intervals between 50 and 150 ms<br>38 A m⁻¹ peak value electric field shielded exposure 10 min and control session | Significant reduction of the power only in the alpha frequency band (8-13 Hz) in parietal and occipital derivations, when analysing sub-groups only in 10 - 10.75 Hz. P / O recordings show significant reductions in the voltage power. | Factors such as physical condition and neurotics were considered as mediators of spherics effectiveness. | Schienle et al., 1996 |

### Evoked potentials after exposure to EMF

| | | | |
|---|---|---|---|
| Visual evoked potentials<br>100 subjects | 5 – 50 Hz pulsed magnetic field<br>up to 100 mT | Phase reversal of components of the visual evoked potential at 60 mT. | Very intense fields. | Silny, 1984;<br>1985; 1986 |
| Auditory evoked potentials<br>6 female and 6 male volunteers | 45 Hz<br>1.26 mT<br>1 s on, 1 s off, 15 min<br>one exposure and one control session | N100 components were shorter, amplitudes were reduced. | | Lyskov et al., 1993a |
| Auditory evoked potentials<br>11 female and 3 male volunteers | 45 Hz<br>1.26 mT<br>10 persons: 1 h continuous field<br>10 persons: 1 h 1 s on/off intermittent field<br>one exposure and one control session | Not affected. | | Lyskov et al., 1993b |

129

**Table 34. Continued**

| | | | | |
|---|---|---|---|---|
| Auditory, visual and somatosensory evoked potentials before, during and after exposure 36 (male and female) subjects | 60 Hz 14.1 or 28.3 µT 45 min | No effect except a reduced amplitude of the somatosensory evoked potential in the lower exposure group. | Double-blind, counterbalanced study. | Graham & Cook, 1999 |

**Event-related potentials after exposure to EMF**

| | | | | |
|---|---|---|---|---|
| Electrodes $C_z$, $P_{3,4}$ for event-related potentials (P300), following auditory or visual stimuli in the Oddball task during exposure 30 male volunteers | 60 Hz 9 kV m⁻¹, 20 µT 18 exposed and sham-exposed over four 6-h sessions, 12 exposed in all sessions | Amplitude of the auditory P300 was increased. Visual ERPs were not affected. | Effects on auditory ERP components were greatest soon after activation of field and after switching off at the end of the session. | Cook et al., 1992 |
| Event-related brain potentials (N200-P300) following auditory stimuli in the Oddball task during exposure 54 male subjects | 3 matched groups of 18 men each, two 6-h sessions, exposure or sham, 60 Hz: a) 6 kV m⁻¹, 10 µT b) 9 kV m⁻¹, 20 µT c) 12 kV m⁻¹, 30 µT | Significant increases of P300 latency in group b), but decrease during sham exposure. | N200-P300 component complex altered in all groups, order of exposure did not affect results. Double blind, counterbalanced study. | Graham et al., 1994 |
| Event-related potentials during performance of the Oddball task, the dichotic listening task and the CNV paradigm after exposure 21 male subjects | 50 Hz 100 µT 30 min, continuous or intermittent head only | Differences in ERP amplitudes were seen during the dichotic listening task. | Some effects were inconsistent between trials. Double-blind studies. | Crasson et al., 1999 |
| Event-related potentials during performance of the Oddball task, the dichotic listening task and the CNV paradigm after exposure 18 male subjects | 50 Hz 100 µT 30 min, continuous or intermittent head only | No effects in ERP amplitudes were seen during the dichotic listening task or in other measures of performance. | Replication and extension of above study by the same group. | Crasson & Legros, 2005 |

a C, F, O & P represent standard EEG recording electrode positions; FFT = Fast Fourier Transform.

### 5.2.5 Sleep

Sleep is a complex biological process controlled by the central nervous system and is necessary for general health and well-being. The possibility that EMFs may exert a detrimental effect on sleep has been examined in two studies. Using the EEG to assess sleep parameters, Åkerstedt et al. (1999) reported that continuous exposure of healthy volunteers to 50 Hz at 1 µT at night caused disturbances in sleep. In this study, total sleep time, sleep efficiency, slow-wave sleep (stage III and IV), and slow-wave activity were significantly reduced by exposure, as was subjective depth of sleep. Graham & Cook (1999) reported that intermittent, but not continuous, exposure to 60 Hz, 28 µT magnetic fields at night resulted in less total sleep time, reduced sleep efficiency, increased time in stage II sleep, decreased time in rapid eye movement (REM) sleep and increased latency to first REM period. Consistent with a pattern of poor and broken sleep, volunteers exposed to the intermittent field also reported sleeping less well and feeling less rested in the morning.

A comparison between these two studies is made difficult because of the differences in the exposure levels used, 1 µT (Åkerstedt et al., 1999) vs. 28 µT (Graham & Cook, 1999) and also of other differences in the design. As to the results, in the Åkerstedt study, results were apparently obtained by low-level continuous exposure, whereas the Graham study failed to elicit such results by continuous exposure, but did produce similar results with intermittent exposures. Further studies with similar designs are needed before any conclusions can be drawn.

A summary of studies on brain electrical activity during sleep is given in Table 35.

#### Table 35. Brain electrical activity during sleep

| Test | Exposure | Response | Comments | Authors |
|------|----------|----------|----------|---------|
| Sleep EEGs, conventional recordings 8 female and 10 male healthy volunteers | 50 Hz 1 µT one night (23:00-07:00) with field on, one night with field off | Significantly reduced slow wave activity and slow wave sleep. Also tendency for reduced total sleep time, sleep efficiency, REM sleep (not statistically significant). | Absolute values were within the normal variability; the observed changes are far from clinical significance. Blind study, balanced design. | Åkerstedt et al., 1999 |
| Sleep EEG, 3 nights (23:00-07:00), $C_z$, $C_4$, $O_z$ 24 male volunteers | 60 Hz 28.3 µT, circularly polarised 8 sham-exposed controls, 7 subjects exposed to continuous fields, 9 to intermittent 1 h on, 1 h off, 15 s on/off cycle | Intermittent exposure to magnetic fields produced significant disturbances in nocturnal sleep EEGs in 6 of 9 persons: decreased sleep efficiency, altered sleep architecture, suppression of REM sleep, lower well-feeling of several subjects in the morning. | No effect was seen during continuous field exposure relative to sham-exposed controls. Double-blind, counter-balanced study. | Graham & Cook, 1999 |

### 5.2.6    Cognitive effects

Despite the potential importance of field-induced effects on attention, vigilance, memory and other information processing functions, relatively few studies have looked for evidence of changes in cognitive ability during or after exposure to low frequency EMFs. These have been reviewed by NIEHS (1998), Cook, Thomas & Prato (2002), Bailey (2001), Crasson (2003) and ICNIRP (2003). While few field-dependent changes have been observed, it is important to consider that this type of study may be particularly susceptible to various environmental and individual factors which may increase the variance of the experimental endpoint and decrease the power to detect a small effect. This may be particularly important, since any field-dependent effects are likely to be small with fields at environmental levels (Sienkiewicz et al., 1993; Whittington, Podd & Rapley, 1996).

The effects of acute exposure to magnetic fields on simple and choice reaction time have been investigated in several recent studies using a wide range of magnetic flux densities (20 $\mu$T – 1.26 mT) and experimental conditions. Some studies did not find any field-dependent effects (Gamberale et al., 1989; Kurokawa et al., 2003b; Lyskov et al., 1993b; Lyskov et al., 1993a; Podd et al., 2002; Podd et al., 1995), although modest effects on speed (Crasson et al., 1999; Graham et al., 1994; Whittington, Podd & Rapley, 1996) and accuracy during task performance (Cook et al., 1992; Kazantzis, Podd & Whittington, 1998; Preece, Wesnes & Iwi, 1998) have been reported. However, Crasson & Legros (2005) were unable to replicate these observations. These data also suggest that effects may depend on the difficulty of the task (Kazantzis, Podd & Whittington, 1998; Whittington, Podd & Rapley, 1996) and that exposure may attenuate the usual improvement seen with practice in reaction time (Lyskov et al., 1993b; Lyskov et al., 1993a; Stollery, 1986)

A few studies have reported subtle field-dependent changes in other cognitive functions, including memory and attention. Using a battery of neuropsychological tests, Preece, Wesnes & Iwi (1998) found that exposure to a 50 Hz magnetic field at 0.6 mT decreased accuracy in the performance of numerical working memory task and decreased sensitivity of the performance in a word recognition task. Similarly Keetley et al. (2001) investigated the effects of exposure to 28 $\mu$T, 50 Hz fields using a series of cognitive tests. A significant decrease in performance was seen with one working memory task (the trail-making test, part B) that involves visual-motor tracking and information processing within the prefrontal and parietal areas of the cortex. Podd et al. (2002) reported delayed deficits in the performance of a recognition memory task following exposure to a 50 Hz field at 100 $\mu$T. Trimmel & Schweiger (1998) investigated the effects of acute exposure to 50 Hz magnetic fields at 1 mT. The fields were produced using a power transformer, and volunteers were exposed in the presence of a 45 dB sound pressure level noise. Compared with a no-field, no-noise condition and noise alone (generated using a tape recording) significant reductions in visual attention, perception and verbal memory performance were observed during

**Table 36. Cognitive effects**

| Test | Exposure | Response | Comments | Authors |
|---|---|---|---|---|
| Reaction time, vigilance, memory and perception speed tested before and after each day 26 experienced power utility linemen. | 50 Hz exposure during workday average exposure 23 μT one day live, one day sham | No difference in performance between exposed and non-exposed days. | Intervention study, not laboratory. | Gamberale et al., 1989 |
| Reaction time (RT) and target-deletion test (TDT) 6 female and 8 male volunteers | 45 Hz 1.26 mT 1 s on, 1 s off cycle, 15 min one exposure and one control session | No significant differences for RT, TDT not affected. | | Lyskov et al., 1993a |
| Reaction time (RT) 11 female and 9 male volunteers | 45 Hz 1.26 mT 10 persons: 1 h continuous field 10 persons: 1 hour 1 s on/off intermittent field one exposure and one control session | RT not directly affected. | Learning to perform the RT test (decrease of RT in repeated trials) affected by exposure . | Lyskov et al., 1993b |
| Reaction time to light flashed at variable intervals during exposure 12 subjects (expt 1) and 24 subjects (expt 2), male and female | Experiment 1: 10.1 or 0.2 Hz 1.1 mT 300 s Experiment 2: 0.2 or 43 Hz 1.8 mT 300 s | No effects found. | Experiment 2 designed to test for possible parametric resonance theory. Double blind studies. | Podd et al., 1995 |
| Reaction time, accuracy and memory recognition | 60 Hz 100 μT 1 s on, 1 s off for 11 min | Effect on memory, not on reaction time or accuracy. | Results different from previous studies (Whittington et al., 1996) | Podd et al., 2002 |

**Table 36. Continued**

| Task / subjects | Exposure | Effects | Comments | Reference |
|---|---|---|---|---|
| Reaction time, accuracy, time perception and visual perception 12 male and 8 female subjects | 50 Hz 22 µT circularly polarised with harmonics and repetitive transients up to 100 µT 55 min | No effects. | | Kurokawa et al., 2003b |
| Reaction time (RT), attention, differential reinforcement of low response rate (DRL) 54 male volunteers | 3 matched groups of 18 men each, two 6-h sessions, exposure or sham, 60 Hz: a) 6 kV m$^{-1}$, 10 µT b) 9 kV m$^{-1}$, 20 µT c) 12 kV m$^{-1}$, 30 µT | Slower reaction time in Oddball task and lower accuracy of DRL in group a) only. | No effect on other measures or in other exposure groups. Double blind, counterbalanced study. | Graham et al., 1994 |
| A visual duration-discrimination task with 3 levels of difficulty 100 male and female subjects | 50 Hz 100 µT intermittent 9 min | Decreased reaction time for the hardest level of performance. | A relaxed significance level (0.15) was used. Double-blind, counter-balanced study. | Whittington, Podd & Rapley, 1996 |
| Rey Auditory Verbal Learning test (with delayed recall) and Digit Span Task 21 male subjects. | 50 Hz 100 µT continuous or intermittent 30 min head only | No effects (reported in discussion). | Double-blind studies. | Crasson et al., 1999 |
| Choice serial reaction time task, time estimation task, interval production task, vigilance task, digit span memory task and Wilkinson Addition task during exposure 54 male subjects | 60 Hz 9 kV m$^{-1}$ and 20 µT 2 x 3 h / day for 4 days | Fewer errors in choice reaction time task. No effects on reaction time, memory or vigilance. | Double-blind, counterbalanced study. | Cook et al., 1992 |

**Table 36. Continued**

| | | | | |
|---|---|---|---|---|
| A visual duration-discrimination task with 3 levels of difficulty. 40 male and 59 female subjects | 50 Hz 100 µT intermittent 7.9 min | Improved accuracy for the hardest level of performance. | A relaxed significance level (0.3) was used. Double-blind, counter-balanced study. | Kazantzis, Podd & Whittington, 1998 |
| Immediate word recall, reaction time, digit vigilance task, choice reaction time, spatial working memory, numeric working memory, delayed word recall and recognition and picture recognition during exposure. 16 (male and female) subjects | 50 Hz or static magnetic fields at 0.6 mT applied to the head. Duration not specified. Current density in head estimated as 2–6 mA m⁻² | Reduced accuracy of word and number recall and performance of choice reaction time task. | Randomised blind cross-over design. | Preece, Wesnes & Iwi, 1998 |
| Duration Discrimination Task and Stroop Colour Word test. 18 male subjects | 50 Hz 100 µT continuous or intermittent 30 min head only | No effect on reaction time and performance accuracy. | Double blind with counter-balanced exposure order. | Crasson & Legros, 2005 |
| Syntactic and semantic verbal reasoning tasks, 5-choice serial reaction time task, and visual search tasks during exposure 76 male subjects | 50 Hz current 500 µA directly applied to head and shoulders 5.5 h / day for 2 days | Increased latency in syntactic reasoning task. | Possible differences between groups. Double-blind procedures with cross over design. | Stollery, 1986; 1987 |
| Rey Auditory Verbal Learning test; Digit Span Memory Task; Digit Symbol Substitution test; Speed of Comprehension Test and Trail Making Test verbal and written tests administered 20 min from exposure onset 30 subjects, both sexes | 50 Hz 28 µT 50 min | Most results indicated no effect, but data suggestive of detrimental effect on short-term learning and executive functioning. | Double-blind cross-over design. | Keetley et al., 2001 |
| Visual discrimination, perception, verbal memory and mood and symptom checklist 66 (male and female) subjects | 50 Hz 1 mT 45dB noise compared to noise alone | Significant reduction in visual attention, perception and verbal memory performance. | Double blind studies. | Trimmel & Schweiger, 1998 |

135

field exposure. The presence of the noise during exposure, however, complicates interpretation of this study.

Generally, while electrophysiological considerations suggest that the central nervous system is potentially susceptible to induced electric fields; cognitive studies have not revealed any clear, unambiguous finding. There is a need for a harmonisation of methodological procedures used in different laboratories, and for dose-response relationships to be investigated. The studies on various cognitive effects from ELF field exposure are summarized in Table 36.

### 5.2.7 Hypersensitivity

It has been suggested that some individuals display increased sensitivity to levels of EMFs well below recommended restrictions on exposure. People self-reporting hypersensitivity may experience a wide range of severe and debilitating symptoms, including sleep disturbances, general fatigue, difficulty in concentrating, dizziness, and eyestrain. In extreme forms, everyday living may become problematical. A number of skin problems such as eczema and sensations of itching and burning have also been reported, especially on the face, and, although there may be no specific symptom profile (see Hillert et al., 2002), increased sensitivity to chemical and other factors often occurs (Levallois et al., 2002). The responses to EMFs are reported to occur at field strengths orders of magnitude below those required for conventional perception of the field (Silny, 1999). These data have been reviewed by Bergqvist & Vogel (1997) and more recently by Levallois (2002), ICNIRP (2003) and Rubin et al. (2005).

In contrast to anecdotal reports, the evidence from double-blind provocation studies (Andersson et al., 1996; Flodin, Seneby & Tegenfeldt, 2000; Lonne-Rahm et al., 2000; Lyskov, Sandström & Hansson Mild, 2001b; Swanbeck & Bleeker, 1989) indicate that neither healthy volunteers nor self-reporting hypersensitive individuals can reliably distinguish field exposure from sham-exposure. In addition, subjective symptoms and circulating levels of stress-related hormones and inflammatory mediators could not be related to field exposure. Similar results were reported in a survey of office workers (Arnetz, 1997). In studies reported by Keisu (1996) and by Toomingas (1996), the outcome of tests on an individual was used therapeutically in the medical handling of the patient. In none of these series was there any reproducible association between exposure and symptoms. Further test series have been performed in Sweden, the UK and in Germany, including an unsuccessful repetition of the Rea et al. (1991) study (see below), but these have not been published in a peer reviewed form. For a review, see Bergqvist & Vogel (1997). These results are consistent with the view that hypersensitivity to EMFs is a psychosomatic syndrome, suggested by Gothe, Odoni & Nilsson (1995).

Not all studies dismiss the possibility of EMF hypersensitivity, however. Two studies have reported weak positive field discrimination (Mueller, Krueger & Schierz, 2002; Rea et al., 1991) and another two studies reported subtle differences in heart rate, visual evoked potentials, electroretinogram amplitudes and electrodermal activity between normal and hypersensitive volunteers (Lyskov, Sandström & Hansson Mild, 2001a; Sandström et al., 1997). The study by Rea et al. (1991) has, however, been criticised on several methodological grounds (ICNIRP, 2003): the selection of individuals, the exposure situation and whether the test was blind or not. There is some morphological evidence to suggest that the numbers and distribution of mast cells in the dermis of the skin on the face may be increased in individuals displaying hypersensitive reactions (Gangi & Johansson, 2000; Johansson et al., 1994; Johansson, Hilliges & Han, 1996). Increased responsiveness was attributed to changes in the expression of histamine and somatostatin and other inflammatory peptides. Similar effects in the dermis have also been reported following provocation tests to VDU-type fields in normal, healthy volunteers (Johansson et al., 2001).

EMF hypersensitivity was addressed by the World Health Organization (WHO) at a workshop held in Prague in October 2004 (WHO, 2005). It was proposed that this hypersensitivity, which has multiple recurrent symptoms and is associated with diverse environmental factors tolerated by the majority of people, should be termed "idiopathic environmental intolerance (IEI) with attribution to EMF". The workshop concluded that IEI incorporates a number of disorders sharing similar nonspecific symptoms that adversely affect people and cause disruptions in their occupational, social, and personal functioning. These symptoms are not explained by any known medical, psychiatric or psychological disorder, and the term IEI has no medical diagnostic value. IEI individuals cannot detect EMF exposure any more accurately than non-IEI individuals, and well-controlled and conducted double-blind studies have consistently shown that their symptoms are not related to EMF exposure *per se*. A summary of hypersensitivity studies is given in Table 37.

### 5.2.8 Mood and alertness

The possible impact of EMFs on mood and arousal has also been assessed in double-blind studies in which volunteers completed mood checklists before and after exposure. No field-dependent effects have been reported using a range of field conditions (Cook et al., 1992; Crasson et al., 1999; Crasson & Legros, 2005; Graham et al., 1994). However, in contrast Stollery (1986) reported decreased arousal in one of two participating groups of subjects when mild (500 μA) 50 Hz electric current was passed through the head, upper arms, and feet. This was done to simulate the internal electric fields generated by exposure to an external electric field strength of 36 kV m$^{-1}$. Also Stevens (2001) reported that exposure to a 20 Hz, 50 μT magnetic field increased positive affective responses displayed to visual stimuli compared with sham-exposure. Arousal, as measured by skin conductance, gave variable results. Table 38 summarizes the studies on effects of ELF field exposure on mood and alertness.

**Table 37. Hypersensitivity**

| Test | Exposure | Response | Comments | Authors |
|---|---|---|---|---|
| Skin symptoms 30 patients | VDU: static electric field 0,2 and 30 kV m$^{-1}$<br>ELF magnetic field: 50 and 800 nT<br>dB/dt: 23 and 335 mT s$^{-1}$ | No response related to exposure. | Heat, reddening, itching, stinging, oedema in exposed and sham exposed situations. | Swanbeck & Bleeker, 1989 |
| Perception and symptoms 17 patients | Fields from VDU, pre-tested as causing symptoms in open provocation prior to double blind sessions. In shielded laboratory. | 16 individuals failed to detect (guess) presence of the fields, symptoms were related to guesses, not to the fields. | | Andersson et al., 1996 |
| Perception and symptoms 15 patients and 26 controls | Fields from VDUs and other objects. Subjects tested in their normal home environment, using a variety of devices. | 15 individuals failed to detect presence of the fields, symptoms were not related to the fields. | | Flodin, Seneby & Tegenfeldt, 2000 |
| Provocation study of stress hormone levels, skin biopsies and facial skin sensations 24 patients and 12 controls | VDUs:<br>5 Hz–2 kHz:<br>12 V m$^{-1}$<br>198 nT<br>2 kHz–400 kHz:<br>10 V m$^{-1}$<br>18 nT<br>30 min / week for 4 weeks | None of the test parameters differed between exposed and sham exposed conditions, but skin symptoms appeared in the open provocation tests. | Double-blind study. | Lonne-Rahm et al., 2000 |

138

**Table 37. Continued**

| | | | | |
|---|---|---|---|---|
| EEG, visual evoked potentials, electrodermal activity, ECG and blood pressure. 20 patients and 20 control subjects | 60 Hz 10 T magnetic field exposure and sham exposure applied randomly during a 40 min period intermittent 15 sec on/off cycle at | Magnetic field exposure had no effect on any of the parameters examined. | Patients reporting EHS differed from control subjects in baseline values. | Lyskov, Sandström & Hansson Mild, 2001b |
| General health survey of 133 office employees. Exploratory study of skin disease, office ergonomics and air quality in 3 office workers reporting EMF hypersensitivity compared to 5 controls | VDUs: 5 Hz–2 kHz ~ 10–15 V m$^{-1}$ 100–150 nT | 10% (13) of general staff reported EMF hypersensitivity; no differences in skin symptoms between EMF hypersensitives and controls in exploratory study. | The authors were not able to attribute EMF hypersensitivity to any particular environmental factor. | Arnetz, 1997 |
| Perception and symptoms in one female patient 10 double-blind tests | Fields from VDU | The discomfort the patient experienced had no correlation to whether or not the monitor actually was on. | The patient reconsidered her own perception of the illness, and in time the symptoms receded completely. | Keisu, 1996 |
| Perception and symptoms in one patient | 50 Hz 34 or 100 µT 1 or 10 s repeated | Positive response when humming of the coils audible, disappeared when "camouflaged" by masking noise. | . | Toomingas, 1996 |
| Symptoms and physiological reactions 100 subjects | Low level magnetic fields (< 1 µT) at varying frequencies (0.1 Hz–5 MHz), in shielded laboratory. | 16 out of 100 individuals reacted repeatedly to fields by several parameters (symptoms, pupil diameter changes etc.). | Not sure whether fully blind study. | Rea et al., 1991 |

**Table 37. Continued**

| | | | |
|---|---|---|---|
| EMF perception<br>49 subjects with EHS and 14 controls | 50 Hz<br>100 V m$^{-1}$  6 µT<br>randomly presented as 2 min<br>block of exposure / sham expo-<br>sure | Perception by 7 subjects, but no dif-<br>ference in perception between sub-<br>jects with or without self-reported<br>EHS. | Mueller,<br>Krueger &<br>Schierz,<br>2002 |
| Electrocardiogram, visual evoked poten-<br>tials (VEP) and electroretinograms<br>10 subjects reporting EMF hypersensiv-<br>ity and 10 controls | Exposure to flickering light at<br>between 25 and 75 flashes per<br>second. No EMF exposure | Higher VEP amplitudes in EMF<br>hypersensitive patients. | Sandström<br>et al., 1997<br><br>Differences between<br>mean age of patients<br>and controls (37 vs 47<br>year). |
| Self-reported symptoms, blood pressure,<br>heart rate, (skin) electrodermal activity,<br>EEGs and visual evoked potentials<br>10 subjects reporting hypersensitivity<br>and 10 controls | No EMF exposure | Differences between patients and<br>controls regarding self-reported<br>symptoms, heart rate, electrical<br>activity of the skin, and visual<br>evoked potential amplitudes. | Lyskov,<br>Sandström<br>& Hansscn<br>Mild, 2001a |
| Immuno-fluorescent staining of mast<br>cells from skin biopsies<br>13 healthy subjects | VDU (TV or PC) exposure for 2<br>or 4 h | Increase in number of mast cells in<br>papillary and reticular dermis in 5<br>subjects. | Johansson<br>et al., 2001 |

140

**Table 38. Mood and alertness**

| Test | Exposure | Response | Comments | Authors |
|---|---|---|---|---|
| Mood Adjective Checklist before and after exposure; Stanford Sleepiness Scale before during and after exposure 30 male subjects | 60 Hz 9 kV m⁻¹ and 20 µT 2 x 3 h / day for 4 days | No effect. | Double-blind, counterbalanced study. | Cook et al., 1992 |
| Alertness Rating Scale, Mood Adjective Checklist before and after exposure 54 male subjects | 60 Hz 6 kV m⁻¹ and 10 µT 9 kV m⁻¹ and 20 µT 12 kV m⁻¹ and 30 µT 2 x 3 h / day for 4 days | No effect. | Double-blind, counterbalanced study. | Graham et al., 1994 |
| State-Trait Anxiety Inventory, Profile of Mood States, Visual Analogue Scales of mood and vigilance before and after exposure 21 male subjects | 50 Hz 100 µT 30 min, continuous or intermittent Head only exposures | No effect. | Double-blind studies. | Crasson et al., 1999 |
| State-Trait Anxiety Inventory, Profile of Mood States, Visual Analogue Scales of mood 18 subjects | 50 Hz 100 µT 30 min, continuous or intermittent Head only exposures. | No effect. | Replicate and extension of Crasson et al., 1999 | Crasson & Legros, 2005 |
| Mood checklist before and after exposure 76 male subjects | 50 Hz current; 500 µA directly applied to head and shoulders 5.5 h / day for 2 days | Decreased arousal in one of two groups; no effect on mood. | Possible differences between groups. Double-blind procedures with cross-over design. | Stollery, 1986 |
| Skin conductance and self-assessed arousal and affective content 20 male, 9 female subjects | 20 Hz 50 µT 5 s with concurrent visual stimulus | No effect on skin conductance and arousal but positive effect of exposure on image content. | Subject blind as to exposure status. | Stevens, 2001 |

141

## Table 39. Depression

| Study base and subject identification | Definition and estimation of exposure | Study design and numbers | RR (95% CI) | Authors |
|---|---|---|---|---|
| Persons who lived near a 132 kV line and persons who lived 3 miles away Questionnaire asking about depression | Distance between home and overhead line | Cross-sectional 132 near line, 9 with depression 94 away from line, 1 with depression | Strong association of depression to proximity to overhead power line. | Dowson et al., 1988 |
| Persons discharged with depression from hospital (England) and controls from electoral list | Measurements at front doors. Average for case and control groups compared | Case-control 359 persons discharged with diagnosis depressive illness | Average measurement cases: 0.23 µT; controls 0.21 µT. | Perry, Pearl & Binns, 1989 |
| Residents in 8 towns along a transmission line right-of-way (ROW) in the US, 1987. A sample was interviewed. Depressive symptoms obtained by CES-D[a] scale. Cut-off for depression was median of score. | Distance from power-line: near vs far Near: properties abutting ROW or towers visible | Cross-sectional 382 persons interviewed | 2.8 (1.6–5.1) | Poole et al., 1993 |
| Male veterans who served in the US army first time 1965-71. Two diagnostic inventories used: the Diagnostic Interview Schedule and the Minnesota Personality Inventory. Life time depression used for this report | Present job identified in interview together with duration Electrical worker | Cross-sectional 183 electrical workers (13 with life-time depression) 3861 non-electrical workers | 1.0 (0.5–1.7) | Savitz & Ananth, 1994 |
| Population of neighborhood near a transmission line in Orange County, CA, USA, 1992. A sample of homes near a power line and one block away from the power line. Depressive symptoms identified through questionnaire CES-D* scale | EMDEX measurements at the front door. Average for homes on easement: 0.486 µT and one block away 0.068 µT | Cross-sectional 152 women | 0.9 (0.5–1.9) | McMahan, Ericson & Meyer, 1994 |
| Finnish twins who had answered the Beck Depression Inventory (BDI) in 1990 | Residential magnetic field estimated from power lines near the homes | Cross-sectional 12063 persons | BDI scores not related to exposure. | Verkasalo et al., 1997 |

[a] CES-D scale: Centre for Epidemiologic Studies-Depression scale.

142

## 5.3 Epidemiological studies

With regard to neurobehavioural effects, epidemiological studies have focussed on depression and suicide. Studies of an association between EMF exposure and neurodegeneration are covered in Chapter 6.

### 5.3.1 Depression

Two early studies relating ELF EMF exposure to depression (Dowson et al., 1988; Perry, Pearl & Binns, 1989) are difficult to interpret because of methodological limitations to the procedures for selection of study subjects, because they did not use validated scales for identification of depressive symptoms (ICNIRP, 2003). Moreover, Perry, Pearl & Binns (1989) also reported unusually high average EMF levels that remain unexplained.

More recent studies used validated depression scales. One of these studies showed a clear association between proximity to power lines and depression (Poole et al., 1993), whereas three more recent studies (McMahan, Ericson & Meyer, 1994; Savitz & Ananth, 1994; Verkasalo et al., 1997) provided little evidence for such an association. The study by Poole et al. (1993) is well designed: it compares subjects on properties abutting a power line right-of-way to subjects further away, and the results appear internally consistent. The investigators report a relative risk of 2.8 (95% CI: 1.6–5.1). McMahan, Ericson & Meyer (1994) employed a similar design and measurements to confirm that the homes close to the line have considerably higher EMF levels than those further away. This study also appears valid but yields a relative risk of 0.9 (95% CI: 0.5–1.9). McMahan, Ericson & Meyer (1994) offer a number of possible explanations for the lack of consistency between these two studies but none of the explanations is convincing (ICNIRP, 2003).

Overall, ICNIRP (2003) conclude that the literature on depressive symptoms and EMF exposure is difficult to interpret because the findings are not consistent. This complexity cannot easily be resolved by suggesting that one type of result can be confined to a group of studies with methodological problems or some other limitation.

A summary of studies on the effects of ELF field exposure on depression is given in Table 39.

### 5.3.2 Suicide

An early case control study carried out in England (Perry et al., 1981; Reichmanis et al., 1979) found significantly higher EMFs in case homes than control homes. However, ICNIRP (2003) considers the study methodologically limited both for the way subjects were selected and for the statistical analysis employed. Subsequent studies have used a range of different approaches to assess exposure, varying from crude techniques based on distance between home and power lines, or on job titles, to more sophisticated approaches based on detailed information about cohorts of utility workers (Baris et al., 1996a; Baris et al., 1996b; Baris & Armstrong, 1990; Johansen & Olsen, 1998a; McDowall, 1986; van Wijngaarden et al., 2000). Only the latter study provides some support for the original findings, although McKinlay et al. (2004) note that the findings were variable. The two more recent occupational study, based on job titles recorded on death certificates, report contradictory results (Järvholm & Stenberg, 2002; van Wijngaarden, 2003). However, the exposure assessments in these studies were not as detailed as in the previous occupational studies listed.

In a review of ICNIRP (2003) it was observed that, despite methodological limitations, particularly relating to the earlier studies, the detailed study by Van Wijngaarden et al. (2000) suggested that an excess risk for suicide might exist.

A summary of the ELF suicide studies is given in Table 40.

Tabel 40. Suicide

| Study base and subject identification | Definition and estimation of exposure | Study design and numbers | RR (95% CI) | Authors |
|---|---|---|---|---|
| Suicide cases and controls in England | Estimates of residential exposure from power lines Measurements at the homes of subjects | Case-control 589 suicide cases | Higher estimated and measured fields at case homes. | Reichmanis et al., 1979 Perry et al., 1981 |
| Male employees in Danish utility companies observed during 1974—93 Cases: deaths from suicide in mortality registry | Employment records and job exposure matrix estimated average exposure level Medium and high exposure | SMR [a] 21 236 males in cohort; exposed cases | 1.4 (non-significant) | Johansen & Olsen, 1998a |
| Persons resident in the vicinity of transmission facilities, in specified areas in the UK, at the time of 1971 Census | Home within 50 meters from substation or 30 meters from overhead line | SMR [a] 8 cases | 0.75 (non-significant) | McDowall, 1986 |
| Deaths in England and Wales during 1970–72 and 1979–83 | Job titles on death certificates Electrical workers in aggregate as well as specific jobs | PMR [b] 495 cases in electrical occupations | No increase for electrical workers. | Baris & Armstrong, 1990 |
| Male utility workers, Quebec, Canada, 1970–88 Cases: deaths from suicide in mortality registry Controls: 1% random sample from the cohort | Job exposure matrix based on Positron measurements was created. E- and B-and pulsed fields from average and geometric means and from cumulative and current exposure | Case-control 49 cases 215 controls | No evidence for effects of magnetic fields. Some support for some electric field indices. | Baris et al., 1996a; 1996b |

144

**Table 40. Continued**

| Male electric utility workers | Jobs and indices of cumulative exposure based on measurement survey | Case-control 36 cases 5348 controls | Electrician: 2.18 (1.25–3.80) Line worker: 1.59 (1.18–2.14) | van Wijn-gaarden et al., 2000 |
|---|---|---|---|---|
| Swedish male electricians in construction industry Swedish death register | Job exposure matrix | Cohort study - 33 719 electricians (0.31 µT) - 72 653 glass and woodworkers (0.27–0.29 µT) - general population | SMR Electricians: 0.58 (0.47–0.71) Glass and woodworkers: 0.81 (0.72–0.91) | Järvholm & Sten-berg, 2002 |
| United States death certificate files for the years 1991 and 1992 | Occupation code; usual occupation and industry on the death certificates | Case-control 11 707 cases 132 771 controls | 1.3 (1.2–1.4) | van Wijn-gaarden, 2003 |

[a] SMR: Standardized Mortality Ratio.
[b] PMR: Proportional Mortality Ratio.

## 5.4 Animal studies

Various animal models have been used to investigate possible field-induced effects on brain function and behaviour. These include effects on neurotransmitter levels, electrical activity, field detection and the performance of learned tasks. Overall, a few field-dependent responses have been tentatively identified but even the most consistent effects appear small in magnitude and transient in nature.

### 5.4.1 Perception and field detection

It is known that animals can detect the presence of low frequency electric fields, possibly as a result of surface charge effects (Weigel & Lundstrom, 1987). Using appropriate behavioural techniques, a number of studies using rats (Sagan et al., 1987; Stell, Sheppard & Adey, 1993; Stern et al., 1983; Stern & Laties, 1985; reviewed in ICNIRP, 2003; NIEHS, 1998; NRC, 1997) indicate that the threshold for field detection is about 3–13 kV m$^{-1}$. Detection thresholds are similar in a variety of other species, with thresholds reported at 5–15 kV m$^{-1}$ in baboons (Orr, Rogers & Smith, 1995a), and 30–35 kV m$^{-1}$ in miniature swine (Kaune et al., 1978).

Detection thresholds for magnetic fields in animals are less clear and show greater variability than those for electric fields (ICNIRP, 2003). Using a conditioned suppression paradigm, Smith, Clarke & Justesen (1994) reported that rats were able to detect ELF magnetic fields as low as 200 µT, although the validity of this result has been questioned by Stern & Justesen (1995).

A summary of studies on perception and detection of fields is given in Table 41.

**Table 41. Perception and field detection**

| Endpoint | Exposure | Response | Comment | Authors |
|---|---|---|---|---|
| **ELF electric fields** | | | | |
| Rats: operant behaviour Electric field acting as cue or discriminative stimulus | 60 Hz up to 55 kV m$^{-1}$ brief daily exposures | Threshold of between 3 and 10 kV m$^{-1}$. | | Stern et al., 1983 Stern & Laties, 1985 |
| Rats: operant behaviour Electric field acting as cue | 60 Hz up to 27 kV m$^{-1}$ brief daily exposures | Threshold of 8 or 13 kV m$^{-1}$ depending on the test protocol. | | Sagan et al., 1987 |
| Rats: effect of air current on operant behaviour Electric field acting as cue | 60 Hz up to 25 kV m$^{-1}$ brief daily exposures | Threshold of 7.5 kV m$^{-1}$ unaffected by wind-induced hair movement. | Detection below threshold increased; results difficult to interpret. | Stell, Sheppard & Adey, 1993 |
| Baboons: operant behaviour Electric field acting as cue | 60 Hz 4–50 kV m$^{-1}$ brief daily exposures | Average threshold of 12 kV m$^{-1}$; range of 5–15 kV m$^{-1}$. | | Orr, Rogers & Smith, 1995a |
| Handford minature swine: drinking behaviour (n=4) Electric fields acts as conditioned stimulus | 60 Hz up to 55 kV m$^{-1}$ brief (20 s) repeated exposures | Threshold of 30–35 kV m$^{-1}$. | | Kaune et al., 1978 |
| **ELF magnetic fields** | | | | |
| Rats: conditioned suppression of operant behaviour | 7, 16, 30, 60 and 65 Hz 200 µT – 1.9 mT 1 h / day, 5 days / week, 5 weeks | All magnetic fields effective as cue for conditioned response suppression. | Temporal rather than magnetic field conditioning? | Smith, Clarke & Justesen, 1994; Stern, 1995 |

### 5.4.2 Arousal and aversion

Initial exposure to power-frequency electric fields in excess of detection thresholds may cause transient arousal and stress responses in rodents and non-human primates (Coelho, Easley & Rogers, 1991; Easley, Coelho & Rogers, 1991; Rosenberg et al., 1983; Rosenberg, Duffy & Sacher, 1981; reviewed in IARC, 2002; ICNIRP, 2003). These responses appear to habituate quickly following prolonged exposure. There is also some evidence that animals may avoid exposure to intense electric fields (e.g. Hjeresen et al., 1980; 1982), and that such fields can elicit aversive behaviours following exposure to high field strengths in rats (Creim et al., 1984) and in non-human primates (Rogers, Orr & Smith, 1995; Stern & Laties, 1989). The results of the latter study indicated that electric fields at levels of up to 65 kV $m^{-1}$ are not highly aversive to non-human primates.

Exposure of baboons to combined 60 Hz electric and magnetic fields at 6 kV $m^{-1}$ and 50 µT or at 30 kV $m^{-1}$ and 100 µT did not produce significant changes in social behaviour (Coelho, Rogers & Easley, 1995) previously seen to be affected by exposure to electric fields alone (Coelho, Easley & Rogers, 1991; Easley, Coelho & Rogers, 1991). While it is possible that the magnetic field may have modulated the electric field-induced responses, it was considered that some of the animals in the later experiment may have become desensitised by prior subthreshold electric field exposure.

Acute exposure to power frequency magnetic fields at up to 3 mT does not appear to induce aversive behaviour (Lovely et al., 1992). Such results suggest that the arousal responses observed using electric fields are not caused by field-induced internal electric fields, and may be attributed to body-surface interactions. One study reported that long-term, intermittent exposure to 50 Hz at 18 mT reduced behavioural responses ("irritability") induced by tactile and somatosensory stimuli in rats (Trzeciak et al., 1993). Another study reported that exposure to specific combinations of static and low frequency fields affected exploratory behaviour in rats (Zhadin, Deryugina & Pisachenko, 1999). Exposure to conditions corresponding to the putative cyclotron resonance for calcium ions reduced this behaviour, and exposure to conditions for magnesium ions increased it.

Studies on arousal and aversion in experimental animals are summarized in Table 42.

## Table 42. Arousal and aversion

| Endpoint | Exposure | Response | Comment | Authors |
|---|---|---|---|---|
| **Arousal and activity** | | | | |
| **ELF electric fields** | | | | |
| Mice: arousal assessed by activity, oxygen consumption, carbon dioxide production during exposure | 60 Hz 10, 25, 35, 50, 75 and 100 kV m⁻¹ Four 1 h exposures at 1 h intervals | Increased arousal during the first exposure to fields of 50 kV m⁻¹ and above; little effect during subsequent exposures. | | Rosenberg et al., 1983; Rosenberg, Duffy & Sacher, 1931 |
| Mice: exploratory activity in open field arena after exposure | 15, 30 and 50 Hz 50, 100, 400 V m⁻¹ 30 min / day for 5 days | No effect. | | Blackwell & Reed, 1985 |
| Baboons: social behaviour in 8 adult males | 60 Hz 30 kV m⁻¹ 12 h / day, 7 days / week for 6 weeks | Initally, exposed animals showed passive affinity (e.g. huddling), tension and stereotypy (e.g. scratching). | Indicative of stress. | Coelho, Easley & Rogers, 1991 |
| Baboons: social behaviour in 8 adult males | 60 Hz 60 kV m⁻¹ 12 h / day, 7 days / week for 6 weeks | Increased initial levels of passive affinity, tension and stereotypy. | Repeat of previous study using higher electric field strength. | Easley, Coelho & Rogers, 1991 |
| **ELF magnetic fields** | | | | |
| Rats: rearing, ambulatory and grooming behaviour in an open field arena after exposure. | 50 Hz 80 µT 4 h at beginning of light (quiet) period or dark (active) period | Increased rearing after exposure in quiet but not active period. No effects on ambulation or grooming. | Effect replicated in 2nd experiment. No sham exposed controls. | Rudolph et al., 1985 |

**Table 42. Continued**

| | | | |
|---|---|---|---|
| Rats: irritability, exploratory (open field) activity and locomotion | 50 Hz<br>18 mT<br>2 h / day for 20 days | Decrease in irritability, no effects on exploratory activity or locomotion. | Trzeciak et al., 1993 |
| Rats: open field behaviour | DC fields of 50 or 500 µT corresponding AC fields set for cyclotron resonance conditions for several ionic species | Reduced locomotor and exploratory behaviour during calcium ion resonance conditions; opposite effect for magnesium. | Zhadin, Deryugina & Pisagina, 1999 |

**ELF Electric and Magnetic Fields**

| | | | |
|---|---|---|---|
| Baboons: social behaviour in 8 adult males | 60 Hz<br>6 kV m⁻¹ and 50 µT<br>30 kV m⁻¹ and 100 µT<br>12 h / day, 7 days / week for 6 weeks | No effects on passive affinity, tension and stereotypy. | Coelho, Rogers & Easley, 1995 |

| | |
|---|---|
| Results contrast with effects of 50 Hz electric fields alone described above. | |

**Avoidance and aversion**

**ELF electric fields**

| | | | |
|---|---|---|---|
| Rats: avoidance behaviour in a shuttlebox (which has exposed and unexposed ends) | 60 Hz<br>25–105 kV m⁻¹<br>45 min / week for 4 weeks or once for 23.5 h | Significant preference for shielded region above 90 kV m⁻¹ (short exposure) or 75 kV m⁻¹ (long exposure). | Hjeresen et al., 1980 |
| Rats: taste aversion to electric field plus flavoured water | 60 Hz<br>50, 101 or 196 kV m⁻¹ (unperturbed fields)<br>20 min | No effect. | Creim et al., 1984 |
| | | Positive control with chemical inducer. | |
| Rats: avoidance behaviour in a shuttlebox | 60 Hz<br>30 kV m⁻¹<br>20 h | Significant preference for shielded region. | Hjeresen et al., 1982 |
| | | Follow on to chronic study. | |

149

**Table 42. Continued**

| | | | |
|---|---|---|---|
| Baboons: behavioural aversion through operant responses (lever press) to terminate exposure | 60 Hz<br>up to 65 kV m$^{-1}$ during testing | Field perceived but did not act as negative (aversive) re-inforcer. | No support for stress effect. | Rogers, Orr & Smith, 1995 |
| Baboons: behavioural aversion through operant responses (lever press) to terminate exposure | 60 Hz<br>90 or 100 kV m$^{-1}$<br>brief exposures | Exposure did not induce lever pressing (field termination) behaviour. | Incandescent lamp as positive control. | Stern & Laties, 1989 |
| **ELF magnetic fields** | | | | |
| Rats: avoidance behaviour in a shuttlebox | 60 Hz<br>3.03 mT<br>1 h | No effect. | | Lovely et al., 1992 |

## 5.4.3  Brain electrical activity

A number of animal studies have investigated if acute exposure to low frequency electric and magnetic fields can affect brain electrical activity demonstrated in the EEG or as evoked potentials following presentation of a sensory stimulus (e.g. Blackwell, 1986; Dowman et al., 1989, reviewed by NIEHS, 1998; Sienkiewicz, Saunders & Kowalczuk, 1991). The results of these studies are somewhat mixed and difficult to interpret, but none suggests any obvious hazard (ICNIRP, 2003). Some of these studies may have been confounded by experimental design: for example, it has long been recognised that recording electrical potentials through electrodes attached to the skull is liable to produce artefacts in the presence of EMFs. Two more recent studies reported significant EEG changes in rabbits during magnetic field exposure (Bell et al., 1992) and in rats following magnetic field exposure (Lyskov et al., 1993c). However, the possibility of an artefact or of false positive results complicates interpretation of both studies (NIEHS, 1998). A summary of studies on brain electrical activity in experimental animals exposed to ELF fields is given in Table 43.

**Table 43. Brain electrical activity**

| Endpoint | Exposure | Response | Comment | Authors |
|---|---|---|---|---|
| **ELF electric fields** | | | | |
| Rats: CNS neuronal activity in anaesthetised animals during exposure | 15, 30 and 50 Hz 100 V m$^{-1}$ (peak–peak) | No overall effect on firing rate; some synchrony at 15 and 30 Hz. | Anaesthesia-depressed responsiveness. | Blackwell, 1986 |
| **ELF magnetic fields** | | | | |
| Rabbits: EEG recordings during exposure | 5 Hz, 100 µT DC + 25 Hz, 64 µT 25 Hz, 1 µT | Increased EEG signal in response to 5 Hz. | Possibility of induction artefact. | Bell et al., 1992 |
| Rats: EEG recordings from Sprague-Dawley rats before and after exposure | 45 Hz 126 µT, intermittent 1.26 mT, 24 h exposure twice, 24 h apart | Dose-dependent increase in significant changes to EEG pattern following exposure. | Induced currents possibly increased due to permanent electrodes. | Lyskov et al., 1993c |
| **Electric & magnetic fields** | | | | |
| Macaque monkeys: auditory, visual and somatosensory evoked potentials recorded during "field off" period. | 60 Hz 3 kV m$^{-1}$ and 10 µT 10 kV m$^{-1}$ and 30 µT 30 kV m$^{-1}$ and 90 µT 3 weeks | Most measures unaffected. Decreased amplitude of late components of somatosensory evoked potentials. | | Dowman et al., 1989 |

151

## 5.4.4    *Neurotransmitter function*

A number of studies have investigated the potential of ELF fields to affect the levels of different neurotransmitters within various regions of the brain. Neurotransmitters are chemical substances released from nerve cells which enable the transmission of information to adjacent nerve cells equipped with appropriate receptors and may also have more widespread effects when released into the circulation. Different neurotransmitter systems are associated with different functions: the main groups are the cholinergic neurotransmitters such as acetylcholine, the biogenic amines comprising the catecholamines, including dopamine, norepinephrine (noradrenaline), epinephrine (adrenaline), and serotonin, the amino acid neurotransmitters such as glutamate and aspartate, and the peptide neurotransmitters such as the opioids. Most groups have important roles in brain function, the latter two almost exclusively so. Altered transmitter levels can be associated with functional changes but interpretation is usually difficult (NIEHS 1999).

These data have been most recently reviewed by ICNIRP (2003). Early studies (e.g. Vasquez et al., 1988; Zecca et al., 1991) reported effects of both acute and chronic exposure to intense electric fields on catecholamine and amino acid neurotransmitter levels in some parts of the brain, but values often stayed within the normal range. More recently, Margonato et al. (1995) reported that chronic exposure to 50 Hz magnetic fields at 5 μT had no effect on levels of norepinephrine, dopamine and its major metabolites, or 5-hydroxytryptamine or its major metabolite in the striatum, hypothalamus, hippocampus or cerebellum. However, in a companion study, Zecca et al. (1998) reported effects on norepinephrine levels in the pineal gland but not elsewhere in the brain following chronic exposure to combined electric and magnetic fields at either 1 kV m$^{-1}$ and 5 μT or 5 kV m$^{-1}$ and 100 μT. In addition, intensity-dependent changes were reported in the opioid receptor system in the frontal cortex, parietal cortex and hippocampus, but not in other brain areas investigated.

Other studies have also investigated field-dependent changes in opioid-related physiology in molluscs and in mammals. In a series of related experiments, Kavaliers, Prato and colleagues (e.g. Kavaliers & Ossenkopp, 1986a; Kavaliers & Ossenkopp, 1986b; Kavaliers, Ossenkopp & Hirst, 1984; Ossenkopp & Kavaliers, 1987) have indicated that various types of ELF magnetic fields may affect the endogenous opioid systems and modulate the response of both groups of animals to the analgesic effects of injected opiates such as morphine (reviewed by Kavaliers et al., 1994; Kavaliers & Ossenkopp, 1991). These responses are complex, and magnetic fields appear to have a differential effect on the functions of different opioid receptor subtypes. There is evidence that the mechanism for these effects may involve changes in calcium ion channel function in mice (Kavaliers et al., 1998) and in protein kinase C activity, nitric oxide (NO) release and NO synthase activity in the land snail *Cepaea nemoralis* (1998; Kavaliers, Ossenkopp & Tysdale, 1991). Further studies with land snails suggest that the field induced analgesic effects depend on the relative direction of the applied fields (Prato et al., 1995) as well as the presence of light (1997; Prato, Kavaliers & Carson, 1996; 2000).

In another series of experiments, it was reported that the acute exposure of rats to a 60 Hz magnetic field at 0.75 mT decreased activity in the cholinergic pathways in the frontal cortex and hippocampus (Lai et al., 1993). These effects were blocked by naltrexone, but not by naloxone methiodide, which was taken as evidence that magnetic fields affected endogenous opioids only within the central nervous system. Further studies showed the changes in cholinergic activity appeared to be mediated by activation of endogenous opioids (Lai, Carino & Ushijima, 1998). There also appears to be some interaction between exposure duration and field intensity, such that longer exposures (3 hours) at lower intensity fields (0.05 mT) could induce changes in cholinergic activity similar to those induced by shorter exposure at higher intensity (Lai & Carino, 1999).

Overall, limited changes in neurotransmitter levels in different parts of the rodent brain have been reported. Although of less direct relevance to human health, similar results have been reported in the molluscan nervous system. The biological significance of the changes seen in mammals is difficult to assess without corroborative changes in brain function and behaviour. However, several studies suggest possible EMF effects on the opioid and cholinergic systems which can be modulated by appropriate antagonists and should be studied further. Studies on the effects of ELF fields on neurotransmitters and analgesia are summarized in Table 44.

### 5.4.5    Cognitive function

Early studies with macaque monkeys reported that exposure to ELF electric fields at well below detection thresholds may affect operant performance (IARC, 2002; ICNIRP, 2003). However, well-conducted studies using baboons found that exposure to 60 Hz electric fields at 30 and 60 kV $m^{-1}$ had no sustained effect on the performance of two operant schedules (Rogers et al., 1995a; 1995b) although initial exposure may contribute towards producing a temporary interruption in responding.

Similarly, studies using 60 Hz electric and magnetic fields (Orr, Rogers & Smith, 1995b) indicated that combined exposure to 6 kV $m^{-1}$ and 50 µT or to 30 kV $m^{-1}$ and 100 µT had no effect on operant performance on a delayed match-to-sample task in baboons. This result is generally consistent with earlier results from other research groups using non-human primates (reviewed by ICNIRP, 2003; NIEHS, 1998; Sienkiewicz, Saunders & Kowalczuk, 1991). However, one study using rats (Salzinger et al., 1990) suggested exposure to 60 Hz fields of 30 kV $m^{-1}$ and 100 µT may exert subtle effects on performance that depend on the time of testing within the light-dark cycle.

**Table 44. Neurotransmitters and analgesia**

| Endpoint | Exposure | Response | Comment | Authors |
|---|---|---|---|---|
| **Neurotransmitters** | | | | |
| **ELF electric field** | | | | |
| Rats: biogenic amine levels in striatum, hypothalamus and hippocampus | 60 Hz 39 kV m$^{-1}$ 20 h / day, 4 weeks | No effects in hippocampus; some changes in striatum and hypothalamus. | | Vasquez et al., 1988 |
| Rats: amino acid levels in striatum | 50 Hz 25 and 100 kV m$^{-1}$ 8–22 h / day, 5–7 days/ week for 320, 640, 1240, or 1408 h | General increase after 320 h exposure; decreased levels after longer periods. | Observed values within normal range. Three replicate experiments. | Zecca et al., 1991 |
| **ELF magnetic field** | | | | |
| Rats: central cholinergic systems in brain | 60 Hz 0.5, 0.75, 1 mT 45 min | Reduced high-affinity choline uptake in frontal cortex and hippocampus. | Effect blocked by central but not peripheral opioid antagonists. | Lai et al., 1993 |
| Rats: biogenic amine levels in 4 regions of the brain | 50 Hz 5 µT 22 h / day, 32 weeks | No effect. | Two replicate experiments. | Margonato et al., 1995 |
| **ELF Electric and Magnetic Fields** | | | | |
| Rats: neurotransmitter and receptor levels in brain and pineal | 50 Hz 5 µT and 1 kV m$^{-1}$ 100 µT and 5 kV m$^{-1}$ 8 h / day, 5 days / week, 8 months | Increase in norepinephrine levels in the pineal gland; changes in the distribution of µ-opioid receptors in the brain. | | Zecca et al., 1998 |

**Table 44. Continued**

**Opioids and analgesia**

**ELF magnetic fields**

| | | | |
|---|---|---|---|
| Land snails: morphine-induced analgesia | 60 Hz<br>100 mT<br>2 h | Exposure-induced reduction in analgesia. | Effect enhanced by PKC activators. | Kavaliers & Ossenkopp, 1991 |
| Land snails: morphine-induced analgesia | 10–240 Hz<br>0–547 µT with parallel static magnetic field | Non-linear dose-response; frequency response relationships seen in analgesia reduction. | Results suggested direct effect of magnetic field. | Prato et al., 1995 |
| Land snails: morphine-induced analgesia | 60 Hz<br>141 µT<br>15 min | Exposure-induced reduction in analgesia. | Effects enhanced by NO releasing agent, and reduced by NO synthase inhibitor. | Kavaliers et al., 1998 |
| Land snails: morphine-induced analgesia | ELF magnetic fields consistent with the PRM for $Ca^{2+}$ or $K^+$ ions | Effects on morphine-induced analgesia consistent with PRM mechanism. | Effects dependent on the presence of light. | Prato, Kavaliers & Thomas, 2000 |
| Mice: morphine-induced analgesia | 0.5 Hz<br>150 µT – 9 mT in mid-light-phase and mid dark phase<br>5–10 days | Reduction in the increased night-time latency to respond to hot-plate. | Exposure system comprised motor-driven, rotating horseshoe permanent magnets. | Kavaliers, Ossenkopp & Hirst, 1984 |
| Mice: stress (restraint) induced analgesia and hyperactivity | 0.5 Hz<br>150 µT – 9 mT<br>30 min in mid-light-phase and mid dark phase | Reduction in the increased night-time latency and day-time activity. | As above; similar effect with opioid antagonist naloxone. | Kavaliers & Ossenkopp, 1986b |
| Mice: opioid-induced analgesia | 0.5 Hz<br>150 µT – 9 mT<br>60 min in mid-light-phase | Inhibition of daytime opioid analgesia. | As above; affects actions of mu, delta and kappa but not sigma agonists. | Kavaliers & Ossenkopp, 1986a |

155

**Table 44. Continued**

| | | | |
|---|---|---|---|
| Mice: morphine-induced analge-sia | 60 Hz<br>50, 100 or 150 µT<br>1 h | Dose-dependant reduction in analgesia. | | Ossenkopp & Kavaliers, 1987 |
| Mice: steroid-induced analgesia | 60 Hz<br>141 µT<br>30 min | Exposure-induced reduction in analgesia. | Effect blocked by calcium chan-nel antagonists. | Kavaliers, Wiebe & Ossenkopp, 1998 |
| Rat: central cholinergic systems in brain | 60 Hz<br>2 mT<br>1 h | Reduced high-affinity choline uptake in frontal cortex and hip-pocampus. | Effect blocked by mu- and delta-opiate antagonists. | Lai, Carino & Ushijima, 1998 |
| Rat: central cholinergic systems in brain | 60 Hz<br>0.5, 1.0, 1.5 or 2.0 mT, 1 h<br>1.0 mT, 30, 45, 60 or 90 min | High-affinity choline uptake in frontal cortex and hippocampus reduced. | Reduction occurs in intensity and duration-dependent manner. | Lai & Carino, 1999 |

Several recent studies using the Morris water maze or radial arm maze have investigated the effects of magnetic fields on spatial memory and place learning. These studies provide evidence that exposure of rats, mice or voles to power frequency fields at ~100 μT and above may modulate task performance (Kavaliers & Ossenkopp, 1993 Kavaliers et al., 1996; Lai, 1996; Lai, Carino & Ushijima, 1998; Sienkiewicz et al., 1998; Sienkiewicz, Haylock & Saunders, 1998). Exposure to complex pulsed magnetic fields may also affect performance (McKay & Persinger, 2000; Thomas & Persinger, 1997). In addition, much evidence has accrued over the last decade that effects may also occur using specific combinations of static and time-varying fields (see Sienkiewicz, Haylock & Saunders, 1998). The mechanism for these effects has been partly explored and the changes in behaviour have been attributed to decreases in cholinergic functions caused by field-induced changes in endogenous opioid activity (Lai, 1996; Lai, Carino & Ushijima, 1998; Thomas & Persinger, 1997).

The conditions to produce any of these phenomena are not well defined, and both deficits and enhancements in performance have been observed and one study did not report any field-dependent effects (Sienkiewicz, Haylock & Saunders, 1996). It is feasible that these differences in outcome may depend on experimental or other variables including the timing and duration of exposure relative to learning (McKay & Persinger, 2000; Sienkiewicz et al., 2001). While these results suggest that the neural representations or processes underlying the performance of spatial memory tasks may be vulnerable to the effects of magnetic fields, some part of the observed outcome may be attributable to changes in arousal (IARC, 2002; ICNIRP, 2003) or in motivation (Thomas & Persinger, 1997). Nevertheless, the transient nature and small magnitudes of the responses do not suggest an obvious deleterious effect.

Two studies using rodents have investigated the effects of magnetic fields on recognition memory. Using the field conditions putatively identified as having an acute effect of spatial memory, Sienkiewicz et al. (2001) found no effects on the performance of an object recognition task by mice. Animals were exposed for 45 minutes to a 50 Hz field at 7.5, 75 or 750 μT. However, Mostafa, Mostafa & Ennaceur et al. (2002) reported that discrimination between familiar and novel objects was impaired in rats following chronic exposure at 200 μT for 2 weeks.

Stern et al. (1996) failed to replicate the results of earlier studies (Liboff, McLeod & Smith, 1989; Thomas, Schrot & Liboff, 1986) suggesting exposure to combined static and power frequency magnetic fields, arranged to simulate the cyclotron resonance conditions for lithium ions, significantly impaired operant performance. The earlier positive results were attributed to possible confounding.

A summary of studies on cognitive function in animals is given in Table 45.

**Table 45. Cognitive function**

| Endpoint | Exposure | Response | Comment | Authors |
|---|---|---|---|---|
| **Spatial memory** | | | | |
| **ELF magnetic fields** | | | | |
| Meadow voles and deer mice: water maze performance | 60 Hz 100 µT 5 min during task acquisition | Enhanced performance opiate-induced reduction abolished by magnetic field exposure in deer mice. | Suggests magnetic field reduces opiate activity. | Kavaliers & Ossenkopp, 1993 Kavaliers et al., 1996 |
| Rats: radial arm maze performance | 60 Hz 750 µT 45 min prior to behavioural testing | Performance reduced. Effect abolished by cholinergic antagonist. | Suggests magnetic field reduces cholinergic activity. | Lai, 1996 |
| Mice: radial arm maze performance | 50 Hz 5, 50 or 500 µT or 5 mT during behavioural testing (up to 15 min) | No effect. | | Sienkiewicz, Haylock & Saunders, 1996 |
| Rats: radial arm maze with operant task at the end of each arm | Pulsed (burst firing pattern for 1 sec every 3 sec) 1–4 µT 5 or 30 min immediately or 30 min after 8 training sessions | Some differences were seen between the exposed and sham exposed animals. | Small number of animals; complex post hoc interpretation of data. | Thomas & Persinger, 1997 |
| Rats: water maze performance | 60 Hz 1 mT 1 h prior to behavioural testing | No effect on performance but retention impaired. | Reduced swim speed. | Lai, Carino & Ushijima, 1998 |
| Mice: radial arm maze performance | 50 Hz 7.5, 75, or 750 µT or 7.5 mT prior to behavioural testing | No overall effect but transiently reduced acquisition rate. | No effect on movement or motivation. | Sienkiewicz et al., 1998; 1998 |
| Rats: complex radial maze performance | A complex low intensity magnetic field of between 200–500 nT for 1 h of a 2 h period between training and testing | Exposure immediately after training impaired spatial memory and those immediately before testing impaired motivation. | | McKay & Persinger, 2000 |

**Table 45. Continued**

| | | | | |
|---|---|---|---|---|
| Mice: spontaneous object recognition task | 50 Hz 7.5, 75, or 750 µT between initial testing and re-testing | No significant field-dependent effects. | | McKay & Persinger, 2000 Sienkiewicz et al., 2001 |
| Rats: spontaneous object recognition task | 50 Hz 200 µT 1 or 2 weeks | Significant decrease in discrimination between familiar and novel objects. | Significant corticosterone elevation in exposed animals. | Mostafa, Mostafa & Ennaceur, 2002 |

**Operant behaviour**

**ELF electric fields**

| | | | |
|---|---|---|---|
| Baboons: multiple FR (fast) and DRL (slow) schedules | 60 Hz 30 or 60 kV m$^{-1}$ 6 weeks during behavioural testing | Exposure on day 1 induced temporary work stoppage. | Rogers et al., 1995a |

**Static and ELF magnetic fields**

| | | | | |
|---|---|---|---|---|
| Rats: multiple FR (fast) and DRL (slow) schedules | Static field of 26 µT plus 60 Hz field of up to 200 µT 30 min prior to operant testing | DRL response impaired; temporal discrimination reduced. | Cyclotron resonance conditions for lithium. | Thomas, Schrot & Liboff, 1986 Liboff, McLeod & Smith, 1989 |
| Rats: multiple FR (fast) and DRL (slow) schedules | Static field of 26 or 27 µT plus 60 Hz field of 50 or 70 µT 30 min prior to behavioural testing | No effect. | Attempted replication of Thomas et al. 1986, | Stern et al., 1996 |

**ELF electric and magnetic fields**

| | | | | |
|---|---|---|---|---|
| Rats: multiple random interval (RI) schedule in adult males exposed perinatally followed by extinction and reconditioning | 60 Hz 100 µT, 30 kV m$^{-1}$ 20 h / day, 22 days in utero and 8 days post-natally | Reduced performance in exposed rats. | Two replicate studies. | Salzinger et al., 1990 |
| Baboons: delayed match-to-sample procedure (light-flash stimulus) | 60 Hz 6 kV m$^{-1}$, 50 µT 30 kV m$^{-1}$, 100 µT 6 weeks during behavioural testing | No effect. | | Orr, Rogers & Smith, 1995b |

## 5.5    Conclusions

Exposure of volunteers to power frequency electric fields causes well-defined biological responses, ranging from perception to annoyance, through surface electric-charge effects. These responses depend on field strength, ambient environmental conditions, and individual sensitivity. The thresholds for direct perception by 10% of volunteers varied between 2 and 20 kV m$^{-1}$, while 5% found 15–20 kV m$^{-1}$ annoying. The spark discharge from a person to ground is found to be painful by 7% of volunteers in a field of 5 kV m$^{-1}$. Thresholds for the discharge from an object through a grounded person depend on the size of the object and therefore require specific assessment.

High field strength, rapidly pulsed magnetic fields can stimulate peripheral or central nerve tissue; such effects can arise during MRI exposure and are used in transcranial magnetic stimulation. Threshold induced electric field strengths for direct nerve stimulation could be as low as a few volts per metre. The threshold is likely to be constant over a frequency range between a few hertz and a few kilohertz. People suffering from or predisposed to epilepsy are likely to be more susceptible to induced ELF electric fields in the CNS. Furthermore, sensitivity to electrical stimulation of the CNS seems likely to be associated with a family history of seizure and the use of tricyclic antidepressants, neuroleptic agents and other drugs that lower the seizure threshold.

The function of the retina, which is part of the CNS, can be affected by exposure to much weaker ELF magnetic fields than those that cause direct nerve stimulation. A flickering light sensation, called magnetic phosphenes or magnetophosphenes, results from the interaction of the induced electric field with electrically excitable cells in the retina. Threshold electric field strengths in the extracellular fluid of the retina have been estimated to lie between about 10–100 mV m$^{-1}$ at 20 Hz. There is, however, considerable uncertainty attached to these values.

The evidence for other neurobehavioural effects in volunteer studies, such as the effects on brain electrical activity, cognition, sleep, hypersensitivity and mood, is less clear. Generally, such studies have been carried out at exposure levels below those required to induce effects described above, and have produced evidence only of subtle and transitory effects at best. The conditions necessary to elicit such responses are not well defined at present. There is some evidence suggesting the existence of field-dependent effects on reaction time and reduced accuracy in the performance of some cognitive tasks, which is supported by the results of studies on the gross electrical activity of the brain. Studies investigating EMF-induced changes in sleep quality have reported inconsistent results. It is possible that these differences may be attributable in part to differences in the design of the studies.

Some people claim to be hypersensitive to EMF. However, the evidence from double blind provocation studies suggests that the reported symptoms are unrelated to EMF exposure.

There is only inconsistent and inconclusive evidence that exposure to ELF electric and magnetic fields causes depressive symptoms or suicide. Thus, the evidence is considered inadequate.

In animals, the possibility that exposure to ELF fields may affect neurobehavioral functions has been explored from a number of perspectives using a range of exposure conditions. Few robust effects have been established. There is convincing evidence that power-frequency electric fields can be detected by animals, most likely as a result of surface charge effects, and may induce transient arousal or mild stress. In rats, the detection range is between 3 and 13 kV m$^{-1}$. Rodents have been shown to be aversive to field strengths greater than 50 kV m$^{-1}$. Other possible field-dependent changes are less well-defined and generally laboratory studies have only produced evidence of subtle and transitory effects. There is some evidence that exposure to magnetic fields may modulate the functions of the opioid and cholinergic systems, and this is supported by the results of studies investigating the effects on analgesia and on the acquisition and performance of spatial memory tasks.

# 6 NEUROENDOCRINE SYSTEM

The pineal and pituitary neuroendocrine glands, both situated in the brain and intimately connected with and controlled by the nervous system, release hormones into the blood stream which exert a profound influence on body metabolism and physiology, particularly during development and reproduction, partly via their influence on the release of hormones from other endocrine glands situated elsewhere in the body. These studies have been reviewed by NIEHS (1998), IARC (2002), McKinlay et al. (2004) and recently by AGNIR (2006).

The hypothesis, first suggested by Stevens (1987), that exposure to EMFs might reduce melatonin secretion and thereby increase the risk of breast cancer has stimulated a number of human laboratory studies and investigations of circulating melatonin levels in people exposed to EMFs in domestic or occupational situations.

## 6.1 Volunteer studies

The majority of studies have investigated the effects of EMF exposure, mostly to power frequencies, on circulating levels of the pineal hormone melatonin (or on the urinary excretion of a metabolite of melatonin). Fewer studies have been carried out on circulating levels of pituitary hormones or other hormones released from other endocrine glands such as the thyroid gland, adrenal cortex and reproductive organs.

### 6.1.1 The pineal hormone: melatonin

Melatonin is produced by the pineal gland in the brain in a distinct daily or circadian rhythm which is governed by day length. It is implicated in the control of daily activities such as the sleep/wake cycle and in seasonal rhythms such as those of reproduction in animals that show annual cycles of fertility and infertility. Maximum serum levels occur during the night, and minimum levels during the day, even in nocturnally active animals. Night-time peak values of serum melatonin in humans, however, can vary up to ten-fold between individuals (Graham et al., 1996). It has been suggested that melatonin has a negative impact on human reproductive physiology, but that any changes are slight compared to those seen in experimental animals (Reiter, 1997). However, the overall evidence suggests that human melatonin rhythms are not significantly delayed or suppressed by exposure to magnetic fields (AGNIR, 2001b; IARC 2002; ICNIRP, 2003; NIEHS, 1998; although see Karasek & Lerchl, 2002).

#### 6.1.1.1 Laboratory studies

Several laboratory studies have been carried out in which volunteers, screened for various factors which might have influenced melatonin levels, were exposed or sham exposed overnight to circularly or horizontally polarized intermittent or continuous power-frequency magnetic fields. No significant effects of exposure on night-time serum melatonin levels were found (Crasson et al., 2001; Graham et al., 1996; Graham, Cook & Riffle,

162

1997; Kurokawa et al., 2003a; Selmaoui, Lambrozo & Touitou, 1996; Warman et al., 2003a). Other studies, using the excretion of the major urinary metabolite of melatonin as a surrogate measures of serum melatonin, also found no effect (Åkerstedt et al., 1999; Crasson et al., 2001; Graham et al., 2001a; Graham et al., 2001b; Selmaoui, Lambrozo & Touitou, 1996). The use of the urinary excretion data complicates interpretation, however, since information regarding any possible phase shift in melatonin production is lost. Griefahn (2001; 2002) found no effect of exposure to 16.7 Hz magnetic fields on hourly saliva melatonin concentration.

Some positive effects have been reported, but these have generally not proved consistent. An initial report (Graham et al., 1996) of a magnetic field-induced reduction of night-time serum melatonin levels in volunteers with low basal melatonin levels was not confirmed using a larger number of volunteers. It is possible that the initial positive findings were due to chance with a relatively small number of subjects. However, the results of a study investigating the effects of night-time exposure to 60 Hz fields for four nights (Graham et al., 2000b) suggested a weak cumulative effect of exposure. Exposed subjects showed more intra-individual variability in the overnight levels of excretion of melatonin or its major metabolite on night 4, although there was no overall effect on levels of melatonin.

Wood et al. (1998) exposed or sham exposed male subjects to an intermittent, circularly-polarised, power-frequency magnetic field at various times during the dusk or night and measured the effect on night-time serum melatonin levels. The results indicated that exposure prior to the night-time rise in serum melatonin may have delayed the onset of the rise by about half an hour and may have reduced peak levels, possibly in a sensitive sub-group of the study population. However, exposure categorisation was made post-hoc (Wood et al., 1998) and the result can only be considered to be exploratory.

### 6.1.1.2 Residential and occupational studies

Several studies of responses have been carried out in people in residential or occupational situations. These are naturally more realistic than laboratory studies but suffer from diminished control of possible confounding factors, such as differences in lifestyle (Warman et al., 2003b). With regard to domestic exposure, one study (Wilson et al., 1990) has examined the possible effects on volunteers exposed at home to pulsed EMFs generated by mains or DC-powered electric blankets over a 6–10 week period. Overall, no effect of exposure was seen on the urinary excretion of the major urinary metabolite of melatonin (aMT6s). However, transient increases in night-time excretion were seen in the periods following the onset of a period of electric blanket use and following the cessation of the period of electric blanket use in seven of 28 users of one type of electric blanket. This observation may, however, be rather weak given the lack of correspondence of the effect with field condition and the fact that responsiveness was only identified following the separate analysis of the excretion data from each of 42 volunteers, of which some analyses may have turned out positive by chance (Hong et al., 2001). In contrast, Hong et al. (2001) found no significant field dependent effects on melatonin rhythms in nine men following 11 weeks of night-time exposure. In this study, the urinary excretion of aMT6s was followed in five urine samples collected each day. This study too, however, exercised very little control over possible confounding by environmental and lifestyle factors.

Several more recent studies relating to residential exposure have been carried out. Davis et al. (2001) reported lower nocturnal levels of melatonin, measured as the excretion of aMT6s, in women with a history of breast cancer to be associated with higher bedroom magnetic field levels, once adjustment had been made for hours of daylight, age, body mass index, current alcohol consumption and the use of certain medications. Levallois et al. (2001) found no relation of night-time excretion of aMT6s to proximity of the residence to power lines or to EMF exposure. There were, however, significantly stronger relations to age and obesity (out of five variables for which the authors investigated effect modification) in women who lived close to power lines than in those who lived more distantly. In a general review of all these studies, IARC (2002) concluded that it was difficult to distinguish between the effects of magnetic fields and those of other environmental factors. In a later study, Youngstedt et al. (2002) found no significant associations between several measures of magnetic field exposure in bed (but not elsewhere) and various measures of the urinary excretion of aMT6s in 242 adults, mostly women, aged 50–81.

A number of other studies have examined urinary metabolite excretion in occupationally exposed workers. For railway workers, Pfluger & Minder (1996) reported that early evening aMT6s excretion (taken as an index of daytime serum melatonin levels) but not early morning excretion was decreased in exposed workers. However, the authors noted that the effects of differences in daylight exposure, which suppresses night-time melatonin, could not be excluded. In a study of electric utility workers, Burch et al. (1998; 1999) found no overall effect of exposure on night-time aMT6s excretion (taken as an index of night-time melatonin levels) when considering mean levels of exposure. The authors did find lower levels of night-time excretion in individuals exposed to temporally more stable magnetic fields, raising some questions as to the interpretation of these data. A reduction in melatonin levels was found to be associated with working near 3-phase conductors and not near 1-phase conductors, indicating a possible role of field polarisation (Burch et al., 2000). Burch, Reif & Jost (1999) also found that reduction of aMT6s excretion was associated with high geomagnetic activity. Juutilainen et al. (2000) found that occupational exposure to magnetic fields produced by sewing machines did not affect the ratio of Friday morning/Monday morning levels of aMT6s excretion, suggesting that weekends without workplace exposure did not change melatonin response. Average Thursday night excretion (Friday morning sample) was lower in exposed compared to control workers.

In a study of a further group of male electrical utility workers, Burch et al. (2002) investigated nocturnal excretion of aMT6s in men with high compared with low or medium workplace 60-Hz exposure. After adjusting for light exposure at work, reduced melatonin levels were found within men with high cellular phone use; the effect was not present in those with medium or no such phone use. Touitou et al. (2003) found no effect on serum melatonin levels or the overnight excretion of urinary aMT6s in workers at a high voltage substations chronically exposed to 50 Hz magnetic fields compared to white collar workers from the same company.

A preliminary study by Arnetz & Berg (1996) of daytime serum melatonin levels in visual display units (VDU) workers (sex not given) exposed to ELF and other frequency electromagnetic fields (values not given) reported a slightly larger decrease during VDU work compared to leisure time. The biological significance of this small daytime effect is not at all clear, given that serum melatonin peaks during the night.

In a study by Lonne-Rahm et al. (2000), 24 patients with electromagnetic hypersensitivity and 12 controls were exposed to a combination of stress situations and electric and magnetic fields from a VDU. Blood samples were drawn for circulating levels of stress-related hormones (melatonin, prolactin, adrenocorticotrophic hormone, neuropeptide Y and growth hormone). In double-blind tests, none of these parameters responded to the fields, neither alone nor in combination with stress levels.

Table 46 summarizes the human melatonin studies.

### 6.1.2 Pituitary and other hormones

Few studies of EMF effects on hormones of the pituitary and other endocrine glands have been carried out. Principal pituitary hormones investigated in EMF studies include several hormones involved in growth and body physiology, particularly thyroid-stimulating hormone (TSH) which controls the function of the thyroid gland and the release of thyroxin; adrenocorticotropic hormone (ACTH), which regulates the function of the adrenal cortex and particularly the release of cortisol; and growth hormone (GH), which affects body growth. Hormones released by the pituitary which have important sexual and reproductive functions have also been studied, particularly follicle stimulating hormone (FSH), luteinising hormone (LH) and prolactin. Both FSH and LH influence the function of the testis and the release of testosterone.

Three laboratory studies have investigated the possible effects of acute exposure to power-frequency magnetic fields and power-frequency electric and magnetic fields on TSH, thyroxin, GH, cortisol, FSH, LH and testosterone in men (Maresh et al., 1988; Selmaoui, Lambrozo & Touitou, 1997) and GH, cortisol and prolactin in men and women (Åkerstedt et al., 1999). Overall, no effects were found.

An occupational study (Gamberale et al., 1989) of linesmen working on "live" or "dead" 400-kV power lines found no effect of combined

**Table 46. Human melatonin studies**

| Endpoint | Exposure | Response | Comment | Authors |
|---|---|---|---|---|
| **ELF magnetic fields** | | | | |
| *Laboratory studies* | | | | |
| Night-time serum melatonin levels | 60 Hz 1 or 20 µT, intermittent 8 h at night | No effect. Possible effect on low melatonin subjects not replicated in larger study. | Well described and well planned double blind study. | Graham et al., 1996 |
| Night-time serum melatonin levels | 60 Hz 20 µT, continuous 8 h at night | No effect. | Well described and well planned double blind study. | Graham, Cook & Riffle, 1997 |
| Night-time serum melatonin levels and excretion of its major urinary metabolite (aMT6s). | 50 Hz 10 µT, continuous or intermittent 9 h at night | No effect. | Well described and well planned double blind study. | Selmaoui, Lambrozo & Touitou, 1996 |
| Night-time serum melatonin levels | 50 Hz 20 µT, sinusoidal or square wave field, intermittent 1.5–4 h at night | Possible delay and reduction of night-time melatonin levels in sub-group. | Double blind study; incomplete volunteer participation. | Wood et al., 1998 |
| Night-time serum melatonin levels | 50 Hz 1 µT during sleep (24.00 to 08.00 h) | No effect. | Double blind study. | Åkerstedt et al., 1999 |
| Night-time serum melatonin levels and excretion of aMT6s. | 60 Hz 28.3 µT, continuous 8 h at night | No effect. | Well described and well planned double blind study. | Graham et al., 2000b |
| Night-time serum melatonin levels and excretion of aMT6s | 50 Hz 100 µT, continuous or intermittent 30 min | No effect. | Well described and well planned double blind study. | Crasson et al., 2001 |

166

**Table 46. Continued**

| | | | |
|---|---|---|---|
| Night-time serum melatonin levels in women | 60 Hz<br>28.3 μT, intermittent<br>8 h at night | No effect. | Well described and well planned double blind study. | Graham et al., 2001a |
| Night-time serum melatonin levels and excretion of aMT6s | 60 Hz<br>127 μT, continuous or intermittent<br>8 h at night | No effect. | Well described and well planned double blind study. | Graham et al., 2001b |
| Night-time serum melatonin levels and excretion of aMT6s | 60 Hz<br>28.3 μT, continuous<br>8 h at night | No effect. | Well described and well planned double blind study. | Graham et al., 2001c |
| Salivary melatonin levels | 16.7 Hz<br>200 μT<br>6 h at night | No effect. | Well described and well planned double blind study. | Griefahn et al., 2001 |
| Salivary melatonin levels | 16.7 Hz<br>200 μT<br>6 h at night | No effect. | Well described and well planned double blind study. | Griefahn et al., 2002 |
| Night-time serum melatonin levels | 50 Hz<br>20 μT, linearly polarised<br>8 h at night | No effect. | Well described and well planned double blind study. | Kurokawa et al., 2003a |
| Night-time serum melatonin levels | 50 Hz<br>200 or 300 μT<br>2 h at night across rising phase of melatonin secretion | No effect. | Well described and well planned double blind study. | Warman et al., 2003a |

**ELF electric and magnetic fields**

*Domestic occupational studies*

| | | | |
|---|---|---|---|
| Early morning excretion of urinary aMT6s | 60 Hz<br>EMFs generated by pulsed AC or DC current supply to electric blankets<br>7–10 weeks at night | No overall effect; transient increases in 7/28 users of one type of blanket. | Realistic, but concomitant lack of control over lifestyle etc. | Wilson et al., 1990 |

167

**Table 46. Continued**

| | | | | |
|---|---|---|---|---|
| Urinary excretion of aMT6s collected 5 times per day | 50 Hz ~1–8 µT, electric 'sheet' over the body 11 weeks at night | No effect. | The only restriction on each subject's usual daily activities were avoiding overeating and strenuous exercise. | Hong et al., 2001 |
| Morning and evening urinary excretion of aMT6s in railway workers. | 16.7 Hz approximately 20 µT mean value in engine drivers | Decreased evening 6-aMT6s levels but no effect on morning levels. No dose-response effect. | Subjects acted as own controls; samples collected early autumn; fully described protocol. | Pfluger & Minder, 1996 |
| Night-time and early morning urinary excretion of aMT6s in electric utility workers | 60 Hz ~0.1–0.2 µT 24 hr at work, home and during sleep | No overall effect with exposure. Temporally more stable fields at home (using calculated index) associated with reduced nocturnal melatonin. | Well described study; some adjustment for age, month of participation and light exposure. | Burch et al, 1998 |
| Post work urinary excretion of aMT6s electric utility workers | 60 Hz occupational exposure over a week | No overall effect. Reduction in aMT6s excretion in workers exposed to more stable fields during work. | Significant interaction with occupational light exposure. | Burch et al., 1999 |
| Night-time urinary excretion of aMT6s in electric utility workers | 60 Hz occupational exposure to magnetic fields | Exposure-related reduction in aMT6s excretion in workers exposed in substations or 3 phase environments for > 2 h. | Adjusted for workplace light exposure. | Burch et al., 2000 |
| Night-time urinary excretion of aMT6s in garment workers | 50 Hz occupational exposure to magnetic fields | Average aMT6s excretion lower in exposed workers compared to office workers. | No difference in Friday to Monday levels | Juutilainen et al., 2000 |
| Night-time urinary excretion of aMT6s | 50 Hz proximity to power lines and/or exposure to domestic EMFs | No overall effect. Significantly stronger association with age and obesity in women living closer to power lines. | Adjusted for confounders. | Levallois et al., 2001 |

168

**Table 46. Continued**

| | | | | |
|---|---|---|---|---|
| Night-time urinary excretion of aMT6s | 60 Hz domestic exposure to magnetic fields | Borderline association with one measure of exposure in a subgroup of women. | Significant association with day length. | Davis et al., 2001 |
| Night-time urinary excretion of aMT6s in electric utility workers | 60 Hz occupational exposure to magnetic fields | Exposure-related reduction in aMT6s excretion in highly exposed workers associated with mobile phone use. | Not present in workers with low or medium phone use. | Burch et al., 2002 |
| 24 hr urinary excretion of aMT6s | 60 Hz domestic exposure to magnetic fields measured in the bedroom only | No significant associations between exposure and excretion. | Potential confounders such as lighting, age and medication taken into account. | Youngstedt et al., 2002 |
| Serum melatonin levels and urinary excretion of aMT6s in high-voltage sub-station workers | Geometric mean fields of 0.1–2.6 μT chronic occupational exposure (1–20 y) | No effect compared to levels in white-collar workers. | Considerable care taken to avoid some confounders, e.g. study participants all non-smokers. | Touitou et al., 2003 |

**ELF and VLF electric and magnetic fields**

*Occupational studies*

| | | | | |
|---|---|---|---|---|
| Morning and afternoon serum melatonin levels in VDU workers during one working and one leisure day. | Exposure details not given | Decrease in serum melatonin during the day was statistically significant at work (-0.9 ng/l) but not leisure (-0.8 ng/l). | Samples collected Oct – Feb. Experimental protocol briefly described. No measured fields; no control over lifestyle etc. | Arnetz & Berg, 1996 |
| Circulating levels of stress-related hormones (melatonin, prolactin, ACTH, neuropeptide Y and growth hormone) | 24 patients with electromagnetic hypersensitivity and 12 controls electric and magnetic fields from a VDU | No effect. | Double blind study. | Lonne-Rahm et al., 2000 |

electric and magnetic field exposure over a working day on daytime levels of serum TSH, cortisol, FSH, prolactin, LH and testosterone. A preliminary study (Arnetz & Berg, 1996) of VDU workers (sex not specified) exposed to ELF electric and magnetic fields (exposure not given) reported elevated ACTH levels at work compared to leisure time; an effect, as the authors note, which is probably attributable to work-related factors other than EMFs.

The studies on the effects of ELF on the human pituitary and endocrine system are summarized in Table 47.

**Table 47. Human pituitary and other endocrine studies**

| Endpoint | Exposure | Response | Comment | Authors |
|---|---|---|---|---|
| **ELF magnetic fields** | | | | |
| *Laboratory studies* | | | | |
| Night-time serum levels of TSH, thyroxin, cortisol, FSH and LH in young men | 50 Hz 10 µT, continuous or intermittent overnight from 23.00 to 08.00 h | No differences between exposed and sham-exposed. | Well designed, double-blind study. | Selmaoui, Lambrozo & Touitou, 1997 |
| Night-time levels of GH, cortisol and prolactin in men and women | 50 Hz 1 µT during sleep (24.00 to 08.00 h) | No effect. | Double blind study. | Åkerstedt et al., 1999 |
| **ELF electric and magnetic fields** | | | | |
| *Laboratory study* | | | | |
| GH, cortisol and testosterone in young men | 60 Hz 9 kV m$^{-1}$ and 20 µT 2 h following 45 min rest | No effect. | Double-blind study. | Maresh et al., 1988 |
| *Occupational studies* | | | | |
| Day-time serum TSH, cortisol, FSH, prolactin, LH, and testosterone in linesmen working on "live" and "dead" 400 kV power lines | 50 Hz 2.8 kV m$^{-1}$ and 23.3 µT 4.5 h during working day | No effect. | Counterbalanced presentation of "live" and "dead" power lines. | Gamberale et al., 1989 |
| Morning and afternoon serum ACTH levels in VDU workers during one working and one leisure day | Exposure details not given. | Increase in serum ACTH during the day was statistically significant at work (0.6 pmol/l). but not leisure (0.1 pmol/l) | Samples collected Oct – Feb. Experimental protocol briefly described. No measured fields; no control over lifestyle etc. | Arnetz & Berg, 1996 |

## 6.2 Animal studies

A large number of studies have been carried out investigating the effects of EMF on circulating melatonin levels in animals, because of the possible links between EMF and breast cancer. The impact of melatonin on reproduction is particularly pronounced in seasonally breeding animals, where the effect varies depending on the length of gestation in order to ensure that the offspring are born in late spring when food is plentiful. Thus, for melatonin, the studies have been subdivided into those on laboratory rodents, which have short gestational periods and seasonally breeding animals and primates, which are more closely related to humans.

### 6.2.1 Melatonin

As indicated above, Stevens (1987) first suggested that chronic exposure to electric fields may reduce melatonin secretion by the pineal gland and increase the risk of breast cancer. This followed reports particularly by Wilson et al. (1981) of a significant overall reduction in pineal melatonin in rats chronically exposed to 60 Hz electric fields and by Tamarkin et al. (1981) and Shah, Mhatre & Kothari (1984) of increased DMBA-induced mammary carcinogenesis in rats with reduced melatonin levels. However, the significance of these observations for humans is not clearly established.

#### 6.2.1.1 Laboratory rodents

Few studies have been carried out using mice. In a study by Picazo et al. (1998) a significant reduction in the night-time serum melatonin levels of mice exposed up to sexual maturity for four generations to power frequency magnetic fields was observed.

A great many more studies have been carried out using rats. The effects of electric fields were investigated before interest turned predominantly to magnetic fields. Several studies by one group of authors (Reiter et al., 1988; Wilson et al., 1981; Wilson et al., 1983; Wilson, Chess & Anderson, 1986) reported that the exposure to electric fields significantly suppressed pineal melatonin and the activity of the N-acetyl-transferase enzyme (NAT) important in the synthesis of melatonin in the pineal gland. This effect was transient, appearing within three weeks of exposure but recovered within three days following the cessation of exposure. Subsequently, however, the same laboratory (Sasser et al., 1991) reported in an abstract that it was unable to reproduce the E-field-induced reduction in pineal melatonin. Another laboratory (Grota et al., 1994) also reported that exposure to power-frequency electric fields had no effect on pineal melatonin levels or NAT activity, although serum melatonin levels were significantly depressed.

Further work used rats to investigate the effect of exposure to power-frequency magnetic fields. An early study by Martínez-Soriano et al. (1992) was inconclusive because of technical difficulties. A more extensive series of tests has been carried out by Kato et al. (1993; 1994a; 1994b; 1994c; 1994d, summarized in Kato & Shigemitsu, 1997). They studied the effects of exposure to circularly- or linearly-polarised power-frequency magnetic fields of up to 250 μT for up to 6 weeks on pineal and serum melatonin levels in male rats. These authors reported that exposure to circularly polarised but not linearly polarised field reduced night-time serum and pineal melatonin levels. However, a major difficulty with the interpretation of many of the studies by this group was that the sham-exposed groups were sometimes treated as a "low dose" exposed groups because they were exposed to stray magnetic fields (of less than 2%) generated by the exposure system. Thus, statistical comparison was sometimes made with historical controls. Such procedures fail to allow for the inter-experimental variability that was reported in replicate studies by Kato & Shigemitsu (1997). Results from four further groups who have investigated magnetic-field effects on serum and pineal melatonin levels in rats (Bakos et al., 1995; Bakos et al., 1997; Bakos et al., 1999; John, Liu & Brown, 1998; Löscher, Mevissen & Lerchl, 1998; Mevissen, Lerchl & Löscher, 1996; Selmaoui & Touitou, 1995; Selmaoui & Touitou, 1999) were inconsistent but mostly negative.

Table 48 summarizes the studies into effects of ELF fields on melatonin in experimental animals.

## 6.2.1.2 Seasonal breeders

Four different laboratories have investigated the effects of EMF exposure on pineal activity, serum melatonin levels and reproductive development in animals which breed seasonally. A series of studies by Yellon and colleagues (Truong, Smith & Yellon, 1996; Truong & Yellon, 1997; Yellon, 1994; Yellon, 1996; Yellon & Truong, 1998) investigated magnetic field exposure of Djungarian hamsters in which the duration of melatonin secretion during the shortening days of autumn and winter inhibit reproductive activity. These authors reported that a brief exposure to a power-frequency magnetic field 2 h before the onset of darkness reduced and delayed the night-time rise in serum and pineal melatonin. In expanded replicate studies no reduction in melatonin was observed and no effect was seen on reproductive development. In contrast to this work, Niehaus et al. (1997) reported that the chronic exposure of Djungarian hamsters to "rectangular" power-frequency magnetic fields resulted in increased testis cell numbers and night-time levels of serum melatonin. However, the results are not easy to interpret: increased melatonin levels in the Djungarian hamster are usually accompanied by decreased testicular activity. Wilson et al. (1999) investigated the effect of exposure to power-frequency magnetic fields on pineal melatonin levels, serum prolactin levels and testicular and seminal vesicle weights in Djungarian hamsters moved to a "short day" light regime in order to induce sexual regression. Night-time pineal melatonin levels were reduced following acute exposure but this effect diminished with prolonged exposure. In contrast, induced sexual regression, as indicated by the testicular and seminal vesicle weights, seemed to be enhanced rather than diminished by prolonged magnetic field exposure, suggesting a possible stress response.

**Table 48. Melatonin studies in laboratory rodents**

| Endpoint | Exposure | Response | Comment | Authors |
|---|---|---|---|---|
| **ELF electric fields** | | | | |
| *Rats* | | | | |
| Night-time pineal melatonin levels and NAT enzyme activity in adult rats | 60 Hz 1.7–1.9 kV m⁻¹ (not 65 kV m⁻¹ due to equipment failure) 20 h per day for 30 days | Reduced pineal melatonin and NAT activity. | Data combined in one experiment because of variability. | Wilson et al., 1981 |
| Night-time pineal melatonin levels and NAT enzyme activity in adult rats | 60 Hz 65 kV m⁻¹ (39 kV m⁻¹ effective) up to 4 weeks | Pineal melatonin and NAT activity reduced within 3 weeks exposure; recovered 3 days after exposure. | | Wilson, Chess & Anderson, 1986 |
| Night-time pineal melatonin levels in adult rats | 60 Hz 10, 65 or 130 kV m⁻¹ during gestation and 23 days postnatally | Night-time peak reduced and delayed in exposed animals. | No simple dose-response relationship. | Reiter et al., 1988 |
| Night-time pineal melatonin levels in adult rats | 60 Hz 65 kV m⁻¹ 20 h per day for 30 days | No effect on night-time peak pineal melatonin. | Meeting abstract, but included because it attempted to replicate earlier studies from this group. | Sasser et al., 1991 |
| Night-time pineal melatonin and NAT activity and serum melatonin in adult rats | 60 Hz 10 or 65 kV m⁻¹ 20 h per day for 30 days | No effect on night-time melatonin and NAT; serum melatonin down after 65 kV m⁻¹. | Similar to Wilson et al. 1986. | Grota et al., 1994 |

173

**Table 48. Continued**

**ELF magnetic Fields**

*Mice*

| | | | | |
|---|---|---|---|---|
| Serum melatonin levels in 4th gen. male mice | 50 Hz 15 µT for 4 generations | Reduced night-time levels. | Experimental procedures not fully described. | Picazo et al., 1998 |
| *Rats* | | | | |
| Serum melatonin levels in adult rats | 50 Hz 5 mT 30 min during the morning for 1, 3, 7, 15 and 21 days | Serum melatonin reduced on day 15; no values for days 1, 7, or 21. | Technical difficulties; brief description of method. | Martinez et al., 1992 |
| Pineal and serum melatonin levels in adult rats | 50 Hz 1, 5, 50 or 250 µT, circularly polarised 6 weeks | Night-time and some daytime reductions in serum and pineal melatonin. | Questionable comparisons to historical controls. | Kato et al., 1993 |
| Serum melatonin levels in adult rats | 50 Hz 1 µT, circularly polarised 6 weeks | Night-time melatonin levels reduced, returning to normal within one week. | Comparison to sham exposed. | Kato et al, 1994d |
| Pineal and serum melatonin levels in adult rats | 50 Hz 1 µT, circularly polarised 6 weeks | Night-time pineal and serum levels reduced. | Comparison to sham exposed and historical controls. | Kato et al., 1994c |
| Serum melatonin levels in adult rats | 50 Hz 1 µT, horizontally or vertically polarised 6 weeks | No effect. | Comparison to sham exposed and historical controls. | Kato et al., 1994b |

**Table 48. Continued**

| | | | | |
|---|---|---|---|---|
| 'Antigonadotrophic' effect of melatonin on serum testosterone in adult rats | 50 Hz circularly polarised 1, 5, or 50 µT for 6 weeks | No effect. | Comparison with sham exposed. | Kato et al., 1994a |
| Night-time serum melatonin levels and pineal NAT activity in adult rats | 50 Hz 1, 10 or 100 µT 12 h once, or 18 h per day for 30 days | Reduced melatonin and NAT activity after 100 µT (acute) and 10 and 100 µT (chronic). | | Selmaoui & Touitou, 1995 |
| Night-time serum melatonin levels and pineal NAT activity in young (9 wks) and aged (23 mos) rats | 50 Hz 100 µT 18 h per day for one week | Reduced melatonin and NAT activity in young rats but not old rats. | | Selmaoui & Touitou, 1999 |
| Night-time excretion of melatonin urinary metabolite in adult rats | 50 Hz 1, 5, 100 or 500 µT 24 h | No significant effects compared to base-line pre-exposure controls. | | Bakos et al., 1995; 1997; 1999 |
| Night-time pineal melatonin levels in non-DMBA treated adult rats | 50 Hz 10 µT 13 weeks | No effect. | A small part of a larger, well planned mammary tumour study. | Mevissen, Lerchl & Löscher, 1996 |
| Night-time serum melatonin, levels in SD rats | 50 Hz 100 µT 1 day, 1, 2, 4, 8 or 13 weeks | No consistent effects on melatonin. | The few positive effects could not be replicated. | Löscher, Mevissen & Lerchl, 1998 |
| Night-time excretion of melatonin urinary metabolite in adult rats | 60 Hz 1 mT continuous for 10 days or 6 weeks intermittent for 2 days | No effect. | | John, Liu & Brown, 1998 |

175

**Table 49. Melatonin levels in seasonally breeding animals**

| Endpoint | Exposure | Response | Comment | Authors |
|----------|----------|----------|---------|---------|
| **ELF magnetic fields** | | | | |
| *Djungarian hamsters* | | | | |
| Night-time pineal and serum melatonin levels | 60 Hz 100 µT 15 min, 2 h before dark | Reduced and delayed night-time peak; diminished and absent in 2nd and 3rd replicates. | Considerable variability between replicate studies. | Yellon, 1994 |
| Night-time pineal and serum melatonin levels; adult male reproductive status | 60 Hz 100 µT 15 min, 2 h before dark; second study over 3-week period | Reduced and delayed night-time peak; diminished in 2nd replicate study; no effect on melatonin-induced sexual atrophy. | Considerable variability between replicate studies. | Yellon, 1996 |
| Night-time pineal and serum melatonin levels; adult male reproductive status | 60 Hz 100 µT 15 min, 2 h before dark for 3 weeks | No effect on pineal or serum melatonin; no effect on melatonin-induced sexual atrophy. | Second part of above paper. | Yellon, 1996 |
| Night-time pineal and serum melatonin levels; male puberty, assessed by testes weight | 60 Hz 100 µT 15 min, 2 h before dark from 16–25 days of age | Reduced and delayed night-time peak; absent in 2nd replicate study. No effect on development of puberty. | Considerable variability in melatonin levels between replicate studies. | Truong, Smith & Yellon, 1996 |
| Night-time pineal and serum melatonin levels | 60 Hz 10 or 100 µT (continuous) or 100 µT (intermittent) 15 or 60 min before or after onset of dark period | No effect. | | Truong & Yellon, 1997 |
| Night-time rise in pineal and serum melatonin levels; testes weight | 60 Hz 100 µT 15 min per day, in complete darkness, for up to 21 days | No effect, even in absence of photoperiodic cue. | | Yellon & Truong, 1998 |
| Night-time pineal and serum melatonin levels; testis cell numbers | 50 Hz 450 µT (peak) sinusoidal or 360 µT (peak) rectangular 56 days | Increased cell number and night-time serum melatonin levels after rectangular field exposure. | Animals on long day schedule; difficult interpretation. | Niehaus et al., 1997 |

176

**Table 49. Continued**

| | | | | |
|---|---|---|---|---|
| Night-time pineal melatonin levels, and testis and seminal vesicle weights in short day (regressed) animals | 60 Hz 100 or 500 T, continuous and/or intermittent starting 30 min or 2 h before onset of darkness; for up to 3 h up to 42 days | Reduced pineal melatonin after 15 min exposure; reduced gonad weight but not melatonin after 42 day exposure. | Authors suggest a stress-like effect. | Wilson et al., 1999 |

**ELF electric and magnetic fields**

*Suffolk sheep*

| | | | | |
|---|---|---|---|---|
| Night-time serum melatonin levels and female puberty, detected by rise in serum progesterone | 60 Hz 6 kV m$^{-1}$ and 4 µT, generated by overhead power lines 10 months | No effect of EMFs; strong seasonal effects. | Two replicate studies; open air conditions. | Lee et al., 1993; 1995 |

The third set of studies of EMF effects on seasonal breeders concerned Suffolk sheep; these have a long gestational period and become reproductively active in the autumn, as day length shortens. In two replicate studies (Lee et al., 1993; 1995), Suffolk lambs were exposed outdoors to the magnetic fields generated by overhead transmission lines for about 10 months. The authors reported no effect of exposure on serum melatonin levels or on the onset of puberty.

Table 49 summarizes the studies into effects of ELF fields on melatonin in seasonal breeders.

### 6.2.1.3 Non-human primates

Non-human primates are close, in evolutionary terms, to humans and share many similar characteristics. Rogers et al. (1995b; 1995a) studied responses in male baboons. Generally, no effect on night-time serum melatonin levels was seen (Rogers et al., 1995a). However, a preliminary study (Rogers et al., 1995b), based on data from only two baboons, reported that exposure to an irregular, intermittent sequence of combined electric and magnetic fields in which switching transients were generated, resulted in a marked suppression of the night-time rise in melatonin. These studies are summarized in Table 50.

**Table 50. Melatonin levels in non-human primates**

| Endpoint | Exposure | Response | Comment | Authors |
|---|---|---|---|---|
| **ELF electric and magnetic fields** | | | | |
| Night-time serum melatonin level in baboons | 60 Hz<br>6 kV m$^{-1}$ and 50 µT, 6 weeks<br>30 kV m$^{-1}$ and 100 µT, 3 weeks | No effect. | | Rogers et al., 1995a |
| Night-time serum melatonin level in baboons | 60 Hz<br>6 kV m$^{-1}$ and 50 µT or 30 kV m$^{-1}$ and 100 µT irregular and intermittent sequence for 3 weeks | Reduced serum melatonin levels. | Preliminary study on two baboons. | Rogers et al., 1995b |

### 6.2.2 The pituitary and other hormones

The pituitary gland, like the pineal gland, is intimately connected to the nervous system. It releases hormones into the blood stream either from specialised neurosecretory cells originating in the hypothalamus region of the brain, or from the cells in the pituitary whose function is under the control of such neurosecretory cells via factors released into a specialised hypothalamic-pituitary portal system. The main pituitary hormones investigated in EMF studies include several involved in growth and body physiology, particularly thyroid-stimulating hormone (TSH), which controls the function of the thyroid gland, adrenocorticotrophic hormone (ACTH), which regulates the function of the adrenal cortex, and growth hormone (GH), which affects body growth, and hormones which have important sexual and reproductive functions, particularly follicle stimulating hormone (FSH), luteinising hormone (LH) and prolactin (or luteotrophic hormone).

#### 6.2.2.1 Pituitary-adrenal effects

The possibility that EMF might act as a stressor has been investigated in a number of studies that have examined possible effects of EMF exposure on the release of hormones involved in stress responses, particularly ACTH and cortisol and/or corticosterone released from the adrenal cortex. For ELF electric fields, Hackman & Graves (1981) reported a transient (minutes) increase in serum corticosterone levels in young rats immediately following the onset of exposure to levels greatly in excess of the electric field perception threshold; however, exposure for longer durations had no effect. A lack of effect of prolonged exposure to ELF fields has been reported by other authors on ACTH levels (Portet & Cabanes, 1988) and on cortisol/corticosterone levels (Burchard et al., 1996; Free et al., 1981; Portet & Cabanes, 1988; Quinlan et al., 1985; Thompson et al., 1995). Two studies, both limited by small numbers of animals, reported positive effects of exposure to power frequency electric (de Bruyn & de Jager, 1994) and magnetic (Picazo et al.,

1996) fields on the diurnal rhythmicity of cortisol/corticosterone levels in mice.

### 6.2.2.2 *Other endocrine studies*

Studies of TSH levels and of the thyroid hormones (T3 and T4), which have a major influence on metabolic functions, have been carried out in three studies. No effect on serum TSH levels was found (Free et al., 1981; Portet & Cabanes, 1988; Quinlan et al., 1985); in addition, no effects were reported on serum thyroxin (T3 and T4) levels in rabbits (Portet & Cabanes, 1988), but T3 levels were reduced in rats (Portet and Cabanes, 1988). Growth hormone levels were reported to increase in rats intermittently exposed for 3 h (Quinlan et al., 1985), but were reported to be unaffected following prolonged (3–18 weeks) electric-field exposure at the same level (Free et al., 1981).

Similarly negative or inconsistent data exist concerning possible effects of ELF field exposure on hormones associated with reproduction and sexual development. Prolactin, FSH, LH and testosterone levels in rats were reported unaffected by exposure to power-frequency electric fields (Margonato et al., 1993; Quinlan et al., 1985); similar results for prolactin were reported by Free et al. (1981), but variable effects on FSH levels were seen during development and serum testosterone levels were reported to be decreased in adults. In contrast, an increase in serum prolactin levels was reported in Djungarian hamsters briefly exposed to ELF magnetic fields (Wilson et al., 1999), and an increase in serum progesterone in cattle exposed to combined electric and magnetic fields (Burchard et al., 1996). In a subsequent study, Burchard et al. (2004) found that continuous exposure to an electric field for 4 weeks had no effect on circulating levels of progesterone, prolactin and insulin-like growth factor.

Table 51 summarizes the studies investigating the effects of ELF fields on hormone levels in experimental animals.

## 6.3    In vitro studies

In vitro studies of exposure to EMFs divide into two types of investigation: effects on the production of melatonin by cells from the pineal gland; and effects on the action of melatonin on cells. Some studies have investigated the effects of static magnetic fields, but these have not been reviewed here.

## Table 51. The pituitary and other hormones

| Endpoint | Exposure | Response | Comment | Authors |
|---|---|---|---|---|
| **ELF electric fields** | | | | |
| *Mice* | | | | |
| Serum levels of corticosterone in adult male mice | 60 Hz 10 kV m$^{-1}$ 22 h per day for 6 generations | Elevated daytime but not night-time levels compared to controls. | Small numbers and variable daytime data. | de Bruyn & de Jager, 1994 |
| *Rats* | | | | |
| Serum levels of TSH, GH, FSH, prolactin, LH, corticosterone and testosterone in young and adult male rats | 60 Hz 100 kV m$^{-1}$ (unadjusted) 20 h per day for 30 and/or 120 days (adults) or from 20–56 days of age (young) | Testosterone levels significantly decreased after 120 days; no other consistent effects in adults; significant changes in FSH levels in young rats. | Variable changes in hormone plasma concentration during development. | Free et al., 1981 |
| Serum corticosterone levels in adult male mice. | 60 Hz 25 or 50 kV m$^{-1}$ 5 min per day up to 42 days | Transient increase in serum levels at onset of exposure. | Positive control group; incomplete presentation of data. | Hackman & Graves, 1981 |
| Serum levels of TSH, GH, prolactin and corticosterone in adult male rats | 60 Hz 100 kV m$^{-1}$, continuous or intermittent 1 or 3 h | Increase in GH levels in rats exposed intermittent for 3 h, but not 1 h; no other effects. | Care taken to avoid extraneous confounding factors. | Quinlan et al., 1985 |
| Serum levels of TSH, ACTH, thyroxin (T$_3$ + T$_4$) and corticosterone in young male rats | 50 Hz 50 kV m$^{-1}$ 8 h per day for 28 days | No significant effects except T$_3$ (but not T$_4$) reduced. | | Portet & Cabanes, 1988 |
| Serum levels of FSH, LH and testosterone in adult male rats | 50 Hz 25 or 100 kV m$^{-1}$ 8 h per day for up to 38 weeks | No significant effects. | Variable data. | Margonato et al., 1993 |
| *Rabbits* | | | | |
| Serum levels of GH, ACTH, thyroxin (T$_3$ + T$_4$) and corticosterone (and cortisol) in 6 week old rabbits | 50 Hz 50 kV m$^{-1}$ 16 h per day from last 2 weeks of gestation to 6 weeks after birth | No significant effects. | | Portet & Cabanes, 1988 |

**Table 51. Continued**

**ELF magnetic fields**

*Mice*

| | | | | |
|---|---|---|---|---|
| Serum cortisol levels in adult male mice | 50 Hz 15 µT 14 weeks prior to conception, gestation and 10 weeks post gestation | Loss of diurnal rhythmicity; daytime levels fell and night-time levels rose. | Small numbers per group. | Picazo et al., 1996 |

*Djungarian hamsters*

| | | | | |
|---|---|---|---|---|
| Serum levels of prolactin in adult male Djungarian hamsters on long or short days | 60 Hz 100 µT 15 min before dark 100 µT, intermittent / continuous 45 min per day before dark for 16–42 days | Prolactin levels elevated 4 h after dark following acute but not chronic exposure. | Incomplete presentation of prolactin data. | Wilson et al., 1999 |

### 6.3.1   Effects on melatonin production in vitro

There are only a few studies that have investigated the effect of magnetic fields on melatonin production in vitro. All used rodents as the source of pineal gland cells but there are marked differences in their methodology. Most used power frequencies (50 or 60 Hz), but the field strength (50 µT–1 mT) and duration (1–12 h) differ between the studies. Direct measures include melatonin content or melatonin release from cells. Indirect measures can be made from the activity of N-acetyltransferase (NAT), an enzyme involved in the synthesis of melatonin, or of hydroxyindole-O-methyltransferase (HIOMT), an enzyme responsible for methylation and hence release of melatonin from the cells. Most of the studies have stimulated pharmacologically the production of melatonin in the isolated glands by the addition of noradrenaline (NA) or isoproterenol.

Lerchl et al. (1991) exposed pineal glands from young rats, removed during the day light period, to a combination of a static field (44 µT) and a low frequency magnetic field (44 µT at 33.7 Hz), the theoretical conditions for cyclotron resonance of the calcium ion. Exposure caused a reduction in NAT activity, melatonin production and melatonin release into the culture medium. Rosen, Barber & Lyle (1998) also used pineal glands from the rat, but this study was different to the other studies in that the pineal gland was separated into individual cells. The overall result was that magnetic field exposure caused a statistically significant 46% reduction in stimulated melatonin release. Chacon (2000) used rat pineal glands to study NAT activity. The enzyme activity decreased by approximately 20% after 1 h exposure to the highest field strength tested (1000 µT) but was not significantly altered by field strengths of 10 or 100 µT. The interpretation of the result may be complicated by the removal of the pineal gland during the rats' dark period, which may have had an effect on melatonin synthesis and a confounding effect on the result.

A study by Brendel, Niehaus & Lerchl (2000) used pineal glands from the Djungarian hamster. It also differed from the previous studies in that the glands were maintained in a flow-system, so that changes of melatonin released from the glands could be monitored throughout the duration of the experiment. The experimental protocol appears to have been well-designed with random allocation of exposure or sham to identical exposure systems and the experiments run blind. The authors concluded that EMF inhibited melatonin production in both the 50 Hz and 16.67 Hz experiments. However there is only one time point in one of four experiments that the melatonin released is statistically different from the sham exposed. Similarly, a study by Tripp, Warman & Arendt (2003) used a flow system to detect changes of melatonin release during the course of the exposure. The exposure was for 4 h to a circularly polarised magnetic fields at 500 μT, 50 Hz. Samples were taken every 30 min; the process used remote collection to avoid potential artefacts involved in manual collection. The glands were not stimulated pharmacologically and no field-dependent changes in melatonin release were detected.

Lewy, Massot & Touitou (2003) used rat pineal glands isolated in the morning and hence during the 12 h light period. The glands were exposed for 4 h to a 50 Hz magnetic field at 1 mT. The activity of enzymes NAT and HIOMT was measured, as well as the release of melatonin into the incubation liquid. In contrast to many other studies, field exposure given simultaneously with NA or 30 min prior to NA administration caused a significant increase (approximately 50%) in melatonin release. There was no change in melatonin release due to field exposure in glands that had not been stimulated by NA.

### 6.3.2    Effects on the action of melatonin in vitro

The main interest in this area was caused by the claim that exposure to magnetic fields can block the inhibitory effect of melatonin on growth of breast cancer cells. The original work was reported by Liburdy et al. (1993) in a study using a human oestrogen-responsive breast cancer cell line (MCF-7). They found that the proliferation of MCF-7 cells can be slowed by the addition of physiological concentrations of melatonin (1 nM). However, if the cells are simultaneously exposed to a 60 Hz, 1.2 μT magnetic field, then the effect of melatonin on the rate of proliferation is reduced. The effects are fairly small and can only been seen after 7 days in culture. They suggested that the magnetic field disrupted either the ligand/receptor interaction or the subsequent signalling pathway. The authors found no effect at a magnetic field strength of 0.2 μT and suggested a threshold between 0.2 μT and 1.2 μT. No effect was seen using field exposure alone. A similar effect of a 60 Hz field was reported by Harland & Liburdy (1997) but using tamoxifen (100 nM) rather than melatonin to bring about the initial inhibition. The effect has been reported in other cell lines, namely a second breast cancer cell line, T47D, (Harland, Levine & Liburdy, 1998) and a human glioma cell line 5F757 (Afzal, Levine & Liburdy, 1998). However, as previously noted (AGNIR, 2001b; NIEHS, 1998), the effect seen in the initial study (Liburdy et al., 1993) was small (10–20 % growth over 7 days) and some concern was noted regarding the robustness of the effect.

Blackman, Benane & House (2001) set out to replicate these findings, using the MCF-7 cells supplied by Liburdy, but with a modified and improved experimental protocol. Melatonin caused a significant 17% inhibition of MCF-7 growth (p < 0.001), even though the standard errors of the estimated growth statistics showed considerable overlap. This reported effect was abolished by exposure to a 60 Hz magnetic field at 1.2 µT, confirming the results of Liburdy et al. (1993). In addition, tamoxifen caused a 25% inhibition in cell numbers, which was reduced to a 13% inhibition by exposure to a 60 Hz magnetic field at 1.2 µT. This result confirmed the results reported by Harland & Liburdy (1997), in which a 40% inhibition was reduced to 25% by EMF exposure. A later study by Ishido (2001) exposed MCF-7 cells (supplied by Liburdy) to 0, 1.2 or 100 µT at 50 Hz for 7 days. Melatonin at concentrations of $10^{-9}$ M or higher induced inhibition of intracellular cyclic AMP which was blocked by exposure to a 50 Hz field at 100 µT. Similarly DNA synthesis, which was inhibited by $10^{-11}$ M melatonin levels, was partially released by exposure at 1.2 µT.

However, although the MCF-7 cell line has undoubtedly provided a useful model to investigate effects on isolated breast cancer cells it is only one possible model in cells that have been separated from their natural environment and therefore its implication for breast cancer in general is limited. The cell line is rather heterogeneous; different subclones show different growth characteristics (e.g. Luben & Morgan, 1998; Morris et al., 1998) raising the possibility that the effects were specific to individual subclone phenotypes. The effects of stronger magnetic fields were studied by Leman et al. (2001) in three breast cancer cell lines that were reported to have different metastatic capabilities: MDA-MB-435 cells, which were considered to be highly metastatic, MDA-MB-231 cells which were considered to be weakly metastatic, and MCF-7 cells, which were considered as non-metastatic. Only the weakly and non-metastatic cells responded to melatonin and optimum inhibition was achieved at 1mM concentration of melatonin (a million-fold higher than used in the Liburdy study). Exposure for 1 h to a pulsed field at 300 µT repeated for 3 days had no effect on growth in either cell line.

The in vitro studies into the effects of ELF magnetic fields on melatonin are summarized in Table 52.

**Table 52. Magnetic field effects on melatonin**

| Endpoint | Exposure | Response | Comment | Authors |
|---|---|---|---|---|
| **Effects on melatonin production in vitro** | | | | |
| NA stimulation of melatonin production and release from rat pineal gland | Static field and 33.7 Hz, 44 µT 2.5 h | Reduced production and release. | Opposite to expected effect of calcium ions. | Lerchl et al., 1991 |
| NA stimulation of melatonin release from rat pineal cells | 60 Hz 50 µT 12 h | Reduced release. | | Rosen, Barber & Lyle, 1998 |
| NAT activity in rat pineal glands | 50 Hz 10, 100 µT or 1 mT 1 h | Decreased NAT activity at the highest exposure level only. | | Chacon, 2000 |
| Isoproterenol stimulation of melatonin production in Djungarian hamster pineal gland | 50 Hz or 16.7 Hz 86 µT 8 h | Melatonin production reduced. | Continuous flow system used allowing temporal resolution of any effect. | Brendel, Niehaus & Lerchl, 2000 |
| Melatonin release from rat pineal gland | 50 Hz 0.5 mT 4 h | No effect on melatonin release. | Continuous flow system used allowing temporal resolution of any effect. | Tripp, Warman & Arendt, 2003 |
| NA stimulated melatonin release from rat pineal gland. | 50 Hz 1 mT 4 h | Melatonin release increase. | | Lewy, Massot & Touitou, 2003 |
| **Effects on cell responses to melatonin or tamoxifen in vitro** | | | | |
| Melatonin inhibition of MCF-7 cell growth | 60 Hz 1.2 µT 7 days | EMF exposure reduced growth inhibition. | Small (10–20%) effect. | Liburdy et al., 1993 |
| Tamoxifen inhibition of MCF-7 cell growth | 60 Hz 1.2 µT 7 days | EMF exposure reduced growth inhibition. | | Harland & Liburdy, 1997 |
| Melatonin or Tamoxifen inhibition of MCF-7 cell growth | 60 Hz 1.2 µT 7 days | EMF exposure reduced growth inhibition by melatonin and tamoxifen. | Standard errors on growth statistics show considerable overlap. | Blackman, Benane & House, 2001 |
| Melatonin inhibition of cAMP and DNA synthesis in MCF-7 cells | 50 Hz 1.2 or 100 µT 7 days | Reduction of melatonin induced inhibition. | | Ishido, 2001 |

184

**Table 52. Continued**

| | | | |
|---|---|---|---|
| Melatonin inhibition of growth of 3 breast cancer cell lines including MCF-7 | 2 Hz pulsed field; pulse width 20 ms 0.3 mT 1 h per day for 3 days | No effect on cell growth. | Leman et al., 2001 |

## 6.4    Conclusions

The results of volunteer studies as well as residential and occupational studies suggests that the neuroendocrine system is not adversely affected by exposure to power-frequency electric and/or magnetic fields. This applies particularly to the circulating levels of specific hormones of the neuroendocrine system, including melatonin, released by the pineal gland, and a number of hormones involved in the control of body metabolism and physiology, released by the pituitary gland. Subtle differences were sometimes observed in the timing of melatonin release or associated with certain characteristics of exposure, but these results were not consistent. It is very difficult to eliminate possible confounding by a variety of environmental and lifestyle factors that might also affect hormone levels. Most laboratory studies of the effects of ELF exposure on night-time melatonin levels in volunteers found no effect when care was taken to control possible confounding.

From the large number of animal studies investigating power-frequency EMF effects on rat pineal and serum melatonin levels, some reported that exposure resulted in night-time suppression of melatonin. The changes in melatonin levels first observed in early studies of electric-field exposures up to 100 kV m$^{-1}$ could not be replicated. The findings from a series of more recent studies which showed that circularly-polarised magnetic fields suppressed night-time melatonin levels were weakened by inappropriate comparisons between exposed animals and historical controls. The data from other magnetic fields experiments in laboratory rodents, covering intensity levels over three orders of magnitude from a few microtesla to 5 mT, were equivocal, with some results showing depression of melatonin but others showing no change. In seasonally breeding animals, the evidence for an effect of exposure to power-frequency fields on melatonin levels and melatonin-dependent reproductive status is predominantly negative. No convincing effect on melatonin levels has been seen in a study of non-human primates chronically exposed to power-frequency fields, although a preliminary study using two animals reported melatonin suppression in response to an irregular and intermittent exposure.

The effects of ELF exposure on melatonin production or release in isolated pineal glands was variable, although relatively few in vitro studies have been undertaken. The evidence that ELF exposure interferes with the action of melatonin on breast cancer cells in vitro is intriguing and there appears to be some supporting evidence in terms of independent replication using MCF-7 cells. However this system suffers from the disadvantage that the cell lines frequently show genotypic and phenotypic drift in culture that can hinder transferability between laboratories.

With the possible exception of transient (minutes duration) stress following the onset of ELF electric field exposure at levels significantly above perception thresholds, no consistent effects have been seen in the stress-related hormones of the pituitary-adrenal axis in a variety of mammalian species. Similarly, mostly negative or inconsistent effects have been observed in amounts of growth hormone, levels of hormones involved in controlling metabolic activity or associated with the control of reproduction and sexual development, but few studies have been carried out.

Overall, these data do not indicate that ELF electric and/or magnetic fields affect the neuroendocrine system in a way that would have an adverse impact on human health and the evidence is thus considered inadequate.

# 7 NEURODEGENERATIVE DISORDERS

A number of studies have examined associations between exposure to electromagnetic fields and Alzheimer disease, motor neuron disease and Parkinson disease. These diseases may be classed as neurodegenerative diseases as all involve the death of specific neurons. Although their aetiology seems different (Savitz, 1998; Savitz, Loomis & Tse, 1998), a part of the pathogenic mechanisms may be common. Most investigators examine these diseases separately. In relation to electromagnetic fields, amyotrophic lateral sclerosis (ALS) has been studied most often.

Radical stress, caused by the production of reactive oxygen species (ROS) and other radical species such as reactive nitrogen species (RNS), is thought to be a critical factor in the modest neuronal degeneration that occurs with ageing. It also seems important in the aetiology of Parkinson disease and ALS and may play a part in Alzheimer disease (Felician & Sandson, 1999). Superoxide radicals, hydrogen peroxide ($H_2O_2$) and hydroxyl radicals are oxygen-centered reactive species (Coyle & Puttfarcken, 1993) that have been implicated in several neurotoxic disorders (Liu et al., 1994). They are produced by many normal biochemical reactions, but their concentrations are kept in a harmless range by potent protective mechanisms (Makar et al., 1994). Increased free radical concentrations, resulting from either increased production or decreased detoxification, can cause oxidative damage to various cellular components, particularly mitochondria, ultimately leading to cell death by apoptosis (Bogdanov et al., 1998).

Several experimental investigations have examined the effect of ELF electromagnetic fields on calcium exchange in nervous tissue and other direct effects on nerve tissue function. A variety of effects of ELF exposure of potential relevance to neurodegenerative disease have previously been reported (Lacy-Hulbert, Metcalfe & Hesketh, 1998). These include small increases (Blackman et al., 1982; 1985), but also decreases (Bawin & Adey, 1976), in $Ca^{2+}$ efflux from brain tissue, in vivo and in vitro, inhibition of outgrowth of neurites from cultured neurons (Blackman, Benane & House, 1993), and an increase in superoxide production from neutrophils (Roy et al., 1995).

It is conceivable that prolonged exposure to ELF fields could alter $Ca^{2+}$ levels in neurons and thus induce oxidative stress through its influence on mitochondrial metabolism. On the other hand, the biological evidence, particularly concerning the response of neurons, is limited.

Neurons can be directly activated by strong electrical currents (see Chapter 5, especially section 5.2.2). Some evidence, discussed in sections 5.1 and 5.2, suggests that ELF exposure might modulate ongoing electrical activity in the CNS, although studies on hormone and neurotransmitter levels have generally reported no effect or only minor influences of ELF exposure (see section 5.4.4). While these effects are unlikely to be damaging, especially in the short term, there is the possibility that prolonged exposure to ELF fields could synchronize certain neurons of high sensitivity (perhaps especially the large motor neurons), possibly leading to voltage-activated $Ca^{2+}$ entry, which could have a damaging effect on the neurons. There might also be an accumulation of extracellular glutamate relative to GABA (gamma-aminobutyric acid), which could have excitotoxic effects on surrounding neurons.

It is possible that even modest cellular effects of ELF fields may exacerbate pathological changes in otherwise compromised neurons. For instance, intercellular transfer of metabolites and ions via gap junctions has been shown to be affected by exposure to 0.8 mT (but not 0.05 mT) magnetic fields (Li et al., 1999).

In contrast to the effect of ELF it has been suggested that exposure to electric shocks may increase the risk for ALS (Haynal & Regli, 1964). Electric currents may damage brain tissue by disturbing the circulation. It has also been speculated that severe electric shocks cause a massive synchronized discharge of neurons, which might release sufficient glutamate to precipitate toxic changes, as outlined above (AGNIR, 2001a). No mechanism has been identified, however, that could provide a coherent explanation of the observed association between exposure to ELF or electric shocks and these neurodegenerative diseases.

## 7.1    Alzheimer disease

### 7.1.1    *Pathology*

Alzheimer disease (AD) is characterized clinically by progressive loss of memory and other cognitive abilities (e.g. language, attention). Its onset is thought to be heralded by a phase of mild cognitive impairment in which cognition is not normal but not severe enough to warrant a diagnosis of dementia. The exact duration of mild cognitive impairment is unclear, but is likely to last at least a few years. Most data on disease duration come from studies of prevalent AD which suggest that disease duration may average seven or more years, although a recent study estimated that disease duration may actually be closer to 3½ years from the onset of the manifestations of dementia. Many persons with AD also develop motor, behavioral, and affective disturbances. In particular, parkinsonian signs, hallucinations delusions, and depressive symptoms are present in half or more of persons with the disease. Data also suggest that these signs are related to increased risk of death and to rate of cognitive decline. Cholinesterase inhibitor therapy, the mainstay of symptomatic treatment, is not known to definitively affect disease course or outcomes.

Although oxidative stress may be involved in the sporadic forms of AD, the evidence is less compelling. Indices of oxidative damage are significantly increased compared with those in age-matched controls (Felician & Sandson, 1999). Inflammatory and immune responses have also been implicated, although it is difficult to know whether these are secondary to the other pathological changes. Cellular responses to increased oxidative stress appear to be a mechanism that contributes to the varied cytopathology of AD.

Inflammation in the CNS often occurs in both Parkinson and Alzheimer diseases and chronic neurological disorders such as brain trauma, ischemic stroke (for a review, see Rothwell, 1997). It has long been known that the extent of inflammatory responses in the CNS is less than observed in the periphery (for review, see Lotan & Schwartz, 1994; Perry, Brown & Gordon, 1987). A cascade of inflammatory responses is orchestrated by microglia (resident macrophages) and astrocytes in the CNS.

The fact that microglia become reactive in the aging brain as the natural death of neurons occurs (Sloane et al., 1999) suggests that interactions between neurons and glia play an important role in controlling inflammatory responses in the CNS. Chang et al. (2001) showed that activation of microglia in the ageing brain was linked to the death of neurons.

### 7.1.2  Epidemiology

Sobel et al. (1995) reported the results of three small case-control studies of AD, two of which had been carried out in Finland and one in the USA. Occupational histories for demented subjects were obtained from the most knowledgeable surrogates and, for non-demented controls, by direct interview. The individuals' primary lifetime occupations were classed blindly by an industrial hygienist as causing low, medium, or high (or medium to high) exposure on the basis of previous knowledge. Dressmakers, seamstresses, and tailors had not previously been classified as occupations with high EMF exposure. The classification of medium to high exposure was confirmed by measurement of the fields produced by four industrial and two home sewing machines.

The first Finnish series consisted in 53 men and women with sporadic AD and 70 with sporadic vascular dementia; the second of 198 men and women admitted to a geriatric institution diagnosed as having AD (sporadic and familial combined) and 298 controls selected in order from the alphabetic listing of patients admitted to the long stay internal medicine wards of the Koskela Hospital in 1978, excluding those with a diagnosis of dementia or mental retardation, psychosis, depression, general or brain arteriosclerosis, Parkinsonism, or multiple sclerosis. The third series consisted in 136 patients admitted to the University of Southern California between 1984 and 1993 with sporadic AD and 106 neuropsychologically normal individuals without any known history of dementia or memory problems in first degree relatives in the communities from which the Alzheimer patients came. The results are summarized in Table 53. The odds ratio for probable medium to high exposure compared to low for the three series combined was 3.0 and was hardly altered (2.9 with 95% CI 1.6–5.4) by adjustment for education and social class and for age at onset, age at examination, and sex. [In this study the newly designated category of dressmakers, seamstresses, and tailors accounted for the greater part of the excess risk from medium to high exposure occupations (23 out of 36 individuals in the AD series and 8 out of

16 in the controls). The limitations of the study are use of different control groups in the three series, particularly patients with vascular dementia who may in fact have had AD; obtaining job histories by questionnaires; lack of validation of exposure of the study population; the measure of high exposures among seamstresses was not confirmed in a later and more extensive study in the US (Kelsh et al., 2003), dependence on proxy respondents for job histories of cases but not for some of the control.]

A further case-control study, based on patients attending an Alzheimer's Disease Treatment & Diagnostic Center in Downey, California, was reported by Sobel et al. (1996) in the following year and may be regarded as constituting a test of the hypothesis formed in the first report. Patients at the Center had been included in several previous studies and information about their primary occupation throughout life was extracted from existing forms. Comparisons were made between 326 patients with probable or definite AD and 152 control patients with cognitive impairment or dementia due to other causes, excluding vascular dementia. These were classified in 20 groups, the largest being head trauma (26) and alcohol abuse (21). These results are also summarized in Table 53. The odds ratio for a primary occupation that caused medium or high exposure to EMF, was 3.93 with 95% CI 1.45–10.56. [Again seamstresses, dressmakers, and tailors combined, in this study, with sewing factory workers and clothing cutters contributed a relatively high proportion of the cases with medium or high exposure. The odds ratios in the study were higher for men than for women, contrary to what had been observed in the previous study. The limitations of this study were that the cases included 24 patients with unclear diagnoses; the controls were not matched by age or gender to the cases and were from the same clinic, which specialized in AD; job histories were obtained by questionnaire; and the exposure of the study population was not validated. The different designs used in this study and in the three other studies of Sobel et al. lead to a diverse collection of relative risks and potential biases].

Table 53. First case-control studies of Alzheimer disease: ELF magnetic field exposure estimated for primary lifetime occupation

| Authors | | No. of subjects (medium or high exposure / total) | | Odds ratio | |
|---|---|---|---|---|---|
| | | Cases | Controls | Univariate | Adjusted |
| Sobel et al., 1995 | Finnish 1 | 6 / 53[a] | 3 / 70 | 2.9 | 2.7 |
| | Finnish 2 | 19 / 198 | 10 / 289 | 3.1** | 3.2*** |
| | University S. California | 11 / 136 | 3 / 106 | 3.0 | 2.4 |
| Sobel et al., 1996 | | 39 / 326 | 8 / 152 | 2.45* | 3.93** |

[a] Data for one patient missing.
* p ≤ 0.05; ** p ≤ 0.01; *** p ≤ 0.001

The findings of subsequent studies, which are summarized in Table 54, present a different picture. Savitz, Loomis & Tse (1998) studied men aged 20 years and over who were certified as having died from amyotrophic lateral sclerosis, AD or Parkinson disease in the period 1985–1991 and had recorded occupations in one of the 25 US states that coded occupational information on the death certificate. Three controls were selected from all other men dying in the same states matched with each of the cases and stratified by year of death and age at death in five broad age groups. AD was given as the cause of 256 deaths and the odds ratio for occupations previously defined as involving electrical work, adjusted for age, period, social class and race was 1.2 with 95% CI 1.0–1.4. [The major limitations of this study are the use of death certificates to assess outcome, particularly since AD is difficult to diagnose and is often underreported on death certificates; the small number of cases, and lack of validation in exposure assessment.]

Feychting et al. (1998) studied 77 men and women with dementia, 55 of whom were classed as having probable or possible Alzheimer disease, diagnosed when a sample of individuals drawn from the twins registered in the Swedish Adoption/Twin Study of Ageing were screened for dementia. If both members of a twin-pair had dementia, one was randomly selected for inclusion in the study. Two groups of controls were drawn from the same original sample of twins who, on testing, were mentally intact. Death and refusal diminished the number of controls available for study and the samples were reinforced by a few additional persons from another Swedish twin study. The occupational history of both cases and controls had been recorded at a structured interview, as part of the mental testing procedure, information about demented subjects being obtained from a surrogate (mostly spouse or offspring). Each subject's primary occupation was defined as that held for the greatest number of years. The relevant information about magnetic field exposure was obtained from the records of a previous study in which work-day measurements had been made for a large number of occupations held by a sample of the population (Floderus et al., 1993; Floderus, 1996). Lack of data for some occupations and lack of occupational histories for housewives reduced the number of cases available for analysis to 41 for all dementia and 27 for Alzheimer disease, and to 150 and 164 for the two control groups. No clear relationship with exposure from the primary occupation was seen for all dementia: the odds ratios for exposures = 0.2 μT were 1.5 (95% CI 0.6–4.0) and 1.2 (95% CI 0.5–3.2) against the two control groups, nor for AD where the odds ratio for exposure = 0.2 μT were respectively 0.9 (95% CI 0.3–2.8) and 0.8 (95% CI 0.3–2.3). There was, however, some evidence of a relationship with exposure from the last occupation held for both categories: the odds ratios for exposure = 0.2 μT were for all dementias 3.3 (95% CI 1.3–8.6) and 3.8 (95% CI 1.4–10.2); and for AD 2.4 (95% CI 0.8–6.9) and 2.7 (95% CI 0.9–7.8). [It is notable that in this study the relationship with magnetic fields is stronger for all dementias than for AD, and hence stronger still for dementias other than AD, which had been used as the controls in some other studies (Sobel et al., 1995; 1996). The limitations are the small number of cases, particularly of AD; possible selection bias due to twins who refused to be examined; potential information biases in the job histories which were obtained for cases from proxy respondents; lack of autopsy confirmation of the diagnosis of AD.]

The results of the two cohort studies with measured exposures for large random samples of men with different occupations in the electricity utility industry provide unbiased tests of the hypotheses that the fields can increase the risk of neurodegenerative disease. The studies were designed to find out if exposure to 50 Hz magnetic fields increased the risk of leukaemia, brain cancer, and some other cancers (Johansen & Olsen, 1998b; Savitz & Loomis, 1995) but the causes of all deaths that occurred over prolonged periods were recorded and the results can provide relevant information. Such a test, however, is limited since these are mortality studies which are limited in investigating causes such as Alzheimer disease which might not be reported consistently on the death certificate.

One study covering 21 000 Danish workers followed for up to 19 years was reported by Johansen & Olsen (1998a). The standardized mortality ratio (SMR) for dementia (senile and presenile combined) was less than unity (0.7) for the total population based on six deaths and still lower for the most highly exposed group (0.4). [As specified previously, the use of death certificates for diagnosis of AD is a major limitation, as is the absence of validation of exposure in the study population.]

The second study covered nearly 140 000 workers employed in five US utilities and followed from 1950 or 6 months after the date of hire, whichever was the later, to the end of 1988 (Savitz, Checkoway & Loomis, 1998). The SMR for AD was 1.0, based on 24 deaths. Information was also obtained on the frequency with which the disease was referred to on the death certificates as a contributory cause and the 56 deaths for which it was mentioned as an underlying or contributory cause were related to the individuals' estimated cumulative exposure in terms of µT-years: that is, the time weighted average exposure multiplied by the number of years exposed. This provides no evidence of any association between exposure and death from AD, expressed as relative risk (RR) per µT-year cumulative exposure, either for career exposure or, for what might be the more relevant, as AD commonly lasts for 5 to 10 years before death, for exposure 10–19 years or 20 or more years before death. [Again, the use of death certificates for diagnosis of AD is a major limitation.]

Recently Li, Sung & Wu (2002) reported that among 2198 elderly individuals aged 65 years or over, there was no increased risk of cognitive impairment due higher levels of exposure to power frequency EMFs from a previous occupation, higher residential exposure or both and therefore little support for a link between cognitive impairment and ELF exposure.

Feychting and colleagues (2003) identified all men and women included in the 1980 Swedish census who were working in 1970 or 1980 and alive on January 1, 1981 and followed them until December 31, 1995. All deaths with neurodegenerative disease listed were identified, although AD

192

and vascular dementia were not separate categories until January 1, 1987, thus the follow-up for these started from that date. Information on subjects' occupational and socioeconomic status (SES) came from census data.

To estimate EMF exposure over the working lifetime, Feychting et al. used Floderus's 1996 job-exposure matrix, which includes some sample occupational 50-Hz magnetic field measurements for the 100 most common jobs held by Swedish men. They also analyzed occupations with the highest estimated EMF exposure in the matrix, plus a group of "electrical occupations" reported earlier by others (Sobel and Savitz) as being associated with higher AD and ALS risk. They calculated person-years of exposure and created groups based on 1st (below 0.11 µT) and 3rd quartiles (0.11 to 0.19 µT), the 90th percentile (0.19 to 0.29 µT) and the 95th percentile (> 0.5 µT). All risk estimates were adjusted for age and SES.

A total of 2 649 300 men and 2 163 346 women were included. Overall, AD was not associated with magnetic field exposure of 0.3 µT or above in men or women. A modest increased risk of AD in men with exposure of 0.5 µT and above in 1970, with a "slightly higher" risk estimate in 1980. Stronger associations were found among men when analyses were limited to mortality before age 75, and even stronger when follow-up was limited to 10 years after the 1980 census. The highest risk ratio (RR) of 3.4 (95% CI 1.6–7.0) was reported for men exposed to 0.5 µT or above in 1980. [The limitations include lack of a complete work history and the reliance on the job-exposure matrix developed for a different study, use of death certificates and reliance on census data for occupation and SES.]

Another investigation in Sweden, by Håkansson et al. (2003) evaluated the relationship between occupational 50-Hz magnetic field exposure and mortality from AD, ALS, Parkinson disease and multiple sclerosis. This population overlapped with a previous study, but focused on highly exposed group of workers (resistance welders) with some exposures in the millitesla range. First, 40 types of occupation where resistance welding could be part of the job description during the study period 1985 to 1994 were identified. Income tax records were used to identify subjects employed at any of the selected work places. A total of 537 692 men and 180 529 women were identified and about 10% of eligible subjects, 53 049 men and 18 478 women, for whom either occupation or exposure data were missing were excluded.

The census data from 1980, 1985 and 1990, which included occupation codes and some job descriptions, were used to identify resistance welders. These 1697 subjects formed the highest exposure group for the analyses. For assignment to other exposure categories, the same Floderus's 1996 job-exposure matrix, plus some additional "exposure information" from a 1993 Swedish study for some rare occupations were used. Further, Håkansson et al. added three other occupations employing mostly women – "domestic service", "computer operator" and "other needlework" – not included in the matrix. They assigned domestic workers to a low exposure categoryandcomputer operators and needleworkers to a high exposure category. As the authors note, overall this cohort was "comparatively young" with a median age of 35. Causes of death were ascertained from the Swedish national death certificate registry. For workers who moved from a higher exposure level job to a lower one during the study period, the higher level was used for analysis. If information on a subject was lacking for a given census period, the earlier data was used.

Håkansson et al. (2003) report elevated relative risk for AD among exposed men and women, with increasing risk with increasing exposure. Exposure-response analysis yielded an RR of 3.2 for each increase of 1 μT. The risk estimate for men and women in the highest exposure category was 4.64 (95% CI 1.40–11.66), but based on only eight cases. [Results rely on small numbers. No effect is seen if only primary cause of death (without contributing cause) is used. Potential confounding from welders' exposure to metals might be present.]

The most recent study (Qiu et al., 2004) is also from Sweden (Stockholm). It evaluates lifetime occupational exposures to magnetic field and Alzheimer disease in a community cohort of individuals 75 years and older. This cohort was dementia-free at the beginning of the follow-up (1987–89) and was followed to 1994–96. Information on occupational history was obtained from a proxy, exposure to magnetic fields was based on the already mentioned job-exposure matrix and some supplementary information focusing on women. Of 931 individuals 202 were diagnosed with AD based on a structured interview, a clinical examination and psychological assessment. For the deceased subjects the diagnosis was made by the examination of medical records by two physicians. Adjustment was made for numerous potential confounders. Increased risk was seen for men in both medium lifetime average occupational exposure (RR = 1.7; 95% CI 0.6–4.5) and high exposure (RR = 2.0; 95% CI 0.7–5.5), but these elevations were not statistically significant and the broad confidence intervals indicate a high level of uncertainty. The risk was slightly higher but less consistent when adjustments for many potential confounders were made. No risk was evident for women. [Limitations include exposure assessment including information on jobs held and relevance of the job-exposure matrix used especially for women.]

When evaluated across all the studies, there is only very limited evidence of an association between estimated ELF exposure and disease risk. This is mainly confined to the first two studies (Sobel et al., 1995; 1996) and it is not clearly confirmed by the later studies (Feychting et al., 1998; Feychting et al., 2003; Qiu et al., 2004; Savitz, Checkoway & Loomis, 1998; Savitz, Loomis & Tse, 1998). The exception might be a study by Håkansson et al. (2003). The two studies that show excess (Sobel et al., 1995; 1996) may have been affected by selection bias. Because the study populations are undefined, there is no way to determine the extent to which the controls are representative with respect to exposure of the population from which the cases originated. The Håkansson et al. results depend on the use of a contributing cause. Use of mortality information for the evaluation of AD is particularly problematic, because this diagnosis is often not reported as an under-

**Table 54. Later studies of Alzheimer disease and dementia unspecified**

| Authors | Exposure (μT) | No. of deaths | Relative risk (95% CI) | Disease |
|---|---|---|---|---|
| Savitz, Loomis & Tse, 1998 | Electrical occupation | 256 | 1.2 (1.0–1.4) | AD |
| Feychting et al., 1998 | Primary occupation 0.2 / < 0.12 | (i) 27 [a] (ii) 27 | 0.9 (0.3–2.8) 0.8 (0.3–2.3) | AD |
| | Last occupation 0.2 / < 0.12 | (i) 29 (ii) 29 | 2.4 (0.8–6.9) 2.7 (0.9–7.8) | AD |
| | Primary occupation 0.2 / < 0.12 | (i) 41 (ii) 41 | 1.5 (0.6–4.0) 1.2 (0.5–3.2) | Dementia |
| | Last occupation 0.2 / < 0.12 | (i) 44 (ii) 44 | 3.3 (1.3–8.6) 3.8 (1.4–10.2) | Dementia |
| Savitz, Checkoway & Loomis, 1998 | Cumulative career | 56 | 0.97 (0.87–1.08) [b] | AD |
| | Cumulative 10–19 y before death | 56 | 0.47 (0.21–1.04) [b] | AD |
| | Cumulative 20 y before death | 56 | 0.97 (0.87–1.09) [b] | AD |
| Johansen & Olsen, 1998a | Any | 6 | 0.7 | Dementia |
| | Most highly exposed | 1 | 0.4 | Dementia |
| Feychting et al., 2003 | Occupation in 1970 (males) | | | AD |
| | Reference (< 0.11) | 178 | | |
| | 3rd quartile (0.12–0.19) | 696 | 1.0 (0.9–1.2) | |
| | 90th percentile ( 0.20–0.29) | 239 | 1.1 (0.9–1.3) | |
| | 95th percentile (> 0.5) | 90 | 1.3 (1.0–1.7) | |
| Håkansson et al., 2003 | Occupational exposure (males & females) | | | AD |
| | Reference (< 0.16) | 7 | | |
| | Medium (0.16–0.25) | 17 | 1.3 (0.5–3.2) | |
| | High (0.25–0.53) | 8 | 2.2 (0.6–6.3) | |
| | Very high ( > 0.53) | 8 | 4.0 (1.4–11.7) | |
| Qiu et al., 2004 | Lifetime average occupational exposure (males & females) | | | AD |
| | Reference (< 0.15) | 69 | | |
| | Medium (0.16–0.18) | 64 | 1.2 (0.9–1.7) | |
| | High ( > 0.10) | 69 | 1.1 (0.7–1.5) | |

[a] (i) & (ii) odds ratios for same cases with two different sets of controls.
[b] Relative risk per μT-year cumulative exposure.

lying cause and is underrepresented as a contributing cause as well. Note that, overall, the studies that did not rely on the death certificates for diagnosis appear to be more positive. This should be considered in the interpretation and development of future studies.

## 7.2　Amyotrophic lateral sclerosis

### 7.2.1　Pathology

Amyotrophic lateral sclerosis (ALS) is characterized clinically by progressive motor dysfunction, including painless muscle wasting and spasticity. Most data on disease duration come from clinic samples which suggest that disease duration may average only two to three years. Signs of the disease depend greatly on where the symptoms begin. Brainstem (bulbar) dysfunction may be the first sign in persons presenting with dysphagia or dysarthria. Alternatively, persons may present with painless wasting and weakness of a limb, or one side of the body. Persons with ALS may develop cognitive and autonomic dysfunction. In particular, a frontal lobe dementia and hypotension may develop. Some data suggest that these signs portend a more malignant course of disease. As the disease progresses, pulmonary function and dysphagia result in the need for artificial respiratory support and the insertion of feeding devices to maintain life. Pathologically, the hallmarks of the disease are degeneration of anterior horn cells, ubiquinated inclusions, hardening (sclerosis) of the white matter in the brain and spinal cord, and degeneration of other motor nuclei. Evidence of degeneration and regeneration in muscle is thought to be secondary to the loss of anterior horn cells. About 10% of ALS cases are familial (Brown, 1997).

Trauma has long been suspected as being a cause of motor neuron disease and specifically of ALS. No clear evidence that it was a cause has, however, ever been obtained, partly, perhaps, because of variation in the reports of the type, location, and timing of the trauma in relation to the onset of the disease and partly because of the probability that the many positive findings were affected by recall bias, patients with the disease being more motivated to recall traumatic events than their corresponding controls.

### 7.2.2　Epidemiology

The results of five case-control studies examining possible etiology of electric shocks and ALS are summarized in Table 55. Four of them specifically noted the prevalence of electric shocks or injuries and four the proportion of people employed in defined electrical occupations. The first study, which gave rise to the hypothesis, was reported from Germany by Haynal & Regli as long ago as 1964. Nine out of 73 patients with ALS had worked in contact with electricity against five out of 150 controls, giving, according to Deapen & Henderson (1986) an odds ratio of 4.1.

No further study was reported until seventeen years later, when Kondo & Tsubaki (1981) described two studies in Japan, one of which involved a substantial number of cases. Both were essentially negative. In the first, information was obtained by personal interview from the spouses of

458 men and 254 women whose deaths were attributed to motor neuron disease, most of whom had ALS (333 men and 178 women) and the findings were compared with those obtained from 216 of the widowers and 421 of the widows, who were used as controls. In the second study, 104 men and 54 women with ALS were interviewed and the findings compared with those in a similarly sized control group matched for sex, age within 5 years, and area of residence, about half of whom were "normal", the others being patients in the same hospitals with relatively mild neurological disease. Very few subjects in either group reported "electrical injuries", that is injuries that resulted in burns, persistent pain, or loss of consciousness, very few were employed in electrical work, and the relative risks were close to unity.

A small study from the UK (Gawel, Zaiwalla & Rose, 1983) reported the findings in response to a questionnaire given to 63 patients with motor neuron disease and 61 undefined controls whose "age and sex distribution ..... was not statistically significant different". Thirteen of the patients had experienced an undefined electric shock against five of the controls and two of the patients had been struck by lightning (one stating that he had been flung to the ground) against none of the controls. The difference between the combined results was statistically significant, but is difficult to interpret in the absence of a clearer description of the method of enquiry. The odds ratio for the combined exposures (4.6) was similar to that of 4.1 for "working in contact with electricity" in Haynal & Regli's (1964) original study.

The fifth, and most important, study was carried out by Deapen & Henderson (1986) in conjunction with the Amyotrophic Lateral Sclerosis Society of America. Histories were obtained from 518 patients with the disease and from a control group of the same size matched for sex and age within 5 years, drawn from individuals nominated by the patients as workmates, neighbours, and other social acquaintances. Information was obtained *inter alia* about the individual's occupation 3 years before the date of diagnosis of the disease (or the corresponding period in the case of the controls) and the occurrence more than 3 years previously of electric shocks severe enough to cause unconsciousness. Odds ratios of 3.8 and 2.8 were calculated respectively for employment in one or other of 19 previously defined electrical occupations and for the occurrence of severe electric shocks. Both were statistically significant. Deapen & Henderson (1986) noted that electric shock was a form of trauma that had been shown to cause demyelinisation, reactive gliosis, and neuronal death in experimental animals, but that previous studies had provided inconsistent results and they were unable to draw any conclusions from their findings, the significance of which they considered to be "not clear". [Limitations of the Deapen & Henderson's study are that the exposure to EMF was assessed from job titles based on responses to the questionnaire; failure to report the criteria for control selection and the potential recall bias inherent in using occupational histories and reports of electric shock.]

A further study of 135 patients with ALS whose disease began under 45 years of age and 85 control patients with multiple sclerosis, is of limited value. Eight of the ALS patients were noted to have experienced electric shocks before the onset of the disease, severe enough "in some cases" to throw the subject to the ground (Gallagher & Sanders, 1987) but the severity of the shocks in the other cases is not defined and no reference is made to the occurrence (or non-occurrence) of shocks in the controls. Cruz et al. (1999) assessed the association between ALS and several risk factors including electrical shocks. They found a positive association for a familial history of ALS but found no association for electrical shocks.

A cohort study of over 4 million people who were born between 1896 and 1940, were registered in the 1960 Swedish census, and were still alive in 1970 was examined. About 1067 men and 308 women with a known occupation who died between 1970 and 1983 and had ALS given as either the underlying cause or a contributory cause of death on their death certificates (Gunnarsson et al., 1991) were identified. The occupations of the ALS subjects were compared with those of an age-stratified control sample of approximately 250 persons drawn from each 5 year birth cohort from 1896–1900 to 1936–1940. Occupations were classified in 90 groups (54 for men and 36 for women) and significant excesses of ALS were observed for only two (male office workers and male farm workers). It was noted, however, that, in agreement with Deapen & Henderson's (1986) findings "there seemed to be an association between ALS and work with electricity" (OR = 1.5 for male electricity workers). [This study can be viewed only as hypothesis generating.]

In 1997 Davanipour et al. found that 28 patients with ALS had had, on average, more intense occupational exposure to ELF fields than 32 controls. In their study, the controls were relatives of the patients and selected to be of similar age and, if possible, of the same gender. Unfortunately the requirements were too stringent and they obtained the two controls intended (one blood and one non-blood relative) for 12 cases and only one control for the remaining eight. Detailed occupational histories were obtained and exposure to ELF electromagnetic fields was classed for each job held in one of five categories, from low to high, and exposure indices were calculated taking into account the numbers of years worked in each job. The odds ratio per unit value of the exposure index (which ranged from 3 to 383) was positive (1.006) but not quite statistically significant (95% CI 0.99–1.01). Gender made little difference to the results and the odds ratio cited is one for all subjects irrespective of sex. Davanipour et al. (1997) considered that recent findings had made the concept that ELF fields were an aetiological factor in the development of ALS more plausible and that, despite the defects of the control group, their findings indicated that "long term occupational exposure to ELF may increase the risk of ALS". [The study is limited by the small sample size and potential control selection bias.]

Table 55. Case-control studies of amyotrophic lateral sclerosis before 1997: electrical employment and electric shocks [a]

| Authors | Exposure | No. of subjects | | Odds ratio |
|---------|----------|-----------------|--|------------|
| | | Cases | Controls | |
| Haynal & Regli, 1964 | Occupation in contact with electricity | 9 / 73 | 5 / 150 | 4.1* |
| Kondo & Tsubaki, 1981 first study [b] | Electric injuries | 2 / 458 (M) 3 / 254 (F | 1 / 216 (M) 2 / 421 (F) | 1.0 |
| Kondo & Tsubaki, 1981 second study | | 6 / 104 (M) 1 / 54 (F) | 7 / 104 (M) 2 / 54 (F) | 1.0 |
| Kondo & Tsubaki, 1981 first study | Occupation electric work | 3 / 458 (M) | 1 / 216 (M) | 1.4 |
| Gawel, Zaiwalla & Rose, 1983 | Struck by lightning Other electric shock | 2 / 63 13 / 63 | 0 / 61 5 / 61 | 4.6* |
| Deapen & Henderson, 1986 | Occupation electricity related | 19 / 518 | 5 / 518 | 3.8* |
| | Electric shock | 14 / 518 | 5 / 518 | 2.8* |

[a] A sixth study (Gallagher & Sanders, 1987) is omitted (see text).

[b] First study was on motor neuron disease, included 333 men and 178 women with ALS; second study limited to ALS. No woman was reported with an electric work occupation in either study, neither was any man in the second study.

* $p \leq 0.05$

Estimates of the risks associated with electric work were also provided in five of the later studies described under Alzheimer disease. These arc summarized in Table 56.

In the Savitz, Loomis & Tse (1998) proportional mortality study, electrical work, as previously defined, was recorded slightly more often for the 114 men with amyotrophic lateral sclerosis than for the 1614 controls, giving an odds ratio of 1.3 adjusted for age, period, social class, and race, which was statistically significant (95% CI 1.1–1.6). [The diagnosis of ALS from death certificates in this study was based on ICD9, which groups ALS with other motor neuron diseases. Other limitations of this study include the fact that only one occupation was taken from death certificates and the absence of data on important confounders, such as familial neurodegenerative diseases or exposure to electric shocks].

Johansen & Olsen's (1998a) cohort study of Danish electricity workers recorded only 14 deaths from ALS, but the SMR (2.0; 95% CI 1.1–3.4) was, nevertheless, statistically significant and was higher, though no longer significant, for men with the highest average exposure of = 0.1 μT (SMR = 2.8; 95% CI 0.8–7.3). In this population the mortality from electricity accidents was 18 times the national average (based on 10 deaths) and 31 times that expected in the group with the highest average exposure.

In a study of the morbidity from neurodegenerative diseases and other disorders of the central nervous system, data on the entire Danish cohort (n = 30 631) were linked to the population-based National Register of Patients, which records more than 99% of all hospital discharges for somatic diseases (Danish National Board of Health, 1981). Data on all 30 631 employees were linked to the Register for follow-up for central nervous system diseases between 1 January 1978 or the date of first employment, whichever came last, and the date of death, emigration or 31 December 1993, whichever came first. Medical records were obtained for cases of ALS and other motor neuron diseases to verify the diagnosis and to obtain information on episodes of electric shocks or other occupational exposure before development of the disease. Men had an increased risk for all motor neuron diseases combined (SIR = 1.89; 95% CI = 1.16–2.93), based on 20 cases, which was confined to the 15 men with a diagnosis of ALS (SIR = 1.72; 95% CI 0.96–2.83). They also had an increased risk for other motor neuron diseases (SIR = 2.75; 95% CI 0.88–6.41) and for demyelinating diseases, with four cases observed (SIR = 1.90; 95% CI = 0.51–4.86) (Johansen, 2000).

The Savitz, Checkoway & Loomis (1998) cohort study of US utility workers recorded 28 deaths from ALS giving an SMR of 0.8. When, however, all the 33 deaths in which ALS was mentioned on the death certificate as either the underlying or a contributory cause of death, were related to the individuals' estimated cumulative exposure in terms of μT-years, that is the time-weighted average exposure multiplied by the number of years exposed, a positive but non-significant association was observed (relative risk per μT-year = 1.03; 95% CI 0.90–1.18). Unlike Alzheimer disease, ALS progresses rapidly over 1 or 2 years and this may be the most relevant association. Should, however, any effect of exposure have a long latent period, it is notable that the only positive relationship for a specific period was that for 20 or more years in the past (relative risk per μT-year = 1.07; 95% CI 0.91–1.26). [Limitations of this study are the modest number of ALS cases, diagnosis from death certificates, and the absence of the data on electric shocks or the family's disease history].

In a previously described study, Feychting et al. (2003) found no increased risk for ALS in any of their analyses, including occupations having the highest EMF exposure. They also analyzed the "electrician" category separately because this job reports the largest number of electric shock accidents in Sweden. When looking at risk for men only by job title alone, Feychting et al. observed an increased risk (statistically significant) of ALS among welders based on 24 cases, and a slightly elevated risk among radio and television assemblers (seven cases) and telephone and telegraph installers/repairmen (six cases), but these were not statistically significant. No risk was observed for electricians.

For ALS Håkansson et al. (2003) report the statistically significant risk estimate RR = 2.2 (95% CI 1.0–4.7) for both men and women in the very high exposure group (based on 13 cases). Additonally, they report an exposure-response relationship with an RR of 1.5 for an increase of 1 μT.

**Table 56. Later studies of amyotrophic lateral sclerosis**

| Authors | Exposure | No. of deaths | Relative risk (95% CI) |
|---|---|---|---|
| Savitz, Loomis & Tse, 1998 | Electrical occupation | 114 | 1.3 (1.1–1.6) |
| Savitz, Checkoway & Loomis, 1998 | Cumulative, career | 33 | 1.03 (0.90–1.18) [a] |
| | Cumulative, 10–19 y before death | 33 | 0.82 (0.40–1.65) [a] |
| | Cumulative, 20 y before death | 33 | 1.07 (0.91–1.26) [a] |
| Johansen & Olsen, 1998a | Any | 14 | 2.0 (1.1–3.4)* |
| | 1.0 µT average | 4 | 2.8 (0.8–7.3) |
| Feychting et al., 2003 | Occupation in 1970 (males) | | |
| | reference group < 0.11 µT | 227 | |
| | 3rd quartile 0.12–0.19 µT | 723 | 0.9 (0.7–1.0) |
| | 90th percentile 0.20–0.29 µT | 210 | 0.8 (0.7–1.0) |
| | 95th percentile > 0.5 µT | 70 | 0.8 (0.6–1.0) |
| Håkansson et al., 2003 | Occupational exposure (males & females) | | |
| | reference < 0.16 µT | 15 | |
| | medium 0.16–0.25 µT | 52 | 1.6 (0.9–2.8) |
| | high 0.25–0.53 µT | 17 | 1.9 (1.0–4.0) |
| | very high > 0.530 µT | 13 | 2.1 (1.0–4.7) |

[a] Relative risk for µT-year cumulative exposure.

\* p < 0.05

Most of these studies do not allow examination of possible confounding from electric shock. It is conceivable that exposure to electric shocks increases ALS risk and, also, clearly work in the utility industry carries a risk of experiencing electric shocks. Some to the reviewed studies did report analyses that indeed linked electric shocks to ALS (Deapen & Henderson, 1986; Gunnarsson et al., 1992; Johansen & Olsen, 1998a), but none of the studies provided an analysis in which the relation between EMF and ALS was studied with control for electric shocks. A crude calculation can be made from the data provided by Deapen and Hendersen, and this seems to indicate the EMF association holds up even after control for electric shock experience.

There is no obvious biological explanation for the epidemiological evidence for a link between severe electric shocks and ALS. However, it is

201

possible that the massive, synchronized discharge of neurons (especially the large motor neurons) might release sufficient glutamate to precipitate excito-toxic changes. It might also trigger more subtle and persistent changes in the excitability of neurons. In many parts of the brain a tetanic burst of impulses arriving at a synapse can lead to a prolonged increase in the efficacy of that synapse and neighbouring synapses in activating the post-synaptic cell (a phenomenon called Long-Term Potentiation or LTP). In many situations, LTP appears to involve activation of the N-methyl-D-aspartate (NMDA) receptor by glutamate. The ionic channel of the NMDA receptor is blocked by intracellular $Mg^{2+}$ at normal intracellular potentials, but this block is released if the cell is substantially depolarised by a preceding burst of impulses. Any impulse that follows a burst will then cause $Ca^{2+}$ influx through the NMDA receptor channel, and this is thought to trigger reactions that lead to an increase in the effectiveness of the synapse, which can last for months (Kandel, Schwartz & Jessell, 1991). If severe electric shocks do pro-duce LTP, the increased excitability of cells might produce cumulative patho-logical changes, perhaps involving $Ca^{2+}$ influx through voltage-activated channels or increased metabolic demand, with spillover of reactive oxygen species.

The pathogenetic mechanisms leading to the selective loss of certain populations of dopaminergic neurons are not clear. It has been suggested that the dopamine transporter and vesicular monoamine transporter proteins, which are heavily expressed in the dopaminergic neurons of the substantia nigra, might act as portals of entry for toxins that are structurally related to monoamines (Speciale et al., 1998; Uhl, 1998).

### 7.3 Parkinson disease, Multiple Sclerosis

#### 7.3.1 Pathology

Parkinson disease is characterized clinically by progressive motor dysfunction, including bradykinesia, gait disturbance, rigidity, and tremor. Most data on disease duration come from clinical samples which suggest that disease duration may average seven or more years. Many persons with Parkinson disease develop cognitive, behavioral, and autonomic signs: visible or measureable indications of changes in responses controlled by the autonomic nervous system, such as skin colour, sweating, pupil diametre and blood pressure. In particular, dementia, hallucinations, delusions, and hypotension develop in many persons with the disease. While the behavioral disturbances and autonomic signs are worsened by the dopaminergic agents commonly prescribed to treat the disease, these agents improve quality of life and probably prolong life. Some data suggest that behavioral disturbances and autonomic signs portend a more malignant course of disease. Pathologically, an important hallmark of the disease is degeneration of the substantia nigra (e.g. neuronal loss) .

### 7.3.2    Epidemiology

Occupation has been considered as a possible cause of Parkinson disease in several studies. The study by Wechsler et al. (1991) included jobs likely to involve relatively high exposures to EMF and reported three of 19 affected men were welders against zero out of nine controls and that two other affected men had worked as electricians or electrical engineers. However, Savitz, Loomis & Tse (1998) found very little evidence of an increased risk in electrical workers. Overall the odds ratio derived from the occupations of 168 men dying from Parkinson disease and 1614 controls was 1.1 (95% CI 0.9–1.2).

In the Danish cohort study (Johansen & Olsen, 1998a), the SMR for Parkinsonism was 0.8, based on 14 deaths and even lower for the more heavily exposed men (0.5). In the US study by Savitz, Loomis & Tse (1998), positive relationships were observed with both cumulative cancer exposure and exposure more than 20 years before death, neither of which were, however, statistically significant (relative risks 1.03 per $\mu$T-year, 95% CI 0.90–1.18, and 1.07 per $\mu$T-year, 95% CI 0.91–1.26). Noonan et al. (2002) reported a positive association with an OR of 1.5 for the highest exposure category for Parkinson disease and magnetic field exposure in electrical workers.

Feychting et al. (2003) found no increased risk for vascular dementia, senile dementia, pre-senile dementia, Parkinson disease, multiple sclerosis or epilepsy for either men or women. Håkansson et al. (2003) also found no increased risk for Parkinson disease or multiple sclerosis (MS) and they observed a decreased RR for epilepsy.

In one Danish study (Johansen et al., 1999) of the risk for MS, data on the entire cohort (n = 31 990) were linked to the files of the Danish Multiple Sclerosis Registry, which was founded in January 1948 as a nationwide program to register all cases of MS in Denmark. All cases of suspected or verified MS are currently notified to the Register from all 22 Danish neurological departments and the two rehabilitation centers of the Danish Multiple Sclerosis Society. Only verified cases of MS were included in the present study. Overall, 32 cases of MS were diagnosed, as compared with 23.7 expected from national incidence rates, to yield a standardized incidence ratio of 1.35 (95% CI 0.92–1.91).

### 7.4    Discussion

Of the four neurodegenerative diseases that have been considered, Parkinson disease and MS have received the least attention in epidemiology. No study has provided clear evidence of an association with above-average exposure to extremely low frequency EMFs and, in the absence of laboratory evidence to the contrary, it seems unlikely that such fields are involved in the disease.

The evidence relating to Alzheimer disease is more difficult to assess. The initial reports that gave rise to the idea suggested that the increased risk could be substantial (Sobel et al., 1995). Despite the fact that the initial report was based on the combined results of three independent studies, it should be regarded only as hypothesis forming, as the greater risk was largely the result of classifying groups of garment workers in the heavily exposed groups that had not previously been so classified. The finding was quickly confirmed (by some of the authors of the original report) in another case-control study and was weakly supported by the proportional mortality ratio of causes of death as recorded on US death certificates. It was not supported, however, by the three studies that could provide quantified estimates of people's exposures. One, a case-control study, that did not show risk associated with the individual's primary occupation, did show a substantial and statistically significant risk with the last recorded occupation, which would have been the association recorded in the death certificate study. Neither of the cohort studies, however, provided evidence of a risk with increasing exposure nor, in the one study that provided the information, any excess mortality in power plant workers as a group. The three more recent studies have provided a mixed evidence as well: one providing a limited evidence for males in the highest exposure group, another (overlapping) study focusing on the resistance welders showed an effect, and a third one showing an effect in males, but not in females. In conclusion, there is only inadequate evidence to suggest that 50/60 Hz fields could cause Alzheimer disease.

More evidence is available for ALS. Eight reports of the relationship between electrical work or the experience of electrical shocks have been published since the original suggestion was made that electric shocks might increase the risk of the disease. Two early studies from Japan, where the prevalence of electrical work (as recorded in the medical history) and of electrical shock was low, failed to provide any support for the hypothesis. The others all provided some support. In three, including one of the two cohort studies with measured exposure, the excess associated with exposure was statistically significant. Electric shocks were recorded only in four early reports, in two of which (one from the UK and one from the US) the prevalence was significantly raised. The two most recent and overlapping studies from Sweden focusing on magnetic field exposure and electric shock are inconsistent, with one showing no effect and the other indicting a relative risk of about 2 in the two highest exposure categories. The epidemiological evidence suggests that employment in electrical occupations may increase the risk of ALS, however, separating the increased risk due to receiving an electric shock from the increased exposure to EMFs is difficult.

In considering a possible causal relationship between neurodegenerative disease and the electrical environment, the relevant exposure has been assumed to be some aspect (e.g. time weighted average, number of exposures above some critical level, etc.) of ELF magnetic fields, contact currents and/or electrical shock[1]. "Contact current" is defined here as an electrical current that

---

1. There are other environmental exposures that can cause electrical effects in the human body, such as the environmental electric field. Except in special circumstances such as near high voltage transmission lines, however, the effect of this source is usually smaller than either of the other two sources.

passes through the body between two points when they are in "contact" with an external electrical system. An electrical shock occurs as "a reflex response to the passage of current through the body" and thus is the result of contact currents large enough to be perceived. Although it is clear from these definitions that contact current and electrical shock are closely related, it may appear that the ELF magnetic field is a distinctly different exposure because ambient magnetic fields, with specific exceptions (e.g. MRI machines) are not nearly large enough to produce neural stimulation. This is not entirely correct. In fact, there are several important connections between the two that should be understood before the possible effects of one exposure can be separated from those of the other.

The first connection is that each exposure can be responsible for inducing an electric field and a corresponding electric current density within the human body. Biophysicists consider *the induced electric field* as the metric most relevant for evaluating biological interactions from EMF or contact current exposure[1]. Thus, a biological effect due to an electric field in the body may be caused by exposure to an ELF magnetic field, a contact current or some other aspect of the electrical environment that can cause an electric field in the body. What might allow one to discern the origin of the effect is recognition that the distribution of the magnitude and orientation within the body of the electric field induced by an ELF magnetic field and that due to a contact current can be significantly different.

It is well known that a time varying ELF magnetic field in the body can cause electric fields and currents to be induced in the body via Faraday's law. This induced electric field is limited by the size of the body and the magnitude of the magnetic field. In fact, it is generally well recognized that the electric fields induced by typical environmental 50/60-Hertz magnetic fields are usually thought to be too small to cause biological effects. Contact currents with commonly experienced amplitudes, on the other hand, have been estimated to produce electric fields in the body that are orders of magnitude larger than induced electric fields from typical levels of ambient magnetic fields. Further, the electric field produced by a magnetic field is larger near the periphery of the body while the electric field produced by contact currents is larger in the path between contact points and hence often in the limbs and the body's interior. These differences in amplitude and spatial distribution within the body may be suggestive of a cause and effect relationship with diseases that have their origin in specific parts of the body. For these reasons, contact currents and the related electrical shocks are important exposures and should be considered when conducting studies of possible health outcomes due to the electrical environment.

The second connection between the ELF magnetic field and contact currents is the fact that environmental magnetic fields may induce voltages

---

1.  Several other mechanisms have been proposed by which ELF magnetic fields might directly interact with the body. However, they are either thought to be implausible or unlikely at environmental field levels.

in electrical systems that in turn cause current, i.e. contact current, in a human body that is in contact with this system. In addition, conducted currents on residential grounding systems may be related to nearby ELF magnetic fields. When either is the case, the amplitudes of the ELF magnetic field and the contact current are related.

The identification of which of these two exposures (if either) is associated with a health outcome, is a very important question. Properly configured studies should be designed to identify the specific exposure responsible for a specific biological effect.

The measurement of magnetic fields is a well-established enterprise. The measurement of electrical contact current and or shock current, however, is not as well advanced. It would require either that the current entering the body during normal life or work be measured or that the circuit contacted by the body be characterized by a simple equivalent circuit. It is only recently that an instrument for measuring the currents entering the body has been developed and it has not been extensively tested. Measurements that lead to a simple equivalent for a circuit that can be contacted by a human, however, have been made. In either case, methodology to allow evaluation of "contact current" exposure should be tested further. If acceptable, it should be used in further studies of the relationship between the electrical environment and neurodegenerative diseases.

Quantitatively, the flow of electricity through the brain is likely to be substantially greater from the use of electro-convulsive therapy for the treatment of psychiatric conditions than from even severe electric shock received occupationally or from non-fatal strikes by lightning. However, no large, long-term study of patients has been reported in sufficient detail to permit the detection of (say) a five-fold risk of a disease that normally causes about one death in 100 adults.

## 7.5    Conclusions

It has been hypothesized that exposure to ELF fields is associated with several neurodegenerative diseases. For Parkinson disease and multiple sclerosis the number of studies has been small and there is no evidence for an association with these diseases. For Alzheimer disease and amyotrophic lateral sclerosis (ALS) more studies have been published. Some of these reports suggest that people employed in electrical occupations have an increased risk of ALS. So far no biological mechanism has been established which can explain this association, although it could have arisen because of confounders related to electrical occupations such as electric shocks. Overall, the evidence for the association between ELF exposure and ALS is considered inadequate.

The few studies investigating the association between ELF exposure and Alzheimer disease are inconsistent. However, the higher quality studies that focused on Alzheimer morbidity rather than mortality do not indicate an association. Altogether, the evidence for an association between ELF exposure and Alzheimer disease is inadequate.

# 8    CARDIOVASCULAR DISORDERS

Concerns about chronic cardiovascular changes resulting from exposure to ELF fields originated from descriptions in the 1960s and early 1970s of the symptoms among Russian high voltage switchyard operators and workers (Asanova & Rakov, 1966; 1972). Further studies carried out in the Russian Federation in the 1980's and 90's reported various functional changes in the cardiovascular system, such as hypertension in workers in 500 kV, 750 kV and 1150 kV power installations (Rubtsova, Tikhonova & Gurvich, 1999). More recent investigations have focused mainly on direct cardiac effects of EMF exposure, mostly related to heart rate variability and subsequent acute cardiovascular events.

## 8.1    Acute effects

Current flow through the human body appears to be necessary in order to result in major cardiovascular effects from EMF exposure, such as the effects due to electric shock (Hocking, 1994). Normally electric shock requires direct electrical contact of a conductor with the body. It may, however, also occur if the body is exposed to very strong electric or magnetic fields (Foster, 1992). Minor effects have also been reported in other situations of low-level EMF exposure. Most human studies on EMF effects on the cardiovascular system have focused on acute rather than long-term effects.

### 8.1.1    *Electrocardiogram changes, heart rate, and heart rate variability*

Silny (1981) found no effects on the electrocardiogram (ECG) in 100 persons exposed to time-varying magnetic fields (5 Hz to 1 kHz, less than 100 mT). Hauf (1989) has performed human tests exposing the subjects to 50-Hz fields (20 kV m$^{-1}$ and 0.3 mT) with a current of 500 µA passing through the body. The experiments did not indicate any significant effects on the heart rate of the subjects. In another study, there were no significant changes in heart rate in persons exposed locally to pulsed magnetic fields up to 2.2 µT by transcranial magnetic stimulation (TMS) (see 5.2.2) (Chokroverty et al., 1995).

In a series of studies carried out by the Midwest Research Institute in the US, effects of ELF fields on the heart rate in humans have been investigated. In a set of studies by Graham et al. (1994), subjects were exposed to different levels of combined electric and magnetic fields (low: 6 kV m$^{-1}$ and 10 µT; medium: 9 kV m$^{-1}$ and 20 µT; high: 12 kV m$^{-1}$ and 30 µT). In the medium group a significantly decreased heart rate was observed, while in the other groups no change was found. In another study by the same group, six physiological parameters were examined at five sampling points with and without exercise (Maresh et al., 1988). During no-exercise sessions the cardiac interbeat interval was increased at two sampling points when subjects were exposed to 60-Hz fields. No other difference between the sham and exposed groups was found. A similar effect was found by another study of the same group (Cook et al., 1992).

In a replication study by Whittington, Podd & Rapley (1996), no effect of a higher magnetic field (100 μT, 50 Hz) on heart rate or blood pressure was found, however. Humans exposed for 1 hour to EMFs under a 400-kV power line exhibited no difference in pulse rate during autonomic function tests (Korpinen & Partanen, 1994a). The same researchers reported that exposure to 50-Hz fields (up to 10 kV m$^{-1}$ and 15 μT for several hours) did not affect the incidence of extrasystoles or arrhythmia (Korpinen & Partanen, 1994b; Korpinen, Partanen & Uusitalo, 1993). A 2% decrease of heart rate was also observed by Sait et al. (1999) after a 100 to 150-s exposure to a 50 Hz, 28 μT magnetic field. From these studies, it can be noted that the positive but inconsistent results from the US Midwest Research Institute of reduced heart rates after exposure to EMF have not been confirmed by other studies. The heart rate effects, where such have been found, are generally of small magnitude, and can currently not serve as an indicator of an acute health effect (Hauf, 1982).

Sastre, Cook & Graham (1998) performed studies on heart rate variability (HRV) of 77 healthy men exposed to 60-Hz magnetic fields of 14.1 μT or 28.3 μT. Statistically significant alterations in HRV were observed during intermittent exposure to the higher field strength, while no effects occurred at the lower field strengths or when the exposure was continuous. A reduction in the power ratio in the low band of the HRV spectra (0.02–0.15 Hz) to the high band (0.16–1.0 Hz) was also observed by Sait, Wood & Sadafi (1999) after a 100 to 150-s exposure to a 50 Hz, 28 μT magnetic field with the exposure conditions already mentioned. In two studies on the same issue, HRV was evaluated during intermittent exposure to 28.3 μT (Graham, Cook & Riffle, 1997; 1998). In the latter study, three different frequencies were used (16, 40, 60 Hz). Exposure to 16 Hz was associated with significant alterations of the HRV spectrum. However, in a later pooled analysis of several studies conducted at the same institute, Graham et al. (1999) reported that this effect occurred only in studies where hourly blood sampling was performed. The authors hypothesised that blood sampling altered the level of subject arousal, allowing EMF interaction to affect HRV. A multi-study analysis indicates that the effect on HRV happens when EMF exposure is accompanied by increases in physiologic arousal, stress, or a disturbance in sleep, such as blood collection, but not otherwise (Graham et al. 2000a).

Recently, Graham et al. (2000e) performed studies using a much higher magnetic field (127.3 μT) and both continuous and intermittent exposure. No alterations in HRV were observed by either exposure condition, and the researchers concluded that, taking into account earlier reports, direct excitation of the human heart is extremely unlikely under exposure to magnetic fields lower than 127.3 μT.

A summary of the studies into the effects of ELF fields on ECG and heart rate is given in Table 57.

**Table 57. Studies of ECG and heart rates after ELF exposure**

| Test | Exposure | Response | Comments | Authors |
|---|---|---|---|---|
| ECG | 5 Hz–1 kHz < 100 mT | No change. | | Silny, 1981 |
| Cardiac inter-beat interval | 60 Hz 9 kV m$^{-1}$, 16 A m$^{-1}$ | Longer cardiac interbeat interval. | | Maresh et al., 1988 |
| Pulse rate | 50 Hz 20 kV m$^{-1}$, 300 µT or combined + 200 and 500 µA-currents at 50 Hz | No change. | Protocol looks confused, mixing haemato-logical and physiological parameters. | Hauf, 1989 |
| Pain, ECG, heart rate | Not defined: mag-neto-stimulation | No pain, no change in ECG and heart rate. | No dosimetry | Nagano et al., 1991 |
| Interbeat interval before, during and after expo-sure 30 male subjects | 60 Hz 9 kV m$^{-1}$, 20 µT 2x3 h day$^{-1}$, 4 days | Interbeat interval longer during and immediately after exposure. | Double-blind, counterbal-anced study. | Cook et al., 1992 |
| Extrasystoles, pulse rate | 50 Hz 0.14–10 kV m$^{-1}$, 1.0-5.4 µT 0.5 h – few hours | No more extrasys-toles in the field than out the field. Small decrease in pulse rate can be due to changes in work load. | | Korpinen, Par-tanen & Uusi-talo, 1993 Korpinen & Partanen, 1994b |
| Interbeat interval before, during and after expo-sure 54 male subjects | 60 Hz 6 kV m$^{-1}$, 10 µT 9 kV m$^{-1}$, 20 µT 12 kV m$^{-1}$, 30 µT | Interbeat interval longer during and immediately after exposure only at the intermediate level of exposure. | Double-blind, counterbal-anced study. | Graham et al., 1994 |
| Pulse rate | 50 Hz 3.5–4.3 kV m$^{-1}$, 1.4–6.6 µT 1 h | No change in pulse rate. | | Korpinen & Partanen, 1994a |
| ECG, systolic and diastolic blood pressure, orthostatic test, valsalva maneu-ver, deep breath-ing test | 50 Hz 3.5–4.3 kV m$^{-1}$, 1.4–6.6 µT 1 h | No change. | CV autonomic tests were per-formed 0.5 h before and after the 1 h-exposure. | Korpinen & Partanen, 1995 |
| Heart rate | pulsed magnetic fields of up to 2.2 µT used in TMS | No change | | Chokroverty et al., 1995 |

209

**Table 57. Continued**

| | | | | |
|---|---|---|---|---|
| Heart rate and blood pressure 100 (male and female) subjects | 50 Hz 100 µT, intermittent 9 min | No effect. | Double-blind, counterbalanced study. | Whittington, Podd & Rapley, 1996 |
| Heart rate variability 33 male subjects (exp 1) 40 male subjects (exps 2 and 3) | 60 Hz 1 or 20 µT, intermittent Overnight (23.00–07.00) | Altered heart rate variability at 20 µT, but not at 1 µT. | Double-blind (all studies) and counterbalanced (exps 2 and 3). | Graham, Cook & Riffle, 1997 Sastre, Cook & Graham, 1998 |
| Heart rate and heart rate variability 18 (pilot study) and 35 subjects (follow-up study) | 50 Hz 28 µT, sinusoidal continuous or intermittent (15 s on-off), or square-wave for 100–150 s | Altered heart rate and heart rate variability by continuous sinusoidal fields, but not by intermittent or square-wave fields. | Blind and counterbalanced. | Sait, Wood & Sadafi, 1999 |
| Heart rate variability 172 male subjects (pooled from 7 studies) | 60 Hz 28.3 or 127.3 µT, intermittent or continuous Overnight | Altered heart rate variability in some conditions. | Blood sampling (for another study) at night was critical for this effect. Double-blind studies. | Graham et al., 1999; 2000e; 2000d |

### 8.1.2 Blood pressure

No changes were observed in blood pressure, neither in subjects exposed to a 50 Hz field (20 kV m$^{-1}$ and 0.3 mT) with a current of 500 µA passing through the body (Hauf, 1989), neither in humans exposed for 1 hour to EMFs under a 400-kV power line (Korpinen & Partanen, 1996), nor in persons exposed locally to pulsed magnetic fields up to 2.2 µT by TMS (Chokroverty et al., 1995). These studies are summarized in Table 58.

**Table 58. Studies of blood pressure after ELF exposure**

| Test | Exposure | Response | Comments | Authors |
|---|---|---|---|---|
| Blood pressure | 50 Hz 20 kV m$^{-1}$, 300 µT or combined + 200 and 500 µA-currents at 50 Hz | No change. | | Hauf, 1989 |
| Blood pressure | pulsed magnetic fields of up to 2.2 µT used in TMS | No change. | | Chokroverty et al., 1995 |
| Blood pressure | 50 Hz 3.5–4.3 kV m$^{-1}$, 1.4– 6.6 µT 1 h | No change. | | Korpinen & Partanen, 1996 |

## 8.2    Long-term effects

Knave et al. (1979) and Stopps, Janischewskyj & Alcock (1979) found no significant effects on cardiovascular function in male workers who were exposed occupationally for more than 5 years to electric fields from 400 kV power lines. Checcucci (1985) found no effect on the cardiovascular system in 1200 workers at high-voltage railway substations (1–4.6 kV m$^{-1}$ and 4–15 µT). In a health survey of 627 railway high-voltage substation workers, Baroncelli et al. (1986) found no difference in the ECG between exposed and control groups. Table 59 gives a summary of these studies.

**Table 59. Studies of cardiovascular effects after long-term ELF exposure**

| Test | Exposure | Response | Comments | Authors |
|------|----------|----------|----------|---------|
| CV parameters and diseases | 50 Hz 400 kV power lines > 5 years | No effect. | Better psychologic performance linked to higher education level, and lower fertility predominant on boys, anterior to the exposure period. | Knave et al., 1979 |
| CV parameters and diseases | 50 Hz 400 kV power lines > 5 years | No effect. | | Stopps, Janischewskyj & Alcock, 1979 |
| CV parameters and diseases | 1–4.6 kV m$^{-1}$, 4–15 µT | No effect. | | Checcucci, 1985 |
| Haematology electro-cardiogram | 50 Hz HV railway substation < 5 kV m$^{-1}$, 15 µT 0, 1, 10 and 20 h / week | No effect. | | Baroncelli et al., 1986 |

Based on the idea put forth by Sastre, Savitz (1999) hypothesized an association between exposure to EMF and cardiovascular disease. This hypothesis was based on two independent lines of evidence. The first was experimental data on heart rate variability described above in which intermittent 60-Hz magnetic fields were found to reduce the normal HRV (Sastre, Cook & Graham, 1998). The second came from several prospective cohort studies which indicated that reductions in some components of the HRV increase the risk for: (1) heart disease (Dekker et al., 1997; Liao et al., 1997, Martin et al., 1987; Tsuji et al., 1996); (2) overall mortality rate in survivors of myocardial infarction (Kleiger et al., 1987; Lombardi et al., 1987; Vaishnav et al., 1994); and (3) risk for sudden cardiovascular death (Malik, Farrell

& Camm, 1990). Thus, they postulated that occupational exposure to EMF will increase the risk for cardiac arrhythmia-related conditions and acute myocardial infarction, but not for chronic cardiovascular disease.

Several studies, published before the specific hypothesis of an effect on HRV was suggested, examined general cardiovascular mortality in relation to EMF (Table 60). In a Canadian retrospective cohort study of 21 744 men employed in an electrical utility company in the province of Quebec between 1 January 1970 and 31 December 1988, the standardised mortality ratio (SMR) for circulatory diseases was below 1 in all job categories and with all exposure levels to magnetic fields, electric fields and pulsed electromagnetic fields (Baris et al., 1996b). Exposure information was obtained from a job-exposure matrix (JEM) constructed on the basis of the last job held in the industry. The JEM was constructed for a larger study of employees in the utility industry in Canada and France (Theriault et al., 1994) and included a measurement protocol of magnetic fields, electric fields and pulsed electromagnetic fields among 466 employees for one week. Among employees exposed to magnetic fields > 0.16 μT, 137 persons died from circulatory diseases (adjusted RR = 0.91; 95% CI 0.73–1.14). The SMRs, when using electric fields and pulsed electromagnetic fields as the exposure variables, were close to those observed for exposure to magnetic fields. [It must be noted that no definition of diagnoses included as "circulatory diseases" are given. Likewise, there is no reference to the quality of the Canadian mortality statistics in this paper, or to what extent it is the underlying cause of death, the contributory cause of death or a combination of the two, which is used as the outcome measurement.]

A retrospective cohort study from the US (Kelsh & Sahl, 1997) of 40 335 men and women employed between 1960 and 1991 in a Californian utility company observed a significantly reduced SMR of 0.62 (95% CI 0.59–0.65) for both sexes combined. This was based on a comparison with the general population of the geographical area of the utility company and included 1561 cases of cardiovascular death (ICD-9, 3900–4489). The risk estimates in different occupational categories were very close to each other and all but the category "Meter readers/Field service" had significantly decreased mortality. Exposure information was primarily based on job title and work environment and included no measurement protocol. Each employee was assigned to one of seven categories based on the occupation held for the longest time. Information on mortality was obtained from three public sources and also from company records, indicating some underreporting to the primary sources. In internal analyses conducted across employment categories and using administrative employees as a reference group, mortality from "Major Cardiovascular" (category not defined) was significantly increased in all categories, the highest RR being 1.71 (95% CI 1.13–2.58) in the "Meter Reader/Field service" category. When stratifying the internal analyses by work employment period (before or after 1960) no clear pattern emerged. [A clear healthy worker effect seems to explain the results of the external analyses. However, no clear explanation can be given for the increased risk of death from "Major Cardiovascular" as no precise and

212

detailed information was available for exposure to known risk factors for these disorders (tobacco smoking, alcohol consumption or physical activity).] A re-analysis of this study cohort (Sahl et al., 2002) is described below.

In a nationwide retrospective cohort study in Denmark of 21 236 men employed in utility companies between 1900 and 1993 the causes of death were ascertained for 1 January 1974 through 31 December 1993, and cause-specific mortality was analysed by latency and estimated levels of exposure to 50 Hz electromagnetic fields (Johansen & Olsen, 1998b). A dedicated job-exposure matrix was designed that distinguished between 25 different job titles held by utility company employees and 19 work areas within this industry. Each of the 475 combinations of job title and work area was assigned an average level of exposure to 50 Hz EMF during a working day, which in turn was grouped into five categories of exposure to ELF fields. The conversion program was constructed by four engineers from the utility companies experienced in the planning and operation of electric utilities in Denmark. The construction of the matrix was based partly on a series of 196 24-hour measurements of 50 Hz EMF among 129 employees in six Danish utility companies and partly on judgements. The individual exposure assignment was based on the characteristics of the first employment held. Overall, 3540 deaths were observed as compared with 3709 expected from national mortality rates, yielding a standardized mortality ratio of 0.96 (95% CI 0.93–0.99). Overall mortality caused by acute myocardial infarction (ICD-8, 410) yielded an SMR of 0.95 (95% CI 0.9–1.0) based on 713 cases. SMR for cardiac sclerosis (ICD-8, 412) was 0.9 (95% CI 0.8–1.0) based on 300 cases and for mortality caused by other heart disorders (ICD-8, 394–402; 413; 420–429; 450 and 782) the SMR was 0.9 (95% CI 0.8–1.0). When analysing the cause-specific mortality by time since first employment or categories of estimated EMF exposure no increased mortality for these disorders appeared. [No information was available about known risk factors for cardiovascular disease. The exposure assessment in this study is based on few measurements and historical records and one cannot exclude that misclassification has taken place. In addition the use of mortality records as the measurement of the outcome may have caused some additional misclassification as the autopsy rates in Denmark has been decreasing in the study period. This study only use external comparisons as the method of analyses and this does not take into account a possible healthy worker effect.] This study cohort was later followed up for risk of pacemaker implantation – summarized below (Johansen et al., 2002).

In a recent follow-up study of Thai employees of the Electricity Generating Authority of Thailand, changes in levels of vascular risk factors over 12 years, and the associations of baseline risk factors with mortality were examined (Sritara et al., 2003). Over the 12-year period, levels of all major vascular risk factors, apart from smoking, worsened in this occupational study population. Although the authors note that the increases appear to exceed those expected from ageing of the cohort alone, very little regarding the impact of exposure on disease and mortality can be inferred from this study.

In the first study conducted with the specific aim to test the hypothesis of an association between EMF and acute cardiovascular disease risk another US retrospective cohort study of utility workers (Savitz et al., 1999) was analysed. It included 138 903 men employed for six months or more between 1950 and 1986. The authors report a significantly increased risk of mortality from arrhythmia-related conditions and acute myocardial infarction among workers with long duration of work (with rate ratios of 1.4–1.5 for the longest employment intervals) and with high exposure to magnetic fields (with rate ratios of 1.6–2.4 in the highest exposure category). As postulated a positive association was seen for acute myocardial infarction (AMI) and an inverse association for chronic cardiovascular disease (CVD). The EMF exposure categories were based on 2842 complete work shift time weighted average magnetic field exposure measurements and information on outcome (death certificate) was obtained from 97% of the deceased men. This cohort was reanalysed by Van Wijngaarden et al. (2001a), however, not providing further information on the hypothesis of an association between EMF exposure and mortality of arrhythmia-related cardiovascular diseases or AMI. Finkelstein (1999) questioned the use of death certificates as a source of information on a diagnosis of loss of autonomic cardiovascular control by Savitz et al. (1999) and pointed out that etiologic conclusions could not be drawn on the basis of death certificate codes (Finkelstein, 1999). Problems in using subtypes of CVD as coded on death certificates, which are of uncertain validity and reliability, are particularly evident in this study where the excess of deaths in acute cardiovascular categories coincides with a deficit of deaths in chronic categories for all exposure groups except the highest group. This either suggests specificity of effect or miscoding. In addition, they could not examine the temporal relation between exposure and outcome in any detail other than to look at jobs (with their estimated mean) and death, but not diagnosis. They also lacked information on other CVD risk factors.

The hypothesis of an association between exposure to EMF and the risk for arrhythmia-related cardiovascular disorders was further addressed in the Danish cohort of utility workers (Johansen et al., 2002). The incidence of severe cardiac arrhythmia as indicated by the need for a pacemaker was investigated by a linkage to the nationwide, population-based Danish Pacemaker Register. The study identified all cases of pacemaker implantation among 24 056 male utility workers between 1982 and 2000 and compared this number with the corresponding numbers in the general population. In addition, the data on utility workers was fitted to a multiplicative Poisson regression model in relation to estimated levels of exposure to 50 Hz electromagnetic fields. Overall, the risk was not increased for severe cardiac arrhythmia among employees in the utility companies, based on 135 men with pacemakers with 140 expected, yielding a risk estimate of 0.96 (95% CI 0.8 –1.1). No clear dose-response pattern emerged with increasing level of exposure to EMF or duration of employment. [The study investigated the risk of a morbidity, which leads to the implantation of a pacemaker. One may also consider that other arrhythmias, which are not associated with a pacemaker implantation, and thus not included here, may be associated with the exposure under study. Furthermore the files of the workers were established years before the events reported to the Danish Pacemaker Registry and were supported by personal data from the nationwide, compulsory pension fund and the public payroll system kept for administrative purposes. The completeness of these registries of employments and pacemaker implantation highly reduces the likelihood of selection and information bias. Comparisons with the general population might have been influenced by the healthy worker effect. This was not the case, however, in the internal comparisons within the cohort of different exposure groups. No control of confounding for other risk factors was made. As mentioned before, the exposure assessment in this study is based on few measurements and historical records and one cannot exclude that misclassification has taken place.]

A re-analysis of the data reported by Kelsh & Sahl (1997) did not confirm the findings from Savitz' study (Sahl et al., 2002). In this cohort of 35 391 male utility workers in southern California, USA, with follow-up from 1960 to 1992, 369 cases of chronic coronary heart disease and 407 cases of myocardial infarct were identified. For cumulative exposure, adjusting for socioeconomic factors, no association was observed with mortality from acute myocardial infarction (rate ratio per $\mu$T-year = 1.01, 95% CI 0.99–1.02) or chronic cardiovascular heart disease (rate ratio per $\mu$T-year = 1.00, 95% CI 0.99–1.02). In this study (Sahl et al., 2002) the analyses were performed by the same methods and analytical models as those used by Savitz et al. (1999) in an attempt to conduct as a close a replication as possible of the Savitz work. In the previous study (Kelsh & Sahl, 1997) men aged > 80 years were excluded, EMF exposure was defined on the basis of the worker's usual occupation as opposed to a detailed occupational history, and different reference groups were used in the internal analyses. One group with a significantly increased mortality from cardiovascular disease, but with low EMF exposure, was assigned to the reference group in the present study (Sahl et al., 2002). This might explain some of the observed changes in risk estimates. [Weaknesses include the inability to control for potentially important factors that may influence mortality due to cardiovascular disease, the use of death certificates to identify the cause of death, and the reliability of the distinction between AMI and chronic cardiovascular heart disease as recorded on the death certificate. Strengths include large number of exposed, improved exposure assessment and an attempt to indirectly examine smoking as a potential confounder.]

A population-based case-control study from Sweden (Ahlbom et al., 2004) investigating risk factors for acute myocardial infarction in the city of Stockholm included information on occupational EMF exposure based on job titles one, five, and ten years prior to diagnosis. The analysis was restricted to the 695 cases and 1133 controls with information on job titles. Of these, 595 cases and 949 controls had jobs that were common enough to have been classified according to a previously developed JEM. The study used two approaches to classify exposure. First, specific individual job titles with presumed elevated EMF exposure were investigated and secondly, the subjects were classified according to a JEM. Both analytical approaches

215

revealed risk estimates for acute myocardial infarction below or close to one. [The strengths of this study include the fact that it is population based, looks at morbidity rather than mortality, the high participation rates and finally the high validity of the AMI diagnoses. This study is the first to include information on potential confounders, in particular blood pressure, serum cholesterol, socio-economic status, and cigarette smoking. The limitations of this study include the use of the previously developed JEM. Although this has been utilized in several other studies and seemingly performed well, its sensitivity and specificity in relation to classification of EMF exposure are not assessed. Thus, it is not entirely inconceivable that non-differential recall bias plays a role. On the other hand, several specific job titles were also analyzed and gave consistent results.]

Another Swedish study of the association between EMF exposure and mortality from heart diseases utilised data from the Swedish twin registry including close to 28 000 twins from two different cohorts of twins in Sweden (Håkansson et al., 2003). These twins were interviewed in 1967 and 1973 and at that time their occupation was recorded. In addition the interview covered information on smoking, alcohol consumption, level of physical activity and body mass index. The analyses were based on the primary and contributory cause of death followed up until 1996 utilizing the previously described exposure matrix (Ahlbom et al., 2004) adjusted for the previously mentioned risk factors. The results did not show an overall increased risk for arrhythmia related death, ischemic heart disease other than AMI or atherosclerosis. A non-significantly increased risk for AMI was observed in the highest exposure group (RR = 1.3; 95% CI 0.9–1.9; exposure level > 0.3 $\mu$T). Since this study was conducted within a twin cohort a sub-analysis that took into account the twin information was conducted. In this analysis the authors observed a larger increase in risk for AMI and magnetic fields in genetically susceptible subgroups (i.e. among the monozygotic twins, one of whom previously had an AMI) for which there is no obvious explanation. [Note that this study included subjects from the general population and its exposure assessment was based on a single question on the subjects' "main occupation" at one point in time in the past.]

The latest study of utility workers examined a cohort of 83 997 workers in the UK employed for at least six months between 1973 and 1982 and followed up from 1973 to 1997 (Sorahan & Nichols, 2004). Estimates were obtained for lifetime exposure and exposures accumulated during the most recent 5 years using comprehensive occupational magnetic field exposure assessment. Causes of death (both underlying and contributing) from cardiovascular diseases were grouped into four categories: (1) arrhythmia related, (2) acute myocardial infarction, (3) atherosclerosis related, and (4) chronic/sub-chronic coronary heart disease. Poisson regression modeling with adjustments for age, sex, calendar time, beginning year of employment, and an indicator for socioeconomic status was used. Only for arrhythmia-related death, the relative risk estimates were greater than one for all exposure categories, however, the estimates were based on small numbers, showed no monotonic trend with increasing exposure, and were not statistically significant. (RR per 10 µT-years = 1.1; 95% CI 0.8–1.6). [Of note in this study is the exposure assessment, which was based on elaborate methods that considered individual job histories, job environments, and local sources of magnetic fields in individual job locations, which is likely to have reduced misclassification.]

**Table 60. Studies of general cardiovascular mortality in relation to EMF**

| Population | Design | Exposure | Outcome | Size | Results (95% CI) | Authors |
|---|---|---|---|---|---|---|
| Workers employed in electrical company between 1970–1988 | Cohort SMR and internal comparisons | Member of cohort, job-exposure matrix | Circulatory disease mortality | Circulatory deaths: 137 Cohort: 21 744 | Highest exposure category: SMR = 0.63 (0.53–0.74) RR = 0.91 (0.73–1.14) | Baris et al., 1996b |
| Utility workers, employed 1 y between 1960–1991, followed - 1992 | Cohort SMR and internal comparisons | Member of cohort, certain occupational categories | CVD mortality | CVD deaths: 1561 Cohort: 40 335 | Total cohort: SMR = 0.62 (0.59–0.65) Linemen: RR = 1.42 (1.18–1.71) | Kelsh & Sahl, 1997 |
| Male utility workers, employed 3 months between 1990–1993, followed 1974–1993 | Cohort SMR | Member of cohort, classification of workplaces based on measurements | CVD mortality | CVD deaths: 713 Cohort: 21 236 | High exposure workplace, AMI: SMR = 0.095 (0.9–1.0) | Johansen & Olsen, 1998b |
| Male utility workers, employed 6 months between 1950–1986, followed - 1988 | Cohort SMR and internal comparisons | Duration of work in jobs with elevated EMF | CVD mortality | CVD deaths: 6802 Cohort: 138 903 | Highest µT-year category, AMI: RR = 1.62 (1.45–1.82) Chronic CHD: RR = 1.0 (0.86–1.77) | Savitz et al., 1999 |
| Male utility workers, employed 3 months between 1990–1993, followed 1974–1993 | Cohort SMR | Member of cohort, classification of workplaces based on measurements | Pacemaker implantation | Implants: 135 Cohort: 24 056 | Highest exposure category total SIR = 1.00 (0.6–1.5) | Johansen et al., 2002 |

**Table 60. Continued**

| Male utility workers in Kelsh & Sahl, 1997 | Cohort SMR and internal comparisons | Duration of work in jobs with elevated EMF | CVD mortality | AMI deaths: 407 CCHD deaths: 369 Cohort: 35 391 | Highest µT-year category, AMI: RR = 0.99 (0.65–1.51) Chronic CHD: RR = 1.19 (0.79–1.77) | Sahl et al., 2002 |
|---|---|---|---|---|---|---|
| Swedish twins responding to job questionnaire in 1967 or 1973 | Cohort Cox analysis | Job-exposure matrix | CVD mortality | Twin cohort: 27 790 | Highest exposure group, AMI: RR = 1.3 (0.9–1.9) | Håkansson et al., 2003 |
| Male population of Stockholm 1992–1993 | Population-based case-control | Job titles, job-exposure matrix | AMI morbidity | 695 and 1133 cases and controls | Highest exposure category: RR = 0.57 (0.36–0.89) | Ahlbom et al., 2004 |
| Utility workers, employed 6 months between 1973–1982, followed – 1997 | Cohort SMR and internal comparisons | Duration of work in jobs and locations with elevated EMF | CVD mortality | CVD deaths: 6802 Cohort: 79 972 | Highest µT-year category, AMI: RR = 1.03 (0.88–1.21) Chronic CHD: RR = 0.92 (0.73-1.16) | Sorahan & Nichols, 2004 |

## 8.3 Discussion

### 8.3.1 Heart rate variability hypothesis

Occupational exposure to electromagnetic fields has been suggested to increase the risk for cardiac arrhythmia-related conditions and acute myocardial infarction (Savitz et al., 1999). This hypothesized association between exposure to EMF and cardiovascular disorders was based on experimental data on HRV (Sastre, Cook & Graham, 1998). These experimental data were obtained in a double-blind laboratory investigation in which exposure to 20 µT of intermittent 60 Hz magnetic fields was found to reduce the normal variation of the HRV (Sastre, Cook & Graham, 1998). However, these findings have not been reproduced, and subsequent studies with volunteers did not always produce consistent results regarding HRV and exposures to magnetic fields. After conducting a multi-study analysis, it was concluded that differences in study design factors related to physiologic arousal might explain the apparent inconsistency (Graham et al., 2000d).

In addition, several prospective cohort studies have indicated that reductions in some components of the variation in heart rate increase: (1) the risk for heart disease (Dekker et al., 1997; Liao et al., 1997; Martin et al., 1987; Tsuji et al., 1996), (2) overall mortality rate in survivors of myocardial infarction (Kleiger et al., 1987; Lombardi et al., 1987; Vaishnav et al., 1994), and (3) the risk for sudden cardiovascular death (Malik, Farrell & Camm, 1990). Changed HRV reflects changed cardiac autonomic control (Akselrod et al., 1981; Willich et al., 1993), suggesting this is a possible mechanism of action of EMF exposure on the heart

Thus, while reduced HRV seems to be predictive for the development and survival from heart disease, it is difficult to explain how the mechanism underlying the transient changes in heart rate variability seen in healthy young men after EMF exposure in controlled settings (Graham et al., 2000a; Sastre, Cook & Graham, 1998; Tabor, Michalski & Rokita, 2004) can also explain deaths from arrhythmia and infarction many years after long-term occupational exposure to ELF fields. Furthermore, the influence of EMF on HRV seems questionable.

### 8.3.2 Epidemiologic evidence

The biologically plausible model described above gave Savitz et al. (1999) the impetus to look at cardiovascular mortality in a cohort of utility workers. As postulated *a priori* Savitz observed an increased risk from AMI and arrhythmia related death, but not from chronic cardiovascular disease (Savitz et al., 1999). The only and limited support for the original observation comes from a study based on data from the Swedish twin registry (Håkansson et al., 2003), which observed a nonsignificantly increased risk for AMI. However, seven other studies failed to support to this hypothesis. The first three of these studies were done before the HRV hypothesis was introduced and were mainly descriptive and did not focus on cardiovascular disease. The other four studies were specifically designed to test this hypothesis from different point of views: two (Sahl et al., 2002; Sorahan & Nichols, 2004) were replications of the original study, and like Savitz et al. (1999), focused on cohorts of utility workers. One study focused specifically on arrhythmia (Johansen et al., 2002); one study investigated cardiovascular morbidity and was the first study to have detailed information on confounding factors and thus an ability to control for them (Ahlbom et al., 2004).

Thus only mortality studies of the association between occupational exposure to EMF and cardiovascular diseases have reported an association (Håkansson et al., 2003; Savitz et al., 1999). Studies of cardiovascular diseases which rely on mortality records as the measure of outcome are limited because the disease under study may not be mentioned on the death certificate, and if so, the accuracy of the diagnosis may not be correct. It is well known that death certificates do not provide the same quality of outcome measure as compared to incidence records which mainly can be obtained in disease registries or prospectively designed cohort or case-control studies. There are limitations to speculating about causal mechanisms of types of CVD as coded on death certificates of uncertain validity and reliability

(Finkelstein, 1999). A recent UK study identified inaccuracy in identifying underlying cause of death on the death certificates and difficulties in differentiating between acute and chronic cardiac causes (Mant et al., 2006). Thus, on balance, the evidence supporting an etiologic relation between occupational EMF exposures has been overturned by more focused and rigorous studies.

## 8.4    Conclusions

Experimental studies of both short- and long-term exposure indicate that, while electric shock is an obvious health hazard, other hazardous cardiovascular effects associated with ELF fields are unlikely to occur at exposure levels commonly encountered environmentally or occupationally. Although various cardiovascular changes have been reported in the literature, the majority of effects are small and the results have not been consistent within and between studies. With one exception, none of the studies of cardiovascular disease morbidity and mortality has shown an association with exposure. Whether a specific association exists between exposure and altered autonomic control of the heart remains speculative. Overall, the evidence does not support an association between ELF exposure and cardiovascular disease.

Haematology is the branch of medicine that is concerned with blood, the blood-forming organs and blood diseases. Studies encompass the growth and development of the leukocyte (white blood cell) populations that form part of the immune system in addition to the erythrocyte (red cell) populations and the non-cellular serum constituents such as serum iron and serum alkaline phosphatase concentrations. Haemopoiesis, the formation of blood cells, occurs primarily in bone marrow, where there is progressive division and maturation from stem cells through to the formation of mature erythrocytes and leukocytes. Erythrocytes and leukocytes circulate in the bloodstream, from which cell populations and other haematological parameters may be readily sampled. However, there is a continual and active exchange of leukocytes with other body compartments such as the lymphoid system. In the adult human body, for example, only about 2% of the total lymphocyte pool is present in the blood and the lymphocyte subset composition can be varied by a number of different factors including disease. Few studies have examined ELF effects either on immune system function or on heamatology. The tables below summarize the results of studies conducted on the immune system and haematology. Only the more significant ones are discussed in the text.

## 9.1     Immune system

The immune system identifies and responds to invading micro-organisms such as viruses, bacteria, and various single-celled or multicellular organisms, and to "foreign" macromolecules including proteins and polysaccharides. Thus, it serves to protect individuals from infectious diseases and can also act against tumour cells, although these responses are fairly weak. Immunological responses are mediated through intercellular signalling pathways via chemical messengers such as cytokines and interleukins.

The first line of defence against pathogens is sustained by relatively nonspecific (natural or innate) parts of the immune system. These are natural killer (NK)-cells, mononuclear phagocytes and granulocytes. The protein "complement system" mediates many of the cytolytic and inflammatory effects of humoral (non-cell-mediated) immunity. These innate responses are followed by the adaptive (or aquired) antigen-specific responses of the immune system. The cells that mediate the antigen-specific (or acquired) responses are the B-lymphocytes, which secrete antibodies (humoral immunity) that circulate in body fluids, and the T-lymphocytes, that can function as cytotoxic cells (cell-mediated immunity) or as helper T-cells which assist in B- or T-cell activation. Activated cytotoxic T-lymphocytes specifically recognise and kill cells having foreign molecules on their surface and are implicated in anti-tumour responses. The acquired immune responses also involve the recruitment and amplification of the responses of the innate parts of the immune system.

### 9.1.1 Human studies

Selmaoui, Lambrozo & Touitou (1996) showed that a one-night (23.00 to 08.00) exposure to either continuous or intermittent (1 hour off and 1 hour with on/off switching every 15 s) 50-Hz, 10-T magnetic fields did not affect immunological parameters (CD3-, CD4-, CD8-lymphocytes, NK-cells and B-cell populations) in 16 healthy men aged 20–30 years as compared to 16 healthy sham-exposed men.

In 2000, Tuschl et al. (2000) published some results on immune parameters of ten workers exposed to the magnetic fields associated with induction heaters (50–600 Hz, up to 2 mT, or 2.8–21 kHz, 0.13–2 mT, for at least two years). Overall, there were no differences between exposed and control subjects in the levels of B- and T-cells, cytokines and immunoglobulins. However, the numbers of NK-cells and oxidative bursts of monocytes, implicated in cytotoxic responses were significantly increased in the exposed group while monocytes had significantly reduced phagocytic activity compared with those from unexposed personnel. The authors considered that overall the non-specific immunity of the exposed subjects was normal and that the most peculiar finding was the increase in NK-cell population.

Recently, the Mandeville group has reported effects of 60 Hz magnetic fields on 60 workers of power utilities (Ichinose et al., 2004). They monitored the activity of ornithine decarboxylase (ODC) in white blood cell, the activity of NK-cells, lymphocyte phenotypes, and differential cell counts. They monitored exposure over three consecutive days before collecting peripheral blood. There was no alteration of NK-cell activity nor of the number of circulating neutrophils, eosinophils, basophils, or T-lymphocytes. However, there was an association between exposure intensity and a decreased ODC activity and lower NK-cell counts.

The production of melatonin, which is known to stimulate the immune system, was quantified on the night preceding immune marker determinations. While no alteration in melatonin levels could be observed in the exposed subjects, the decrease in ODC activity, counts of NK- and B-cells, and monocytes were strongest for the workers with lowest melatonin production. According to the authors, the health consequences associated with these changes are not known.

Using a cross-section approach, Chinese scientists investigated the effects of ELF fields on the immune system. Zhu and coworkers (2002; 2001) systematically explored its effects on red blood cell, platelets and white blood cells of peripheral blood taken from people who were working with the electric railway system. They reported that the fields (50 Hz, 0.01–0.938 mT, or 0–12 kV m$^{-1}$) decreased the number of white blood cells and the level of IgA and IgG (Immunoglobulins A and G) antibodies. They also found that the percentage of lymphocytes showing DNA damage was higher in the exposed group than in the control group. The authors concluded that ELF fields might induce DNA damage in lymphocytes, then cause apoptosis of these cells, and further result in the decrease of cell number and immuno-globulin level in the blood.

Dasdag et al. (2002) compared blood cell counts, hematocrit and lymphocyte surface antigens of a group of 16 welders with that of a group of 14 healthy male control subjects. Although CD4 and CD8 levels were decreased in the welders and the hematocrit increased, the authors concluded that the differences were not clinically significant and that the results were not suggestive of an ELF effect on immunologic parameters.

Table 61 summarizes the studies on immune responses in humans exposed to ELF fields.

**Table 61. Immune system responses in humans**

| Test | Exposure | Results | Comments | Authors |
|------|----------|---------|----------|---------|
| Numbers of CD3+, CD4+, CD8+ lympho-cytes, of NK- cells and B- cells Healthy young men exposed: n=16 sham-exposed: n=16 | 50 Hz 10 µT Continuous or intermittent (1 h off, 1 h with on/off switch-ing every 15 s) Exposure for one night (23:00 to 08:00). | No effect with either exposure protocol. | Well con-trolled study. Low power. | Sel-maoui, Lam-brozo & Touitou, 1996 |
| Number of B- and T-cells, levels of cytokines and immunoglobulins Numbers of NK cells and oxidative bursts of mono-cytes Monocyte phagocytic activity Workers exposed to induction heaters (n=10) | 50–600 Hz up to 2 mT or 2.8–21 kHz 0.13–2 mT Exposure for at least two years | No effect on B- and T-cells, cytokines and immunoglobu-lins. Increase in NK cells and in bursts of monocytes. Decreased phago-cytic activity. | | Tuschl et al., 2000 |
| Activity of ornithine decarboxylase (ODC) in white blood cells Activity of NK cells Lymphocyte phenotypes Differential cell counts Power-utility workers (n=60) | 60 Hz Personal mag-netic field monitor for 3 consecutive working days | Decreased ODC activity. No alteration of NK activity. No change in num-ber of circulating neutrophils, eosino-phils, basophils, and T-lymphocytes, lower NK-cell counts | | Ichinose et al., 2004 |

223

**Table 61. Continued**

| | | | | |
|---|---|---|---|---|
| Numbers of blood cells, levels of immunoglobulins, levels of DNA damage in lymphocytes (comet assay) Daily exposed workers: n=192 Unexposed control workers: n=106 | 50 Hz 0-12 kV m$^{-1}$, 0.01-0.92 mT 4.59±2.64 h / day, 9.72±3.09 year | Increase in red blood cells, platelets, and haemoglobin. Decrease in white blood cells and lymphocytes. Decrease in IgA and IgG. Increase in DNA damage of lymphocytes. | | Zhu, Way & Zhu, 2001 |
| Numbers of blood cells, levels of immunoglobulins, levels of DNA damage in lymphocytes (comet assay) Daily exposed workers: n=33 Unexposed control workers: n=106 | 50 Hz 1.69-3.25 kV m$^{-1}$, 0.245-0.938 mT 4.59±2.64 h / day, 9.4±3.2 year | Increase in red blood cells and platelets. Decrease in white blood cells and lymphocytes. Decrease in IgA and IgG. Increase in DNA damage of lymphocytes. | Extension of Zhu et al., 2001 | Zhu et al., 2002 |
| Red blood cells; hemoglobin; hematocrit; platelets; total white blood cells; neutrophils; lymphocytes; eosinophils; and CD3, CD4, CD8, and CD4/CD8 Male welders: n=16 Male controls: n=14 | Welders exposed 3-4 hours per day per week and for at least 10 years | CD4, CD8 lower, hematocrit higher in welders. Differences "not clinically significant". | | Dasdag et al., 2002 |

## 9.1.2 Animal studies

Animal studies have been carried out using several approaches: some authors have examined the responsiveness of the whole immune system, while other used blood cell counts and standard in vitro tests on cells taken from the peripheral blood or spleen of exposed animals. This section discusses all experiments done with exposure of the animals even if the tests on their immune cells were done in vitro. Many of these studies have been previously reviewed by ICNIRP (2003) and the general conclusion was that "there is little consistent evidence on any inhibitory effect of power-frequency EMF exposure on various aspects of immune system function".

The Löscher group (Mevissen et al., 1996) had reported a decreased spleen T-lymphocyte proliferation in rats chronically exposed to 50 Hz magnetic fields. In a follow-up study, the same authors (Mevissen et al., 1998) found that this proliferation was initially increased, after 2 weeks, but then decreased, after 13weeks, compared to sham-exposed animals.

Later, the same group (Häussler et al., 1999) reported on two independent experiments on the ex vivo production of interleukins (ILs) by mitogen-stimulated splenic lymphocytes from female Sprague-Dawley rats exposed to 100 µT 50 Hz magnetic fields. In the first experiment, the rats were treated with DMBA and exposed or sham-exposed for 14 weeks. There was no difference between exposed and sham-exposed groups in the level of production of IL-1 by mitogen-activated splenic B-cells. In the second experiment, rats were exposed for 1 day, 1 week, or 2 weeks, followed by collection and activation of spleen lymphocytes. There was no difference in IL-1 or IL-2 production from stimulated B- or T-cells. According to the authors, these negative findings suggested that the reported changes in T-cell proliferation in response to magnetic field exposure (Mevissen et al., 1996; 1998) was not mediated via alterations in IL production.

In another experiment, Thun-Battersby, Westermann & Löscher (1999) exposed female Sprague-Dawley rats to a 50 Hz, 100 µT field for periods of 3 or 14 days or 13 weeks. They performed analyses of T-lymphocyte subsets and other immune cells: NK- cells, B-lymphocytes, macrophages, and granulocytes in blood, spleen and mesenteric lymph nodes. They also detected proliferating and apoptotic cells in the compartments of spleen tissue. No effect was found on different types of leukocytes, including lymphocyte subsets for any of the exposure durations. The authors concluded that exposure did not affect lymphocyte homeostasis, but did not exclude that functional alterations in T-cell responses to mitogens and in NK-cell activity, as described in some studies of exposed rodents, may be one of the mechanisms involved in the carcinogenic effects of magnetic field exposure observed in some models of co-carcinogenesis, such as the DMBA model used by this group.

A number of tests of NK-cell activity have been carried out, mainly on exposed mice. House et al. (1996) reported that the NK-cell activity of young B6C3F(1) female mice was reduced in some experiments after exposure to continuous or intermittent 60 Hz magnetic fields (2–1000 µT) but not in male mice nor in male or female rats. The authors later did the experiment with older female mice, and observed a similar decrease in NK-cell activity at 1000 µT but not at the lower field intensities (House & McCormick, 2000). They concluded that the inhibition of NK-cell activity caused by exposure was consistent across their experiments but had little biological significance, as it was not associated with an increase in neoplasms in separate investigations with the same type of exposure.

Arafa et al. (2003) investigated the bioeffects of repeated exposure to 50 Hz high-strength (20 mT) magnetic fields on some immune parameters in mice. The animals were exposed daily for 30 minutes three times per week for 2 weeks. Immune endpoints included total body weight, spleen/body weight ratio, splenocytes viability, total and differential white blood cell (WBC) counts, as well as lymphocyte proliferation induced by phytohaemagglutinin, concanavalin-A and lipoploysaccharide. Magnetic field exposure decreased splenocyte viability, WBC count, as well as mitogen-induced lymphocyte proliferation (by approximately 20%).

The authors also tested the effects of two distinct anti-radical compounds: L-carnitine and Q10. Both drugs were given 1 h prior to each ELF exposure. L-carnitine, but not Q10 attenuated the adverse effects of exposure on the vast majority of the immune parameters tested. It was speculated by the authors that the effect of L-carnitine was due to its anti-ROS properties.

Ushiyama & Ohkubo (2004) and Ushiyama et al. (2004) studied the acute and subchronic effects of whole-body exposure to 50 Hz magnetic field on leukocyte-endothelium interaction using a dorsal skinfold chamber technique in conscious BALB/c mice. They perfomed an acute exposure experiment by exposing for 30 min at 0, 3, 30 and 30 mT and a subchronic exposure experiment by continuous exposure for 17 days at 0, 0.3, 1 and 3 mT. The intra-microvascular leukocyte adherence to endothelial cells significantly increased at 30 mT in the acute exposure and at 3 mT in the subchronic exposure conditions. In a companion study Ushiyama et al. (2004), however, they failed to find changes in serum tumour necrosis factor-$\alpha$ (TNF-$\alpha$) and IL-1 $\beta$ levels under exposure to subchronic exposure to 30 mT.

The effect of long-term exposure to ELF electric and magnetic fields on the thymocytes of rats was studied by Quaglino et al. (2004). The 2-month-old Sprague-Dawley rats were exposed or sham exposed for 8 months to 50 Hz fields (1 kV m$^{-1}$, 5 $\mu$T or 5 kV m$^{-1}$, 100 $\mu$T). Simultaneous exposure to continuous light and ELF fields did not change significantly the rate of mitoses compared to sham-exposed rats, but the amount of cell death was significantly increased. The conclusion of the authors was that, in vivo, stress, such as that caused by continuous exposure to light and ELF exposure can act in synergy to cause a more rapid involution of the thymus and suggested that this could be responsible for an increased susceptibility to the potentially hazardous effects of ELF-EMF.

Table 62 summarizes the studies on immune system responses found in experimental animals.

### 9.1.3    Cellular studies

Jandova et al. (1999; 2001) found that the adherence of leukocytes taken from cancer patients to solid surfaces (such as glass surfaces or plastic materials) was increased after 1 hour of exposure to a 50 Hz sinusoidal magnetic field (1 mT and 10 mT), while it was decreased in T-lymphocytes taken from healthy donors. The leukocyte surface properties manifest cell-mediated immunity, since, in the presence of antigens, leucocytes taken from cancer patients exhibit less adherence than leucocytes from healthy humans. The authors concluded that the response of cell-mediated immunity was altered by external magnetic field exposure and hypothesized about different biophysical mechanisms, among which were the free radical reactions.

**Table 62. Immune system responses in animals**

| Biological endpoint | Exposure conditions | Results | Comments | Authors |
|---|---|---|---|---|
| **T-cell proliferation** | | | | |
| Spleen lymphocyte proliferation Swiss-Webster mice | 60 Hz 100 kV m$^{-1}$ 90–150 days | No effect. | | Morris & Phillips, 1982 |
| Spleen T-lymphocyte proliferation Sprague-Dawley rats | 50 Hz 50 µT 13 weeks | Decreased T-cell proliferation | | Mevissen et al., 1996 |
| Spleen T-lymphocyte proliferation Sprague-Dawley rats | 50 Hz 100 T 13 weeks | Increase in T-cell proliferation after 2 weeks; decrease after 13 weeks; no effect on B-cells | | Mevissen et al., 1998 |
| Peripheral blood lymphocyte proliferation Baboons | Pilot study: 60 Hz 9 kV m$^{-1}$, 20 µT 5 weeks Main study: 60 Hz 30 kV m$^{-1}$, 50 µT 5 weeks | Reduced B-lymphocyte response in pilot study. No effect in main study. | Considerable heterogeneity in results of sham exposed animals. | Murthy, Rogers & Smith, 1995 |
| **T-cell function** | | | | |
| Ex vivo production of interleukins (ILs) by mitogen-stimulated splenic lymphocytes Female Sprague-Dawley rats treated with DMBA | 50 Hz 100 µT 14 weeks 1 day, 1 week, 2 weeks | No effect on production of IL-1. No difference in IL-1 or IL-2-production by stimulated B- or T-cells. | | Häussler et al., 1999 |

**Table 62. Continued**

| | | | | |
|---|---|---|---|---|
| T-lymphocyte subsets; NK-cells, B-lymphocytes, macrophages and granulocytes in blood, spleen and mesenteric lymph nodes; proliferating and apoptotic cells in the compartments of spleen tissue. Sprague-Dawley rats | 50 Hz 100 µT 3 or 14 days or 13 weeks. | No effects. | | Thun-Battersby, Westermann & Löscher, 1999 |
| Delayed-type hypersensitivity to oxazolone. B6C3F1 mice | 60 Hz 2, 200, 1000 µT continuous, 1000 µT intermittent (1 h on/off) 13 weeks | No consistent effect. | Generally well described study. | House et al, 1996 |
| Resistance to Listeria monocytogenes infection. Mice (BALB/C) | 60 Hz 2, 200, 1000 µT continuous, 1000 µT intermittent (1 h on/off) 4 or 13 weeks | No effect. | Experimental and control data not shown. | House et al, 1996 |
| Long-term effects on IL-1 and IL-2 activity. Sheep | 60 Hz transmission lines 1.07, 3.5 µT 12–27 mo | No effect. | | Hefeneider et al, 2001 |
| **NK-cell activity** | | | | |
| Spleen and blood NK cells SENCAR mice treated with DMBA and TPA | 60 Hz 2 mT 6 h / day, 5 days / week, 21 weeks | No significant effect. | | McLean et al, 1991 |

**Table 62. Continued**

| | | | | |
|---|---|---|---|---|
| Spleen natural killer cells BALB/C mice | 0.8 Hz (pulsed) 10–120 mT 10 h / day, 5 days | Enhanced activity at 30 mT and above. | | de Seze et al., 1993 |
| NK-cell activity Young mice and rats | 60 Hz 2–1000 µT, continuous or intermittent | Reduced NK-cell activity in some experiments in female mice but not in male mice nor in male or female rats. | Generally well described study, replicate experiments. | House et al., 1996 |
| NK-cell activity Older mice | Repeat of above study | Reduced NK-cell activity. | | House & McCormick, 2000 |
| Spleen NK-cells F344 rats | 60 Hz 2, 200, 1000 µT continuous, 1000 µT intermittent (1 h on/off) 6 or 13 weeks | No consistent effect in males or females. | Generally well described study, replicate experiments. | House et al., 1996 |
| Spleen NK-cells F344 rats | 60 Hz 20 µT–2 mT 20 h / day, 6 weeks | Trend for enhanced activity with exposure. | Fully described study; but significant effects with control rather than sham comparison. | Tremblay et al., 1996 |
| **Macrophage activity** | | | | |
| Peritoneal macrophages F344 rats | 60 Hz 20 µT–2 mT 20 h / day, 6 weeks | Trend for enhanced hydrogen peroxide release with exposure. | Fully described study; but significant effects with control rather than sham comparison. | Tremblay et al., 1996 |
| **Antibody cell activity** | | | | |
| Circulating antibody levels to keyhole limpet haemocyanin Immunised Swiss Webster mice | 60 Hz 100 kV m$^{-1}$ 30 or 60 days | No effect. | | Morris & Phillips, 1982 |

**Table 62. Continued**

| Endpoint / Model | Exposure | Effect | Comment | Reference |
|---|---|---|---|---|
| Antibody-forming spleen cells Immunised BALB/C mice | 60 Hz 500 µT 5 h on three alternate days | No effect. | | Putinas & Michaelson, 1990 |
| Antibody-forming spleen cells Immunised BALB/C mice | 0.8 Hz (pulsed) 10–120 mT 10 h / day, 5 days | No effect. | | de Seze et al., 1993 |
| Antibody-forming spleen cells Immunised B6C3F1 mice | 60 Hz 2, 200, 1000 µT continuous 1000 µT intermittent (1 h on/off) 3 or 13 weeks | No effect. | Generally well described study; positive controls. | House et al., 1996 |
| Body weight, spleen/body weight ratio, splenocytes viability, total and differential WBC counts, lymphocyte proliferation induced by PHA, Con-A and LPS Effect of anti-radical compounds L-carnitine and Q10 Mice | 50 Hz 20 mT 30 min / day, 3 days /week, 2 weeks | Decreased splenocyte viability, WBCs count, and mitogen-induced lymphocyte proliferation. Only L-carnitine attenuated the effects of exposure. | | Arafa et al., 2003 |
| Leukocyte-endothelial interaction BALB/c mice | 50 Hz 0, 3, 10 and 30 mT 30 min | Increased leukocyte adherence at 30 mT. | | Ushiyama & Ohkubo, 2004 |
| Leukocyte-endothelial interaction; serum TNF-alpha and IL-l beta BALB/c mice | 50 Hz 0, 0.3, 1 and 3 mT continuous for 17 days | Increased leukocyte adherence at 3 mT, no change in serum TNF-alpha and IL-l beta levels. | | Ushiyama et al., 2004 |
| Rate of mitosis in thymocytes 2-month-old Sprague-Dawley rats | 50 Hz 1 kV m$^{-1}$, 5 µT 5 kV m$^{-1}$, 100 µT 8 months | No change in rate of mitoses; cell death significantly increased. | | Quaglino et al., 2004 |

Ikeda et al. (2003) studied the immunological functions of human peripheral blood mononuclear cells (PBMCs) from healthy male volunteers. They assessed the activities of NK and lymphokine activated killer (LAK) cells and the production of interferon-$\gamma$ (IFN-$\gamma$), tumour necrosis factor-$\alpha$ (TNF-$\alpha$), interleukin-2 (IL-2), and interleukin-10 (IL-10). The PBMCs were exposed for 24 hours to linearly (vertical), or circularly, or elliptically polarised fields, at 50 and 60 Hz (2–500 $\mu$T for the vertical field and 500 $\mu$T for the rotating fields). They found no effect of exposure on the cytotoxic activities and the cytokines production of human PBMCs.

The Simko-group in Germany has been very active in recent years studying the effects of 50 Hz, 1 mT magnetic fields on various immune cells. The effects on the production of free radicals was studied by Lupke, Rollwitz & Simko (2004) in monocytes from the blood of human umbilical cord and in human Mono Mac6 cells. In monocytes a significant increase of superoxide radical anion production was observed (up to 40%) and an increase in ROS release (up to 20%) upon 45-min exposure of monocytes. The increases were even larger in Mono Mac6 cells.

Rollwitz, Lupke & Simko (2004) gave some evidence of the cell-activating capacity of ELF magnetic fields by reporting a significant increase in free radical production after exposure of mouse bone marrow-derived (MBM) promonocytes and macrophages. The superoxide anion radicals were produced in both types of cells. The authors suggested that the NADH-oxidase pathway was stimulated by exposure, but not the NADPH pathway.

The same research group (Simko & Mattsson, 2004) has concluded that some of the effects of ELF magnetic field exposure might be caused by increasing levels of free radicals. They considered four different types of processes: (i) direct activation of macrophages (or other immune cells) by short-term exposure leading to phagocytosis (or other cell specific responses) and consequently, free radical production, (ii) exposure-induced macrophage activation including direct stimulation of free radical production, (iii) increase in the lifetime of free radicals under exposure leading to long-term elevation of free radical concentrations, (iv) long-term exposure leading to a durable increase in the level of free radicals, subsequently causing an inhibition of the effects of the pineal gland hormone melatonin. However, there are no well-established data showing that free radical production is affected by ELF magnetic field exposure.

Table 63 summarizes the results of ELF in vitro studies on immune system responses.

**Table 63. Immune system in vitro studies**

| Biological endpoint | Exposure conditions | Results | Authors |
|---|---|---|---|
| Adherence assay Leukocytes taken from venous blood of normal donors and cancer patients | 50 Hz 1 and 10 mT (measurements gave 1.02 and 9.52 mT, respectively) 1 h Test tubes placed in the center of a coil. Exposure performed at 37°C. Sham exposure not mentioned. | Decreased adherence in normal leukocytes which normally are adherent. Increased adherence in cancer leukocytes that are usually not adherent to solid surfaces. Similar effect for longer exposure duration (2, 3 and 4 h tested but no data shown). | Jandova et al., 1999; 2001 |
| Several CD markers and transcription and expression of CD4. | 50 Hz 24, 48, 72 h | Slight effect on CD4, CD14 and CD16 receptor expression, other CD receptors not affected. | Conti et al., 1999 |
| Peripheral blood mononuclear cells CD4 expression | 50 Hz, pulsed (2 msec. impulse duration) generated by a BIOSTIM apparatus 1.5 mT 24, 48 and 72 hours | DNA CD4+ expression increased mRNA CD4+ expression increased in resting cells exposed for 24 h, but not 48 or 72 h Increase in percentage cell cycle progression in S phase | Felaco et al., 1999 |
| Activity of NK and LAK cells; production of IFN-gamma, TNF-alpha, IL-2, and IL-10 PBMCs from healthy male volunteers | 50 and 60 Hz linearly (vertical), circularly, or elliptically polarised magnetic fields 2–500 µT (vertical field) 500 µT (rotating fields) 24 h | No effects. | Ikeda et al., 2003 |
| Monocytes from blood of human umbilical cord and human Mono Mac6 cells Production of free radicals | 50 Hz 1 mT 45 min | Increase in superoxide radical anion production in monocytes; increase in ROS release upon 45-min exposure of monocytes (larger in Mono Mac6 cells). | Lupke, Rollwitz & Simko, 2004 |
| Mouse bone marrow-derived (MBM) promonocytes and macrophages Production of free radicals | 50 Hz 1 mT 45 min to 24 hours | Increase of free radical production: superoxide anion radicals were produced in both types of cells. | Rollwitz, Lupke & Simko, 2004 |

## 9.2     Haematological system

Haematological parameters include: leukocyte and erythrocyte counts, haemoglobin concentration, reticulocyte and thrombocyte counts, bone marrow cellularity and prothrombin times, serum iron and serum alkaline phosphatase concentrations and serum triglyceride values. Most studies have included assessments of the differential white blood cell count, that is, the overall concentration of white cells (leukocytes) and their various subgroups. However, the importance of small alterations of the levels of circulating leukocytes is not clear as there is a continual and active exchange with other body compartments such as the lymphoid system which can be affected by a number of different factors including disease.

### 9.2.1     Human studies

Very few studies have been performed on volunteers and none in recent years.

Selmaoui et al. (1996) exposed or sham exposed 32 male volunteers to 10 μT, 50 Hz horizontally polarised magnetic fields between 23.00 and 08.00 on two separate days. Blood samples were taken from each subject at 3-hourly intervals from 11.00 to 20.00 and hourly from 22.00 to 08.00. One month later, the exposed group was subjected to an intermittent 10 μT, 50 Hz magnetic field between 23.00 and 08.00. In the intermittent regimen, the magnetic field was turned on for one hour and off for the next hour; during the on-period, the field was cycled on and off every 15 s. Counts of all cell types showed a strong circadian rhythm with the possible exception of neutrophils and NK-cells; However, values in the group exposed continuously and in those exposed intermittently were always very similar to values in the sham exposed groups. Moreover, inter- and intra-individual variations were so high that small effects due to exposure were unlikely to be detected.

Bonhomme-Faivre et al. (1998) monitored a few subjects exposed for 8 hours per day for more than 1year in their hospital laboratory to 50 Hz, 0.2–6.6 μT magnetic fields. CD3 and CD4 lymphocyte counts were significantly lower than those measured in six control workers, but NK-cell counts were increased. Since exposure levels were measured at ankle level, the whole-body exposure of the individuals was unknown and no health consequences could be attributed to field exposure.

These studies are summarized in Table 64.

### 9.2.2     Animal studies

Boorman et al. (1997) exposed Fischer 344/N rats and B6C3F1 mice to 60 Hz magnetic fields (2200 and 1000 μT) for 8 weeks (18.5 h per day, 7 days per week). An additional group of rats and mice was exposed intermittently (1 h on and 1 h off) to 1000 μT magnetic fields. There were no haematological alterations that could be attributed to magnetic field exposure.

**Table 64. Human haematological studies**

| Biological endpoint | Exposure conditions | Results | Comments | Authors |
|---|---|---|---|---|
| Counts of all blood cell types | 50 Hz 10 µT 23.00 to 08.00 on two separate days | No effect but strong inter and intra-individual variations. | Well controlled study. Low power. | Selmaoui et al., 1996 |
| CD3 and CD4 lymphocytes and NK counts | 50 Hz 0.2–6.6 µT at ankle level 8 h / day, 1 year | Decrease in CD3 and CD4 and increase in NK cells. | Dosimetry not provided. Low number of subjects (6 exposed, 6 controls). | Bonhomme-Faivre et al., 1998 |

Zecca et al. (1998) assessed haematological variables before exposure and at 12-week intervals during exposure up to 32 weeks. Male Sprague-Dawley rats (64 animals per group) were exposed for 8 h per day, 5 days per week for 32 weeks at 50 Hz (5 µT and 1 kV m$^{-1}$, and 100 µT and 5 kV m$^{-1}$). Blood samples were collected at 0, 12, 24, and 32 weeks. No pathological changes were observed under any exposure conditions in animal growth rate, in morphology and histology of the tissues collected from the liver, heart, mesenteric lymph nodes, testes and bone marrow or in serum chemistry.

Three studies were performed by Korneva et al. (1999) in male CBA mice exposed to 50 Hz, 22 µT magnetic fields for 1 h, at the same time of day, for 5 successive days. In the first study, spleen colony formation was examined and the number of colony-forming units was not higher than in sham-exposed animals. Significant changes were seen in the thymus weight and thymus index of exposed animals when compared to sham-exposed animals. In a second study, mice were given a sublethal dose of X-rays (6 Gy) followed 2 h later with the same magnetic field exposure as above. The number of colonies per spleen showed a consistent, significant increase with exposure and the number of colony forming units per femur was decreased. In the third study, bone marrow was taken from mice that had been exposed in still the same way, and injected into mice that had been exposed to a lethal dose of X-rays (9 Gy). The number of colony forming units per femur in the recipient mice was significantly reduced at days 1 and 4 after injection.

A summary of these studies is presented in Table 65.

**Table 65. Animal haematological studies**

| Biological end-point | Exposure conditions | Results | Comments | Authors |
|---|---|---|---|---|
| Differential white blood cell count Swiss-Webster mice and Sprague-Dawley rats | 60 Hz 100 kV m⁻¹ 15 (rats only), 30, 60 or 120 days | No consistent effects seen in replicate studies. | Replicate studies; some results variable. | Ragan et al., 1983 |
| Differential white blood cell and bone marrow progenitor cell count CBA/H mice | 50 Hz 20 mT 7 days | No effect. | | Lorimore et al., 1990 |
| Splenic lymphocyte subgroup analysis B6C3F1 mice | 60 Hz 2, 200, 1000 µT continuous 1000 µT intermittent (1 h on/off) 4 or 13 weeks | No effect. | Generally well described study. | House et al., 1996 |
| Differential white blood cell count F344 rats | 60 Hz 20 µT–2 mT 20 h / day, 6 weeks | Trend for reduced T-cell count with exposure; reduced total, cytotoxic and helper T-cells. | Fully described study; significant effects with control rather than sham comparison. | Tremblay et al., 1996 |
| Differential white blood cell count Sprague-Dawley rats | 50 Hz 100 µT 3 days, 14 days or 13 weeks | No effect. | Extensive lymphocyte sub-set analysis. | Thun-Battersby, Westermann & Löscher, 1999 |
| Differential white blood cell count Baboons | Pilot study: 60 Hz 9 kV m⁻¹, 20 µT 5 weeks Main study: 60 Hz 30 kV m⁻¹, 50 µT | Reduced helper T-lymphocyte count in pilot study; no effect in main study. | Considerable heterogeneity in sham exposed results. | Murthy, Rogers & Smith, 1995 |
| Haematology Fischer rats and B6C3F1 mice | 60 Hz 1000 or 2200 µT continuous 1000 µT Intermittent (1 h on, 1 h off) 18.5 h / day, 7 days / week, 8 weeks | No effect. | | Boorman et al., 1997 |

**Table 65. Continued**

| | | | |
|---|---|---|---|
| Blood cells count before exposure, at 12, 24 and 32 weeks of exposure Morphology and histology of different organs (liver, heart, mesenteric lymph nodes, testes, bone marrow) Groups of 64 rats sham-exposed | 50 Hz 5 µT, 1 kV m$^{-1}$ 100 µT, 5 kV m$^{-1}$ 8 h / day, 5 days / week, 32 weeks | No effects. | Zecca et al., 1998 |
| Spleen colony formation Bone marrow injected to mice exposed to 9 Gy X-rays Male CBA mice | 50 Hz 22 µT 1 h / day, same time of day, 5 successive days 6 Gy X-rays followed after 2 h by same exposure as above | No effect of EMF alone. Increase in number of colonies per spleen; decrease in colony forming units per femur. Number of colony forming units per femur significantly reduced in the recipient mice. | Korneva et al., 1999 |
| Total and differential white blood cell counts Mice | 50 Hz 20 mT 30 min / day, 3 days / week, 2 weeks | Decreased white blood cells count. | Arafa et al., 2003 |

### 9.2.3 Cellular studies

Only one paper has been published recently on the effects on cells of the haematopoietic system: Van Den Heuvel et al. (2001) studied the effects of 50 Hz, 80 µT magnetic fields on the proliferation of different types of stem cells, including haemopoietic cells. The cytotoxic effects of exposure were investigated on the proliferation of undifferentiated murine 3T3 cells using the neutral red test. Magnetic fields had no cytotoxic effect on this cell line.

When exposed to the same fields, a reduction in the proliferation and differentiation of the granulocyte-macrophage progenitor (CFU-GM) grown from the bone marrow of male and female mice was shown compared to non-exposed cells. Stromal stem cell proliferation (CFU-f) from female mice showed a reduction while CFU-f from male mice did not decrease. The authors concluded that these effects on CFU-f are equivocal.

Table 66 summarizes the results of ELF in vitro studies.

**Table 66. Cell proliferation studies**

| Biological endpoint | Exposure conditions | Results | Authors |
|---|---|---|---|
| Cell numbers and colony following efficiency Mouse haemopoetic progenitor cells FDCP mix A4 | Nulled fields, 50 Hz vertical fields, Ca2+ ion cyclotron resonance conditions at 50 Hz 0.006, 1 and 2 mT 2 hours immediately after seeding 1, 4 or 7 days, one hour after seeding | No effects. | Reipert et al., 1997 |
| Cell number K562 myeloid leukaemia cells | 50 Hz 0.2–200 µT up to 24 h | No effects. | Fiorani et al., 1992 |
| $^3$H-thymidine uptake CCRF-CEM human lymphoblastoid cells | 72 Hz pulsed 3.5 mT 0.5–24 h | No effects. | Phillips & McChesney, 1991 |
| Proliferation Stem cells Undifferentiated murine 3T3 cells | 50 Hz 80 µT 4 days | No effects. | Van Den Heuvel et al., 2001 |
| Proliferation and differentiation of the granulocyte-macrophage progenitor | 50 Hz 80 µT 7 days | Reduction in proliferation and differentiation. | Van Den Heuvel et al., 2001 |
| Stromal stem cell proliferation | 50 Hz 80 µT 10 days | Decrease in female mice and no change in male mice. | Van Den Heuvel et al., 2001 |

## 9.3    Conclusions

Evidence for the effects of ELF electric or magnetic fields on components of the immune system is generally inconsistent. Many of the cell populations and functional markers were unaffected by exposure. However, in some human studies with fields from 10 µT to 2 mT, changes were observed in natural killer cells, which showed both increased and decreased cell numbers, and in white blood cell counts, which showed no change or decreased numbers. In animal studies reduced natural killer cell activity was seen in female, but not male mice or in rats of either sex. White blood cell counts also showed inconsistency, with decreases or no change reported in different studies. The animal exposures had an even broader range of 2 µT to 30 mT. The difficulty in interpreting the potential health impact of these data is due to the large variations in exposure and environmental conditions, the relatively small numbers of subjects tested and the broad range of endpoints.

There have been few studies carried out on the effects of ELF magnetic fields on the haematological system. In experiments evaluating differ-

237

ential white blood cell counts, exposures range from 2 µT to 2 mT. No consistent effects of acute exposure to magnetic fields or to combined electric and magnetic fields have been found in either human or animal studies.

Overall therefore, the evidence for effects of ELF electric or magnetic fields on the immune system and haematological system is considered inadequate.

# 10    REPRODUCTION AND DEVELOPMENT

The effects of exposure to low frequency EMFs on fertility, reproduction, prenatal and postnatal growth and development have been investigated in epidemiological and laboratory studies for a number of years.
Epidemiological studies have examined reproductive outcome in relation to
visual display terminal use, and to residential exposure, especially in relation
to electrically heated beds. Experimentally, this issue has been addressed in
studies of effects on mammalian and non-mammalian species, particularly
birds. Several comprehensive reviews are available (e.g. AGNIR, 1994;
Brent et al., 1993; Brent, 1999; Huuskonen, Lindbohm & Juutilainen, 1998;
IARC, 2002; ICNIRP, 2003; Juutilainen, 2003; Juutilainen & Lang, 1997;
McKinlay et al., 2004; NIEHS, 1998).

## 10.1    Epidemiology

### 10.1.1    Maternal exposure

#### 10.1.1.1 Video display terminals

A number of epidemiological studies have investigated possible
association of adverse pregnancy outcome with the use of video display terminals during pregnancy (for reviews, see Brent et al., 1993; Delpizzo, 1994;
IARC, 2002; Juutilainen, 1991; Parazzini et al., 1993; Shaw, 2001; Shaw &
Croen, 1993). The electromagnetic fields emitted by video display terminals
include ELF as well as higher frequencies up to 100 kHz. In general, these
studies have not suggested increased risks for spontaneous abortion, low
birth weight, pre-term delivery, intrauterine growth retardation, or congenital
abnormalities. However, most of the studies did not include any measurements of ELF field exposure. The average exposure of a video display operator is typically low (around 0.1 µT), so these studies are not informative for
assessing possible effects associated with higher exposures. Lindbohm et al.
(1992) carried out measurements of the field emissions of displays used by
the study subjects, and observed an increased odds ratio (3.4; 95% CI: 1.4–
8.6) for spontaneous abortions among women who used the few video display terminal types that had unusually high ELF magnetic field emissions
(> 0.9 µT peak-to-peak value). Another study that included ELF field measurements (Schnorr et al., 1991) did not report any association with field
exposure. The strongest fields to which subjects were exposed in this study
were weaker than those in the Lindbohm study.

#### 10.1.1.2 Electrically heated beds

Electric blankets and electrically heated waterbeds can significantly
increase exposure to ELF magnetic and electric fields, because they are used
close to the body for long time periods. Electric blankets produce fields up to
about 2.2 µT and the users of waterbeds are exposed to flux densities of 0.3–
0.5 µT (Bracken et al., 1995; Florig & Hoburg, 1990; Kaune et al., 1987).
The use of these devices may also result in increased maternal heat stress.

The first suggestion of harmful effects of electric blankets and heated waterbeds came from the study by Wertheimer & Leeper (1986). They examined seasonal patterns of foetal growth and spontaneous abortion rate among the users of heated beds, and reported that these outcomes were associated with conception in the winter months, and hence with use of bed heating. This study, however, has been criticized for several methodological shortcomings (Chernoff, Rogers & Kavet, 1992; Hatch, 1992). The findings of the studies on electrically heated beds and birth defects have been mostly negative. The use of electric blankets or heated waterbeds was not related to neural tube defects, oral cleft defects, or urinary tract defects (Dlugosz et al., 1992; Milunsky et al., 1992; Shaw et al., 1999). In the study of Li, Checkoway & Mueller (1995) electric blanket use was not associated with an increased risk of urinary tract anomalies. However, in a subgroup of women (37 cases, 85 controls) with a history of sub-fertility, an odds ratio of 4.4 was observed (95% CI: 0.9-23).

All the above studies were retrospective and assessment of exposure was usually based on self-reported data on the use of heated beds. Thus, incomplete information of exposure level (which varies between different types of electric blankets and waterbeds) and biased reporting of exposure may have influenced the findings. These difficulties were partly overcome in a prospective study (Bracken et al., 1995). In this study, exposure was estimated by measurements of magnetic fields produced by electric blankets and waterbeds and using interview data on hours of daily use. Low birth weight and intrauterine growth retardation were not related to use of electrically heated beds during pregnancy. The same group also examined the occurrence of spontaneous abortion in women who used electric blankets or electrically heated waterbeds (Belanger et al., 1998). The use of electric blankets did result in an increased risk ratio (1.8; 95% CI: 1.1–3.1), whereas the use of waterbeds or wire codes indicating elevated ELF field exposure were not associated with increased risk. In another prospective study (Lee et al., 2000), no increased risks of spontaneous abortions were found for users of electric blankets (OR = 0.8; 95% CI: 0.6–1.2) or waterbeds (OR = 1.0; 95% CI 0.7–1.3). No increase of risk with increasing setting-duration combination of electrically heated bed use was observed. The adjusted odds ratio for the twenty women who used electric blankets at high setting for 1 hour or less was 3.0 (95% CI: 1.1–8,3), but there were no spontaneous abortions among the women (n = 13) who used a high setting for 2 hours or more.

Overall, the studies on electrically heated beds have not provided convincing evidence for an association with adverse pregnancy outcomes. This view is supported by reviews from the UK Advisory Group on Non-Ionising Radiation (AGNIR, 1994) and more recently from the Health Council of the Netherlands (HCN, 2004). There is some indication of different patterns of results for waterbeds and electric blankets. For use of waterbeds during pregnancy, the risk estimates have generally been close to 1.0, while higher (and in some cases statistically significant) risk estimates have been reported for electric blankets, particularly among those women who used the high power setting of electric blankets. This pattern of results could be interpreted to reflect the higher magnetic fields produced by electric blankets (compared to waterbeds), or higher thermal stress experienced by the users of electric blankets.

Table 67 summarizes the results of epidemiological studies investigating various reproductive outcomes in humans exposed to different ELF sources.

**Table 67. Epidemiological studies on reproductive outcome**

| Endpoint | Study population | Exposure (EB: electric blankets; WB: electrically heated water beds) | Relative risk (95% CI) | Authors |
|---|---|---|---|---|
| Miscarriage Low birth weight | 673 cases, 583 controls | EB WB | not determined | Wertheimer & Leeper, 1986 |
| Miscarriage | Prospective study, n = 2967 | EB, use at conception | 1.74 (1.0–3.2) | Belanger et al., 1998 |
| | | EB, use at interview | 1.61 (0.8–3.2) | |
| | | EB, high setting at conception | 1.65 (0.6–4.9) | |
| | | EB, high setting at interview | 2.05 (0.7–4.7) | |
| | | WB, use at conception | 0.59 (0.3–1.1) | |
| | | WB, use at interview | 0.63 (0.4–1.1) | |
| | | WB, high setting at conception | 0.59 (0.3–1.1) | |
| | | WB, high setting at interview | 0.49 (0.2–1.1) | |
| Miscarriage | Prospective study, n = 5144 | EB | 0.8 (0.6–1.2) | Lee et al., 2000 |
| | | EB, high setting | 1.6 (0.6–3.3) | |
| | | WB | 1.0 (0.7–1.3) | |
| | | WB, high setting | 1.0 (0.7–1.5) | |
| Low birth weight Intrauterine growth retardation | Prospective study, n = 2967 | EB or WB, low setting [a] | 1.2 (0.5–2.8) | Bracken et al., 1995 |
| | | EB or WB, high setting [a] | 1.2 (0.6–2.5) | |
| | | EB or WB, low setting [a] | 0.8 (0.4–1.7) | |
| | | EB or WB, high setting [a] | 1.6 (1.0–2.6) | |
| Neural tube defects Oral cleft defects | 535 cases, 535 controls | EB | 0.9 (0.5–1.6) | Dlugosz et al., 1992 |

241

**Table 67. Continued**

| | | | | |
|---|---|---|---|---|
| | | WB | 1.1 (0.6–1.9) | |
| | | EB | 0.7 (0.4–1.2) | |
| | | WB | 0.7 (0.4–1.1) | |
| Neural tube defects | Cohort, n = 23491 | EB | 1.2 (0.5–2.6) | Milunsky et al., 1992 |
| Neural tube defects | Two studies, 1455 cases, 1754 controls in total | EB (study 1) | 1.8 (1.2–2.6) | Shaw et al., 1999 |
| | | EB (study 2) | 1.2 (0.6–2.3) | |
| | | WB (study 1) | 1.2 (0.8–1.8) | |
| | | WB (study 2) | 1.2 (0.8–1.9) | |
| CLP, isolated [b] | | EB | 0.8 (0.5–1.5) | |
| | | WB | 1.0 (0.7–1.5) | |
| CLP, multiple [c] | | EB | 1.3 (0.5–3.4) | |
| | | WB | 1.8 (1.0–3.2) | |
| Urinary tract anomalies (UTA) UTA, subfertile women | 118 cases, 369 controls 37 cases, 85 controls | EB | 1.1 (0.5–2.3) | Li, Checkoway & Mueller, 1995 |
| | | WB | 0.8 (0.3–2.7) | |
| | | EB | 4.4 (0.9–23) | |

[a] Exposure during 3rd trimester. Odds ratios were lower for exposures estimated for earlier periods of pregnancy.

[b] Cleft lip with/without cleft palate, no other (or only minor) anomalies.

[c] Cleft lip with/without cleft palate with at least one accompanying major anomaly.

### 10.1.1.3 Other residential and occupational exposure

Several studies have investigated residential ELF exposures other than heated beds. Wertheimer & Leeper (1989), using an approach similar to their earlier study on electric blankets and waterbeds (Wertheimer & Leeper, 1989), reported that monthly rate of foetal loss was correlated with monthly increase of heating degree days (= need of heating) in homes with ceiling cable heat (which was reported to expose the occupants to magnetic fields of about 1 µT), but not in homes without such heating. No association with pregnancy outcome has been seen in studies that have assessed magnetic field exposure using wire codes (a method of classifying dwellings based on proximity to visible electrical installations, widely used in epidemiological studies on childhood cancer – see Chapter 11) or proximity to power lines.

Measurement-based exposure assessment has been used in five studies. One study showed a suggestive association (OR = 5.1; 95% CI: 1.0–26) between early pregnancy loss and magnetic fields above 0.63 μT measured at the front door (Juutilainen et al., 1993). The preclinical miscarriages studied by Juutilainen et al. may be etiologically different from the clinically observed miscarriages investigated in the other studies. Fields above 0.2 μT measured in residences were not associated with miscarriages, low birth weight or pre-term delivery (Savitz & Ananth, 1994). These two studies had small numbers of exposed women, and used spot measurements to characterize the magnetic field levels of the subjects' homes. Spot measurements have been shown to be correlated with personal exposure, but their use may result in significant misclassification (Eskelinen et al., 2002). A prospective study (Bracken et al., 1995) used a wrist-worn meter to assess personal average exposure during seven days. Exposure to fields above 0.2 μT was not statistically significantly associated with low birth weight or intrauterine growth retardation.

Another prospective cohort study assessed the association of personal measured ELF magnetic field exposure with spontaneous abortion (Li et al., 2001). The association with time-weighted average (TWA) magnetic field exposure was not significant. However, a significantly increased risk (OR = 1.8; 95% CI: 1.2–2.7) was found when the exposure metric used was maximum exposure above 1.6 μT. The association was stronger for early miscarriages (<10 weeks of gestation). Analysis of dose-response showed weakly rising risk with magnetic field "dose", measured as the product of field level and duration above 1.6 μT (in μTs). The association was more pronounced (OR = 2.9; 95% CI: 1.6–5.3) among those women who indicated that the measurement (by body-worn meter) had been taken on a "typical day", possibly reflecting lower exposure misclassification among these subjects. The risk was further increased for subjects who had a history of difficulties during pregnancy.

A nested case-control study with personal exposure measurements (Lee et al., 2002) reported findings that were in certain respects similar to those of Li et al. (2001). In the study by Lee et al. miscarriages did not show a significant associated with TWA magnetic fields (although a suggestive step function response was seen with higher TWA quartiles). Statistically significant associations, and dose response trends with increasing exposure quartiles, were found for two personal exposure metrics – maximum exposure and rate-of-change of the magnetic field – but the value of these metrics has not yet been established.

Lee et al. (2002) also conducted a prospective substudy of 219 participants of the same parent cohort. The results of the prospective substudy were consistent with those of the case-control study, suggesting increased miscarriage risk associated with high rate-of-change and maximum field values. Unlike the nested study results, the personal TWA exposure at home (but not total 24-h TWA exposure) showed a significantly increased risk for fields above 0.2 μT (OR = 3.0; 95% CI: 1.1–8,4).

Savitz (2002) hypothesized that the apparent association with peak exposures and magnetic field variability might be explained by lower mobility of subjects who experience nausea, which is known to be less common among women who will miscarry. In their response, Li & Neutra (2002) provided evidence against this hypothesis using data from the prospective study by Li et al. (2001). However, McKinlay et al. (2004) noted that the parameter that provided evidence of a risk – namely maximum magnetic fields – was not chosen *a priori* on the basis of aetiological plausibility (Li & Neutra, 2002). In addition, the results were sensitive to the choice of breakpoint, which was made on the basis of the observations; and the study was not a standard prospective study as more than half of the miscarriages (and all those at all strongly related to maximum field exposure) occurred before the measurements were made. McKinlay et al. (2004) also note that the compliance rate was low and the possibility of selection bias was not excluded. Analyses of four data sets from the Li et al. (2001) study indicate that the magnitude of the maximum, but not the 95th or 99th percentile, is affected by the sampling rate of the meter and the mobility of the wearer (Mezei et al., 2006). This supports the hypothesis proposed by Savitz that the differential mobility of cases and controls could affect the maximum magnetic field measured.

Finally, in a case-control study in France, Robert et al. (1996) looked at congenital abnormalities in relation to distance from power lines. For distance < 50 m the odds ratios was 1.3 (95% CI: 0.5–3.2) and for distance < 100 m it was 1.0 (95% CI: 0.5–2.0). However, this was based on only two cases and since the entire study involved only 11 cases and 22 controls, its statistical power was limited.

Overall, the studies on residential ELF magnetic field exposure have provided some limited evidence for increased miscarriage risk associated with magnetic field exposure. This association is stronger for maximum value and variability of the magnetic field than for time-weighted average field level, but risk estimates above 1.0 were also reported for high TWA magnetic fields. One study provided evidence that the effect might be stronger for early miscarriages, and one study suggested effects on very early (pre-clinical) foetal loss. There is no evidence (but also very few data) of increased risks of adverse pregnancy outcomes other than miscarriage.

The results of epidemiological studies on reproductive outcomes in people exposed to ELF fields in their homes are summarized in Table 68.

**Table 68. Epidemiological studies on reproductive outcome and exposure to residential ELF magnetic fields assessed by measurements, wire codes or distance to power line**

| Study population | Outcome | Exposure [a] | Risk estimate and 95% CI | Authors |
|---|---|---|---|---|
| 257-396 pregnancies | Miscarriage | Home spot measurement 0.2 μT | 0.8 (0.3–2.3) | Savitz & Ananth, 1994 |
| | | High wire code | 0.7 (0.3–1.9) | |
| | Low birth weight | High wire code | 0.7 (0.2–2.3) | |
| | Preterm delivery | Home spot measurement 0.2 μT | 0.7 (0.1–4.0) | |
| | | High wire code | 0.2 (0.0–1.5) | |
| Prospective study, n = 2967 | Miscarriage | Very high wire code | 0.37 (0.2–1.1) | Belanger et al., 1998 |
| Prospective study, n = 969 | Miscarriage (MC) | Personal TWA 0.3 μT | 1.2 (0.7–2.2) | Li et al., 2001 |
| | | Personal 24-h maximum 1.6 μT | 1.8 (1.2–2.7) | |
| | | Total sum above 1.6 μT 476 μTs | 2.0 (1.2–3.1) | |
| | MC before 10 weeks | Personal 24-h maximum 1.6 μT | 2.2 (1.2–4.0) | |
| | MC after 10 weeks | Personal maximum 1.6 μT | 1.4 (0.8–2.5) | |
| 155 cases, 509 controls | Miscarriage | Very high wire code | 1.2 (0.7–2.1) | Lee et al., 2002 |
| | | Home spot measurement 0.2 μT | 1.1 (0.5–2.2) | |
| | | Personal TWA 0.128 μT | 1.7 (0.9–3.2) | |
| | | Personal 24-h maximum 3.51 μT | 2.3 (1.2–4.4) | |
| | | Personal rate-of-change 0.094 μT | 3.1 (1.6–6.0) | |
| Prospective study, n = 219 | Miscarriage | Home spot measurement 0.2 μT | 3.1 (1.0–9.7) | |
| | | Personal TWA 0.2 μT | 1.9 (0.6–6.1) | |
| | | Personal 24-h maximum 2.69 μT | 2.6 (0.9–7.6) | |

**Table 68. Continued**

| | | | | |
|---|---|---|---|---|
| | | Personal rate-of-change 0.069 µT | 2.4 (0.9–6.6) | |
| 89 cases, 102 controls | Early pregnancy loss | Home spot measurement 0.25 µT | 1.1 (0.6–2.3) | Juutilainen et al., 1993 |
| | | Home spot measurement 0.63 µT | 5.1 (1.0–26) | |
| Prospective study, n = 2967 | Low birth weight | Very high wire code | 0.83 (0.3–2.1) | Bracken et al., 1995 |
| | | Personal TWA 0.2 µT | 1.35 (0.3–6.1) | |
| | Intrauterine growth retardation | Very high wire code | 0.75 (0.4–1.6) | |
| | | Personal TWA 0.2 µT | 1.16 (0.4–3.1) | |
| 11 cases, 22 controls | All abnormalities | Distance to power line 100 m | 0.95 (0.5–2.0) | Robert et al., 1996 |
| | | Distance to power line 50 m | 1.25 (0.5–3.2) | |

[a] In many studies, the results were reported for several different exposure levels. The highest exposure levels were selected for this table.

### 10.1.2 Paternal exposure

Reproductive outcomes have also been occasionally related to paternal magnetic field exposure. Buiatti et al. (1984) reported that cases with infertility reported radioelectric work as their usual occupation more often than the controls. No association was observed between semen abnormalities and job titles linked to magnetic field exposure (Lundsberg, Bracken & Belanger, 1995). Schnitzer, Olshan & Erickson (1995) reported an excess of birth defects in the children of electronic equipment operators. Increased frequency of abnormal pregnancy outcome (congenital malformations and fertility difficulties) was observed among high-voltage switchyard workers (Nordström, Birk & Gustavsson, 1983). No significant increase of abnormal birth outcome was found for offspring of power-industry workers (Tornqvist, 1998). Two studies suggested an association between magnetic field exposure and decreased male/female ratio in the offspring (Irgens et al., 1997; Mubarak, 1996).

The results of the studies on paternal exposure are inconclusive and share the methodological limitation that occupation is used as a surrogate for electromagnetic field exposure. While some studies indicated increased risks associated with electrical occupations, there is very little evidence for a causal role of ELF fields in these associations.

## 10.2 Effects on laboratory mammals

### 10.2.1 Electric fields

Several studies have addressed effects of 60 Hz electric fields on reproduction and development in rats, using field strengths from 10 kV m$^{-1}$ to 150 kV m$^{-1}$ (for review, see IARC, 2002). The studies involved large group sizes and exposure over multiple generations. In general, the studies did not report any consistent adverse effects. For example, malformations were increased and fertility was decreased in one experiment (Rommereim et al., 1987). These effects were not confirmed in further studies by the same group (Rommereim et al., 1990; 1996).

Exposure to 50 Hz electric fields at 50 kV m$^{-1}$ did not induce significant effects on growth and development in eight-week-old male rats exposed 8 h per day for 4 weeks, or rabbits exposed 16 h per day from the last two weeks of gestation to six weeks after birth (Portet & Cabanes, 1988).

Sikov et al. (1987) conducted a three-generation study on Hanford Miniature swine. The exposed group was kept in a 60 Hz, 30 kV m$^{-1}$ electric field for 20 h per day, 7 days per week. Two teratological evaluations were performed on the offspring of the $F_0$ generation. Malformations were decreased in the first teratological evaluation (significant only if analysed by foetus), but increased in the second evaluation. Increased malformations were also found among offspring of the $F_1$ generation at 18 months, but not in another offspring 10 months later. The inconsistency of the results makes it impossible to conclude that there is a causal relationship between ELF electric field exposure and developmental effects in swine.

### 10.2.2 Magnetic fields

#### 10.2.2.1 Effects on prenatal development

Several studies have investigated effects of low frequency magnetic fields on prenatal development of rodents, and have been reviewed previously (Huuskonen, Lindbohm & Juutilainen, 1998; IARC, 2002). The magnetic flux densities varied from 2 µT to 30 mT. In general, the results do not show any consistent effects on gross external or visceral malformations or increase of foetal loss. The only findings that show some consistency are increases in minor skeletal alterations in several experiments in rats (Huuskonen, Juutilainen & Komulainen, 1993; Mevissen, Buntenkotter & Löscher, 1994; Ryan et al., 2000; Stuchly et al., 1988) and mice (Huuskonen et al., 1998b; Kowalczuk et al., 1994). However, in many other studies in rats (Chung et al., 2003; Negishi et al., 2002; Rommereim et al., 1996) and mice (Chiang et al., 1995; Frolen, Svedenstal & Paulsson, 1993; Ohnishi et al., 2002; Wiley et al., 1992) this effect was not observed. The lowest flux density reported to induce this kind of effect was 13 µT (Huuskonen, Juutilainen & Komulainen, 1993; Huuskonen et al., 1998b). Skeletal variations are relatively common findings in teratological studies and often considered biologically insignificant. Some of the groups concluded that the increased skeletal changes observed in their studies resulted from statistical fluctuation rather than effects of the magnetic field exposure. Another possible explanation is that these findings indicate subtle developmental effects similar to the developmental instability reported by Graham et al. (2000c) in Drosophila (see 3.2). The use of low frequency magnetic fields for facilitating bone healing (for review, see IARC, 2002) may imply effects on growth and development of bone tissue.

Table 69 summarizes the results of ELF studies on prenatal development in mammals.

Table 69. Low frequency magnetic fields and prenatal development in mammals

| Animal strain | Frequency waveform | Flux density (μT) | Exposure time (days) | Findings [a] | Other findings, notes | Authors |
|---|---|---|---|---|---|---|
| CBA/Ca mouse | 50 Hz sinusoidal | 12.6, 126 | 0–18 | M- S+ R- | | Huuskonen et al., 1998b |
| CD-1 mouse | 50 Hz sinusoidal | 20 000 | 0–17 | M- S- R- | Body weight and length increased. | Kowalczuk et al., 1994 |
| Swiss Webster mouse | 15.6 kHz sawtooth | 40 (p-p) | 5–16 | M+ S- R- | Combined exposure with cytosine arabinoside. | Chiang et al., 1995 |
| CBA/S mouse | 20 kHz sawtooth | 15 (p-p) | 0–18 1–18 4–18 6–18 | M- S- R+ | | Frolen, Svedenstål & Paulsson, 1993 |
| CBA/S mouse | 20 kHz sawtooth | 15 (p-p) | 0–4.5 0–6 | M- R- | Number of dead fetuses increased, weight and length decreased. | Svedenstål & Johanson, 1995 |
| CBA/S mouse | 20 kHz sawtooth | 15 (p-p) | 0–18 | M- S- R- | | Huuskonen et al., 1998a |
| CBA/Ca mouse | 20 kHz sawtooth | 15 (p-p) | 0–18 | M- S+ R- | | Huuskonen et al., 1998b |
| CD-1 mouse | 20 kHz sawtooth | 3.6, 17, 200 (p-p) | 0–17 | M- S- R- | | Wiley et al., 1992 |
| Wistar rat | 50 Hz sinusoidal | 12.6 | 0–20 | M- S+ R- | | Huuskonen, Juutilainen & Komulainen, 1993 |

248

**Table 69. Continued**

| Wistar rat | 50 Hz sinusoidal | 30 000 | 0–19 | M- S+ R- | | Mevissen, Buntenkotter & Löscher, 1994 |
|---|---|---|---|---|---|---|
| SD rat | 60 Hz sinusoidal | 0.6, 1000 | 0–20 | M- S- R- | | Rommereim et al., 1996 |
| SD rat | 60 Hz sinusoidal | 2, 200, 1000 | 6–19 | M- S- R- | | Ryan et al., 1996 |
| SD rat | 60, 180 or 60+180 Hz sinusoidal | 200 | 6–19 | M- S+ R- | | Ryan et al., 2000 |
| SD rat | 50 Hz sinusoidal | 7, 70, 350 | 0–7 8–15 | M- S- R- | | Negishi et al., 2002 |
| ICR mouse | 50 Hz sinusoidal | 500, 5000 | 0–18 | M- S- | Exposure before mating. | Ohnishi et al., 2002 |
| SD rat | 60 Hz sinusoidal | 5, 83.3, 500 | 6–20 | M- S- R- | Visceral variations decreased, resorptions increased nonsignificantly . | Chung et al., 2003 |
| Wistar rat | 10 kHz sinusoidal | 95, 240, 950 | 0–22 | M- S- R- | | Dawson et al., 1998 |
| SD rat | 18 kHz, sawtooth | 5.7, 23, 66 (p-p) | 0–21 | M- S+ R- | Exposure before mating. | Stuchly et al., 1988 |
| Wistar rat | 20 kHz, sawtooth | 15 (p-p) | 0–20 | M- S+ R- | | Huuskonen, Juutilainen & Komulainen, 1993 |
| ICR mouse | 20 kHz, sawtooth | 6.25 µT (peak) | 2.5–15.5 | M- R- | | Kim et al., 2004 |

[a] M=major external or visceral malformations; S=minor skeleton anomalies; R=resorptions; + positive finding; - no statistically significant difference from controls.

Effects of a 50 Hz, 20 mT magnetic field on postnatal development and behaviour of prenatally exposed CD1 mice were studied by Sienkiewicz et al. (1994). Three possible field-dependent effects were found: the exposed animals performed the air-righting reflex earlier (about 2 days), the exposed males were significantly lighter in weight at 30 days of age and the exposed animals remained on a Rota-rod for less time as juveniles. A reduction in running time on a Rota-rod which was found in juvenile mice may represent a magnetic field-induced impairment in motor coordination during adolescence.

Seven pregnant CD1 mice were exposed for the period of gestation to a vertical, sinusoidal, 50 Hz, magnetic field at 5 mT and eight control animals were sham-exposed. Ten males per group were tested at 82–84 days of age for deficits in spatial learning and memory in radial arm maze. No effects on performance were observed (Sienkiewicz, Larder & Saunders, 1996).

Chung, Kim & Myung (2004) exposed Sprague-Dawley rats (24 per group) for 21 h per day from gestational day 6 through lactational day 21 to 60 Hz magnetic fields at flux densities of 5, 83.3 or 500 µT. Growth, physical development, behaviour, and reproductive performance of the offspring was evaluated. A fraction of the $F_1$ pups were evaluated for visceral and skeletal abnormalities, and the $F_2$ foetuses were evaluated for external visible malformations. The behavioural tests included righting reflex, negative geotaxis, traction test, papillary reflex, acoustic startle response, Rota-rod test, open field test and water-filled T-maze test. The statistically significant findings included decrease of anogenital distance in males of the 5 µT group and females of the 5 and 500 µT groups, performance in the open field test in males of the 5 µT group, performance in one of the tests performed with the water maze with the females of the 5 µT group, changes in some organ weights, and increased incidence of visceral variations in the 83.3 µT group. However, as these findings showed no dose-response relationship and a high number of statistical comparisons were performed, they are most probably chance findings.

### 10.2.2.3 Multi-generation studies

A reproductive assessment by continuous breeding (RACB) study on the toxicity of 60 Hz magnetic fields was conducted by Ryan et al. (1999). The RACB protocol permits the evaluation of reproductive performance over multiple generations. Groups of Sprague-Dawley rats, 40 breeding pairs per group were exposed continuously for 18.5 hours per day to sinusoidal 60 Hz magnetic fields at field strengths of 0, 2, 200 or 1000 µT or to an intermittent (1 hour on, 1 hour off) field at 1000 µT. No exposure-related toxicity was observed in any of the three generations examined. Foetal viability and body weight were similar in all groups, and there were no differences in any measure of reproductive performance (litters per breeding pair, percent fertile pairs, latency to parturition, litter size, and sex ratio). Teratological examinations were not performed.

### 10.2.2.4 Effects on mammalian embryos in vitro

Huuskonen, Juutilainen & Kumolainen (2001) studied the effects of 13 µT, 50 Hz magnetic fields on the development of preimplantation CBA/S mouse embryos. The development of the embryos was followed for eight days (up to the blastocyst stage). Significantly fewer embryos died at the 5–8-cell and >8-cell stages in the exposed group than in the control group, but no differences were seen in other developmental stages. There was no overall difference in survival, and no abnormalities or effects on developmental rate were observed. In contrast, Beraldi et al. (2003) reported significantly decreased survival in cultured mouse embryos exposed to 50 Hz fields at 60, 120 or 220 µT. The effect (tested at 60 µT) was more pronounced in embryos obtained by in vitro fertilization than in those resulting from natural breeding. No effects were observed on the morphology or developmental rate of the embryos.

### 10.2.2.5 Effects of paternal exposure

Possible effects of 50 Hz magnetic fields on the fertility of male Sprague-Dawley rats were investigated by Al-Akhras et al. (2001). Ten males per group (13 in the control group) were exposed to a sinusoidal, 50 Hz magnetic field at 25 µT for 90 days before they were mated with unexposed females (two females per male). The number of pregnancies decreased significantly from 24/26 (92%) in the control group to 10/20 (50%) in the exposed group. The effect persisted in a second mating after 45 days, but not at 90 days after removal from the magnetic field. Number of implantations per litter and viable foetuses per litter were not significantly affected. Effects on fertility in females (10 animals per group) were also evaluated in the same study. The 90-day exposure resulted in a statistically significant decrease of pregnancies, from 100% in the controls to 6/10 in the exposed females. The mean number of implantations per litter also decreased from 9.9 to 4.7 and the mean number of viable foetuses per litter from 9.6 to 4.3. These differences were statistically significant, but the numbers of animals in the groups were small.

In another study with similar design, the same investigators reported no adverse effects on fertility and reproduction in Swiss mice (Elbetieha, Al-Akhras & Darmani, 2002).

Picazo et al. (1995) exposed young male and female OF1 mice until adulthood to a sinusoidal 50 Hz, 15 µT magnetic field. The animals were then mated, and the offspring were kept under the same experimental conditions until they acquired sexual maturity. A significant increase of testis size and weight and of testosterone levels was observed in male offspring that had been exposed compared with a control group. However, complete spermatogenesis occurred in both control and exposed animals.

The effects of a 50 Hz, 1.7 mT sinusoidal magnetic field on mouse spermatogenesis (De Vita et al., 1995) was examined by flow cytometry. Groups of five male hybrid FI mice (C57Bl/Cne x C3H/Cne) were exposed for 2 or 4 hours, and measurements were performed at 7, 14, 21, 28, 35, and 42 days after exposure. The only statistically significant difference was a decrease in elongated spermatids at 28 days after treatment in the animals exposed for 4 h.

Kato et al. (1994b) reported no effects of circularly polarized 50 Hz magnetic fields at 1, 5 or 50 µT on plasma testosterone concentration in male Wistar-King rats.

## 10.3 Effects on non-mammalian species

### 10.3.1 Bird embryos

#### 10.3.1.1 Development

Delgado et al. (1982) reported that weak pulsed ELF magnetic fields (0.12–12 µT; 10, 1000 or 1000 Hz) affected the early development of chicken embryos examined after 48 h of incubation. After this initial finding, the same research group published several papers reporting similar effects (Leal et al., 1989; Ubeda et al., 1983; Ubeda et al., 1994; Ubeda, Trillo & Leal, 1987).

The initial results of Delgado were not replicated in an independent study (Maffeo, Miller & Carstensen, 1984). A large well-designed international study ("Henhouse project") aimed at replicating Delgado's results has been carried out in six separate laboratories (Berman et al., 1990). Identical equipment and standardized experimental procedures were used. While the combined data showed a significant (p < 0.001) increase of abnormal embryos in the exposed group, the results were not consistently positive – only two laboratories found a statistically significant increase of abnormalities.

One of the laboratories that participated in the Henhouse project has reported a large additional investigation using pulsed waveforms and 50 Hz sinusoidal fields (Koch et al., 1993). Several different strains were tested to investigate possible strain-specific differences in sensitivity to magnetic fields. No significant magnetic field effects were observed.

Studies by Juutilainen and co-workers (1986) showed that the percentage of abnormalities was increased in chick embryos exposed during their first two days of development to 100 Hz magnetic fields with a pulsed, sinusoidal and rectangular waveforms. In another series of experiments with sinusoidal waveform, similar effects were found in a wide range of frequencies (Juutilainen & Saali, 1986). The effects of 100 Hz sinusoidal fields with a field strength of 1 A m$^{-1}$ were confirmed in experiments with a large number of eggs (Juutilainen, 1986). Further experiments showed similar effects also at 50 Hz (sinusoidal), and indicated a threshold at 1.3 µT (Juutilainen, Läära & Saali, 1987).

Apart from the series of experiments by Juutilainen and colleagues, there have been few other studies on sinusoidal fields. Cox et al. (1993) attempted to partly replicate the findings of Juutilainen et al. No difference from control embryos was observed in 200 embryos exposed to a 10 µT, 50 Hz magnetic field.

Farrell et al. (1997) conducted an extensive series of experiments on the effects of pulsed and sinusoidal magnetic fields on chick embryo development, involving a total of more than 2500 embryos. Both 60 Hz, 4 µT sinusoidal fields and a 100 Hz field with 1 µT peak amplitude (similar to the field used in the Henhouse project) were used. Overall, the abnormality rate was more than doubled by magnetic field exposure, and the effect was statistically significant for both 100 Hz and 60 Hz fields.

Quail embryo development has been reported to be affected by exposure to ELF magnetic fields (Terol & Panchon, 1995). The exposures were 50 or 100 Hz with rectangular waveform and intensities of 0.2, 1.2, 3.3 and 3.2 µT, and the embryos were examined at 48 h. There was a significant increase in embryonic deaths and abnormal development in the 100 Hz group, but not in the 50 Hz group.

### 10.3.1.2 Interaction with known teratogens

Pafkova & Jerabek (1994) reported that exposure to a 50 Hz, 10 mT magnetic field modified the embryotoxic effect of ionizing radiation on chick embryos examined at day 9 of development, although no effects of magnetic fields alone were detected. Embryotoxicity was expressed as the sum of embryonic deaths and malformations. Exposure to the magnetic field prior to the X-ray treatment seemed to protect the embryos from X-ray induced toxicity, while an enhancement of the embryotoxicity was seen when the magnetic field exposure followed the X-ray irradiation. The effects were seen consistently in several experiments and were statistically significant. The same group has also shown a similar protective effect of 50 Hz, 10 mT magnetic field exposure against subsequent exposures to the chemical teratogens insulin and tetracyclin (Pafkova et al., 1996).

Another research group has reported that the survival of chicken embryos exposed to UV-radiation is modified by exposure to a 60 Hz, 8 µT magnetic field (Dicarlo et al., 1999). Similarly to Pafkova's findings, the direction of the effect (enhancement or protection) depended on the exposure protocol. In this case magnetic field exposure always preceded UV exposure, but short exposure (2 h) seemed to protect the embryos, while longer exposure (96 h) increased the UV-induced mortality.

### 10.3.2 Other non-mammalian species

Exposure to sinusoidal magnetic fields has been reported to delay the development of fish embryos at 60 Hz, 0.1 mT (Cameron, Hunter & Winters, 1985), sea urchin embryos at 60 Hz, 0.1 mT (Zimmerman et al., 1990), and fish embryos at 50 Hz, 1 mT (Skauli, Reitan & Walther, 2000). No malformations were found in these studies.

Graham et al. (2000c) studied the effects of 60 Hz magnetic fields on "developmental stability" in *Drosophila melanogaster*. Developmental stability is a concept that describes the ability of an organism to maintain a consistent phenotype under given genetic and environmental conditions (this relatively new concept is potentially a useful tool for detecting weak environmental effects (Graham et al., 2000c). An individual with low developmental stability has reduced ability to correct disturbances in development. The standard measure of developmental instability is fluctuating asymmetry, random deviations from perfect bilateral symmetry. This measure has been shown to respond to environmental agents such as DDT, lead, and benzene.

253

Another measure of developmental instability is the frequency of phenodeviants in a population. Graham et al. exposed the fruit flies for their entire lives, egg to adult, to 60 Hz fields at 1.5 or 80 μT. The magnetic field exposures caused a significant reduction in body weight. The flies exposed to 80 μT showed reduced developmental stability measured both by fluctuating asymmetry (asymmetrical wing veins) and frequency of phenodeviants (fused abdominal segments). Mirabolghasemi & Azarnia (2002) have reported increased abnormalities in adult *D. melanogaster* flies after exposure of larvae to a 11 mT, 50 Hz field.

## 10.4    Conclusions

On the whole, epidemiological studies have not shown an association between adverse human reproductive outcomes and maternal or paternal exposure to ELF fields. There is some evidence for increased risk of miscarriage associated with measured maternal magnetic field exposure, but this evidence is inadequate.

ELF electric fields of up to 150 kV m$^{-1}$ have been evaluated in several mammalian species, including studies with large group sizes and exposure over several generations. The results consistently show no adverse developmental effects.

The exposure of mammals to ELF magnetic fields of up to 20 mT does not result in gross external, visceral or skeletal malformations. Some studies show an increase in minor skeletal anomalies, in both rats and mice. Skeletal variations are relatively common findings in teratological studies and often considered biologically insignificant. However, subtle effects of magnetic fields on skeletal development cannot be ruled out. Very few studies have been published which address reproductive effects and no conclusions can be drawn from them.

Several studies on non-mammalian experimental models (chick embryos, fish, sea urchins and insects) have reported findings indicating that ELF magnetic fields at microtesla levels may disturb early development. However, the findings of non-mammalian experimental models generally carry less weight in the overall evaluation of developmental toxicity than those of corresponding mammalian studies.

Overall the evidence for developmental effects and for reproductive effects is inadequate.

# 11    CANCER

The possibility that exposure to low frequency EMFs increases the risk of cancer has been subject to much epidemiological and experimental research over the last two decades and has been widely reviewed by national and international expert groups (e.g. AGNIR, 2001b; Ahlbom & Feychting, 2001; IARC, 2002; ICNIRP, 2003; NIEHS, 1998). The association between childhood leukaemia and residential ELF magnetic fields, first identified by Wertheimer & Leeper (1979) and subsequently found in a number of epidemiological studies, has driven experimental and epidemiological research and risk assessment forwards in this area and led to the classification of ELF magnetic fields by the International Agency for Research on Cancer (IARC) as a "possible human carcinogen" (IARC, 2002). This evaluation of the carcinogenicity of EMFs is of particular relevance to this Environmental Health Criteria document. However, a number of relevant studies have been published following this assessment.

A cancer is an uncontrolled growth of cells that may invade and disrupt surrounding tissues and spread through the body via the blood and lymphatic vessels. In contrast to normal cells, malignant cells in vitro commonly show persistent and autonomous proliferation in absence of any proper attachment (immortalisation and "anchorage free" growth). Carcinogenesis itself is a multi-stage process and is classically divided into two principal stages: initiation, which is the induction of irreversible changes (mutations in genes), and promotion, which is reversible and needs to be sustained by repeated stimuli to the initiated cell. Promotion then stimulates further development (outgrowth) into a tumour. Because of the low energy levels in molecular interactions, it is physically highly implausible that ELF fields cause direct genetic damage (i.e. damage DNA molecules from which genes are made). However, it has been theorised that ELF may enhance such damage from other sources (e.g. endogenous radicals), or that epigenetic (non-genotoxic) interference in signal transduction may enhance cancer formation (see section 11.4). Once the potential for full malignancy has been established in a primary tumour, the progression of the disease may be influenced by other factors such as immune surveillance and hormonal dependency. It has also been hypothesised that ELF fields may interfere with these factors that play a role in a "late-stage" of tumour development (see Chapter 6 on the neuroendocrine system and Chapter 9.1 on the immune system).

This chapter reviews the experimental and epidemiological evidence concerning ELF exposure and the risk of cancer, focussing on studies published subsequent to the IARC assessment in 2002. In contrast to other chapters, the experimental evidence is discussed before the epidemiological evidence. In particular, the section discussing childhood leukaemia presents a detailed risk assessment, drawing on the other evidence presented and leads on to chapters on overall risk assessment and protective measures.

255

## 11.1    IARC 2002 evaluation: summary

Since the first report suggesting an association between residential ELF magnetic fields and childhood leukaemia was published in 1979, dozens of increasingly sophisticated epidemiological studies have examined this association (see Tables 1 and 2 from IARC, 2002). In addition, there have been numerous comprehensive reviews, meta-analyses, and two pooled analyses. In one pooled analysis based on nine well-conducted studies, virtually no association was noted for exposure to ELF magnetic fields below 0.4 µT and an odds ratio of around 2 was seen, indicating an twofold excess risk, for exposure above 0.4 µT (Ahlbom et al., 2000). The other pooled analysis included 15 studies based on less restrictive inclusion criteria and used 0.3 µT as the highest cut-point (Greenland et al., 2000). A relative risk of 1.7 for exposure above 0.3 µT was reported. The two analyses are in close agreement. In contrast to these results for ELF magnetic fields, evidence that electric fields are associated with childhood leukaemia is insufficient for firm conclusions but does not suggest any risk.

The association between childhood leukaemia and estimates of time-weighted average exposures to magnetic fields is unlikely to be due to chance, but bias may explain some of the association. In particular, selection (including participation) bias may account for part of the association in some of the studies. Case-control studies which relied on in-home measurements are especially vulnerable to this bias, because of the low response rates in many studies. Studies conducted in the Nordic countries, which relied on historical calculated magnetic fields, are not subject to any selection bias yet identified, but risk estimates are imprecise due to low numbers of exposed subjects. There have been dramatic improvements in the assessment of exposure to electric and magnetic fields over time, yet all of the studies are subject to misclassification. Non-differential misclassification of exposure (similar degrees of misclassification in cases and controls) is likely to result in bias towards the null. Bias due to unknown confounding factors is very unlikely to explain the entire observed effect. However, some bias due to confounding is quite possible, which could operate in either direction. It cannot be excluded that a combination of selection bias, some degree of confounding and chance could explain the results. Conversely, if the observed relationship were causal, the exposure-associated risk could also be greater than what is reported.

With regard to other childhood cancers, no consistent relationship has been reported in studies of childhood brain tumours or cancers at other sites and residential ELF electric and magnetic fields. However, these studies have generally been smaller and of lower quality and associations can not be ruled out for all those outcomes.

Numerous studies of the relationship between electrical appliance use and various childhood cancers have been published. In general, these studies provide no discernible pattern of increased risks associated with increased duration and frequency of use of appliances. Since many of the studies collected information from interviews that took place many years after the time period of etiological interest, recall bias is likely to be a major problem. Studies on parental occupational exposure to ELF electric and magnetic fields in the preconception period or during gestation are methodologically weak and the results are not consistent.

Concerning adult cancer risk and residential exposures, the evidence was considered sparse and methodologically limited, and although there had been a considerable number of reports, a consistent association between residential exposure and adult leukaemia and brain cancer was not established. For breast and other cancers, the existing data were not considered adequate to test for an association with electric or magnetic fields. Concerning studies of occupational exposure, most had focused on leukaemia and brain cancer. There was no consistent finding across studies of an exposure-response relationship and no consistency in the association with specific sub-types of leukaemia or brain tumour. Evidence for cancers at other sites was not considered adequate for evaluation.

In general, the animal studies, which included a number of life-time studies and studies of animals predisposed to develop cancer, and in vitro studies of cellular processes implicated in carcinogenesis, did not support the hypothesis that ELF EMFs were carcinogenic.

In summary, taking this information into consideration, the overall IARC (2002) evaluation for the carcinogenicity of EMFs was:

- There is *limited* evidence in humans for the carcinogenicity of extremely low-frequency magnetic fields in relation to childhood leukaemia.

- There is *inadequate* evidence in humans for the carcinogenicity of extremely low-frequency magnetic fields in relation to all other cancers.

- There is *inadequate* evidence in humans for the carcinogenicity of static electric or magnetic fields and extremely low-frequency electric fields.

- There is *inadequate* evidence in experimental animals for the carcinogenicity of extremely low-frequency magnetic fields.

- No data relevant to the carcinogenicity of extremely low-frequency electric fields in experimental animals were available.

Leading to the conclusion that:

- Extremely low-frequency magnetic fields are *possibly carcinogenic to humans (Group 2B)*.

- ...extremely low-frequency electric fields are *not classifiable as to their carcinogenicity to humans (Group 3)*.

**Table 70. Case–control studies of childhood leukaemia and exposure to ELF magnetic fields [a] [b]**

| Study area, population | Exposure | # cases | OR (95% CI) | Comments | Authors |
|---|---|---|---|---|---|
| Denver, CO, USA 155 deceased cases, 155 controls aged 0–19 y | *Wire code [c]* LCC HCC | 92 (126 controls) 63 (29 controls) | | No risk estimates presented; lack of blinding for the exposure assessment; hypothesis-generating study. | Wertheimer & Leeper, 1979 |
| Los Angeles County, CA, USA 211 cases, 205 controls aged 0–10 y | *Wire code* UG/VLCC (baseline) OLCC OHCC VHCC | 31 58 80 42 | 1.0 0.95 (0.53–1.7) 1.4 (0.81–2.6) 2.2 (1.1–4.3) | Matched analysis, no further adjustments; low response rates for measurements; no wire coding of subjects who refused to participate. | London et al., 1991 |
| 164 cases, 144 controls aged 0–10 y | *Mean magnetic fields (24-h bedroom measurement)* < 0.067 µT (baseline) 0.068–0.118 µT 0.119–0.267 µT ≥ 0.268 µT | 85 35 24 20 | 1.0 0.68 (0.39–1.2) 0.89 (0.46–1.7) 1.5 (0.66–3.3) | | |
| Sweden (corridors along power lines) 39 cases, 558 controls aged 0–15 y | *Calculated historical magnetic fields* < 0.1 µT (baseline) 0.1–0.19 µT ≥ 0.2 µT | 27 4 7 | 1.0 2.1 (0.6–6.1) 2.7 (1.0–6.3) | Adjusted for sex, age, year of diagnosis, type of house, Stockholm county (yes/ no); in subsequent analysis also for socioeconomic status and air pollution from traffic; no contact with subjects required. | Feychting & Ahlbom, 1993 |

# Table 70. Continued

| Location | Exposure | n | OR (95% CI) | Comments | Reference |
|---|---|---|---|---|---|
| Denmark 833 cases, 1666 controls aged 0–14 y | *Calculated historical magnetic fields* | | | Adjusted for sex and age at diagnosis; socioeconomic status, distribution similar between cases and controls; no contact with subjects required. | Olsen, Nielsen & Schulgen, 1993 |
| | < 0.1 µT (baseline) | 829 | 1.0 | | |
| | 0.1–0.24 µT | 1 | 0.5 (0.1–4.3) | | |
| | ≥ 0.25 µT | 3 | 1.5 (0.3–6.7) | | |
| Norway (census wards crossed by power lines) 148 cases, 579 controls aged 0–14 y | *Calculated historical magnetic fields* | | | Adjusted for sex, age and municipality, socioeconomic status, type of house, and number of dwellings; no contact with subjects required. | Tynes & Haldorsen, 1997 |
| | < 0.05 µT (baseline) | 139 | 1.0 | | |
| | 0.05–< 0.14 µT | 8 | 1.8 (0.7–4.2) | | |
| | ≥ 0.14 µT | 1 | 0.3 (0.0–2.1) | | |
| Lower Saxony and Berlin (Germany) 176 cases, 414 controls aged 0–14 y | *Median magnetic fields (24-h bedroom measurement)* | | | Adjusted for sex, age and part of Germany (East, West), socioeconomic status and degree of urbanization; information on a variety of potential confounders available; low response rates. | Michaelis et al., 1998 |
| | < 0.2 µT (baseline) | 167 | 1.0 | | |
| | ≥ 0.2 µT | 9 | 2.3 (0.8–6.7) | | |
| Canada: five provinces, subjects living within 100 km of major cities 351 cases, 362 controls aged 0–14 y | *Wire code* | | | Adjusted for age, sex, province, maternal age at birth of child, maternal education, family income, ethnicity and number of residences since birth; information on a variety of potential confounding factors available; relatively low response rates for personal monitoring portion; children with Down syndrome excluded. | McBride et al., 1999 |
| | UG (baseline) | 79 | 1.0 | | |
| | VLCC | 73 | 0.70 (0.41–1.2) | | |
| | OLCC | 77 | 0.76 (0.45–1.3) | | |
| | OHCC | 83 | 0.64 (0.38–1.1) | | |
| | VHCC | 39 | 1.2 (0.58–2.3) | | |
| 293 cases, 339 controls aged 0–14 y | *Personal monitoring (48-h)* | | | | |
| | < 0.08 µT (baseline) | 149 | 1.0 | | |
| | 0.08–< 0.15 µT | 67 | 0.57 (0.37–0.87) | | |
| | 0.15–< 0.27 µT | 45 | 1.1 (0.61–1.8) | | |
| | ≥ 0.27 µT | 32 | 0.68 (0.37–1.3) | | |

**Table 70. Continued**

| | | | | | |
|---|---|---|---|---|---|
| England, Wales and Scotland 1073 cases, 1073 controls aged 0–14 y | *Time-weighted average magnetic fields (1.5–48-h measurement)* | | | Adjusted for sex, date of birth and region, socioeconomic status; information on a variety of potential confounders available; low reponse rates. | UKCCSI, 1999 |
| | < 0.1 µT (baseline) | 995 | 1.0 | | |
| | 0.1–< 0.2 µT | 57 | 0.78 (0.55–1.1) | | |
| | ≥ 0.2 µT | 21 | 0.90 (0.49–1.6) | | |
| | 0.2–< 0.4 µT | 16 | 0.78 (0.40–1.5) | | |
| | ≥ 0.4 µT | 5 | 1.7 (0.40–7.1) | | |
| West Germany 514 cases, 1301 controls aged 0–14 y | *Median magnetic fields (24-h bedroom measurement)* | | | Adjusted for sex, age, year of birth, socioeconomic status and degree of urbanization; information on a variety of potential confounders available; low response rates; relatively long time lag between date of diagnosis and date of the measurement. | Schüz et al., 2001 |
| | < 0.1 µT (baseline) | 472 | 1.0 | | |
| | 0.1–< 0.2 µT | 33 | 1.2 (0.73–1.8) | | |
| | 0.2–< 0.4 µT | 6 | 1.2 (0.43–3.1) | | |
| | ≥ 0.4 µT | 3 | 5.8 (0.78–43) | | |
| | *Night-time magnetic fields* | | | | |
| | < 0.1 µT (baseline) | 468 | 1.0 | | |
| | 0.1–< 0.2 µT | 34 | 1.4 (0.90–2.2) | | |
| | 0.2–< 0.4 µT | 7 | 2.5 (0.86–7.5) | | |
| | ≥ 0.4 µT | 5 | 5.5 (1.2–27) | | |
| Nine mid-western and mid-Atlantic states, USA 408 cases, 408 controls aged 0–14 y | *Wire code* | | *Matched* | Unmatched analysis additionally adjusted for age, sex, mother's education and family income; information on a variety of potential confounding factors available; wire coding of subjects who refused to participate; relatively low response | Linet et al., 1997 |
| | UG/VLCC (baseline) | 175 | 1.0 | | |
| | OLCC | 116 | 1.1 (0.74–1.5) | | |
| | OHCC | 87 | 0.99 (0.67–1.5) | | |
| | VHCC | 24 | 0.88 (0.48–1.6) | | |

# Table 70. Continued

| 638 cases, 620 controls aged 0–14 y | Time-weighted average (24-h bedroom measurement plus spot measurements in two rooms) | | | rates for measurements in controls; only acute lymphoblastic leukaemia; children with Down syndrome excluded from this study (Schüz et al., 2001). |
|---|---|---|---|---|
| | | | *Unmatched* | |
| | < 0.065 μT (baseline) | 267 | 1.0 | |
| | 0.065–0.099 μT | 123 | 1.1 (0.81–1.5) | |
| | 0.100–0.199 μT | 151 | 1.1 (0.83–1.5) | |
| | ≥ 0.200 μT | 83 | 1.2 (0.86–1.8) | |
| | | | *Matched* | |
| | | 206 | 1.0 | |
| | | 92 | 0.96 (0.65–1.4) | |
| | | 107 | 1.2 (0.79–1.7) | |
| | | 58 | 1.5 (0.91–2.6) | |

[a] Source: (IARC, 2002).

[b] In this table, only studies that contributed substantially to the overall summary are considered and only results that were part of the analysis strategy of IARC are presented. Exposure metrics and cut-points vary across studies.

[c] UG, underground wires; VLCC, very low current configuration; OLCC, ordinary low current configuration; OHCC, ordinary high current configuration; VHCC, very high current configuration; LCC, low current configuration; HCC, high current configuration.

Note that in the IARC procedure, the term "limited evidence of carcinogenicity" means that a positive association has been observed for which a causal interpretation is considered credible, but that chance, bias or confounding could not be ruled out with reasonable confidence. The term "inadequate evidence of carcinogenicity" indicates that either the available studies are of insufficient quality, consistency or statistical power to permit a conclusion, or that no data on cancer are available.

In Tables 70 and 71 the key studies discussed by IARC (2002) are summarized.

### Table 71. Pooled analysis of total leukaemia in children [a]

| Authors | 0.1–< 0.2 µT [b] | 0.2–< 0.4 µT | ≥ 0.4 µT | Observed [c] | Expected | Continuous analysis |
|---|---|---|---|---|---|---|
| **Measurement studies** | | | | | | |
| Canada McBride et al., 1999 | 1.3 (0.84–2.0) | 1.4 (0.78–2.5) | 1.6 (0.65–3.7) | 13 | 10.3 | 1.2 (0.96–1.5) |
| Germany Michaelis et al., 1998 | 1.2 (0.58–2.6) | 1.7 (0.48–5.8) | 2.0 (0.26–15) | 2 | 0.9 | 1.3 (0.76–2.3) |
| New Zealand Dockerty et al., 1998; 1999 | 0.67 (0.20–2.2) | 4 cases, 0 controls | 0 cases 0 controls | 0 | 0 | 1.4 (0.40–4.6) |
| United Kingdom UKCCSI, 1999 | 0.84 (0.57–1.2) | 0.98 (0.50–1.9) | 1.0 (0.30–3.4) | 4 | 4.4 | 0.93 (0.69–1.3) |
| USA Linet et al., 1997 | 1.1 (0.81–1.5) | 1.0 (0.65–1.6) | 3.4 (1.2–9.5) | 17 | 4.7 | 1.3 (1.0–1.7) |
| **Calculated field studies** | | | | | | |
| Denmark Olsen, Nielsen & Schulgen, 1993 | 2.7 (0.24–31) | 0 cases 8 controls | 2 cases 0 controls | 2 | 0 | 1.5 (0.85–2.7) |
| Finland Verkasalo et al., 1993 | 0 cases/ 19 controls | 4.1 (0.48–35) | 6.2 (0.68–57) | 1 | 0.2 | 1.2 (0.79–1.7) |
| Norway Tynes & Haldorsen, 1997 | 1.8 (0.65–4.7) | 1.1 (0.21–5.2) | 0 cases 10 controls | 0 | 2.7 | 0.78 (0.50–1.2) |
| Sweden Feychting & Ahlbom, 1993 | 1.8 (0.48–6.4) | 0.57 (0.07–4.7) | 3.7 (1.2–11.4) | 5 | 1.5 | 1.3 (0.98–1.7) |

**Table 71. Continued**

**Summary** [d]

| | | | | | | |
|---|---|---|---|---|---|---|
| Measurement studies | 1.1 (0.86–1.3) | 1.2 (0.85–1.5) | 1.9 (1.1–3.2) | 36 | 20.1 | 1.2 (1.0–1.3) |
| Calculated field studies | 1.6 (0.77–3.3) | 0.79 (0.27–2.3) | 2.1 (0.93–4.9) | 8 | 4.4 | 1.1 (0.94–1.3) |
| All studies | 1.1 (0.89–1.3) | 1.1 (0.84–1.5) | 2.0 (1.3–3.1) | 44 | 24.2 | 1.2 (1.0–1.3) |

[a] Source: (IARC, 2002).

[b] Relative risks (95% CI) by exposure level and with exposure as continuous variable (relative risk per 0.2 µT) with adjustment for age, sex and socioeconomic status (measurement studies) and residence (in East or West Germany). The reference level is < 0.1 µT.

[c] Observed and expected case numbers at ≥ 0.4 µT, with expected numbers given by modelling the probability of membership of each exposure category based on distribution of controls including covariates.

[d] From Ahlbom et al. (2000).


## 11.2    Epidemiological studies

### 11.2.1   Childhood leukaemia

Since childhood leukaemia is the outcome for which the epidemiological evidence is the most consistent it has attracted particular attention, especially following the IARC (2002) assessment. This section provides an update on studies that have been published since the IARC classification and discusses possible interpretations.

### 11.2.1.1 Epidemiology

Leukaemias are cancers of the blood and bone marrow. The classification of leukaemias is conventionally based on the cell types of origin (lymphocytes, myelocytes, monocytes) and on the rate at which the disease progresses (acute and chronic). Leukaemia is the most common childhood malignancy, constituting more then a third of all childhood cancers. Acute lymphocytic leukaemias (ALL) account for 75% of all cases of childhood leukaemia. Acute myeloid leukaemia (AML) accounts for most non-ALL childhood leukaemias; only a fraction of childhood leukaemia cases are diagnosed with other subtypes.

#### 11.2.1.1.1 Incidence

For children under 15 years of age, the estimated number of new leukaemia cases in 2000 was approximately 49 000 globally, translating into an incidence rate of about 3 cases per 100 000 (IARC, 2000). The incidence of childhood leukaemia in different regions of the world is given in Table 72.

Table 72. Global incidence of childhood leukaemia in 2000

| Region | Population 0-14 year olds [a] | New cases [b] | Incidence (per 100 000) |
|---|---|---|---|
| Africa | 339 631 000 | 3 848 | 1.13 |
| Asia | 1 119 233 000 | 31 062 | 2.78 |
| Europe | 127 382 000 | 4 878 | 3.83 |
| Latin America | 165 828 000 | 6 367 | 3.84 |
| North America | 68 083 000 | 2 841 | 4.17 |
| Oceania | 8 018 000 | 283 | 3.53 |
| World | 1 828 175 000 | 49 000 | 2.68 |

[a] Estimates for 2000: International Association of Cancer Registries (IARC, 2000).

[b] Estimates for 2000: United Nations - World Population Prospects (UN, 2002).

There are marked differences in leukaemia rates among various regional and ethnic groups. In the USA, the highest rates are observed among Hispanics in Los Angeles and Filipinos, Chinese, and Japanese in California and Hawaii. Moderate-to-high rates occur among Caucasians; for African-Americans, rates are significantly lower. The white-to-black ratio of overall leukaemia incidence rates is about 2 throughout various age groups (Linet & Devesa, 1991). Within the United States, there are also clear regional differences, with rates ranging from 2.2–5.6 per 100 000 for boys and 1.4–6.3 per 100 000 for girls (Linet & Devesa, 1991).

International comparisons of overall childhood leukaemia incidence rates indicate a 4–6-fold variability. The highest overall incidence rates of over 6 cases per 100 000 per year have been reported in Costa Rica and among the non-Maori population in New Zealand (Kinlen, 1994; Linet & Devesa, 1991). High incidence rates have also been reported in the Scandinavian countries, Australia, Hong Kong, and the Philippines; rates range between 4.5 and 5.5 cases per 100 000 annually, similar to rates reported among Hispanic males in Los Angeles (Kinlen, 1994; Linet & Devesa, 1991). Intermediately high incidence rates have been observed in European countries, such as Germany, Great Britain, France, and Hungary, as well as in Japan and China and among Jews in Israel (Bhatia et al., 1999; Greenberg & Shuster, 1985; Kinlen, 1994; Linet & Devesa, 1991). Low incidence rates occur in India, among Kuwaitis in Kuwait, and among black children in Africa (Bhatia et al., 1999; Greaves & Alexander, 1993; Greenberg & Shuster, 1985). Although absolute rates vary, the sex ratio of incidence rates and the patterns of age-specific rates are similar among the various countries, except that the early childhood peak in ALL incidence is apparently absent among African children. There is, however, a significant international variation between ALL and non-ALL ratios. As in the United States, the large majority of cases in European and Latin-American countries have ALL, whereas in many Asian countries, such as China, the Philippines, and India, the proportion of non-ALL cases is higher, composing close to 50% of childhood leukaemia cases (Greaves & Alexander, 1993).

Whether the wide international variation in childhood leukaemia incidence rates represents real differences in incidence rates or reflects only differences in completeness of case ascertainment and registration is controversial. Alternative explanations are that inherited genetic factors may predispose certain ethnic groups to childhood leukaemia, or some so-far-unidentified environmental factors or higher socioeconomic status may predispose children in more developed nations to a higher risk of leukaemia. Incidence rates for leukaemia are consistently 10–50% higher among boys than among girls (Gurney et al., 1995; Linet & Devesa, 1991; Zahm & Devesa, 1995). This difference results primarily from higher rates of the most common type of leukaemia, ALL, among boys (Gurney et al., 1995; Linet & Devesa, 1991; Rechavi, Ramot & Ben-Bassat, 1992). Others types of leukaemia do not clearly show such a strong predominance in males. For example, gender-specific AML incidence rates tend to be similar overall.

Incidence rates for ALL cases have a characteristic age pattern. During the first couple of years of life incidence rates dramatically increase, reaching a peak at 2–3 years of age, followed by a slow decline until about age 10, when the rate stabilizes. AML incidence has a different age distribution: the highest incidence rate occurs during the first 2 years of life and lower rates later in childhood (Ries et al., 2001).

Development of the characteristic peak of ALL incidence in early childhood was first shown from mortality data in the 1920s in Britain (Cartwright & Staines, 1992; Milham & Ossiander, 2001). In the United States, this peak was shown to develop about 3–4 decades earlier among white children (in the 1920s and 1930s) than among black children (in the 1960s) (Bhatia et al., 1999; Greaves & Alexander, 1993; Milham & Ossiander, 2001).

### 11.2.1.1.2 Etiology

Leukaemia results from chromosomal alterations and mutations that disrupt the normal process by which lymphoid or myeloid progenitor cells differentiate. The underlying triggers for molecular damage may be inherited at conception, may occur during fetal development or during infancy. Most likely, there is an accumulation of a series of detrimental genetic changes over time (Bhatia et al., 1999). Subtypes of AML and ALL are frequently characterized by genetic alterations, including changes in chromosome number (hyperdiploidy or hypodiploidy) and chromosomal translocations that may involve chimeric or fusion genes (Greaves, 2002; Lightfoot, 2005). There is strong evidence that these rearrangements may originate *in utero*. Other data suggest that the conversion of the preleukemic clone to overt disease is low. The implication is that the development of childhood ALL is a multistep process requiring at least one prenatal event in combination with additional prenatal and/or postnatal events. While the "first hit", the initiating *in utero* event, is believed to be common, the "second hit",

265

possibly occurring postnatally, is rare, and therefore acts as the rate-determining step in the development of the disease. However, although there have been significant advances in diagnostic techniques and improvements in treatment, the etiology of leukaemia in children still remains unclear.

A wide variety of factors have been hypothesized to be involved in the etiology of childhood leukaemia. Among environmental exposures possibly associated with childhood leukaemia, ionizing radiation is a generally accepted risk factor (Bhatia et al., 1999). The list of chemical agents for which some evidence points to a link with leukemogenesis includes solvents, pesticides, tobacco smoke, and certain dietary agents. The possible role of viral or other infectious agents in triggering leukaemia development has also been hypothesized (Mezei & Kheifets, 2002) and has received support from a recently published study (Gilham et al., 2005) carried out as part of the United Kingdom Childhood Cancer Study (UKCCS) into the aetiology of childhood leukaemia. More recently, Kinlen's hypothesis of population mixing (perhaps involving rare reactions to infectious vectors) has received additional support (e.g. Dickinson & Parker, 1999). Generally accepted associations, however, explain only 10% of childhood leukaemia incidence (Kheifets & Shimkhada, 2005), leaving the majority with unexplained etiology.

### 11.2.1.2 Trends and ecologic correlations

Despite the well known pitfalls of using ecological correlations to infer causality, assumed rapid increase in magnetic field exposures and lack of corresponding increase in leukaemia incidence has been used as an argument against causal association between magnetic fields and childhood leuekmia. For completeness, historical changes in exposures are presented and compared to changes in childhood leukaemia rates. As expected, however, when this comparison is made, there is, in fact, relatively little that can be deduced.

#### 11.2.1.2.1 Trends in exposures

Magnetic fields are produced by currents in electricity systems. The electricity consumed in most countries has increased dramatically over the twentieth century (this is a statement of the obvious, as there was no public electricity supply anywhere before the late 1800s). It is natural to assume this increase in electricity use has led to an increase in currents in electricity circuits and hence an increase in magnetic fields. This approach has been followed by, e.g., Jackson (1992), Olsen, Nielsen & Shulgen (1993), Petridou et al. (1993), Kraut, Tate & Tran (1994) and Sokejima, Kagamino & Tatsumura (1996), who all assumed average magnetic fields are proportional to a measure of per capita electricity consumption.

It is possible to criticise this assumption. For instance, the increase in electricity use will have been accommodated partly by building new circuits rather than by increasing the load on existing circuits, and there may have been other changes in engineering practice which affect the link between magnetic fields and electricity consumption. Unfortunately, there are no historical measurements that allow this to be tested, and instead, modelling is required. Swanson (1996), for the UK, broke down average exposure into three main components and considered these separately, taking account of changes in engineering practice. The conclusion was that in the UK, average exposure to magnetic fields from 1949 to 1989 had increased by slightly more than per capita electricity consumption – a factor of 4.5 compared to 3.2. Importantly, Swanson recognised a number of uncertainties in this modelling, but showed that the likely effect of the uncertainties was to make the estimated increase an underestimate rather than an overestimate. Note however, that average exposure to magnetic fields in the UK seemed to have stabilized around 1970 and has remained relatively constant ever since.

It is still possible to postulate changes in electricity distribution practices in other countries that break or reduce the link in those countries between consumption and exposure. For instance, it has been suggested that the decreasing use of "knob and tube" wiring in homes in the USA has reduced exposures (Leeper et al., 1991). However, whether this is significant is speculative. The only available evidence supports a working assumption that average exposures have risen by an amount comparable to that of electricity consumption.

### 11.2.1.2.2 Trends in incidence

There is general agreement that in most countries where data are available (in practice, westernised countries only), childhood cancer registration rates for most but not all cancer types as recorded in registries appear to have risen during the twentieth century (Draper, Kroll & Stiller, 1994). In the UK, a large country with a good national registry, childhood cancer registration rates have risen by 35% from 1962 to 1998, an average of 0.8% per year (Cancer Research UK, 2004). For earlier periods, before registries existed but when most childhood cancers and certainly leukaemia were almost always fatal, mortality can be used as a surrogate for incidence. However, any increase in registration (or incidence or mortality rates) could be caused by (a) the survival of children long enough to get cancer, who in earlier years would have died of other causes such as infections; (b) improved diagnosis of cancer; and (c) improved registration efficiency. The improved diagnosis affects the distinction between different types of leukaemia, but should apply less to total leukaemia rates (Draper, Kroll & Stiller, 1994). These factors almost certainly account for some of the increase in registration rates, but it seems likely that there is a genuine increase in some childhood cancer incidence rates as well. In the US, a very slight overall increase in childhood leukaemia incidence was described for the period from the mid-1970s to the late 1990s, indicating an estimated annual increase of 0.5% for all leukaemias and 1.1% for ALL (Linet et al., 1999; Ries et al , 2001). However, Linet et al. (1999) concluded that this modest increase was confined to short intervals in the mid 1980s, and the pattern suggests that reporting or diagnostic changes, rather than environmental influences, were responsible.

Another relevant phenomenon, decribed earlier, is the appearance of a peak in childhood ALL incidence in children aged 2–4 in the early twentieth century. There is some evidence this peak appeared earlier in more industrialised countries, and also appears differently in different ethnic groups.

### 11.2.1.2.3 Comparison of trends in incidence and exposure

Suppose that magnetic fields are a risk factor for childhood leukaemia, that average exposure to magnetic fields has increased over time and that all other risk factors did not change over time. Then the childhood leukaemia incidence rate would have increased as a consequence of the increase in average exposure, and the size of the increase in incidence rate would be a measure of the fraction of leukaemia incidence attributable to magnetic field exposure.

The calculations presented in the appendix, based on the pooled analyses of the epidemiological data on magnetic field exposure and childhood leukaemia incidence, and again taking the hypothetical case of a causal relationship, suggest that the attributable fraction for magnetic field exposure ranges from 0.5% in a low-exposure country such as the UK to 5% in a high-exposure country such as the USA. Increases at the lower end of this range are essentially indistinguishable from the random fluctuations in incidence-rate data. Further, numerous other factors are suspected to be linked to the development of childhood leukaemia. The assumption that all those other risk factors have remained unchanged is implausible, and it would take only a small change in those factors to mask any change in effects, if any, of magnetic field exposure. Furthermore, reliable incidence data in most countries is available only from about 1970, a time where the exponential increase in exposure may have ceased. Therefore, while available data on incidence rates are compatible with the attributable fraction derived from the pooled analyses, they are also compatible with the alternatives of no cases attributable to magnetic fields or of a larger fraction being attributable. It is therefore impossible to draw any conclusions from a comparison of trends in exposures and incidence rates.

Milham & Ossiander (2001) have suggested that the appearance of the peak incidence at around age 3 in childhood ALL is linked with electrification and therefore with exposures. Again, the data are compatible with this hypothesis. However, many other features of society have also changed with progressive industrialisation, and there is in addition considerable uncertainty whether this peak appeared as a consequence of improved survival from other causes. Therefore, it is not valid to claim this as evidence of a link between EMFs and cancer (Kheifets, Swanson & Greenland, 2006).

### 11.2.1.3 New data

Two studies have been published since the IARC evaluation: Kabuto et al. (2006) in Japan and Draper et al. (2005) in the UK.

Kabuto et al. (2006) conducted a study of ALL and AML in children aged 15 years or less and diagnosed between 1999 and 2002 in the catchment area consisting of 18 prefectures and covering 10.7 million (53.5%) of the total 20.0 million children aged 0–15 years in Japan. For each case, up to 3 controls were selected matched on gender, age and residential area. Exposure assessment included 5-min magnetic field measurements in a room where a child spends the longest time daily, as well as in four corners of the house and at an entrance, and 1-week measurements made in the child's bedroom. The distance from each house to the closest overhead power transmission line (22–500 kV) located within 100 meters was measured. Measurements were done in the current house. Based on the family's residential history the length of stay at the current house for the period from conception to the date of diagnosis was assessed. In order to reduce possible information bias due to seasonal variation of magnetic field levels, measurements for each set of case and controls were made close in time and within 2.6 days on average; four sets with more than 100 days between the measurements were excluded. The main exposure metric consisted of a weekly arithmetic mean magnetic fields in the child's bedroom, categorized with cut-off points of 0.1, 0.2, and 0.4 µT for comparability with the pooled analysis. From 1439 childhood leukaemia cases diagnosed in all Japan, request for participation was sent to 781 (ALL+AML) cases living in the catchment area through the child's physicians. Among them 381 cases agreed to participate, but an additional 60 were later excluded due to change of residence after diagnosis, missing measurements, or lack of controls. The final analysis was based on 251 ALL and 61 AML cases and 495 and 108 controls, respectively (9 additional cases and 31 controls were lost due to matching). All conditional logistic regression analyses were adjusted for mother's education as an indicator of socio-economic status. When compared with children who were exposed to magnetic fields < 0.1 µT, the odds ratio for exposure 0.4 µT was 2.63 (95% CI: 0.77–8.96) for all leukaemia combined. No elevation in risk was observed below 0.4 µT. The risk was higher for ALL: OR = 4.73 (95% CI: 1.14–19.7) and the risk was not increased (no cases in the highest category) for AML. [The results are roughly consistent with those of the pooled analyses, but are limited by the small sample size leading to a broad range of uncertainty. The low response rate was a limitation of this study. Thus the addition of this study to the database will not add much as far as the overall results are concerned.]

In the study by Draper et al. (2005), 33 000 children from birth to 14 years old who had a cancer diagnosis in England, Scotland, or Wales between 1962 and 1995 were identified from various cancer registries. One control for each case matched on gender, birth date within 6 months, and birth registration district was selected. The final data set included 9700 matched case-control pairs for leukaemia who had a known birth address that allowed mapping in relation to transmission lines. The postal code at birth was used to identify subjects within 1 km of a 275- or 400-kV transmission line and a few 132-kV lines. Exposure was based on the shortest distance to any line that had existed in the year of birth. When possible, previous line locations were recreated. A distance-dependent excess risk was observed for leukaemia (ranging from RR = 1.36 for distance-to-line 500–599 m to RR = 1.67 for distance of 0–49 m, compared to distance greater than 600 m). Adjustment for the deprivation index did not change the results. [Given its large size the risk estimates in the paper should be stable. Furthermore, because contact with the subject was not necessary, selection bias due to the differential participation among cases and controls, which plagued some of the previous studies, has been avoided. Thus the dependence of the results on the chosen control group and observation of the excess risk so far from the power lines, both noted by the authors and others, is surprising. Furthermore, distance is known to be a very poor predictor of magnetic field exposure, and therefore, results of this material based on calculated magnetic fields, when completed, should be much more informative.]

### 11.2.1.4 Evaluating epidemiological evidence: possible explanations

The consistent association observed between childhood leukaemia and average magnetic field exposure above 0.3–0.4 µT can be due to chance, selection bias, misclassification and other factors which confound the association, or can be a true causal relationship. Each of these interpretations will be discussed in turn below.

#### 11.2.1.4.1 Random error

In the earlier studies only very small numbers were included, particularly for the very-high exposed categories. These studies were thus subject to substantially potentail random error. However, recent pooled analyses are based on large numbers including for children in the highly exposed categories and as a consequence these pooled analyses are unlikely to be substantially affected by random error.

#### 11.2.1.4.2 Systematic error

*Selection bias*

Since practically all epidemiological studies of ELF and childhood leukaemia have been case-control studies, it has been proposed that control selection bias – a common and potentially serious problem of all case-control studies – may be fully or, at least, partially responsible for the consistently described epidemiological association between ELF magnetic fields and childhood leukaemia. In a case-control study, control selection bias occurs when the ratio of the selection probabilities of exposed and unexposed cases is different than the ratio of the selection probabilities of exposed and unexposed controls. The overall requirement of the controls is that they are representative of the source population of the cases.

Low participation rates alone or even selection or response rates that are associated only with disease or only with exposure do not result in selection bias; selection bias develops only if the selection/inclusion probabilities are differential for cases and controls based on their exposure status.

Low subject participation rates in a case-control epidemiological study, however, may allow for a significantly greater potential for control selection bias to occur. A particular problem arises with hospital-based case-control studies and with studies that use methods such as random digit dialing for selection of controls. The problems arise because of a possible difference between the source population of the cases and the source population of the controls.

Subject participation rates differed greatly in previous epidemiological studies of ELF and childhood leukaemia. Participation rates often depended on the type of study and the way study subjects were recruited. Registry-based studies, where subjects were not contacted, were able to include 94–100% of the selected subjects. Studies requiring interviews and in-home measurements generally had significantly lower participation rates (68–37% of eligible subjects), while matching in a case-control study frequently resulted in further decrease in the number of subjects included in the analysis; in one study only 31% and 9% of the eligible cases and controls, respectively, were included. Clearly, in practice the potential for bias is lower in registry-based studies and higher for studies with interviews and measurements. While some studies do in fact report response rates, accurate response rates are not available for all studies. Even for studies reporting response rates, it is frequently difficult to compare them due to non-uniform reporting.

It is hypothesized that selection bias may occur through socio-economic status (SES) or residential mobility; either because relative participation is lower for low SES controls than cases, and low SES children are more likely to be highly exposed than are high SES children; or high mobility controls are both less likely to be included and more likely to have high exposure, leaving group of controls which were included with lower exposure levels than would be in a representative group of children without leukaemia. Under these scenarios, selection bias upwardly biases the effect estimate (Mezei & Kheifets, 2006).

Some evidence supports this hypothesis. Several studies showed that higher participation tended to be related to higher socio-economic status (Hatch et al., 2000; Michaelis et al., 1997; Spinelli et al., 2001). Others showed that lower SES and higher residential mobility (Gurney et al., 1995; Jones et al., 1993) were associated with higher wire codes and perhaps higher residential exposure. However, it should also be noted that the effect of selection bias introduced by this procedure could be reduced by controlling for SES in the analyses, which most studies have done. No study was able to determine exposure among non-participants. A few studies compared, however, exposure distribution between subjects who partially participated in a study to those who fully participated. Hatch et al. (2000) found that full participants were less likely to live in homes with high wire codes (VHCC) or high measured fields (measurements at front door above 0.2 µT). Savitz et al. (1988) compared subjects with and without magnetic field measurements among those with wire code classification. They found that subjects without field measurement were more likely to live in homes with higher wire codes.

Most of the available information on SES and mobility, however, is either based on ecological studies or studies of wire code. It is unknown, at present, to what extent measured fields are correlated with participation, SES or mobility. The strongest evidence for the role of control selection bias comes from a USA study, in which exclusion of partial participants from analyses tended to increase the relative risk estimates for childhood leukaemia (Hatch et al., 2000).

Evidence against the role of selection bias comes from Ahlbom et al's (2000) pooled analysis. Taking advantage of the fact that studies conducted in the Nordic countries relied on historical calculated magnetic fields and are thus not subject to selection bias, investigators compared risk estimates in Nordic studies (OR = 2.1, 95% CI: 0.9–4.9) to the rest of the world (OR = 1.9, 95% CI:1.1–3.2) and found similar estimates. Calculated field studies, however, included only eight exposed cases, five of which were from the Swedish study. Furthermore, a sensitivity analysis which excluded from the pooling one study at a time showed that exclusion of the North American studies, for which suspicion of selection bias is strongest, did not change the overall results. Another argument against selection bias is that there is a lack of consistent association in studies of childhood brain tumours and residential magnetic fields. Many of the leukaemia studies included in the pooled analysis examined brain tumours as well and there is no reason to think that selection bias will affect one outcome and not the other. However, brain tumour studies have generally been smaller and some of lower quality; and a pooled analysis of brain tumour studies is yet to be conducted.

Pursuit of whether and how selection bias might impact effect estimates from case-control studies remains a high priority, both to understand the association between exposure to ELF magnetic fields and childhood leukaemia, and because of an impact it might have on the field of epidemiology, where similar study designs are widely used.

*Misclassification bias*

All of the difficulties with ELF exposure assessment are likely to have led to substantial exposure misclassification, which, in turn, is likely to interfere with detection of an association between exposure and disease. Almost certainly, measurement errors in both measured and calculated fields are not only present in all studies but they also vary considerably from study to study (Greenland & Kheifets, 2006). Target exposure, often described as the average exposure during the period prior to disease diagnosis, is not measured consistently among studies. Furthermore, because the biologically relevant exposure remains unknown, it is unknown whether, or how much, the measured exposure reflects the relevant exposure.

It is generally assumed that misclassification in ELF and leukaemia studies is non-differential, except perhaps in studies using personal exposure measurements (Green et al., 1999b; McBride et al., 1999); this means that exposure misclassification does not differ by disease status. Non-differential misclassification independent of diagnostic errors translates into a bias of the effect estimate towards the null in most situations, although misclassification in middle categories can lead to the distortion of the dose-response curve.

Pooled analyses point to an association between ELF magnetic fields and leukaemia at levels of exposure greater than 0.3 or 0.4 µT. Since there is no established gold standard for the biologically relevant exposure, both sensitivity and specificity cannot be determined for measurements used in ELF assessment. It is known, however, that the specificity is particularly important for rare exposures; even a small decrease in specificity (less than 5%) can reduce a relative risk of 5 to the observed relative risk of approximately 2 (Schüz et al., 2001). A similar reduction in sensitivity has only a small effect on the risk estimate. For magnetic fields, identifying the unexposed as such is difficult.

It is concluded that while misclassification is likely to be ever present, it is unlikely to provide an explanation for the entire observed association. It does, however, introduce a lot of uncertainty into the potential dose response. For example, it is very possible that the apparent threshold may have resulted from smooth monotonic relation together with random measurement error.

## Confounding

Since the early days of EMF research, investigators searched for possible confounding that would explain the observed association. The hypothesized confounders of the relation between ELF magnetic fields and childhood leukaemia include SES, residential mobility, residence type, viral contacts, environmental tobacco smoke, dietary agents, and traffic density (Kheifets & Shimkhada, 2005). None of these variables have been found to confound the association, although some have been identified as potential risk factors. For a factor to be a confounder it has to exert an effect considerably larger than the observed association and be strongly correlated with exposure (Kheifets & Shimkhada, 2005). Owing to limited knowledge of the etiology of childhood leukaemia and an absence of strong risk factors, it is not surprising that substantial confounding has not been identified. The same observation, however, makes it difficult to exclude a possibility of some (yet to be identified) confounder or of the combination of a number of factors. The pooled analysis by Ahlbom et al. (2000) looked at the possible effect of a number of putative risk factors. However, for none of them did adjustment move the relative risk estimate by more than 2%.

## Multiple bias modeling

With such small relative risks as are seen in the context of ELF magnetic fields and childhood leukaemia, it is conceivable that a combination of the biases can explain the observed associations. In pooled analyses, where random error is not the only source of uncertainty, uncertainty from biases can be modeled using multiple-bias modeling. Multiple-bias modeling is used to systematically integrate the major sources of uncertainty into the results to provide a more unbiased estimate of an effect and can be used as a tool to better understand the impact of the different types of biases on the effect estimate. Using multiple-bias modeling, Greenland (2005) concludes that while selection bias is present, it is unlikely to explain the association; that confounding is probably less important than selection bias; and that allowing for misclassification tends to increase the point estimate of risk, but also increases the standard deviation even more, resulting in less certainty that there is a positive association, but a higher certainty that the effect if present is larger than the observed association. In other words, misclassification greatly increases uncertainty, making both no association and a strong association more plausible. Based on one set of plausible assumptions, Greenland calculates posterior probabilities of 2–4% that the combination of misclassification, selection bias, confounding and random error (i.e. the net impact) explains the association. Other plausible assumptions would yield different results, however, and the sole point of this analysis is that, after taking account of all major uncertainty sources, due to limitations in the design, studies completed through 2003 are not decisive and further studies of similar design (such as the new English and Japanese studies) would add little information.

*Possible interaction mechanisms*

The absence of a clearly elucidated, robust, and reproducible mechanism of interaction of low level magnetic fields with biological systems deprives epidemiologic studies of focus in their study designs and hinders their interpretation. Based on known physical principles and a simplistic biological model, many authors have argued that average magnetic fields of 0.3–0.4 µT are orders of magnitude below levels that could interact with cells or tissues and that such interactions are thus biophysically implausible (see Chapter 4). The various mechanisms discussed include forces on magnetic particles, free radical generation, and "resonant" type interactions. Particular hypotheses directed towards childhood leukaemia include the suggestion reviewed by Kavet (2005) that contact currents generated when a person touches a conducting object at a different electrical potential to ground might be of sufficient magnitude to affect bone marrow, which is more extensively distributed in the limbs of children than in adults. In addition, Henshaw and Reiter (2005) raise the suggestion that EMF exposure may increase the risk of childhood leukaemia through the disruption of the night-time secretion of melatonin by the pineal gland (the experimental evidence for melatonin suppression by EMF exposure is discussed in Chapter 6). None of these hypotheses have however received experimental confirmation.

*11.2.1.4.3 Magnetic fields as a putative factor*

Epidemiologic studies of magnetic fields have consistently shown associations with childhood leukaemia, but lack of a known mechanism at such low energy levels and negative animal data suggest that the association is not causal. This section discusses some of the issues that would arise making the "worst-case" assumption that the associations were causally related to magnetic field exposure.

*Time-weighted average*

In the absence of a known biophysical mechanism, which would yield a known etiologically relevant metric of exposure, the metric of choice used in most epidemiological studies has been the time-weighted average field. In many cases this has been assessed at diagnosis or over a period of, for example, one year prior to diagnosis. Further, most studies have assessed the field present over the general volume of the subject's home, or specifically in the bedroom, and used this as an estimate of the subject's exposure. This approach neglects the contribution to exposure from local sources within the home (e.g. domestic electrical appliances) and from sources outside the home. Other studies used personal dosimeters to estimate exposure from all sources, for a time interval such as a week (e.g. McBride et al., 1999).

The assessment of average personal exposure by the surrogate of average field in the home is clearly an approximation. It is, however, likely to be a better approximation for younger children, who spend more time at home, than for older children, who spend time outside the home and may have significant appliance use, and for adults, who may have significant occupational exposure as well. It is the exposure of younger children which is most relevant for studies of childhood leukaemia. Concentration on the field in the bedroom probably improves the approximation because of the time spent there sleeping. Some studies have included partial assessments of exposure from appliances believed most likely to contribute to average exposure and from schools. Others have assessed previous years and previous residences in order to approximate lifetime exposure rather than exposure at diagnosis. However, all such attempts are inevitably imperfect, particularly exposure to appliances, which so far has been only examined one at a time leading to large misclassification. The pooled analysis of Ahlbom et al. (2000) removed such extra contributions, finding its elevated risk ratio just with the 24 or 48 hour average field in the home.

The calculated-field studies calculate the field in the home from just one source, the high-voltage power line, ignoring the other sources such as low-voltage wiring, which in homes not near high-voltage power lines would be the main source. This clearly introduces an extra element of misclassification, which may be even greater if the historical loads or other data used in the calculation are imperfect. The size of the misclassification depends, however, on the relative sizes of the fields included (power line) and not included (low-voltage wiring).

It is worth mentioning that epidemiologic data appear to be not only consistent, but also specific. For cancer, the observed association seems to be limited to leukaemia, and even more specifically to childhood leukaemia. Several explanations can be advanced to explain the lack of an association with adult leukaemia. One possibility is that exposure assessment methods used are much better in capturing exposure of children than that of adults: as mentioned, children spend more time at home and do not have occupational exposures. Another possibility is that children are more vulnerable to magnetic fields due to, for example, timing of exposure relevant to their development or predisposition due to an initiating event which occurred *in utero*.

*Other correlated magnetic field exposures*

The exposure most often used, implicitly or explicitly, in epidemiological studies, time-weighted average, is attractive for the pragmatic reason that it is probably the easiest to measure. However, it is also attractive because there is a class of biophysical mechanisms, those for which the effect produced is proportional to the magnitude of the field without regard to its direction, for which this indeed is the appropriate metric. Nonetheless, the metric of time-weighted average of the field has the major problem that the level of field at which an elevated risk appears, of the order of a microtesla or less, is well below the levels that can be regarded as plausible from biophysical arguments. Further, it is unlikely that any biophysical mechanism would produce an exactly linear effect over several orders of magnitude. It can also be argued that when the metric used is the average of a quantity (the field experienced by a person) which varies over, say, five orders of magnitude, it would be strange if any risk appeared in the comparatively narrow range between 0.1 and 0.3 or 0.4 $\mu$T.

The fact that the studies which have used time-weighted average field as a metric have found an elevated risk gives a particular status to this metric. Any other metric must, if it is to explain the observed association, be sufficiently correlated with time-weighted average, and the weaker the correlation, the stronger the risk with the "true" metric must be. Consideration of metrics and exposures raises a number of problems in interpretation of epidemiological studies. However, there is currently no alternative metric of exposure which is any more attractive, and the fact remains that the metric used so far, time weighted average, for all its problems, does seem to be associated with an elevated risk. Thus, the attributable fraction calculations given in the appendix are based on the arithmetic and geometric means of the time-weighted average field.

### 11.2.2 Adult cancer

Since the IARC (2002) review, several new studies have been published, many of which have focused on either residential or occupational exposures to ELF magnetic fields and breast cancer. This review updates the IARC evaluation by including studies published from 2001 (subsequent to the IARC monograph) through to January 2005 (for consistency studies published up to 2001 which were included in the IARC monograph are not reproduced here). The main focus is on breast cancer for which data in the previous review were considered inadequate for evaluation. Many of the issues of bias, confounding and other sources of error discussed in 11.2.1.4 in relation to studies of childhood leukaemia are also relevant to the interpretation of the studies of cancers in adults.

## 11.2.2.1 Breast cancer

### 11.2.2.1.1 Residential exposure

Table 73 lists the studies published since 2001 on residential exposure (including appliance use) to ELF electric and magnetic fields and adult cancers – seven of these studies concern breast cancer.

**Table 73. Residential studies of adult cancer by exposure category subsequent to IARC (2002)**

| Outcome | Exposure | | | | | |
|---|---|---|---|---|---|---|
| | Electric blanket | Other appliances | Proximity +/- wire codes | Calculated fields | Spot measurements | Combined occupational and residential |
| *Breast* | | | | | | |
| McElroy et al., 2001 | • | | | | | |
| Davis, Mirick & Stevens, 2002 | • | • | • | | • | |
| Kabat et al., 2003 | • | | | | | |
| Schoenfeld et al., 2003 | | | • | | • | |
| London et al., 2003 | | | • | | • | |
| Zhu et al., 2003 | • | • | | | | |
| Kliukiene, Tynes & Andersen, 2004 | | | | • | | • |
| *Acute myeloid leukaemia* | | | | | | |
| Oppenheimer & Preston-Martin, 2002 | • | • | | | | |
| *Hematological cancers* | | | | | | |
| Tynes & Haldorsen, 2003 | | | | • | | • |
| *Malignant melanoma* | | | | | | |
| Tynes, Klaeboe & Haldorsen, 2003 | | | | • | | • |
| *Brain cancer* | | | | | | |
| Kleinerman et al., 2005 | • | • | | | | |

The design and results of the studies of residential exposure and breast cancer discussed below are summarized in Table 74.

*General residential exposure*

Davis, Mirick & Stevens (2002) conducted a case-control study in the greater Seattle, Washington area. Eligible cases were Caucasian women aged 20 to 74 years selected from the local cancer registry, diagnosed between November 1992 and March 1995 and resident of King or Snohomish County (chosen to ensure representation of urban, suburban and rural areas). Controls were identified through random digit dialing, frequency matched to the cases by 5-year age group and county of residence. Response rate was 78% among cases and 75% among controls. Exposure to magnetic fields was estimated by both direct measurement and wire-code configuration. Continuous 48-hour measurements of magnetic field in the bedroom of each person's current residence were done using an EMDEX II meter set to record broadband (40–800 Hz) and harmonic (100–800 Hz) magnetic fields at 15-s intervals. Three variables based on broadband magnetic field measurements were constructed averaged over two nights: (1) mean nighttime (10 pm to 5 am) bedroom magnetic field; (2) proportion of nighttime bedroom magnetic field measurements $\geq 0.2$ µT; and (3) short-term variability in the nighttime bedroom magnetic field based on grouping of measurement data into 10-min intervals. The wire-coding scheme of Wertheimer and Leeper (1979) was used to classify the participant's current residence and all previous residences occupied for at least six consecutive months within the greater Seattle metropolitan area in the 5 and 10 years prior to diagnosis. Wire codes were ordered (1–5) according to their respective in-home nighttime mean magnetic field measurements using data from the controls. In addition a questionnaire gave data on use of electrical appliances in the home. The magnetic field analyses included 744 (of 813) cases and 711 (of 793) controls. Mean nighttime broadband magnetic field levels of less than 0.16 µT were observed with 90% of both cases and controls and 76% had no measurements above 0.20 µT (mean nighttime broadband magnetic fields were 0.080 µT for cases and 0.071 µT for controls). None of the metrics of mean nighttime magnetic field exposure was associated with breast cancer risk; for the highest quartile (=58%) of the percentage of magnetic field measurements $\geq 0.20$ µT (percentiles estimated among controls with at least one measurement $\geq 0.20$ µT), the adjusted odds ratio was 1.1 (95% CI: 0.7–1.8). For the mean nighttime bedroom broadband magnetic field treated as a continuous variable, the adjusted odds ratio per 0.1 µT was 1.04 (95% CI: 0.97–1.12). No associations were found after stratification by age, menopausal or estrogen receptor status. There was also no association with wire codes either from current configuration or a weighted score for wire codes at residences over the previous 5 or 10 years. For wire codes at home of diagnosis (or reference date for controls), the odds ratio for very high versus very low current configuration was 0.8 (95% CI: 0.5–1.3).

278

**Table 74. Epidemiological studies of residential exposures to magnetic fields and breast cancer and leukemia, published subsequent to IARC (2002)** [a]

| Study area, population | Exposure metrics | Exposure categories | OR (95% CI) | # cases | Comments | Reference |
|---|---|---|---|---|---|---|
| *Breast cancer* | | | | | | |
| King or Snohomish County, Seattle, WA, USA | 48-h measurements of 40–800 Hz magnetic fields in bedroom of current residence. | % Mean nighttime bedroom magnetic field > 0.20 µT | Adjusted | | Data not presented for mean nighttime bedroom magnetic field > 0.20 µT. 90% of cases and controls had mean nighttime broadband magnetic field levels < 0.16 µT; 76% had no measurements > 0.20 µT, limiting statistical power to detect effects at higher exposure levels. | Davis, Mirick & Stevens, 2002 |
| *Cases:* Caucasian women aged 20–74 y identified from cancer registry (Nov 1992 – March 1995). | | | | | | |
| 744 of 813 cases included. | Estimation of magnetic fields from maps and wire coding based on current residence and residences in past 10 y. | Ref.: 0% | | | | |
| *Controls:* obtained by random-digit dialling, frequency matched on age and county of residence. | | < 0.7 | 0.6 (0.4–1.0) | 25 | | |
| | | 0.7–8.9 | 1.2 (0.8–1.9) | 44 | | |
| 711 of 793 controls included. | | 8.9–58 | 1.1 (0.7–1.7) | 45 | | |
| | Electric appliance use from questionnaire. | ≥ 58 | 1.1 (0.7–1.8) | 42 | | |
| Los Angeles County, CA, USA | 7-d measurements of 40–800 Hz magnetic fields in bedroom of current residence. | Mean nighttime bedroom broadband magnetic field (µT) | Adjusted | | 91% of cases and 92 % of controls had mean nighttime broadband magnetic field levels less than 0.20 µT, limiting statistical power to detect effects at higher exposure levels. | London et al., 2003 |
| *Cases:* | | | | | | |
| Breast cancer cases from tumor registries (1993–1999), , nested within a cohort of African Americans, Latinas and Caucasians, aged 45–74 at recruitment, selected primarily licensed drivers. | Wiring configuration codes in homes occupied over the previous 10 y. | Ref.: < 0.1 | | | | |
| | | 0.10–0.19 | 1.3 (0.8–2.1) | 56 | | |
| | | 0.20–0.29 | 1.1 (0.4–2.8) | 11 | | |
| | Electric appliance use from questionnaire (not reported). | 0.30–0.39 | 2.1 (0.6–7.5) | 8 | | |
| 743 (of 751) cases with wire configuration codes and 347 with 7-d bedroom measurements. | | 0.40 | 1.2 (0.5–3.0) | 12 | | |
| *Controls:* Random selected by (frequency matched on ethnicity) from cohort members free of breast cancer at baseline. | | | | | | |

279

**Table 74. Continued**

699 (of 702) controls with wire codes and 286 with magnetic field measurements.

| Study | Methods | Exposure | Risk estimate (95% CI) | No. of cases | Comments | Reference |
|---|---|---|---|---|---|---|
| Long Island, NY, USA<br>*Cases:*<br>Selected from cases aged < 75 y in the Long Island Breast Cancer Study Project (LIBCSP) (663 approached, 576 participated), with residence in same property ≥ 15 y.<br>*Controls:* Selected from LIBCSP controls recruited by random digit dialling (< 65 y) or from Health Care Financing Administration files (≥ 65 y) (702 approached, 585 participated) | Spot and 24-h measurements of 40–800 Hz magnetic fields. Wiring maps used to classify homes according to modified method of Wertheimer and Leeper. Electric appliance use from questionnaire (reported in Kabat et al. (Kabat et al., 2003). | 24-h bedroom broadband magnetic field (µT)<br>Ref: < 0.041<br>0.041–0.081<br>0.082–0.171<br>≥ 0.172 | Adjusted<br><br>1.0 (0.7–1.4)<br>1.0 (0.7–1.4)<br>1.0 (0.7–1.4) | <br><br>148<br>140<br>139 | Data not presented for mean 24-h or spot magnetic field measurements > 0.20 µT. | Schoenfeld et al., 2003 |
| Norway<br>*Cases:*<br>All incident cancer cases (n=1830) from cancer registry (1980–96), from cohort aged ≥ 16 years living within corridor of 40 m (33 kV) to 300 m (420 kV) from power lines.<br>*Controls:*<br>Two controls per case from same cohort (n=3658). Matched on age and municipality. | Calculations of power line magnetic fields. Data on migration between municipalities (1967–85) and between and within municipalities (1986–96). Occupational exposure estimated from job-exposure matrix based on job title provided at decennial census. | Calculated TWA residential fields (5 most recent years) (µT)<br>Ref.: < 0.05<br><br>All ages<br>0.05–0.19<br>≥ 0.20<br><br>< 50 y<br>0.05–0.19<br>≥ 0.20<br>≥ 50 y<br>0.05–0.19 | <br><br><br><br>1.5 (1.1–1.8)<br>1.6 (1.3–2.0)<br><br><br><br>1.8 (1.1–2.8)<br>1.8 (1.2–2.8) | <br><br><br><br>121<br>158<br><br><br><br>37<br>56 | Numbers of cases ≥ 0.20 µT reported at all ages, < 50 y and ≥ 50 y do not tally. | Kliukiene, Tynes & Andersen, 2004 |

# Table 74. Continued

| | | | OR (95% CI) | Cases | | Reference |
|---|---|---|---|---|---|---|
| | | ≥ 0.20 | 1.3 (1.0–1.8) | 84 | | |
| | | ER+, all ages | | | | |
| | | 0.05–0.19 | 1.6 (1.2–2.0) | 112 | | |
| | | ≥ 0.20 | 1.2 (0.8–1.9) | 38 | | |
| | | | 1.6 (1.1–2.4) | 49 | | |

*Leukaemia*

| | | | OR (95% CI) | Cases | | Reference |
|---|---|---|---|---|---|---|
| Norway | See Kliukiene et al. (2004) above | Calculated TWA residential fields (10 most recent years) (µT) | | | Same cohort as Kliukiene et al. (2004) above. | Tynes & Haldorsen, 2003 |
| *Cases:* All incident cancer cases (n=295) from cancer registry (1980–96), from cohort of Norwegian population aged ≥ 16 y living within corridor of 40 m (33 kV) to 300 m (420 kV) from high-voltage power lines. | | Ref.: < 0.05 | | | | |
| | | All leukaemia | | | | |
| | | 0.05–0.19 | 1.6 (0.8–3.1) | 17 | | |
| | | ≥ 0.20 | 1.3 (0.7–2.5) | 19 | | |
| | | ALL: 0.05–0.19 | 1.0 (0.1–11.0) | 1 | | |
| *Controls:* Two controls per case from same cohort. Matched on age, gender and municipality | | ≥ 0.20 | 1.3 (0.2–8.0) | 3 | | |
| | | CLL: 0.05–0.19 | 4.2 (1.0–17.9) | 6 | | |
| | | ≥ 0.20 | 3.0 (0.9–10.0) | 7 | | |
| | | AML: 0.05–0.19 | 1.5 (0.4–5.0) | 5 | | |
| | | ≥ 0.20 | 2.2 (0.6–8.4) | 5 | | |
| | | CML: 0.05–0.19 | 2.4 (0.4–15.0) | 3 | | |
| | | ≥ 0.2 | 0.2 (0.0–2.0) | 1 | | |

[a] OR: odds ratio; CI: confidence interval; ER+: estrogen-receptor-positive; Ref.: reference group with exposure level indicated, ALL: acute lymphocytic leukaemia; CLL: chronic lymphocytic leukaemia; AML: acute myeloid leukaemia; CML: chronic myeloid leukaemia; TWA: time weighted average.

London et al. (2003) carried out a nested case-control study of residential exposure to magnetic fields among a cohort of African Americans, Latinas and Caucasians resident in Los Angeles County, aged 45–74 at recruitment, selected primarily from the file of licensed drivers. Incident breast cancer cases from 1993 to 1999 were ascertained by linkage to state tumour registries. Controls were frequency matched on ethnicity from cohort members free of breast cancer at baseline. Wiring configuration codes were derived according to the scheme of Wertheimer and Leeper (1979) in homes occupied at time of diagnosis (or reference date for controls) and over the previous 10 years. Seven-day measurements of magnetic fields in the bedroom were obtained using an EMDEX II meter, to include both broadband (40–800 Hz) and harmonic (100–800 Hz) magnetic fields sampled at 120-s intervals. The primary magnetic field measurement metric was the nighttime mean based on questionnaire response for each participant concerning usual times of going to bed, obtained separately for weekdays and weekends. Three variables based on magnetic field measurements (separately for broadband and harmonic fields) over nighttime hours for seven days were constructed: (1) mean nighttime bedroom magnetic field; (2) proportion of nighttime bedroom magnetic field measurements $\geq 0.4$ µT; and (3) short-term variability in the nighttime bedroom magnetic field. Wire configuration codes for address at diagnosis (cases) or reference date (controls) were available for 743 (of 751) cases and 699 (of 702) controls, and 7-day measurements of magnetic fields in the bedroom for 347 cases and 286 controls. Mean nighttime broadband magnetic field levels less than 0.20 µT were found with 91% of cases and 92% of controls, and 86% of both cases and controls had no measurements above 0.40 µT (mean nighttime broadband magnetic fields were 0.097 µT for cases and 0.099 µT for controls). None of the metrics of mean nighttime magnetic field exposure (broadband or harmonic fields) was associated with breast cancer risk; adjusted odds ratios compared with mean nighttime bedroom broadband exposure < 0.10 µT were 1.1 (95% CI: 0.43–2.8) for mean nighttime bedroom broadband exposure 0.20–0.29 µT (11 cases), 2.1 (95% CI: 0.58–7.5) for 0.30–0.39 µT (8 cases), and 1.2 (95% CI: 0.50–3.0) for mean nighttime bedroom broadband exposure $\geq 0.40$ µT. For mean nighttime bedroom broadband magnetic field treated as a continuous variable, adjusted odds ratio per 0.1 µT was 1.00 (95% CI: 0.94–1.07). No associations were found after stratification by age, menopausal or estrogen receptor status, or other potential effect modifiers. There was also no association with wire codes either from current configuration or a weighted score for wire codes at residences over the previous 10 years; for wire codes at home of diagnosis (reference), adjusted odds ratio for very high versus very low current configuration was 0.76 (95% CI: 0.49–1.18).

Schoenfeld et al. (2003) carried out a case-control study of EMF exposure (EBCLIS) within the Long Island Breast Cancer Study Project (LIBCSP) of women under 75 years at enrollment, identified between August 1996 and June 1997, who had lived in the same Long Island home for at least 15 years. Cases were selected from the 1354 LIBCSP cases (663 approached, 576 participated, response 87%). Controls were selected from 1426 LIBCSP controls (69% participation) who were recruited by random digit dialling (< 65 years) or from Health Care Financing Administration files (≥ 65 years) (702 approached, 585 participated, response 83%). Both spot (front door, bedroom and most lived-in room) and 24-hour measurements (bedroom and most lived-in room) were collected using EMDEX II meters programmed to record both broadband (40–800 Hz) and harmonic (100–800 Hz) magnetic fields sampled at 3-s intervals for the spot measurements and 15-s intervals for the 24-hour measurements. Ground-current magnetic field measurements were also obtained. Wiring maps were obtained and used to classify homes according to the modified method of Wertheimer and Leeper (Wertheimer & Leeper, 1979). Questionnaire data on electrical appliance use was reported in Kabat et al. (2003). Mean 24-hour broadband magnetic fields in the bedroom were 0.16 µT for cases and 0.14 µT for controls. None of the exposure metrics was associated with risk of breast cancer. For 24-hour measurements in the bedroom, adjusted odds ratio for highest quartile (≥ 0.172 µT) versus lowest quartile (< 0.041 µT) broadband magnetic field was 0.97 (95% CI: 0.69–1.4) and for the mean of the spot measurements it was 1.15 (95% CI: 0.82–1.6) (highest quartile ≥ 0.145 µT; lowest quartile < 0.034 µT). For estimated personal exposure ≥ 0.200 µT (based on mean 24-hour broadband measurements in bedroom and most lived-in room and test-load coefficient for most lived-in room) compared with < 0.039 µT, adjusted odds ratio was 1.08 (95% CI: 0.77–1.5). For the wire code configuration, adjusted odds ratio for very high current configuration compared with underground/very low current configuration was 0.90 (95% CI: 0.54–1.5).

Kliukiene, Tynes & Andersen (2004) carried out a nested case-control study of female breast cancer within a nationwide cohort in Norway. This comprised all women aged 16 or over who on November 1, 1980, or on January 1 of at least one of the years between 1986 and 1996 were living in a residence within a defined corridor near high-voltage power lines (corridor distances ranging from 40 m for 33 kV lines to 300 m for 420 kV lines). The cohort included around 5% of all women in Norway during 1980–1996; cases (n = 1830) with invasive breast cancer were identified for this period from the national cancer registry. Two controls per case (3658 in total) were selected randomly from the cohort according to the following criteria: born within 5 years of the case, free of breast cancer and alive at time of diagnosis, and from the same municipality as the case at entry into the cohort. Data on migration between municipalities (1967–1985) and between or within a municipality (1986–1996) were obtained. Exposure to magnetic fields from the high-voltage lines was estimated from 1967 based on residential address, utilising a computer program (Teslaw) developed at SINTEF Energy, Norway, taking account of height of the towers, distance between phases, ordering of phases, distance between power line and a house, and mean load on the power line during each year that a study participant lived in the house. Distances of houses from the power lines were checked on maps for the half of the corridor nearest the line. Time-weighted average residential exposure to magnetic fields from the lines was estimated, both from 1967 and for the last 5 years before diagnosis of a case. Occupational exposure was estimated – on a scale from 1 (< 4 h exposure at > 0.1 µT per week) to 3 (≥ 24 h exposure at > 0.1 µT per week) – based on a job-exposure matrix from information on job title provided at decennial census, for the period January 1, 1955 (based on 1960 census) until date of diagnosis (assuming working age 18–67 years). A cumulative category x years occupational exposure measure was then calculated. For combined residential and occupational exposure (based on 1296 cases and 2597 controls with available data), women were considered exposed if time weighted average residential exposure = 0.05 µT and occupational exposure > 30 category-years. For residential exposure in most recent 5 years, odds ratio (all ages) for time weighted average exposure ≥ 0.20 µT compared with < 0.05 µT was 1.6 (95% CI: 1.3–2.0); odds ratio at < 50 years was 1.8 (95% CI: 1.2–2.8) and at 50 years 1.6 (95% CI: 1.2–2.0). Odds ratios for time weighted average exposure of 0.05–0.19 µT were similar to those for ≥ 0.20 µT (Table 74). For ≥ 0.20 µT, odds ratio for the total period (all ages) was 1.4 (95% CI: 1.0–1.8). For women with highest estimated occupational exposure compared with the lowest, odds ratio (all ages) was 1.1 (95% CI: 0.9–1.4). For combined residential and occupational exposure, odds ratio (all ages) was 1.3 (95% CI: 0.8–2.1) based on 26 cases. There was no statistically significant increase when residential and occupational exposures were considered together, but numbers were small. [No measurements of magnetic fields were undertaken for persons included in the study. Occupational data were available for 71% of cases and controls. There was only limited control for confounding: age at birth of first child, education, type of residence.]

*Use of electric blankets*

Studies of electric blanket use and breast cancer are summarized in Table 75. McElroy et al. (2001) reported a case-control study of female residents of Wisconsin, Massachusetts (excluding residential Boston) and New Hampshire, aged 50–79. Cases with a new diagnosis of breast cancer reported between January 1992 and December 1994 were eligible. Data for 5685 (83%) cases were available. Controls in each state were randomly selected from two sampling frames: women aged 50–64 years were selected from lists of licensed drivers; those 65–74 years from a roster of Medicare beneficiaries; 5951 (78%) completed the study interview. The analysis was limited to 1949 cases and 2498 controls with available data who were interviewed between June 1994 and July 1995, when data on electric blanket or mattress cover use was elicited by telephone interview. The adjusted odds ratio for ever-users compared with never-users was 0.93 (95% CI: 0.82–1.1). For electric blanket or mattress cover use considered as a continuous variable, adjusted odds ratio per 12 months of use was 1.0 (95% CI: 0.98–1.0). [Although results are not separately presented by menopausal status, 93% of cases and controls were postmenopausal.]

The case-control study of residential exposure to ELF magnetic fields by Davis, Mirick & Stevens (2002) discussed above and summarized in Table 74, included questionnaire data on use of an electric bed-warming device. For ever versus never use, the adjusted odds ratio was 1.1 (95% CI: 0.8–1.3). For hours of use included as a continuous variable, the adjusted odds ratio was 1.0 (95% CI: 1.0–1.0).

The Long Island Breast Cancer Study Project (LIBCSP) discussed above (Schoenfeld et al., 2003) also included information on electric blanket use; more detailed information on electric blanket use was included in the case-control study of EMF exposure (EBCLIS) within LIBCSP (Schoenfeld et al., 2003, summarized in Table 74) (Kabat et al., 2003). The results for LIBCSP and EBCLIS are presented separately, stratified by menopausal status; data for 1324 (out of 1354) LIBCSP cases and 1363 (out of 1426) LIBCSP controls, and 566 (out of 576) EBCLIS cases and 557 (out of 585) EBCLIS controls are included. Adjusted odds ratios for ever versus never use for pre/post menopausal women were 1.2 (95% CI: 0.9–1.6) and 1.0 (95% CI: 0.8–1.3), respectively, for LIBCSP, and 1.1 (95% CI: 0.6–1.9) and 0.9 (95% CI: 0.7–1.3), respectively, for EBCLIS. The EBCLIS study also provided data on estrogen (ER) and progesterone receptor (PR) status. For ER+/PR+, adjusted odds ratio for ever versus never use was 1.2 (95% CI: 0.9–1.5) based on 125 cases. [The EBCLIS cases are a subset of the LIBCSP cases, therefore the results are not independent of each other.]

Zhu et al. (2003) report a case-control study among African-American women aged 20–64 living in one of three Tennessee counties, with telephone service at time of the study; 304 cases (of 670 eligible women, 45%) with first histological diagnosis of breast cancer during 1995–98, identified through the Tennessee Cancer reporting system, were included. Controls were selected through random digit dialling, frequency matched to cases by 5-year age range and county; 305 women (73% of eligible women identified) were included. Information on use of electric bedding devices was obtained by telephone interview. For ever versus never use, adjusted odds ratio was 1.4 (95% CI. 0.9–2.2), and it was 1.4 (95% CI: 0.6–3.4) and 1.2 (95% CI: 0.6–2.1) for pre/post-menopausal women respectively. [Participation rate among cases was low (45%), mainly reflecting lack of physician consent. 205/304 (67%) cases and 213/305 (70%) controls provided data on use of electrical bedding devices. Overall data on only 30% of eligible cases and 51% of eligible controls was included, limiting the interpretation of the study.]

**Table 75.** Studies of use of electric blankets and risk of breast cancer in women, published subsequent to IARC (2002) [a]

| Subjects | # cases/ controls | Ever use [b] | | Use through the night [c] | | Long-term use [d] | | Authors |
|---|---|---|---|---|---|---|---|---|
| | | OR (95% CI) | # cases | OR (95% CI) | # cases | OR (95% CI) | # cases | |
| Mostly post-menopausal | 1949/ 2498 | 0.93 (0.82-1.1) | 834 | NR | NR | 0.98 (0.80–1.2) | 248 | McElroy et al., 2001 |
| Pre- and postmeno-pausal | 720/ 725 | 1.1 (0.8–1.3) | 302 | NR | NR | NR | NR | Davis, Mirick & Stevens, 2002 |
| LIBCSP: Premeno-pausal | 472/ 503 | 1.2 (0.9–1.6) | 171 | NR | NR | 1.4 (0.7–2.6) | 25 | Kabat et al., 2003 |
| Postmeno-pausal | 852/ 860 | 1.0 (0.8-1.3) | 279 | NR | NR | 0.8 (0.5–1.3) | 36 | |
| EBCLIS: Premeno-pausal | 146/ 131 | 1.1 (0.6–1.9) | 58 | 1.3 (0.6–2.6) | 32 | 1.1 (0.3–3.5) | 11 | |
| Postmeno-pausal | 420/ 426 | 0.9 (0.7–1.3) | 149 | 1.0 (0.7–1.5) | 78 | 0.9 (0.5–1.7) | 23 | |
| Pre- and postmeno-pausal | 205/ 213 | 1.4 (0.9–2.2) | 73 | 1.7 (1.0–3.0) | 56 | 4.9 (1.5–15.6) | 16 | Zhu et al., 2003 |

[a] OR: odds ratio; CI: confidence interval; NR: not reported.

[b] Defined as ever use by McElroy, Kabat and Zhu; any use during the last 10 years by Davis.

[c] Defined as use through the night by Kabat; on most of the time by Zhu.

[d] Defined as use for ≥ 5 years by McElroy; longer than 10 years for premenopausal women and 15 years for postmenopausal women by Kabat; longer than 10 years by Zhu.

11.2.2.1.2  Occupational exposure

*Cohort studies*

Pollan, Gustavsson & Floderus (2001) reported on risk of male breast cancer from an extended follow-up (to 1989) among the national

Swedish cohort study of workers, which previously had been followed up to 1984 (Floderus, Stenlund & Persson, 1999). The base population comprised 1 779 646 men aged 25–59 in 1971, who were gainfully employed at the 1970 census and who were also recorded at the 1960 census, followed through end 1989 (31 668 842 person-years). Follow up was through the national cancer registry; 250 cases of breast cancer were reported in the cohort. Occupations classified as "Services and military work" had a significant excess risk; within-cohort RR for this group was 1.8 (95% CI: 1.2–2.8). Among production workers, significant excess risks were found for "Other metal processing workers", RR = 5.3 (95% CI: 1.3–21) based on 2 cases and for "Machinery repairers", RR = 2.1 (95% CI: 1.2–3.6) based on 14 cases. Exposures to ELF magnetic fields were assessed by linking occupations to a job-exposure matrix covering the 100 most common occupations among Swedish men; for these occupations, exposure levels had been estimated based on at least four full-shift measurements. Ten further comparatively rare occupations with "definitely high" exposures but less than four measurements were added. Five exposure groups were identified based on the geometric mean of work-day mean values for an occupational group, with cut-offs at 25th, 50th, 75th and 90th centile points: $\geq 0.12$ µT (reference group), 0.12–0.16 µT, 0.16–0.22 µT, 0.22–0.30 µT, > 0.30 µT. [Inclusion of only the 100 most common occupations for the analysis by exposure categories – with addition of 10 other occupations with "definitely high" exposures – reduced the person-years by 16%, though the number of men included in these analyses is not given.] Two hundred three cases were included in the analyses. Compared with the reference group, relative risks were 1.4 (95% CI: 0.95–2.0), 1.3 (95% CI: 0.82–1.9), 1.6 (95% CI: 1.0–2.6) and 0.92 (95% CI: 0.53–1.6) respectively. [Relative risk estimates are adjusted only for age, period and "geographical area" – counties were grouped into five classes based on their Standardised Incidence Ratio. There may be some overlap with the cases included in Håkansson et al. (2002), below, for the years 1985–89.]

Håkansson et al. (2002) reported a cohort study of cancer incidence among workers in industries using resistance welding in Sweden. All companies and workplaces where resistance welding might take place were identified for the years 1985–94; all workers ever employed at these workplaces during that period were then identified from tax returns. Information on occupation was obtained from censuses of 1980, 1985 and 1990 and from tax returns; resistance welders thus identified were assigned to the highest exposure category. Where someone changed job, the job with the highest exposure category was used; if information was missing for a particular census, that from the previous census was used. A job exposure matrix supplemented by additional information for some rare occupations and for women, was used to classify jobs into "Low" (< 0.164 µT), "Medium" (0.164–0.250 µT), "High" (0.250–0.530 µT) and "Very High" (> 0.530 µT) exposure to ELF magnetic fields based on the geometric mean of average workday mean values, with cutoffs based on 25th, 75th and 90th centile values. Seventy-five percent of people assigned to the "Very High" exposure category were

287

resistance welders. After exclusion of people without information on occupation or where exposure could not be estimated, data for 646 694 individuals (484 643 men and 162 051 women) were included. Cancer incidence cases from 1985–94 were obtained from the national cancer registry and mortality data from the national deaths registry. Within-cohort relative risk estimates were estimated using Cox regression with the "Low" exposure category as reference. There was no excess risk of breast cancer among women; in the "Very High" exposure category, relative risk (37 cases) was 1.1 (95% CI: 0.8–1.5). For men, numbers were small; relative risk in the "Very High" exposure category was 3.8 (95% CI: 0.3–43.5) based on 2 cases. [Classification into exposure categories was mainly on the basis of a job exposure matrix; details of the basis of measurement of workday values of average exposure to ELF magnetic fields are not provided. The results are unadjusted for potential occupational confounders other than inclusion of one dichotomous variable: blue collar workers vs. others.]

Kliukiene, Tynes & Andersen (2003) reported a follow up of breast cancer cases among Norwegian female radio and telegraph operators, based on the cohort reported in Tynes et al. (1996). These authors reported follow up of the cohort from 1961 to the end of 1991; Kliukiene, Tynes & Andersen (2003) extend the follow up to end May 2002. [The report of Tynes et al. (1996) was not included in the IARC (2002) monograph, presumably because the main focus is RF exposure rather than exposure to ELF magnetic fields. However, for completeness, Kliukiene, Tynes & Andersen (2003) is shown in Table 76, as spot measurements of ELF magnetic fields were obtained.] The cohort comprises 2619 women certified as radio and telegraph operators between 1960 and 1980 (98% of whom worked on Norwegian merchant ships). Spot measurements of ELF magnetic fields were made on two ships, when the transmitter was active and when it was shut down – they ranged from < 0.02 µT to about 6 µT, depending on the position occupied by the radio operator and whether or not the transmitter was active; normal exposure of the body was stated as about 0.1–0.2 µT (Tynes et al., 1996). Breast cancer cases were identified through the national cancer registry. There were 99 incident cases of breast cancer. Standardised Incidence Ratio (SIR) was calculated with reference to the Norwegian female population; SIR was 1.3 (95% CI: 1.1–1.6). Similar risks were observed for women < 50 years (44 cases) and ≥ 50 years (55 cases). A nested case-control study based on the same cohort is also reported in Kliukiene, Tynes & Andersen (2003), though as the focus is presumed exposure mainly to RF, results are not reported here. [Tynes et al. (1996) note that "ELF magnetic field levels at the operator's desk were comparable to those in normal working places in Norway, and the background level in the radio room was comparable to levels measured in Norwegian homes".]

*Case-control studies*

Band et al. (2000) report results of a case-control study in Canada focused generally on occupational risks of breast cancer, without a specific focus on ELF magnetic fields. However, they do report risks for occupations

288

with presumed exposure to ELF magnetic fields. [Although published in 2000, this study was not included in the IARC monograph (2002); for completeness, it is included here.] Cases, identified through the British Columbia cancer registry, were women aged < 75 years with breast cancer diagnosed between June 1, 1988 and June 30, 1989. Controls, matched by 5-year age groups, were selected randomly from the electoral roll. Information on job history and various potential confounders was obtained by questionnaire. The study included 1018 women with breast cancer (318 pre-menopausal, 700 post-menopausal) from a total of 1489 cases (68.4%), and 1025 out of 1502 (68.2%) controls; after exclusion of cases and controls with no matches or missing data there were 995 cases and 1020 controls. An excess of breast cancer was observed among electronic data-processing equipment operators; the odds ratio among all women (pre-and post-menopausal combined) was 3.1 (95% CI: 1.6–5.8) based on 24 cases. [As noted, there was no particular focus on ELF magnetic fields and no attempt was made to classify occupations by potential exposure to ELF magnetic fields.]

In a report from the Carolina Breast Cancer Study in the USA, Van Wijngaarden et al. (2001a) give results of a case-control study of occupational exposures to magnetic fields. Cases aged 20–74 years were identified through the North Carolina cancer registry, diagnosed from May 1, 1993 to September 30, 1995, and then stratified sampling was done to obtain equal numbers among younger and older black women and younger and older non-black women. Controls were sampled from lists of motor vehicle license holders (to age 65) and health care financing (above 65 years), frequency matched by race and five-year age group. Overall, response rates were 74.4% among cases and 52.8% among controls (Moorman et al., 1999); the report of Van Wijngaarden et al. (2001a) is based on 843 (of 861) cases and 773 (of 790) controls with adequate information on job history and duration. Occupational exposure to magnetic fields was estimated from the time-weighted average in six broad occupational groups and a homemaker category, based on 217 measurements done for a sample of 202 participants, using a personal average magnetic field exposure meter (AMEX 3-D). Individual exposure assignment was based on the longest and (where available) second-longest held occupation, the numbers of years worked and (where available) hours per work-week, to yield estimated µT-years of occupational exposure. Overall, risks of breast cancer by estimated cumulative exposure to magnetic fields (in comparison with 0–0.59 µT-years as reference) were > 0.59–0.90 µT-years (207 cases): OR = 1.4 (95% CI: 1.1–1.8); > 0.90–1.27 µT-years (143 cases): OR = 1.1 (95% CI: 0.8–1.5); > 1.27–2.43 µT-years (140 cases): OR = 1.0 (95% CI: 0.8–1.4); >2.43 µT-years (79 cases): OR = 1.2 (95% CI: 0.8–1.7). The risk estimates mostly showed a similar pattern by latency of exposure, whether pre- or post-menopausal and by estrogen receptor (ER) status (either ER positive or ER negative), although generally higher risks were found for pre-menopausal women, ER+, with latency > 10–20 years (in comparison with zero occupational exposure as reference): > 0–0.16 µT-years (38 cases): OR = 2.0 (95% CI: 1.1–3.9); > 0.16–0.40 µT-years (73 cases): OR = 2.0 (95% CI: 1.1–3.6); > 0.40–0.52 µT-years (28 cases): OR =

1.6 (95% CI: 0.8–3.2); > 0.52 T-years (38 cases): OR = 2.1 (95% CI: 1.1–4.0).

Labreche et al. (2003) report results of a case-control study of occupational exposure to electromagnetic fields and female breast cancer in Montreal, Canada. Cases ages 50–75 at diagnosis were identified from records of pathology departments and cancer registries from the 18 major hospitals in the greater Montreal area that treat breast cancer, between 1996 and 1997. Controls were selected from the same hospitals over the same period, with 32 different types of cancer (excluding inter alia brain and central nervous system, and leukaemia). Details on all occupations held over the working lifetime were obtained by interview. Duration of exposure to ELF magnetic fields in hours per working day was assigned by hygienists based on a four-category scale: "no exposure" (< 0.2 µT); "low exposure" (0.2–< 0.5 µT); "medium exposure" (≥ 0.5–< 1.0 µT); and "high exposure" (≥ 1.0–10 µT). Response rates were 81.1% for cases and 75.7% for controls; the report of Labreche et al. (2003) focuses on 556 (of 608) postmenopausal cases and 600 (of 667) controls. Combining time spent at "medium" and "high" exposures, across the interquartile range of exposures (6000 hours), for any period of lifetime working, the OR (adjusted for a range of potential confounders) was 1.1 (95% CI: 0.9–1.4); for a lag period of 10 years before diagnosis, the OR was 1.2 (95% CI: 1.0–1.5); and for exposures before age 35 years, the OR was 1.4 (95% CI: 1.0–2.0). The OR were around 10% larger with additional adjustment for working in the textile industry. For sub-analysis by receptor status, for exposures before age 35 years, OR were 1.6 (95% CI: 1.0–2.4) and 0.8 (95% CI: 0.4–1.5) for progesterone receptor positive (PR+) and negative (PR-) tumours respectively, and 1.5 (95% CI: 1.0–2.3) and 0.8 (95% CI: 0.3–2.1) for estrogen receptor positive (ER+) and negative (ER-) tumours respectively. [Exposure assessment was relatively crude based on job title with four classes of exposure, not supported by measurements.]

In other studies (not shown in the tables) Koc & Polat (2001) report a case series of 11 male patients with breast cancer (of a total of 196 breast cancer cases (5%)), admitted to a regional hospital in eastern Turkey from 1990–2000, four of whom worked for the Turkish Institution of Electricity. These four cases were stated to be among 13 male breast cancer cases in the records of the Turkish Institution of Electricity from 1996 to 2000; estimated male breast cancer rate among these workers was stated as 0.3%. [The report is anecdotal and no case verification data, information on possible exposures to ELF electromagnetic fields, nor data on denominators are given. However, rates for male breast cancer and among electrical workers in eastern Turkey seem very high.] Gardner et al. (2002) reported results from the Shanghai Breast Cancer Study in China, a case-control study of female breast cancer among 1458 cases and 1556 age-matched population controls, focussing on occupational risks. Although electrical occupations were not combined in the tables, it was noted that there was no increase in risk among electrical workers. In a case-control study of 1642 women with breast cancer (1494 population-controls) at ages 20–44 years in the USA, Teitelbaum et al. (2003) report breast cancer risks by occupation. Although there was no specific focus on exposure to electromagnetic fields, no significant excess risks were reported among occupations thought to have potential exposure to electromagnetic fields.

A recent study of Forssén et al. (2005) included 20 400 cases of female breast cancer (identified through the regional cancer registry) and 116 227 controls from women gainfully employed in Stockholm or Gotland County in Sweden between 1976 and 1999. Exposure assessment was based on information about occupation obtained from the population censuses from 1960 to 1990. Information about magnetic field exposure was obtained from a job-exposure matrix derived from an electromagnetic field measurement programme performed in Stockholm County between March 2001 and October 2002. It included 49 of the most common occupations among women in Stockholm County (around 85% of the gainfully employed women in 1980 census). Measurements were made using an Emdex Lite personal monitor, carried on a belt for 24 hours; volunteers also completed a diary from which exposures at work could be estimated. Between five and 24 participants were measured in each occupation category. Exposure was estimated as the geometric mean of the time weighted average. At all ages, compared with reference (< 0.10 μT), the OR (adjusted for age, socio-economic status and year of diagnosis) was 1.0 (95% CI: 1.0–1.1) (11 369 cases) for 0.10–0.19 μT; 1.0 (95% CI: 0.9–1.1) (3243 cases) for 0.20–0.29 μT; and 1.0 (95% CI: 0.9–1.1) (814 cases) for ≥ 0.30 μT. Adjusted odds ratios were similar (all non-significant) at < 50 and ≥ 50 years, and for estrogen receptor positive and negative cases. Whereas earlier studies reported some positive results, this study was largely negative and was larger, had a better exposure matrix (based on measurements collected from women) and had more data available for female occupations than the earlier studies. [Some overlap of cases is likely with Floderus, Stenlund & Persson (1999) and possibly with Forssén et al. (2000).]

### 11.2.2.2 Leukaemia and brain cancer

#### 11.2.2.2.1 Residential exposure

One residential study of haematological cancers, one study of electric blanket use and acute myeloid leukaemia, and one study of electric appliance use and brain cancer have been published since the IARC (2002) review (Table 73). Tynes & Haldorsen (2003; see Table 74) report results of risk of haematological cancers (leukaemia, lymphoma and multiple myeloma) with proximity to a high voltage power line, based on a nested case-control study from the Norwegian national cohort. This cohort was described above with respect to female breast cancer (Kliukiene, Tynes & Andersen, 2004; see Table 74), though in Tynes & Haldorsen (2003) both men and women were included. For exposure to magnetic fields during the last 10 years before diagnosis, odds ratio for time weighted average exposure 0.05–0.19 μT (compared with < 0.05 μT) was 1.6 (95% CI: 0.8–3.1) (17 cases), and for ≥ 0.20 μT it was 1.3 (95% CI: 0.7–2.5) (19 cases). For chronic lymphocytic leukaemia, there was borderline significant excess risk at 0.05–0.19 μT, OR

= 4.2 (95% CI: 1.0–17.9) (6 cases); none of the other leukaemia sub-types had significant excess (based on small numbers). For all leukaemias over all years, the OR were 1.3 (95% CI: 0.7–2.5) (18 cases) for 0.05–0.19 µT, and 1.5 (95% CI: 0.8–3.0) (15 cases) for ≥ 0.20 µT. There was no association found with occupational exposure to magnetic fields. [Limitations of the study are noted with respect to Kliukiene, Tynes & Andersen (2004) above.]

Electric blanket and electric appliance use

Oppenheimer & Preston-Martin (2002) reported results of a case-control study of acute myeloid leukaemia and electric blanket use in Los Angeles County, USA. Four hundred twelve cases (of 726 eligible, 57%) ages 30–69 years at diagnosis were identified from the local cancer registry between January 1987 and June 1994, together with neighbourhood controls (matched on birth year ± 5 years, race and gender, 55% response rate). Information on electric blanket use, use of electric waterbeds and occupation was obtained by interview of cases (or proxy respondent, 49% of cases) and controls. The OR for use of an electric blanket regularly was 0.8 (95% CI: 0.6–1.1) and it was 0.9 (95% CI: 0.7–1.2) for use of electric blanket or electrically heated waterbed regularly. [Response rates for both cases and controls were around 55%. 252 of 412 (61%) cases reported less than one year total use of electric blankets. There were proxy respondent in 49% of cases.]

Kleinerman et al. (2005) report the results of a case-control study of brain cancer and acoustic neuroma with respect to use of 14 electrical appliances. Cases (n = 782, 92% of eligible) and hospital controls (n = 799, 86% of eligible) were recruited from 1994–98 from hospitals serving as regional referral centres for the diagnosis and treatment of brain tumours, in three areas in the USA: Boston, Massachusetts; Phoenix, Arizona and Pittsburgh, Pennsylvania. Controls were selected from patients admitted to the same hospitals for a variety of conditions including injuries and non-malignant diseases. Information on residential exposure to electrical appliances was obtained by self-administered questionnaire (completion of questionnaire was aided where necessary). Response rates for the questionnaire were 86.7 % for cases (n = 678) and 85.9% for controls (n = 686), yielding overall response rates of 79.8% for cases and 73.9% for controls. For any use of hair dryers (at least three times throughout life), significantly raised odds ratios (adjusted for age, gender, income, education, race, centre, distance from centre, date of interview and help completing the questionnaire) were found for glioma among males and females combined (OR = 1.7, 95% CI: 1.1–2.5) and among males (OR = 1.7, 95% CI: 1.1–2.7). There was also a significant excess of meningioma associated with "ever" use of an electric shaver among males (OR = 10.9, 95% CI: 2.3–50), based on two non-exposed and 35 exposed cases. There were no significant findings for "ever" use of 12 other appliances, for glioma, meningioma and acoustic neuroma. Odds ratios for meningioma associated with use of an electric shaver among males were higher with increasing duration of use: compared with never users, OR were 3.9 (95% CI: 0.6–26) (1–8 years, 4 cases), 15.6 (95% CI: 2.8–85) (9–28 years, 12 cases) and 16.3 (95% CI: 3.0–89) (≥ 29 years, 15 cases).

Cohort studies

Two cohort studies giving results on leukaemia and brain cancer were published since 2001 subsequent to the IARC (2002) monograph, as well as two further studies giving results on brain cancer. In the study by Håkansson et al. (2002) described in the section on breast cancer, above (Table 76), there was no excess leukaemia risk among men; among women, numbers were small (relative risk in the "Very High" exposure category was 1.8 (95% CI: 0.4–8.5) based on 2 cases). There was no excess risk of cancers of the nervous system among men, though in men < 30 years, there was excess risk of astrocytoma grades I-II in the "High" (RR = 10, 95% CI: 1.2–83.3) and "Very High" (RR = 9.8, 95% CI: 1.1–86.2) exposure categories. For women, relative risk of nervous system tumours in the "Very High" category was 1.9 (95% CI: 0.9–3.9); for all astrocytomas, there was a significant linear trend of increasing risk across exposure categories (p = 0.004); relative risk in the "Very High" exposure category was 3.0 (95% CI: 1.1–8.6) based on 5 cases.

A retrospective cohort mortality study of personnel working in 500 kV and 750 kV power installations was carried out for the period from 1970 to 1992. The cohort consisted of 1532 cohort subjects, who contributed 24 000 person-years. At the end of the observation period, 1319 persons were alive, 141 died, and 72 were lost from the follow-up. Cause-specific standardized mortality rates (SMR) of the general population were used for the comparison. The overall SMR (reflecting all causes of death) was not elevated (SMR = 0.61). The study did not reveal any excess of either all cancers or of cardiovascular diseases, with SMRs of 0.89 and 0.54, respectively. This data have been interpreted as "a healthy worker effect" (Gurvich et al., 1999). The standardized relative mortality risk ratio (SRR) resulting from of all types of cancer was low (SRR = 0.80; 95% CI: 0.57–1.09), as it was for accidents, traumas and poisonings (SRR = 0.67; 95% CI: 0.46–0.93), and suicides (SRR = 0.45; 95% CI: 0.16–0,98). The SRRs of death from leukaemia in men (SRR = 2.03; 95% CI: 0.23–7.31) and of death from brain cancer (SRR = 1.3; 95% CI: 0.64–3.7) were non-significantly increased (Rubtsova, Tikhonova & Gurvich, 1999). These studies were published in Russian and not included in the IARC (2002) review.

Van Wijngaarden et al. (2001b) report a re-analysis of mortality among electrical utility workers in the USA, based on the cohort among five companies reported by Savitz & Loomis (1995) (not shown in Table 76; see Table 29 in IARC (IARC, 2002). For leukaemia, the previously reported association between experience as an electrician and leukaemia was no longer observed (RR = 1.2, 95% CI: 0.7–2.1, based on 15 cases). [The reported results are not directly comparable, as Savitz & Loomis (1995) give results stratified by duration of employment, whereas Van Wijngaarden et al. (2001b) give overall results only, allowing for two year lag]. Compared with the original report, occupations with presumed minimal exposure to any hazardous occupational agents were included in the referent group, whereas previously, the referent group consisted of occupations with minimal exposure to magnetic fields only. This resulted, for example, in auto mechanics, heavy vehicle operators, material handlers and labourers being excluded from the referent group in Van Wijngaarden et al. (2001b), while technical workers, craft supervisors and service workers, who were considered exposed in the previous analysis, were included in the referent group in Van Wijngaarden et al. (2001b). For brain cancer, an excess was still observed among electricians in the revised analysis (RR = 1.7, 95% CI: 1.0–3.0, based on 17 cases).

Navas-Acien et al. (2002) give findings for incidence of brain cancer of an extended follow-up (to 1989) among the national Swedish cohort study of male workers, which previously had been followed up to 1984 (Floderus, Stenlund & Persson, 1999), and is described above with respect to male breast cancer (Pollan, Gustavsson & Floderus, 2001). Exposure to ELF magnetic fields was assessed by linking occupations to a job-exposure matrix covering the 100 most common occupations among Swedish men; for these occupations, exposure levels had been estimated based on at least four full-shift measurements. Ten further comparatively rare occupations with "definitely high" exposures but less than four measurements were added. Four exposure groups were identified based on the geometric mean of workday mean values for an occupational group, with lowest cut-off at $33^{rd}$ centile point and highest at the $90^{th}$ centile point. Navas-Acien et al. (2002) include 1 516 552 men ages 25–64 years; 2859 gliomas and 993 meningiomas were reported in the study cohort. For gliomas, compared with exposures < 0.13 µT the OR at 0.13–0.20 µT was 1.1 (95% CI: 1.0–1.2); at 0.20–0.30 µT, the OR was 1.1 (95% CI: 1.0–1.3); and at > 0.30 µT, the OR was 1.1 (95% CI: 0.9–1.2). There was no association with risk of meningioma (data not given). [This is the same base population and same period of follow-up as described above in Pollan, Gustavsson & Floderus (2001) though numbers in the cohort differ between the two reports.]

Wesseling et al. (2002) give results of a national cohort study of Finnish women born from 1906 to 1945, who reported an occupation in the 1970 census. Findings are reported for incidence of cancer of the brain and nervous system, 1971 to 1995, based on linkage to the national cancer registry (80% with histological diagnosis). Occupations were coded according to the longest held during the year. Women from the two highest social classes and farmers were excluded, giving a base population of 413 877 women, with 693 incident brain and nervous system cancers over the follow-up period. Expected numbers were based on incidence rates of the economically active female population, stratified by 5-year birth cohort, follow-up period and social class (lower two social classes only) to yield standardized incidence ratios (SIR). Occupational exposure to ELF magnetic fields was assessed using a job-exposure matrix designed by a team of exposure-assessment experts, based on job title for occupations held from 1960 to 1984 (to allow for latency), categorised as "unexposed", "low" or "medium/high" exposure. The classification was based on a cut-point of 0.8 µT, judged to be the "median of the intensity distribution of job titles with non-zero intensity".

294

For "low" exposure (≥ 0.8 μT), SIR (adjusted for year of birth, period of diagnosis and job turnover rate) was 1.1 (95% CI: 0.9–1.2); for "medium/high" exposure (> 0.8 μT) the SIR was 1.4 (95% CI: 0.9–2.1). [The exposure assessment was based on job title only, not supported by measurements. Subtypes of brain and nervous system tumours were not analysed.]

Case-control studies

Four case-control studies have reported on occupation and leukaemia risk and four on risk of brain cancer since the IARC (2002) monograph. Five of these studies (four for leukaemia and one for brain cancer) are included in Table 77. Bethwaite et al. (2001) report a case-control study of acute leukaemia among electrical workers in New Zealand. Cases ages 20–75 years at diagnosis were identified from six tertiary referral centres in New Zealand between January 1, 1989 and April 30, 1991, covering 92% of cases notified to the national cancer registry. Controls were selected at random from population registers of the catchment areas of the participating hospitals. Information on occupational history was obtained by telephone questionnaire or from next-of-kin (21 cases); exposure to ELF magnetic fields was assigned from a job-exposure matrix based on previous field measurements (using EMDEX meters) obtained from workers during their entire shifts for different occupational tasks, in an unspecified number of Los Angeles, Seattle and New Zealand workplaces. A "task-weighted" exposure estimate was then calculated based on current job tasks, and based on "historical" job tasks estimated for 15–20 years previously. Overall 100 cases and 199 controls were included with response rates of 86% and 78%, respectively. Any electrical work was associated with an OR of 1.9 (95% CI: 1.0–3.8) based on 26 cases, adjusted for age, education and gender. Among the electrical occupations, telephone line workers had adjusted OR of 5.8 (95% CI: 1.2–28) (6 cases) and welders/flame cutters an adjusted OR of 2.8 (95% CI: 1.2–6.8) (14 cases). Based on the job-exposure matrix for historical exposures, compared with < 0.21 μT (Reference): for 0.21–0.50 μT, adjusted OR was 0.5 (95% CI: 0.1–2.4) (2 cases); for 0.50–1.0 μT, OR was 2.9 (95% CI: 0.7–11.4) (5 cases); and for > 1.0 μT, OR was 3.2 (95% CI: 1.2–8.3) (15 cases) (p-value for trend = 0.002). For current exposures: for 0.21–0.50 μT, adjusted OR was 0.6 (95% CI: 0.2–2.3) (3 cases); for 0.50–1.0 μT, OR was 1.5 (95% CI: 0.2–14.6) (1 case); and for > 1.0 μT, OR was 4.0 (95% CI: 1.6–9.8) (18 cases) (p-value for trend < 0.001). For leukaemia sub-types, a significant trend was apparent only for acute non-lymphoblastic leukaemia. [The job-exposure matrix depended on measurements obtained from a previous study in the USA as well as New Zealand.]

**Table 76. Cohort studies of breast cancer, leukaemia and brain cancer in occupational groups with assumed or documented exposure to ELF magnetic fields, published subsequent to IARC (2002)**

| Study area, population | Exposure metrics | Exposure categories | # cases | RR (95% CI) [a] | Comments | Authors |
|---|---|---|---|---|---|---|
| Sweden<br>National working population of men aged 25–59 in 1971, based on employment at 1970 census (n=1 779 646).<br>Within cohort RR, 1971–1989. | Job–exposure matrix. Geometric mean of work-day mean values for an occupational group. | *Male breast cancer*<br>Mean exposure (µT):<br>< 0.12 (ref)<br>0.12–0.16<br>0.16–0.22<br>0.22–0.30<br>> 0.30 | 203 | <br><br><br>1.4 (1.0–2.0)<br>1.3 (0.8–1.9)<br>1.6 (1.0–2.6)<br>0.9 (0.5–1.6) | Extended follow up (to 1989) of cohort reported in Floderus et al. (1999). RR adjusted for age, period and geographical area. | Pollán, Gustavsson & Floderus, 2001 |
| Sweden<br>National working population of men aged 25–64 in 1971 based on employment at 1970 census (n=1 516 552).<br>Within cohort RR, 1971–1989. | Job–exposure matrix. Geometric mean of work-day mean values for an occupational group. | *Glioma*<br>Mean exposure (µT):<br><0.13 (ref)<br>0.13–0.20<br>0.20–0.30<br>> 0.30 | 2859 | <br><br><br>1.1 (1.0–1.2)<br>1.1 (1.0–1.3)<br>1.1 (0.9–1.2) | Extended follow up (to 1989) of cohort reported in Floderus et al. (1999). RR adjusted for age, period, geographical area and size of town. (See Pollán et al. (2001) above) | Navas-Acien et al., 2002 |
| Sweden<br>Workers in industries using resistance welding.<br>Within-cohort RR | Job exposure matrix; classification into Low (< 0.164 µT), | Men<br>*Breast*<br>Mean exposure:<br>Low (ref) | 1 | | In men < 30 y, excess risk of astrocytoma grades I-II in High (RR=10, 95% CI 1.2–83.3) and Very high | Håkansson et al., 2002 |

**Table 76. Continued**

| | | Cases | RR (95% CI) | |
|---|---|---|---|---|
| (n=646 694, 484 643 men and 162 051 women), 1985-94. | Medium (0.164–0.250 µT), High (0.250–0.530 µT) and Very High exposure (> 0.530 µT) based on geometric mean of average workday mean values. | | | (RR=9.8, 95% CI 1.1–86.2) exposure categories. |
| | Medium | 7 | 2.9 (0.4–23.4) | In women, for all astrocytomas, significant linear trend of increasing risk across exposure categories (p=0.004); relative risk in Very high exposure category was 3.0 (95% CI, 1.1–8.6) (5 cases). Unadjusted for potential occupational confounders other than dichotomous blue collar workers/others. |
| | High | 2 | 3.1 (0.3–34.2) | |
| | Very high | 2 | 3.8 (0.3–43.5) | |
| | *Leukaemia* | | | |
| | Low (reference) | 54 | | |
| | Medium | 45 | 0.8 (0.6–1.1) | |
| | High | 26 | 0.8 (0.5–1.3) | |
| | Very high | 26 | 0.9 (0.6–1.5) | |
| | *Nervous system* | | | |
| | Low (reference) | 105 | | |
| | Medium | 256 | 0.9 (0.7–1.1) | |
| | High | 90 | 1.2 (0.9–1.6) | |
| | Very high | 47 | 0.8 (0.5–1.1) | |
| | Women | | | |
| | *Breast* | | | |
| | Low (reference) | 402 | | |
| | Medium | 492 | 1.0 (0.9–1.2) | |
| | High | 221 | 1.1 (0.9–1.3) | |
| | Very high | 37 | 1.1 (0.8–1.5) | |
| | *Leukaemia* | | | |
| | Low (reference) | 11 | | |
| | Medium | 16 | 1.1 (0.5–2.4) | |
| | High | 12 | 2.0 (0.4–12.3) | |
| | Very high | 2 | 1.8 (0.4–8.5) | |

297

**Table 76. Continued**

| | | | | | |
|---|---|---|---|---|---|
| Finland<br>National working population of women aged 25-64 in 1970 based on employment at 1970 census (blue-collar occupations).<br>SIR (n=413 877), 1971–75. | Job–exposure matrix based on expert review. | *Nervous system*<br>Low (reference)<br>Medium<br>High<br>Very high<br><br>*Brain and nervous system*<br>Low ( 0.8 µT)<br>Medium/high (> 0.8 µT) | 51<br>76<br>40<br>9<br><br>693 | <br>1.2 (0.8–1.7)<br>1.6 (1.0–2.4)<br>1.9 (0.9–3.9)<br><br>(SIR)<br>1.1 (0.9–1.2)<br>1.4 (0.9–2.1) | Adjusted for year of birth, period of diagnosis, job turnover rate. | Wesseling et al., 2002 |
| Norway<br>Female radio and telegraph operators.<br>SIR (n=2619), 1961–2002. | Spot measurements on two ships (range: < 0.02 µT - about 6 µT). | *Female breast* | 99 | (SIR)<br>1.3 (1.1–1.6) | Unadjusted for potential occupational confounders. | Kliukiene, Tynes & Andersen, 2003 |

[a] RR: relative risk; CI: confidence interval; SIR: standardized incidence ratio.

Bjork et al. (2001) report a case-control study of 255 adult patients with chromosome positive chronic myeloid leukaemia cytogenetically analysed at a university hospital in southern Sweden between 1976–93, in relation to occupational exposure to ELF electromagnetic fields. Three population-based controls were selected per case, matched on age, gender and county (one of whom was randomly selected for interview). A lifelong occupational history (all jobs held for at least one year) was obtained by telephone interview. Two hundred twenty six cases (of 255, 89%) and 251 controls (of 349, 72%) were included; information for 182 cases (81%) and 35 controls (14%) was obtained from next-of-kin proxy respondents. Exposure to ELF magnetic fields was based on a job-exposure matrix using 8-hr arithmetic means from measurements obtained elsewhere for different occupations (Floderus, Persson & Stenlund, 1996), for jobs held 20 years or less from time of diagnosis. For the 55 cases with reported occupational exposure to ELF magnetic fields, OR was 1.7 (95% CI: 1.0–2.8). Compared with < 0.23 µT, OR at "low" exposure (0.23–0.30 µT) was 2.0 (95% CI: 1.0–4.1) (25 cases); at "moderate" exposure (> 0.30–0.50 µT), OR was 1.6 (95% CI: 0.8–3.4) (22 cases); at "high" exposure (> 0.50 µT), OR was 1.2 (95% CI: 0.4–3.1) (8 cases). People with 15–20 years occupational exposure to electromagnetic fields had OR 2.3 (95% CI: 1.2–4.5) (35 cases) compared with those with zero occupational exposure. Classification of ELF magnetic fields was uncertain for 20 cases. [Exposure assessment relied on measurements/job-exposure matrix from Floderus, Persson & Stenlund (1996), obtained for Swedish men only. No new measurements were done for this study.]

In the study of Oppenheimer & Preston-Martin (2002) discussed above with respect to use of electric blankets, having at least one of nine specified exposures in electrical occupations was associated with an OR of 1.0 (95% CI: 0.8–1.5), based on 133 cases of acute myeloid leukaemia.

Willett et al. (2003) reported results of a case-control study of people newly diagnosed with acute leukaemia at ages 16–69 years, between April 1, 1991 and December 31, 1996, in two health authorities and two counties in England. Controls matched on year of birth (±2 years), gender and ethnic group were randomly selected from the same general practitioner lists as the case. Eight hundred thirty eight cases (of 1066 eligible, 79%) were included and 1658 controls (of 3227 eligible and contacted, 51.4%). Occupational histories for all jobs held for at least six months were obtained by interview from cases (107 of 838 (13%) from proxy respondents) and controls. Willett et al. (2003) restrict analyses to Caucasians aged 20 or more two years prior to diagnosis, totalling 764 cases and their 1510 individually matched controls. A job exposure matrix was constructed based on job title to classify individuals as either "probably ever" exposed or "never" exposed, allowing for a two-year lag period before diagnosis. "Probable" exposure was associated with an OR of 1.0 (95% CI: 0.8–1.2). Excess risk among those "probably" exposed was confined to acute lymphoblastic leukaemia among women: OR = 3.5 (95% CI: 1.2–10.2) based on 13 cases. For all electrical workers, OR was 0.7 (95% CI: 0.5–1.1). [Exposure assessment was weak, based only on job title, not supported by measurements. The response rate was only 50% among controls. There was no prior hypothesis formulated to suggest excess risk among women only, or for acute lymphoblastic leukaemia.]

Villeneuve et al. (2002) report results from the Canadian National Enhanced Cancer Surveillance System that collected data on 543 malignant brain cancer cases (63% response rate among eligible cases) among men, between January 1994 and August 1997. [Data were not collected from proxy respondents among those who had died (23%), a potential source of bias if exposure is related to survival.] Population-based controls (65% response rate) were frequency matched to the cases by age and gender; a random sample of 543 matched controls was then selected. Mailed questionnaires were used to obtain information on all jobs held for at least one year (followed up in some cases by telephone interview to clarify responses). Each occupation was assigned an exposure value (< 0.3, 0.3–< 0.6, and ≥ 0.6 μT) based on a time-weighted average magnetic flux density for full-time workers, based on expert review, and taking account of questionnaire data on job duties and employment location. Field measurements [numbers not given] were also done for some occupations that could not readily be classified, using a Drexel Corporation Magnum 310 magnetic field monitor. For all brain cancers, compared with < 0.3 μT as reference, the highest average occupational exposure ever received ≥ 0.3 μT was associated with an OR of 1.1 (95% CI: 0.8–1.5) (133 cases), and for ≥ 0.6 μT with an OR of 1.4 (95% CI: 0.8–2.4) (42 cases) [Note: the second exposure category is a subset of the first, and therefore these results are not independent.] Odds ratios were higher for the subset of glioblastoma multiforme cases: ≥ 0.3 μT: OR = 1.5 (95% CI: 0.9–2.5) (55 cases); ≥ 0.6 μT: OR = 5.5 (95% CI: 1.2–24.8) (18 cases). [Exposure assessment was based on expert review, supplemented by an unspecified number of measurements for some occupations.]

Three further case-control studies of occupation and risk of brain cancer have been reported since the IARC (2002) monograph (De Roos et al., 2003; Krishnan et al., 2003; Schlehofer et al., 2005). These are not shown in the tables as there was no specific focus on exposure to ELF electromagnetic fields, and occupations with the potential for such exposures were not separately grouped. Krishnan et al. (2003) and De Roos et al. (2003) both found a non-significant excess risk of glioma among welders and cutters (based on small numbers): OR = 3.0 (95% CI: 0.3–28.6) for longest-held occupation (Krishnan et al., 2003); OR = 2.1 (95% CI: 0.6–7.5) with > 5 years working in the occupation (De Roos et al., 2003). The latter authors also reported an excess risk among electricians and electronic equipment repairers with up to five years working in the occupation: OR = 3.3 (95% CI: 1.0–10.6) based on 10 cases; and among male (but not female) computer programmers and analysts with > 5 years working in the occupation: OR = 3.8 (95% CI: 1.2–12.3) based on 11 cases (De Roos et al., 2003). Schlehofer et al. (2005) found no significant excess risks for work in the electrical/electronics industry (OR = 0.8, 95% CI: 0.6–1.2 for males based on 54 cases, and OR = 0.9, 95% CI: 0.4–1.8 for females based on 13 cases) nor for occupational exposure to non-ionizing radiation (OR = 0.8, 95% CI: 0.6–1.0 for males based on 167 cases, and OR = 1.1, 95% CI: 0.8–1.5 for females based on 109 cases).

Table 77. Case–control studies of occupational groups with assumed or documented exposure to ELF magnetic fields, published subsequent to IARC (2002)

| Study area, population | Exposure assessment | Exposure categories | # cases | RR (95% CI) [a] | Comments | Reference |
|---|---|---|---|---|---|---|
| **Female breast cancer** | | | | | | |
| Canada<br>Electronic data-processing equipment operators<br>Cancer registry; electoral roll (controls)<br>995 cases and 1020 controls (1988–89) | Questionnaire; occupation | | 24 | 3.1 (1.6–5.8) | Matched on age. | Band et al., 2000 |
| USA<br>Cancer registry; population controls<br>843 cases and 773 controls (1993–95) | Questionnaire; job-exposure matrix | TWA [b] (µT-years):<br>0–0.59 (ref)<br>> 0.59–0.90<br>> 0.90–1.27<br>> 1.27–2.43<br>> 2.43 | 264<br>207<br>143<br>140<br>79 | <br>1.4 (1.1–1.8)<br>1.1 (0.8–1.5)<br>1.0 (0.8–1.4)<br>1.2 (0.8–1.7) | Matched on age and race. | van Wijngaarden et al., 2001a |
| Canada<br>18 major hospitals; hospital-based controls<br>556 cases and 600 controls (1996–97) | Questionnaire; job titles graded at four levels of exposure | Time spent at "medium and high" work-time exposure (0.5–10 µT):<br>All periods | <br><br><br><br>NR [c] | (per 6000 hours)<br><br><br><br>1.1 (0.94–1.4) | Adjusted for range of potential confounders. | Labreche et al., 2003 |

301

**Table 77. Continued**

| | | | | | |
|---|---|---|---|---|---|
| | | Lag of 10 years before diagnosis | NR | 1.2 (0.98–1.5) | Adjusted for age, education, gender. Bethwaite et al., 2001 |
| | | Before age 35 years | NR | 1.4 (0.98–2.0) | |

**Leukaemia**

| | | | | | |
|---|---|---|---|---|---|
| New Zealand<br>Six major tertiary referral centers; population controls<br>110 cases (acute leukaemia) and 199 population controls (1989–91) | Telephone interview; job-exposure matrix based on measured magnetic fields | Exposure (µT):<br>Past<br>< 0.21 (ref)<br>0.21–0.50<br>0.50–1.0<br>> 1.0<br>*Current*<br>< 0.21 (ref)<br>0.21–0.50<br>0.50–1.0<br>> 1.0 | <br><br>88<br>2<br>5<br>15<br><br>88<br>3<br>1<br>18 | <br><br><br>0.5 (0.1–2.4)<br>2.9 (0.7–11.4)<br>3.2 (1.2–8.3)<br><br><br>0.6 (0.2–2.3)<br>1.5 (0.2–14.6)<br>4.0 (1.6–9.8) | Adjusted for age, education, gender. Bethwaite et al., 2001 |
| Sweden<br>University hospital in southern Sweden; population controls<br>226 cases (chromosome positive chronic myeloid leukaemia) and 251 matched controls (1976–93) | Telephone interview (81% of cases proxy respondent); job-exposure matrix for jobs held within 20 y of diagnosis; 8-h arithmetic means based on Floderus et al. (1996) | Mean exposure (µT):<br>< 0.23 (ref)<br>0.23–0.30<br>> 0.30–0.50<br>> 0.50 | <br>151<br>25<br>22<br>8 | <br><br>2.0 (1.0–4.1)<br>1.6 (0.8–3.4)<br>1.2 (0.4–3.1) | Matched on age, gender, county | Bjork et al., 2001 |

**Table 77. Continued**

| | | | | | | |
|---|---|---|---|---|---|---|
| USA<br>Cancer registry; matched neighbour-hood controls<br>412 cases with acute myeloid leu-kaemia and matched controls (1987–94) | Personal interview (49% of cases proxy respondent); electri-cal occupations | At least one of nine specified exposures in electrical occu-pations | 133 | 1.0 (0.8–1.5) | Matched on age, race, gender | Oppenhe-imer & Pre-ston-Martin, 2002 |
| England<br>Cancer registry; matched population-based controls<br>764 cases (acute leukaemia) and 1510 matched controls (1991–96) | Personal interview (13% of cases proxy respondent); a) occu-pations with "proba-ble" exposure, b) electrical occupations | "Probable" expo-sure<br>All electrical workers | 120<br><br>31 | 1.0 (0.8–1.2)<br><br>0.7 (0.5–1.1) | Adjusted for depri-vation | Willett et al., 2003 |
| **Brain cancer** | | | | | | |
| Canada<br>Cancer registry; matched population-based controls<br>543 cases (malignant brain cancer) and 543 matched controls | Mailed question-naires on all jobs held for at least one year; time-weighted aver-age magnetic flux density for full-time workers, based on expert review | TWA exposure (μT):<br>All brain cancers<br>< 0.3 (ref)<br>0.3<br>0.6<br><br>Astrocytomas<br>< 0.3 (ref)<br>0.3<br>0.6 | <br><br>410<br>133<br>42<br><br><br>163<br>51<br>12 | <br><br><br>1.1 (0.8–1.5)<br>1.4 (0.8–2.4)<br><br><br><br>0.9 (0.6–1.4)<br>0.6 (0.3–1.5) | Frequency matched on age and gender. 0.3 μT and 0.6 μT groups not inde-pendent | Villeneuve et al., 2002 |

**Table 77. Continued**

| | | |
|---|---|---|
| Glioblastoma multiforme | | |
| < 0.3 (ref) | 143 | |
| 0.3 | 55 | 1.5 (0.9–2.5) |
| 0.6 | 18 | 5.5 (1.2–24.8) |
| Other | | |
| < 0.3 (ref) | 92 | |
| 0.3 | 23 | 1.1 (0.6–2.1) |
| 0.6 | 9 | 1.5 (0.5–4.2) |

[a] RR: relative risk; CI: confidence intervals.

[b] TWA: time weighted average.

[c] NR: not reported.

## 11.2.2.3 Other cancers

A number of studies concerning exposure to ELF electromagnetic fields in relation to other cancer sites have been published since the IARC (2002) monograph. These data are not included in the tables, but are summarized briefly here.

### 11.2.2.3.1 Residential exposure

McElroy et al. (2002) carried out a case-control study of endometrial cancer and electric blanket use in Wisconsin, USA. Cases diagnosed from 1991 to 1994 were identified through the statewide cancer registry; 745 cases (87% of eligible cases) participated. Controls were selected randomly from lists of licensed drivers (age < 65 years) and from Medicare beneficiary files (65–79 years); 2408 controls with intact uterus were eligible for analysis (85% response rate for controls completing the study interview). Information on use of electric blankets and mattress covers was elicited by telephone interview from June to December 1994; analysis was limited to the 148 cases and 659 controls interviewed during this period with complete information. With adjustment for possible confounders, comparing "ever" users with "never" users: OR = 1.0 (95% CI: 0.7–1.6) (68 cases). [Controls overlapped with those selected for a parallel study of electric blanket use and breast cancer discussed above (McElroy et al., 2001; see Table 75.)]

Tynes, Klaeboe & Haldorsen (2003) examined the risk of malignant melanoma with proximity to a high voltage power line, based on a nested case-control study from the Norwegian national cohort. This cohort was described above with respect to female breast cancer (Kliukiene, Tynes & Andersen, 2004; see Table 74) and leukaemia (Tynes & Haldorsen, 2003; see Table 74); in Tynes, Klaeboe & Haldorsen (2003) both men and women were included. For residential exposure in the most recent five years (men and women combined), the odds ratio for time weighted average exposure 0.05–0.19 µT (compared with < 0.05 µT) was 2.9 (95% CI: 1.9–4.4) (56 cases), and for ≥ 0.20 µT, it was 2.1 (95% CI: 1.5–3.0) (64 cases). For all years, the OR were 1.9 (95% CI: 1.2–2.8) (44 cases) and 1.9 (95% CI: 1.2–2.8) (44 cases) respectively. For exposures ≥ 0.20 µT, the estimated OR tended to be higher in women than men. For men and women with highest estimated occupational exposure to ELF electromagnetic fields compared with the lowest, the odds ratio was 1.2 (95% CI: 0.8–1.8). [No measurements of magnetic fields for persons included in the study were undertaken. There was only limited control for confounding, based on routine data: education, type of building and number of dwellings.]

Tynes & Haldorsen (2003) reported risks for lymphoma and multiple myeloma as well as leukaemia, already discussed above (Table 74). For lymphoma, for residential exposure to magnetic fields in the most recent 10 years, the odds ratio for time-weighted average exposure 0.05–0.19 µT (compared with < 0.05 µT) was 0.9 (95% CI: 0.4–1.9) (9 cases), and for ≥ 0.20 µT, it was 1.8 (95% CI: 0.7–4.6) (10 cases). For multiple myeloma, the corresponding ORs were 2.0 (95% CI: 0.1–32.0) (2 cases) and 4.0 (95% CI: 1.0 16.0) (4 cases) respectively.

## 11.2.2.3.2 Occupational exposure

Three studies have reported on occupation and risk of Non-Hodgkin lymphoma (NHL). Cano & Pollan (2001) carried out an analysis of occupation and risk of NHL within the cohort of Swedish workers (followed up to 1989) discussed above with respect to male breast cancer (Pollan, Gustavsson & Floderus, 2001) and brain cancer (Navas-Acien et al., 2002). There was no specific focus on ELF magnetic fields. For workers ascribed to electrical and electronic work, relative risk for men was not reported, as the within-cohort RR was < 1.2; for women, RR was 1.3 (95% CI: 0.8–2.1). Fabbro-Peray, Daures & Rossi (2001) reported a case-control study of environmental and occupational risk factors and NHL in Languedoc-Roussillon in southern France. Four hundred forty-five cases and 1205 population controls were included. Exposure to ELF fields was not specifically investigated, though there was an excess risk associated with daily welding (occupational), with an adjusted OR of 2.6 (95% CI: 1.4–5.1). There was no excess risk associated with work as an electrician or electrical engineer. Band et al. (2004) carried out a case-control study of occupation and NHL in British Columbia, Canada, based on 782 incident cases and matched controls. There was no specific focus on exposure to ELF electromagnetic fields, and occupations with the potential for such exposures were not separately grouped. However, excess risks of NHL (among many occupations and histological subtypes examined) based on small numbers of cases were reported for electrical engineers (OR = 3.2; 95% CI: 1.2–8.0, 4 cases), systems analysts and computer programmers (OR = 3.8; 95% CI: 1.2–12.4, 3 cases) and electrical equipment installing and repairing (OR = 2.0; 95% CI: 1.1–3.5, 10 cases); welding and flame cutting was associated with excess risk of diffuse small cell cleaved tumours (OR = 3.6; 95% CI: 1.5–9.0, 4 cases).

In addition to breast cancer, leukaemia and brain cancers (Table 76), Håkansson et al. (2002) reported on risks of a number of other cancer sites among a cohort of workers in industries using resistance welding in Sweden. Borderline significant excess risk was noted for kidney cancer among men with "Very High" exposure (> 0.530 µT) compared with "Low" exposure (< 0.164 µT): OR = 1.4 (95% CI: 1.0–2.0) based on 62 cases. There was also a borderline significant excess of cancer of the urinary organs (excluding kidney) among men in the "Medium" exposure group: OR = 1.3 (95% CI: 1.0–1.5) (367 cases), but not at higher exposures. None of the other cancer sites showed a significant excess for either men or women.

Van Wijngaarden et al. (2001b) report an excess mortality from all cancers and lung cancer among electrical utility workers, consistent with previous findings from this cohort reported in Savitz & Loomis (1995) and Savitz et al. (1997). Charles et al. (2003) investigated risk of prostate cancer mortality in the same cohort, using a nested case-control design. There were 387 cases and 1935 controls [129 controls were used more than once and 32 cases were used as controls for prior cases]. Exposure to EMF was based on a job-exposure matrix that used personal EMF measurements from workers assigned to one of 28 occupational categories (Savitz & Loomis, 1995). The group average measurement was assigned to individual workers; cumulative exposure to EMFs was obtained by multiplying intensity by duration across all jobs ($\mu$T-years); exposures were categorized to $<$ 25th percentile, 25th–$<$ 50th percentile, 50th–$<$ $75^{th}$ percentile, 75th–$<$ $90^{th}$ percentile, and $\geq$ $90^{th}$ percentile. Allowing for five-year lag, in comparison with the lowest exposure group, age-matched and race–adjusted OR were 1.11 (95% CI: 0.8–1.6) (94 cases) for 0.6–$<$ 1.3 $\mu$T-years; 1.0 (95% CI: 0.7–1.3) (94 cases) for 1.2–$<$ 2.4 $\mu$T-years; 1.2 (95% CI: 0.8–1.7) (66 cases) for 2.4–$<$ 4.3 $\mu$T-years; and 1.6 (95% CI: 1.0–2.3) (47 cases) for $\geq$ 4.3 $\mu$T-years. The ORs were similar when total career exposure was considered rather than allowing for five-year lag period.

Baumgardt-Elms et al. (2002) carried out a case-control of testicular cancer study among 269 incident cases and 797 matched controls in Germany. No excess risks were found for a variety of occupations including work near high-voltage electrical transmission installations, visual display units or complex electrical environments.

Fincham et al. (2000) investigated occupational risk factors for thyroid cancer in a case-control study in Canada (1272 cases, 2666 population-based controls; response rates 80% and 60%, respectively). Occupations possibly associated with electromagnetic fields, based on self-reported job title, were included for which the OR (adjusted for age, gender and cigarette smoking) was 1.6 (95% CI: 0.8–3.2) (19 cases). [Although published in 2000, this paper was not included in the IARC (2002) monograph; it is included here for completeness. There was no external validation of EMF exposure.]

### 11.2.3 Epidemiology: conclusions

The IARC classification was heavily influenced by the associations observed in epidemiological studies on childhood leukaemia. The classification of this evidence as limited has not changed with addition of two childhood leukaemia studies published after 2002. Since publication of the IARC monograph the evidence for other childhood cancers remains inadequate.

Subsequent to the IARC monograph a number of reports have been published concerning the risk of female breast cancer in adults associated with ELF magnetic field exposure. These studies are larger than the previous ones and less susceptible to bias, and overall are negative. With these studies, the evidence for an association between ELF exposure and the risk of breast cancer is weakened considerably and does not support an association of this kind.

In the case of adult brain cancer and leukaemia, the new studies published after the IARC monograph do not change the conclusion that the overall evidence for an association between ELF and the risk of these diseases remains inadequate.

For other diseases and all other cancers, the evidence remains inadequate.

## 11.3    Carcinogenesis in laboratory animals

A variety of animal model systems and experimental designs have been used to investigate the possibility that EMF might affect the process of carcinogenesis. The results of these studies are summarized in Table 78. Recently published reviews of these studies include those of Boorman et al. (2000c; 2000a), McCann (2000), IARC (2002) and ICNIRP (2003). Long-term rodent bioassays are suited to studying carcinogens that are effective only with chronic/long term exposure. In bioassays, large numbers of animals are exposed over most of their lifetime to several levels of the agent being tested. The animals are monitored for tumour incidence, multiplicity, type, and time of appearance. Chemically-induced or radiation-induced tumours in rodents have been widely used as models for mammary cancer, and liver tumours (e.g. Pattengale & Taylor, 1983; Russo & Russo, 1996). With some human cancers, however, such as malignant melanoma, spontaneous brain tumours and the most common form of childhood leukaemia, acute lymphoblastic leukaemia, the animal models available do not closely resemble human disease.

### 11.3.1    Rodent bioassays

Several studies have looked at the effect of EMF exposure alone on tumour incidence; such studies are potentially capable of revealing whether EMFs could act as a complete carcinogen or serve to increase the incidence of spontaneous tumours. Often, inbred strains of mice and rats are for genetic reasons particularly prone to certain cancers and some studies have examined EMF effects on the incidence of these particular tumours. In addition, transgenic animals – e.g. with activated oncogenes or silenced tumour suppressor genes – are being increasingly used to investigate any effects on carcinogenesis and cancer development.

#### 11.3.1.1   Large scale, life-time studies

Four large-scale, long-term studies have been performed on the effects of power-frequency magnetic field exposure for two years on the spontaneous tumour incidences in rats and mice. Two large studies on Fischer (F344) rats (Mandeville et al., 1997; Yasui et al., 1997) investigated the effects on spontaneous cancers of bone marrow and blood cells (haematopoietic cells), mammary, brain and skin tumours. Two more recent studies on 1000 mice (male and female) (McCormick et al., 1999) and 1000 rats (male and female) (Boorman et al., 1999a) were in line with the two earlier studies. The overall results did not show any consistent increase in any type of cancer.

In the more recent study on rats (Boorman et al., 1999b), thyroid C-cell adenomas and carcinomas were significantly elevated in two groups of male animals exposed at 2 µT.

308

In mice, EMF exposure resulted in a slight but significant reduction in tumour incidence in some groups (McCormick et al., 1999). In two groups of female mice and in one group with male and female mice, the overall incidence of malignancies was decreased. Incidences of lymphomas and lung adenomas were found to be significantly decreased in only a few exposure groups but not in others.

The exposure of mice before and during pregnancy to power-frequency magnetic fields had no effect on mortality and the subsequent incidence of cancer in their offspring during the 78 week follow-up period (Otaka et al., 2002).

### 11.3.1.2 Leukaemia/lymphoma

Lymphoma and leukaemia are neoplasias of white blood cells (leukocytes) of the immune system. Neoplastic lymphocytic proliferation in the mouse may occur as a lymphoma (involving primarily lymph nodes and splenic white pulp) and/or as a leukaemia (involving primarily bone marrow, peripheral blood and splenic blood) but this distinction can be, at times, rather difficult and somewhat arbitrary (Pattengale, 1990). An overview is given in Table 78.

As indicated above, these animal models of childhood acute lymphoblastic leukaemia have limited direct relevance for human disease. In particular, although some phenotypic similarities have been suggested (e.g. Pattengale, 1994), the agedependent appearance of murine thymic lymphomas does not recapitulate that of childhood acute lymphoblastic leukaemia and its indirect mechanism of induction has no known human counterpart (Fry & Carnes, 1989; Hoyes, Hendry & Lord, 2000; UNSCEAR, 1993). There are various transgenic mouse models of leukaemia which develop a disease having some similarities to childhood acute lymphoblastic leukaemia: for example, BCR/ABL p190 mice (Griffiths et al., 1992), an E-BCL-2 mouse (Gibbons et al., 1999), mice incorporating the Pim-1 transgene (Kroese et al., 1997; Verbeek et al., 1991) and a TEL-JAK2 mouse model (Carron et al., 2000). Two studies (Harris et al., 1998; McCormick et al., 1998) have used the Eμ-Pim-1 transgenic model referred to above.

Fam & Mikhail (1996) reported a high incidence of lymphoma in CFW mice, reported to have a low background incidence of this disease, exposed over three successive generations to an intense (25 mT) "travelling" power-frequency magnetic field. [A travelling field is described by Fam & Mikhail (1993) as a basic principle of operation of linear synchronous motors used for example in the propulsion of magnetic levitation trains.] However, control animals, which were not sham-exposed, were exposed to stray ELF magnetic fields of up to 50 μT. There were also too few animals in the first generation to draw any rigorous conclusions. However, there was a highly significant excess of lymphomas observed in the third generation of the exposed group compared to the control group. According to some reviewers, the pathology figures presented in the paper were more indicative of age-related lymphocytic infiltrates (McCann, Kavet & Rafferty, 2000) or hyperplasia (Boorman et al., 2000c) than neoplasia. IARC (2002) note that the study was difficult to interpret.

A lack of effect of prolonged exposure to continuous or intermittent power-frequency magnetic fields on the incidence of lymphoma was reported following the prolonged 18-month exposure of transgenic (Eμ-Pim-1) mice which are predisposed to spontaneously develop thymic lymphoblastic (T-cell) lymphoma and non-lymphoblastic (B-cell) lymphoma (Harris et al., 1998). Similarly, McCormick et al. (1998) reported a lack of effect of exposure to power-frequency magnetic fields for 23 weeks on the incidence of spontaneous lymphoma in heterozygous TSG-p53 knockout mice, which lack one copy of the p53 tumour suppressor gene and have a low incidence of spontaneous lymphoma. More recently, Sommer & Lerchl (2004) reported that prolonged exposure to power frequency magnetic fields had no effects on the incidence of thymic lymphoblastic lymphoma in a strain of mouse genetically predisposed to this disease.

### 11.3.1.3 Brain tumours

Several large scale studies have reported a lack of effect of ELF magnetic field exposure on brain tumour incidence (see above), but generally, the number of tumours reported has been too low to allow a meaningful conclusion to be drawn. However, a recently developed model of spontaneous medulloblastoma in Ptch-knockout mice (Hahn, Wojnowski & Miller, 1999), and more particularly, a knockout mouse model of astrocytomas (Reilly et al., 2000), a leading cause of brain cancer in humans, may prove useful in the further investigation of these effects.

### Table 78. Animal cancer studies

| Animal model | Exposure | Response | Comment | Reference |
|---|---|---|---|---|
| *Large scale life-time studies* | | | | |
| Male and female B6C3F1 mice | 60 Hz 2, 200 µT or 1 mT continuous 1 mT intermittent 2 y | No effect on incidence of most tumours; slight overall reduction in female mice exposed at higher 'doses'. | Well designed, fully described experiment. | McCormick et al., 1999 |
| Male and female F344 rats | 50 Hz 500 µT or 5 mT 2 y | No effect on tumour incidence except fibroma of subcutis. | Fibroma levels similar to historical controls. | Yasui et al., 1997 |
| Female F344 rats | 60 Hz 2, 20, 200 µT or 2 mT 2 y | No effect on tumour incidence. | Site-specific incidence close to historical controls. | Mandeville et al., 1997 |

310

**Table 78. Continued**

| | | | | |
|---|---|---|---|---|
| Male and female F344 rats | 60 Hz 2, 200 µT or 1 mT continuous 1 mT intermittent 2 y | No effect on incidence of most tumours; significant increase in thyroid C-cell tumours in males. | Well designed, fully described experiment. | Boorman et al., 1999b |
| Male C3H/ HeJ mice and female C57BL/6J mice | 50 Hz 500 µT or 5 mT for 7 wk (males) before mating and 2 wk (both groups) during mating and up to parturition | No effect on tumour incidence in offspring over 78 wk follow-up. | | Otaka et al., 2002 |

*Leukaemia/lymphoma*

| | | | | |
|---|---|---|---|---|
| Leukaemia-prone female AKR mice for 5 generations | 12 Hz or 460 Hz 6 mT, pulsed 1 h wk$^{-1}$ until death | No effect on survival time, spleen and thymus weight. | Experiment procedures not completely described. | Bellossi, 1991 |
| Male and female CFW mice over three generations | 60 Hz 25 mT 'travelling' field continuous | Highly significant increase in lymphoma incidence in 3rd generation. | Poor experimental set up and design; possible stress; lack of age-matched controls in 2nd generation. | Fam & Mikhail, 1993; 1996 |
| Eµ-Pim-1 transgenic mice prone to two types of lymphoma | 50 Hz 1, 100, 1000 µT continuous 1000 µT intermittent 18 mo | No effect on thymic lymphoblastic or on non-lymphoblastic lymphoma. | Increase in positive control group. | Harris et al., 1998 |
| Heterozygous TSG-p53 knockout mice prone to low incidence of lymphoma | 60 Hz 1 mT continuous 18.5 h d$^{-1}$, 23 wk | No significant effect on lymphoma incidence. | Small numbers of mice; low incidence of tumours. | McCormick et al., 1998 |
| AKJ/R mice, which carry the AK virus, are predisposed to lymphoma | 50 Hz 1 or 100 µT 38 wk from 4–5 wk of age | No significant effect of exposure on lymphoma incidence. | | Sommer & Lerchl, 2004 |

## 11.3.2  EMF exposure combined with carcinogens

A number of studies have examined the possible promotional, co-promotional or co-carcinogenic effects of ELF magnetic fields on the induction by chemicals, or by ionising or UV radiation, of pre-neoplastic lesions in the liver, leukaemia/lymphoma, mammary tumours and skin tumours.

### 11.3.2.1  Liver pre-neoplastic lesions

The induction of pre-neoplastic lesions (foci) in the rat liver is considered to indicate an early response to carcinogenic agents and is used as a medium term bioassay for carcinogenesis (IARC, 1992). Two studies found no promotional effect resulting from exposure to power-frequency magnetic fields on the number of chemically-initiated preneoplastic liver lesions, in contrast to the effect of a known liver tumour promoter (Rannug et al., 1993b) and a lack of any co-promotion effect on liver foci formation in rats treated with a chemical liver-tumour initiator and a promoter (Rannug, Holmberg & Mild, 1993).

### 11.3.2.2  Leukaemia/lymphoma

Other studies have examined promotional effects on neoplasms of the haematopoietic system.

The co-promotion study by McLean et al. (1991) of power-frequency magnetic field effects on chemically-induced skin tumours in mice (described below) reported increased numbers of exposed mice with enlarged spleens and extremely high blood mononuclear cell counts. The authors suggested that these effects might be associated with development of leukaemia.

Svedenstål & Holmberg (1993) found no effect of near life-time exposure to pulsed 20 kHz magnetic fields on the incidence of lymphomas in X-irradiated mice; unfortunately, unexpectedly high levels of X-ray-induced thymic lymphomas in the control animals rendered the study insensitive to any promotional effect. In contrast, the study of Heikkinen et al. (2001) had adequate power to detect an effect of 50 Hz magnetic fields on the incidence of lymphomas induced by X-rays in mice. Complete histopathology was done to investigate possible effects on tumours in other tissues. The incidence of lymphomas was 30% in the X-ray-exposed control animals, and was not increased by EMF exposure (22%). Furthermore, EMF exposure did not increase the incidence of any other neoplasm. Babbit et al. (2000) conducted a large study on the effect of life-time EMF exposure on X-ray induced lymphomas and other haematopoietic neoplasias in 2660 mice. This study showed no significant effect. Analyses of brain tissue from the same experiment (Kharazi, Babbitt & Hahn, 1999) also showed no effect of the EMF exposure, but the low numbers of brain tumours observed limited the power of this analysis.

Other studies reported mostly the absence of any effect of EMF exposure on chemically-induced leukaemia/lymphoma incidences. While

Shen et al. (1997) found no effect on thymic lymphoma incidences, they reported more animals with dense liver metastases in the EMF-exposed group. However, this difference was not maintained when moderate and dense metastases were combined. McCormick et al. (1998) found no effect on chemically induced lymphoblastic lymphoma in Pim-1 transgenic mice, except for a group of males that was continuously exposed to 1 mT. Notably, survival in this group was significantly increased, and the lymphoma incidence was significantly decreased.

### 11.3.2.3 Mammary tumours

The induction of mammary tumours in female rats has been used as a standard assay in the investigation of potential carcinogenesis, often using carcinogens such as DMBA as an initiator and promoter in the two-stage initiator/promoter model of carcinogenesis. Four groups of workers have investigated the effects of ELF magnetic field exposure on the incidence and the development of chemically-induced mammary tumours.

Beniashvili, Bilanishvili & Menabde (1991) found an increased incidence and shortened tumour latency with EMF exposure for 3 h per day, but not with 0.5 h per day. The experimental details were, however, presented very briefly, which hinders evaluation of the study. Similar results have been reported in a series of medium-term studies of magnetic field effects on DMBA-induced mammary tumour incidence carried out by Löscher and colleagues (Baum et al., 1995; Löscher et al., 1993; Löscher et al., 1994; Löscher & Mevissen, 1995; Löscher, Mevissen & Häußler, 1997; Mevissen et al., 1993a; Mevissen et al., 1993b; Mevissen et al., 1996; Mevissen & Häußler, 1998; Mevissen, Lerchl & Löscher, 1996). These authors reported significant increases by chronic EMF exposure in the incidence of palpable tumours (detected during exposure) and macroscopically visible tumours (detected during post-mortem examination) (Löscher et al., 1993; Mevissen, Lerchl & Löscher, 1996). They found a linear dose-response relationship over the flux-density range 0.3–1.0 µT up to 100 µT (Löscher & Mevissen, 1995). No significant effect on tumour incidence could be found following a full histopathalogical analysis for exposure at 100 µT (Baum et al., 1995; Löscher et al., 1994). Löscher & Mevissen (1995) argued that magnetic field exposure does not alter the incidence of neoplastic mammary lesions but accelerates tumour growth, thus enhancing the number of tumours macroscopically visible when the rats are sacrificed. In addition, Baum et al. (1995) reported that there was a statistically significant increase in the number of rats with mammary gland adenocarcinomas that had been exposed to 100 µT. However, the total number of malignant tumours in the exposed group was not significantly increased.

A replicate study at 100 µT (Mevissen & Häußler, 1998) reported that the incidence of macroscopically-visible tumours in the sham-exposed group was almost double the incidence in the earlier study. This was carried out at a different time of the year and seasonal influences were reported to occur (Mevissen & Häußler, 1998). A re-analysis of all of these data showed

313

a statistically significant linear correlation between increase in tumour incidence and magnetic flux density (Mevissen & Häußler, 1998). More recently, these authors (Thun-Battersby, Mevissen & Löscher, 1999) reported a significantly increased incidence of mammary tumours following 100 μT exposure for 27 weeks following initiation by a single dose of 10 mg DMBA.

In an attempted replication study of the 100 μT exposure by Löscher (1994), Anderson et al. (1999) and Boorman et al. (1999a) found no evidence that magnetic field exposure was associated with an earlier onset or an increased multiplicity or incidence of mammary tumours. There were, however, clear differences in the responsiveness to DMBA of the rats used in the replication study (Anderson et al., 1999; Boorman et al., 1999a) compared to those used by Löscher and colleagues and and there was a variety of differences in the experimental protocols (Anderson et al., 2000; Löscher, 2001). Ekström, Hansson Mild & Holmberg (1998) found no effect on DMBA-induced mammary tumour incidence in the same rat strain following prolonged exposure to intermittent power-frequency magnetic fields. There were no statistically significant differences in the number of tumour bearing animals and no differences in the total number of tumours between the different groups. In addition, the rate of tumour appearance was the same in all groups.

In their most recent study (Fedrowitz, Kamino & Löscher, 2004), the Löscher group tested the hypothesis that the different results are explained by the use of different sub-strains of Sprague Dawley rats. Exposure to a 100 μT, 50 Hz magnetic field enhanced mammary tumour development in one sub-strain, but not in another that was obtained from the same breeder. The tumour data were supported by the finding that exposure to an ELF magnetic field increased cell proliferation in the mammary gland of the sensitive sub-strain, but no such effect was seen in the insensitive sub-strain.

### 11.3.2.4 Skin tumours

Mouse skin models, in which repeated topical applications of single carcinogens to shaved skin on the back of mice causes the induction of epithelial tumours within 20 weeks (IARC, 1992) has been used to examine the initiating and promoting activities of a large range of chemicals. Three groups have examined the effect of magnetic fields on chemically induced skin tumours.

Exposure to ELF magnetic fields did not act as a tumour promoter on DMBA-treated mice, nor as a co-promoter on mice that were treated with DMBA followed by weekly applications of the tumour promoter tetradecanoyl phorbol acetate (TPA) (McLean et al., 1991). In the latter experiment the papilloma incidence in the sham-exposed group was very high, greatly limiting the sensitivity of the experiment. In a later study by the same group (Stuchly et al., 1992) the similar treatment, but with sub-optimal doses of TPA, increased the rate of tumour incidence, but did not affect the final number of tumours. Two replicate studies by the same authors (McLean et al.,

1997) did not confirm this increase in the rate of tumour incidence. The authors concluded that the studies did not support a role for EMFs as a strong copromoter in this mouse skin tumour model. This conclusion is supported by the work of Sasser et al. (1998) who, in an attempted replication and extension of the study by Stuchly et al. (1992), also found no effect of EMF exposure on the rate of chemically-induced skin tumour development or tumour incidence. In addition, DiGiovanni et al. (1999), expanding on the study by Sasser et al. (1998), found no evidence of exposure on early markers of skin tumour promotion using the same initiation-promotion model in SENCAR mice.

In one study, the same design was prolonged to 52 weeks (McLean et al., 1995). TPA treatment was discontinued after 24 weeks. There was no increase in total tumours or papillomas, but squamous cell carcinomas were increased in the EMF exposed animals. The authors concluded that EMF exposure may accelerate progression to malignancy.

No effect of long-term exposure to continuous or intermittent power-frequency magnetic field on chemically-induced skin tumour incidence in mice was reported by Rannug et al. (1993a; 1994). A statistically significant increase was seen in the number of skin tumour bearing animals and in the cumulative number of tumours in the pooled data from two intermittently exposed groups compared to the pooled data from animals exposed continuously (Rannug et al., 1994). Based on this comparison the authors suggested that intermittent exposure is more effective than continuous exposure. However, this interpretation is doubtful, since the results in both of these pooled groups were not significantly different from those in their respective controls.

Kumlin et al. (1998b) reported that exposure to continuous or intermittent, variable ELF magnetic fields had no significant effect on the final incidence of UV radiation-induced skin tumours in normal and transgenic mice which overexpress the human ornithine decarboxylase (ODC) gene. However, the authors reported an earlier onset of skin tumours in the animals exposed to magnetic fields and UV radiation compared to those exposed to UV radiation alone. In a more recent article, the same group (Kumlin et al., 2002) investigated the suppression of apoptosis as a possible mechanism for magnetic field effects on skin tumorigenesis and the synergy of UV radiation and magnetic field. Female mice were exposed at 50 Hz, 100 µT and to UV from lamps emitting simulated solar radiation. The authors concluded that the ELF magnetic field exposure may inhibit apoptosis caused by exposure to UV radiation.

### 11.3.2.5 Brain tumours

Several large-scale studies have reported no effect of exposure to ELF fields on brain tumour incidence (Boorman et al., 1999b; Kharazi, Babbitt & Hahn, 1999; Mandeville et al., 1997; Yasui et al., 1997), but generally, the number of tumours has been too low to allow a meaningful conclusion to be drawn. Mandeville et al. (2000) studied the effect of 60 Hz magnetic

315

fields on chemically induced tumours of the neural system in rats in which the chemical carcinogen N-ethyl-N-nitrosourea (ENU) was fed transplacentally. The authors considered that the neural tumours induced in this rat model are a reasonable model of neural tumours in humans. The number of tumour-bearing animals varied from 38% to 60%, but tended to be lower in the exposed groups. Overall, magnetic-field exposure had no statistically significant effect on the number of animals bearing neurogenic tumours or on the survival of the rats. Small changes in tumour incidence were seen in the exposed groups, but were of borderline significance (0.1>p>0.05). The results are consistent with the view that ELF magnetic fields do not have a promoting effect on neurogenic tumours in female rats exposed transplacentally to ENU.

Table 79 presents a summary of the results of animal cancer studies with combined exposure to EMF and carcinogens.

### 11.3.3    Transplanted tumours

Few studies have investigated the effect of ELF magnetic fields on the growth of transplanted tumours; the results are almost wholly negative.

No effect of life-time exposure on the development of leukaemia in mice implanted with mouse leukaemia cells was reported by Thomson, Michaelson & Nguyen (1988). Sasser et al. (1996), Morris et al. (1999), and Anderson et al. (2001) reported no effect of exposure on the development of large-granular-lymphocytic (LGL) leukaemia in rats following the injection of LGL cells derived from rats of the same strain. However, enlarged spleens appeared earlier and survival was significantly depressed in a positive-control group exposed to 5 Gy gamma radiation prior to leukaemia cell injection.

Devevey et al. (2000) examined the effect of chronic exposure to 50 Hz magnetic fields on acute myeloid leukaemia (AML) in rats, the most frequent type of leukaemia reported in studies of occupational ELF magnetic field exposure. This animal model was regarded by the authors as a reasonable model of human AML. No significant differences were seen in survival between exposed and unexposed leukaemic groups. Similarly, in the terminal stage of leukaemia when the rats were sacrificed, there were no differences in white blood cell count, the differential white blood cell count, the degree of bone marrow infiltration, or bone marrow differential cell count. Thus, exposure had no significant effect on leukaemia progression.

### 11.3.4 Genotoxicity in animals

Lai & Singh (2004) used the comet assay to investigate induction of DNA damage in brain cells of rats exposed to 60 Hz magnetic fields. They reported significantly increased DNA strand breaks after exposure to a 10 µT magnetic field for 24 or 48 h. The effect was seen in both the alkaline and neutral versions of the comet assay and, although the effect was small, it was seen in several separate experiments. Exposure for 48 h caused a larger increase than exposure for 24 h.   The effects were blocked by treatment with

**Table 79. Animal cancer studies: EMF combined with known carcinogens**

| Animal model | Exposure | Response | Comment | Authors |
|---|---|---|---|---|
| *Pre-neoplastic lesions* | | | | |
| Partial hepatectomy plus DENA initiated liver lesions in Sprague-Dawley rats | 50 Hz<br>0.5–500 T<br>~ 20 h wk-1, 12 wk | No effect. | Increase in positive control group. | Rannug et al., 1993b |
| Partial hepatectomy plus DENA and phenobarbital induced liver lesions in Sprague-Dawley rats | 50 Hz<br>0.5 or 500 µT<br>~ 20 h wk-1, 12 wk | Slight inhibitory effect. | Detailed description of experimental protocol. | Rannug, Holmberg & Mild, 1993 |
| *Lymphoma/leukaemia* | | | | |
| Lymphoma or leukaemia in SENCAR mice painted with DMBA and TPA | 60 Hz<br>2 mT<br>6 h d-1, 5 d wk-1, 21 wk | Larger spleens and increased mononuclear cells in spleen. | Leukaemia / lymphoma insufficiently identified. | McLean et al., 1991 |
| X-ray induced lymphoma in CBA/S mice | 20 kHz<br>sawtooth field, 15 µT pk-pk<br>until death | No effect of exposure. | Experiment unable to detect increase. | Svedenstål & Holmberg, 1993 |
| X-ray induced lymphoma in CBA/S mice | 50 Hz<br>variable 1.3–130 µT<br>24 h d-1, 1.5 y | No effect on incidence of lyphoma or other neoplasms. | Well designed, fully described experiment. | Heikkinen et al., 2001 |
| DMBA-induced thymic lymphoma in Swiss mice | 50 Hz<br>1 mT<br>3 h d-1, 6 d wk-1, 16 wk | No effect on tumour incidence. | Inconsistent effect on metastatic infiltration. | Shen et al., 1997 |
| ENU-induced lymphoblastic lymphoma in Pim1 transgenic mice. | 60 Hz<br>2, 200 µT or 1 mT continuous<br>1 mT intermittent (1 h on/off)<br>18.5 h d-1, 23 wk | No effect except decreased incidence in 1 mT continuous group. | Small numbers per group. | McCormick et al., 1998 |

317

**Table 79. Continued**

| | | | | |
|---|---|---|---|---|
| γ-radiation-induced lymphomas in C57BL/6 female mice | 60 Hz, circularly polarised 1.42 mT 18 h d-1, up to 29 mo | No effect on incidence of haemopoietic neoplasms including lymphoma. | Large scale study (2660 mice), rigorously monitored. | Babbitt et al., 2000 |
| *Mammary tumours* | | | | |
| NMU-induced mammary tumours in female rats (unidentified strain) | 50 Hz 20 µT 0.5 or 3 h d-1, 2 y | Increased incidence in 3 h d-1 group, plus increased malignancy. | Experimental procedures not adequately described. | Beniashvili; Bilanishvili & Menabde, 1991 |
| DMBA-induced mammary tumours in female Sprague-Dawley rats | 50 Hz 0.3–1.0 µT 13 wk | No effect on visible or histologically identified tumour incidence. | Well designed, fully described experiment. | Mevissen et al., 1993b Löscher et al., 1994 |
| DMBA-induced mammary tumours in female Sprague-Dawley rats | 50 Hz 10 µT 13 wk | No effect on incidence of visible tumours at autopsy. | Well designed, fully described experiment. | Mevissen, Lerchl & Löscher, 1996 |
| DMBA-induced mammary tumours in female Sprague-Dawley rats. | 50 Hz 50 µT 13 wk | Increased incidence of visible tumours at autopsy. | Well designed, fully described experiment. | Mevissen et al., 1996 |
| DMBA-induced mammary tumours in female Sprague-Dawley rats | 50 Hz 100 µT 13 wk | Increased incidence of visible tumours; increased malignancy. | Well designed, fully described experiment; low incidence visible tumours in sham. | Baum et al. 1995 Löscher et al., 1993 |
| DMBA-induced mammary tumours in female Sprague-Dawley rats | 50 Hz 100 µT 13 wk | Increased incidence of visible tumours at autopsy. | Replicate of above experiment. | Mevissen & Häußler, 1998 |

**Table 79. Continued**

| | | | | |
|---|---|---|---|---|
| DMBA-induced mammary tumours in female Sprague-Dawley rats | 50 Hz 30 mT 13 wk | Opposite results in replicate studies but no overall effect. | Well designed, fully described experiment; small numbers. | Mevissen et al., 1993a |
| DMBA-induced mammary tumours in female Sprague-Dawley rats | 50 Hz 100 µT 27 wk | Increased mammary tumour incidence. | Well designed, fully described experiment. | Thun-Battersby, Mevissen & Löscher, 1999 |
| Ornithine decarboxylase (ODC) activity in mammary glands of female Sprague-Dawley rats | 50 Hz 100 µT 1 d 1, 2, 8 or 13 wk | Increased ODC activity in thoracic complex after 2 wk but not 1, 8 or 13 wk. | Well designed, fully described experiment; variable ODC data. | Mevissen, Häußler & Löscher, 1999 |
| DMBA-induced mammary tumours in female Sprague-Dawley rats | 50/60 Hz 100 or 500 µT 13 or 26 weeks | No effect. | Replication and extension of study by Löscher et al., 1993 | Anderson et al., 1999 Boorman et al., 1999a |
| DMBA-induced mammary tumours in female Sprague-Dawley rats | 50 Hz 250 or 500 µT intermittent 21 wk | No effect. | Somewhat brief description of experimental protocol, analysis and results. | Ekström, Mild & Holmberg, 1998 |
| *Skin tumours* | | | | |
| Sub-carcinogenic DMBA initiated or DMBA and sub-optimal (1 µg) TPA induced skin tumours in SENCAR mice | 60 Hz 2 mT 6 h d-1, 5 d wk-1, 21 wk | No tumours in DMBA treated mice; for DMBA plus TPA, test insensitive due to 90% incidence in controls. | Detailed description of experimental protocol. | McLean et al., 1991 Stuchly, Lecuyer & McLean, 1991 |
| DMBA and sub-optimal (0.3 µg) TPA induced skin tumours in SENCAR mice | 60 Hz 2 mT 6 h d-1, 5 d wk-1 wk 2 – wk 23 of age | No consistent effect in replicate studies. | 3 replicate studies; some heterogeneity in results. | McLean et al., 1997 Stuchly et al., 1992 |

**Table 79. Continued**

| | | | | |
|---|---|---|---|---|
| DMBA and sub-optimal (0.3 µg) TPA induced skin tumours in SENCAR mice | 60 Hz 2 mT 6 h d-1, 5 d wk-1 wk 24 – wk 52 of age | Increase in malignant conversion of papillomas to carcinomas. | Continuation of study by Stuchly et al., 1992 | McLean et al., 1995 |
| DMBA and sub-optimal (0.85-3.4 nmol) TPA induced skin tumours in SENCAR mice | 60 Hz 2 mT 6 h d-1, 5 d wk-1, 23 wk | No effect. | Repeat and extension of study by Stuchly et al., 1992 | Sasser et al. 1998 |
| Early markers of skin tumourigenesis in DMBA and sub-optimal TPA-treated SENCAR mice | 60 Hz 2 mT 6 h d-1, 5 d wk-1, for 1, 2 and 5 wk of promotion | No effect on epidermal thickness, mitotic index, or ODC activity. No consistent effect on PKC activity. | Extension of study by Sasser et al., 1998. | DiGiovanni et al., 1999 |
| DMBA-induced skin tumours in NMRI mice | 50 Hz 50 or 500 µT ~ 20 h d-1, 2 y | No effect on skin tumour incidence. | Increase in positive control group. | Rannug et al., 1993a |
| DMBA-induced skin tumours in SENCAR mice | 50 Hz 50 or 500 µT, continuous or intermittent ~ 20 h d-1, 2 y | No effect of continuous or intermittent exposure compared to control groups. | Increase in positive control group. | Rannug et al., 1994 |
| UVR-induced skin tumours in transgenic (K2) and non-transgenic mice | 50 Hz continuous at 100 µT variable 1.3–130 µT 10.5 mo | No effect on final tumour incidence but earlier appearance in exposed mice. | | Kumlin et al., 1998b |
| *Brain tumours* | | | | |
| ENU-induced tumours of the nervous system of female F344 rats | 60 Hz 2, 20, 200 or 2000 µT 20 h d-1, 65 wk | No effect of magnetic field exposure. | Exposure to ENU and magnetic fields began *in utero.* | Mandeville et al., 2000 |

a radical scavenger, a nitric oxide synthase inhibitor and an iron chelator, suggesting involvement of free radicals and iron in the effects of magnetic fields. The same authors have previously reported similar effects after short (2 h) exposure to much higher magnetic flux densities of 0.1 to 0.5 mT (Lai & Singh, 1997a; 1997b). Another group did not find increased DNA damage (measured by the neutral comet assay) in brain cells of mice after 2 h or 5 day exposures at 0.5 mT, but reported a significant increase after 14 days of exposure (Svedenstål et al., 1999). They also reported an increase in DNA damage in mice kept for 32 days outdoors under a power line, where the average magnetic field was approximately 8 μT (Svedenstål, Johanson & Hansson Mild, 1999). However, close control of exposure and environmental parameters is difficult under these conditions.

No effects of ELF magnetic fields have been seen after long-term exposures in other rodent genotoxicity models, such as the dominant lethal assay in mice (Kowalczuk et al., 1995), sister chromatid exchange in rats and micronuclei in mice (Abramsson-Zetterberg & Grawe, 2001; Huuskonen et al., 1998a; Huuskonen et al., 1998b).

### 11.3.5 Non-genotoxic studies

Only a few animal studies have investigated effects relevant to the non-genotoxic mechanisms of cancer, and the results are inconclusive. Changes in the activity of ornithine decarboxylase (ODC) have been reported in various tissues of rodents after short-term exposure to ELF magnetic fields (Kumlin et al., 1998a; Mevissen, Häußler & Löscher, 1999; Mevissen, Kietz-mann & Löscher, 1995) but not after long-term exposures (Kumlin et al., 1998a; Mevissen, Häußler & Löscher, 1999; Sasser et al., 1998). Other stud-ies have reported increases in the cell proliferation markers bromodeoxyuri-dine and Ki-67 in rat mammary gland (Fedrowitz, Westermann & Löscher, 2002), and inhibition of UV radiation-induced apoptosis in mouse skin (Kumlin et al., 2002).

### 11.3.6 Animal studies: conclusions

There is currently no adequate animal model of the most common form of childhood leukaemia, acute lymphoblastic leukaemia. Three inde-pendent large-scale studies of rats provided no evidence of an effect of ELF fields on the incidence of spontaneous mammary tumours. Most studies report no effect of ELF fields on leukaemia or lymphoma in rodent models. Several large-scale long-term studies in rodents have not shown any consis-tent increase in any type of cancer, including haematopoietic, mammary, brain and skin tumours.

A substantial number of studies have examined the effects of ELF fields on chemically induced mammary tumours in rats. Inconsistent results were obtained that may be due in whole or in part to differences in experi-mental protocols, such as the use of specific substrains. Most studies on the effects of ELF field exposure on chemically-induced or radiation-induced leukaemia/lymphoma models were negative. Studies of pre-neoplastic liver lesions, chemically-induced skin tumours and brain tumours reported predominantly negative results. One study reported an acceleration of UV-induced skin tumourigenesis by ELF fields.

Two groups have reported increased levels of DNA strand breaks in brain tissue following in vivo exposure to ELF magnetic fields. However, other groups, using a variety of different rodent genotoxicity models, found no evidence of genotoxic effects. The results of studies investigating non-genotoxic effects relevant to cancer are inconclusive.

Overall there is no evidence that ELF exposure alone causes tumours. The evidence that ELF field exposure can enhance tumour development in combination with carcinogens is inadequate.

## 11.4 In vitro carcinogenesis studies

Experimental models used to study carcinogenesis involve both animal and cellular models. The first approach is highly pertinent in that all regulation mechanisms are present and animals are treated over their lifetime with the agent tested. In this context, human and animal studies are of greater importance than cellular models for health risk evaluation, but they cannot usually be used to investigate mechanistic events underlying the carcinogenesis processes. On the other hand, in spite of limitations linked to the absence of regulation mechanisms that exist only in vivo, cellular or in vitro models can be useful for the investigation of many of the numerous molecular aspects of carcinogenesis. Cellular models also allow for the use of either normal primary cells, immortalised cell lines, or mutant cells that can over-express, or are silent for numerous genes, all of these being very informative. Direct and indirect effects can be studied. Genotoxicity assays are devoted to the exploration of direct damage to DNA related to initiation potential; they include the detection of immediate damage, such as DNA fragmentation, and the detection of permanent damage, mainly by means of conventional cyto-genetic assays: mutation, chromosomal aberration, micronuclei, and sister chromatid exchange. Alterations in DNA repair capability of cells that can result in mutations can also be studied. In vitro models can also be helpful to study other epigenetic or physiological changes (gene expression, signal transduction pathways, proliferation, apoptosis, and production of reactive free radicals, etc.).

The characteristics of cancerous cells are mainly (i) an exaggerated growth potential resulting from non-physiological stimulation pathway (mutations resulting in the activation or overexpression of one or several actors (genes and proteins) in the signal transduction cascades, overexpression of growth (factors, receptors, etc.); (ii) the loss of responsiveness to physiological inhibitors of cell growth (inactivation of mechanisms involved in the cell cycle control, loss of responsiveness to differentiation signals, inactivation of gap-junctional intercellular communications, etc.); (iii) the capability to escape from the apoptotic process (inactivation of physiological inducers of apoptosis, autocrine secretion of growth factors, over-expression of physiological inhibitors of apoptosis, etc.); (iv) acquirement of unlimited potential for cell division; (v) the capability for promoting neo-angiogenesis; (vi) invasiveness and metastatic capabilities. Thus not only mutagenesis but also many cross-talking processes involving numerous specific genes/proteins are involved in carcinogenesis.

In this section the main emphasis of the review is of the more recent work, especially reports published since the IARC monograph (2002).

### 11.4.1 Genotoxic effects

#### 11.4.1.1 Genotoxic effects of ELF magnetic fields alone

Most studies have shown no genotoxic effects after exposure to ELF magnetic fields in several types of mammalian cells, including human cells (reviews by Murphy et al., 1993 and Cantoni et al., 1995; Cantoni et al., 1996; Fairbairn & O'Neill, 1994; ICNIRP, 2003; Livingston et al., 1991; McCann, Kheifets & Rafferty, 1998; Miyakoshi et al., 2000c; Reese, Jostes & Frazier, 1988; Simko et al., 2001). Magnetic flux densities and exposure durations studied ranged to up to 400 mT, and from 0.5 to 48 hours, respectively. However, other studies have shown genotoxicity in cellular models. Most of the studies used exposure to field strength above 1 mT and exposure prolonged to several days or weeks (Ding et al., 2001; Nordenson et al., 1992; Simko et al., 1998; Simko, Kriehuber & Lange, 1998).

Stronati et al. (2004) and Testa et al. (2004) exposed blood cells from four or five healthy donors to 50 Hz magnetic fields for 2 and 48 h, respectively. Four cytogenetic assays (chromosomal aberrations, micronucleus test, sister chromatid exchange, and comet assay, as well as the cytokinesis-blocked proliferation index) were carried out in these experiments. No damage to DNA and no alteration of lymphocyte proliferation were observed in non-mitogen-stimulated human blood cells.

In a series of papers from the Rüdiger group, it was reported that exposure to 50 Hz magnetic fields induced DNA damages in human fibroblasts, as evaluated with the comet assay. Ivancsits et al. (2002a) showed that intermittent exposure (50 Hz, 24 hours) induced not only single strand breaks and alkali damage but also double strand breaks, while continuous exposure did not. The intermittence schedule that gave rise to the highest level of damages was 5 min on/10 min off, no damage being observed with off-time greater than 20 min. Moreover, a threshold of 35 μT was found in cells from a single donor with a dose-dependent trend up to 2000 μT. In further studies, it was found that the maximum of damage was obtained in fibroblasts after 15–19 h of exposure (Ivancsits et al., 2003b), and that cells from elderly donors were found to be slightly more responsive (Ivancsits et al., 2003a). After the peak of the damage, the effect declined within the next hours and background level was almost recovered at 24h of exposure. According to another study of the same group, the maximum effect of 50 Hz magnetic fields is similar to that of exposure to 4.8 kJ m$^{-2}$ UV, and human fibroblasts were also found to be more sensitive to vanadate treatment as compared to human lymphocytes (whole blood) and isolated lymphocytes (Ivancsits et al.,

2002b). When exposure was stopped after 15 h, the effect was found fully reversible within 6 h for both DNA single and double strand breaks (Ivancsits et al., 2003b). In those studies, cells from each donor were tested in only one to two independent experiments for each exposure conditions, which limits the statistical power of the studies. Several independent laboratories are undertaking replication studies. In the first published replication study, Scarfi et al. (2005) used the same human fibroblast cell line, the same exposure system and the same experimental protocol, but were not able to replicate the findings. The DNA strand breaks detected by the assays used have been critically re-evaluated in a subsequent publication (Crumpton & Collins, 2004). The exposure conditions producing maximum strand break levels (1 mT, 5 min on/10 min off) were also reported to induce a significant increase of micronuclei and chromosomal aberrations in fibroblasts (Winker et al., 2005).

Del Re et al. (2003; 2004) used a bacterial test system (Tn10 transposon in *E. coli*) to investigate the transposition activity (genetic rearrangement), cell proliferation, and cell viability after exposure to either continuous or pulsed 50 Hz magnetic fields at various flux densities (50, 100, 200, 500 and 1000 µT) for 58 h. No effect on proliferation (number and morphometric characters of colonies) was seen. While exposure to continuous magnetic fields decreased the transposition activity and increased the bacterial viability, square-pulsed fields had opposite effects with a 40% decrease in viability (reproductive cell death). In both cases, the effect on transposition was dependent of the intensity of the magnetic flux density with no effect observed at 50 µT and a maximum 30% decrease and 20% increase in transposition activity observed after exposure to continuous wave and pulsed fields, respectively.

Wolf et al. (2005) reported increased cell proliferation, changes in cell cycle and increased DNA damage, assessed by the comet assay, in HL-60 leukaemia cells and two fibroblast cell lines exposed to 50 Hz magnetic fields at 0.5–1 mT up to 72 hours. The increase in DNA strand breaks showed two peaks at 24 and 72 h, while no increase was seen at 48 h. A similar time-dependent pattern of oxidative DNA damage was observed by measuring 8-hydroxydeoxyguanine (8-OhdG) adducts. Involvement of magnetic field effects on free radical species was supported by changes seen in intracellular levels of reactive oxygen species measured by a fluorescent probe, and in the expression of proteins that are involved in redox-mediated signals (NFκB p65 and p50). Also, the magnetic field effects were suppressed by pre-treatment of the cells with the antioxidant α-tocopherol. The results of this study are internally consistent, and effects seen on different endpoints support each other. Independent replication of the key findings would be useful to assess their repeatability.

### 11.4.1.2 Combined genotoxic effects

In its 2002 evaluation on the carcinogenicity of ELF magnetic fields, IARC mentioned that "several groups have reported that ELF magnetic fields enhance the effects of known DNA- and chromosome-damaging agents such as ionizing radiation" (Hintenlang, 1993; Lagroye & Poncy, 1997; Miyakoshi et al., 1999; Simko et al., 2001; Walleczek, Shiu & Hahn, 1999). The effects of combined exposure to magnetic fields and either chemical or physical agents have been further investigated in a number of studies.

Three groups have investigated DNA alterations following exposure to ionising or UV radiation and 50/60 Hz magnetic fields.

Stronati et al. (2004) and Testa et al. (2004) irradiated human lymphocytes with 1 Gy of X-rays immediately after exposure to a 50 Hz magnetic field at 1 mT for 2 and 48 h, respectively. Using chromosome aberration, micronucleus, sister chromatic exchange and comet assay, they showed no alterations of X-rays-induced damage after exposure to ELF magnetic fields. In those studies, the magnetic field strength was lower and/or the schedule of exposures (pre-exposure to 50 Hz magnetic field) was different from the conditions tested by Miyakoshi et al. (2000b) who previously reported interactions between ionising radiation and high-strength 50 Hz magnetic fields (400 mT).

Lloyd and colleagues (Hone et al., 2003; Lloyd et al., 2004) also found no difference in the frequency of 2 Gy gamma-radiation-induced chromosome aberrations observed in non-mitogen-stimulated human blood lymphocytes exposed to 50 Hz magnetic fields (230, 470 or 700 µT) for 12 h, as compared with cells sham-exposed after gamma irradiation. Exposure conditions were similar to those used by Walleczek, Shiu & Hahn (1999) who previously reported that exposure to 60 Hz magnetic fields could potentiate mutations in the *hprt* gene induced by ionising radiation.

Zmyslony et al. (2004) investigated the potential interaction between UV-A irradiation (150 J m$^{-2}$, 5 min) and 50 Hz magnetic fields (40 µT, 5 or 60 min,) in rat lymphocytes. DNA single strand breaks and alkali labile sites were assessed using the comet assay. Exposure to 50 Hz magnetic fields alone did not cause DNA damage as compared to unexposed samples. However, a 60 min, but not a 5 min exposure to the magnetic field, significantly enhanced the damage induced by UV radiation as shown by the increased values in several parameters such as tail length (1.7-fold increase), percentage of DNA in the comet tail (2-fold increase), and tail moment (3-fold increase).

Six other papers reported on the effects on DNA damage of co-exposure to 50Hz magnetic fields and chemicals. The mutation frequency was determined by Suri et al. (1996) in cells exposed to a 60 Hz, 3 mT magnetic field, after or concurrently with one of two carcinogens, NMU (N-methylnitrosurea) and menadione (2-methyl-1,4-naphthoquinone). While menadione is known to act through a free radical mechanism, NMU does not However, no enhancement of the mutation frequency was observed with either carcinogen.

Verheyen et al. (2003) exposed phytohemagglutinin (PHA)-stimulated human lymphocytes to 50 Hz magnetic fields and vinblastine. Lymphocytes were first exposed to the ELF field for 24 h at 80 or 800 µT, with or without a subsequent 48 h co-exposure to vinblastine at different doses (0–15 ng ml$^{-1}$). The endpoint was the frequency of micronucleated binucleated cells assessed in samples from six healthy donors per group. Based on the micro-nucleus assay, two additional parameters: nuclear division index (NDI) and apoptosis, were evaluated in the samples. A significant increase in the frequency of micronuclei and apoptosis, along with a significant decrease in the NDI were found at all doses of vinblastin tested. The 50 Hz magnetic fields alone did not elicit any significant effect, except on the NDI (significant 20% increase at 800 µT), nor did the ELF fields affect the vinblastine-induced responses. The small number of the samples and the lack of sham-exposed controls limit the significance of the conclusions that can be drawn from the study.

Cho & Chung (2003) exposed PHA-stimulated human lymphocytes treated with benzo(a)pyrene (BP, 0–15 µg ml$^{-1}$) alone or exposed to 60 Hz, 800 µT magnetic fields and BP for 24 hr. A series of samples was further treated with BP alone for an additional 48 h. The frequencies of micronuclei and sister chromatid exchanges were assessed. The proliferation and replication indexes were determined from the micronucleus and sister chromatid exchange assays, respectively. In contrast to BP, 60 Hz magnetic fields did not induce more micronuclei or sister chromatid exchanges as compared to sham-exposed cells. Co-exposure of cells to BP and an 0.8 mT magnetic field for 24 h did not affect the damage induced by BP. When co-exposure was followed by BP exposure for 48 h, significant increases in the frequency of micronuclei and sister chromatid exchanges, compared to BP treatment for 72h alone, were observed, while no effects were noted on cell proliferation.

Robison et al. (2002) exposed different cell lines, HL60, HL60R (HL60 with mutated retinoic acid receptor-alpha gene) and Raji cells to 60 Hz, 150 µT magnetic field for 24 h before treatment with 1 mM H$_2$O$_2$. Repair was assessed using the alkaline comet assay within the following 15 min. The DNA repair rate was significantly decreased (about 20% after 15 min repair time) in the magnetic-field-exposed leukaemic cell lines (HL60, HL60R cells) as compared to their non-exposed counterparts. No effect was seen in the Raji lymphoma cell line and Raji cells were also less sensitive to other stresses (see section 11.4.3).

Pasquini et al. (2003) investigated the effect of 1 or 24 h exposure of Jurkat cells to a 5 mT, 50Hz magnetic field, either alone, or with benzene, or with two genotoxic metabolites: hydroquinone (1,4-benzenediol) and 1,2,4-benzenetriol. No effect of 1 h exposure to magnetic fields alone was observed. Exposure for 24 h caused a two-fold increase in micronuclei, with no effect on proliferation. There were no additional effects of field exposure on metabolite-induced damage.

Koyama et al. (2004) investigated the mutational effects of hydro-gen peroxide (H$_2$O$_2$, 1 µM for 4 h) in the presence and absence of a 60 Hz magnetic field at 5 mT, using pTN89 plasmids. Mutations were assessed in the *supF* gene carried by these plasmids in *Escherichia coli*. Exposure to the magnetic field did not induce any mutations, but significantly increased the mutation frequency induced with $H_2O_2$ treatment (2.5-fold increase compared to $H_2O_2$ plus sham-exposure), while no difference in the mutation spectrum or the mutational hotspots could be observed between both groups. These data suggest that magnetic fields may potentiate the damage induced by $H_2O_2$, for instance through an enhancement in the formation of the product 8-OhdG which is known to be genotoxic.

The results of in vitro studies on genotoxic effects of ELF magnetic fields alone or in combination with genotoxic chemicals are summarized in Table 80.

### 11.4.2  *Expression of oncogenes and cancer-related genes*

Oncogene expression has been extensively investigated under exposure to ELF magnetic fields. The first reports of an effect of ELF magnetic fields on gene expression came from the Goodman group, who showed an upregulation of the c-myc proto-oncogene in human HL60 cells under exposure ranging from 0.57 to 570 µT. The effect was shown to be a "window effect" (maximum effect at 5.7 µT, no effect at lower and higher levels of exposure), dependent on $Ca^{2+}$. An "EMF-responsive element" (EMRE), required for the induction of c-myc expression, was identified in the c-myc promoter and corresponded to nCTCTn sequences (Goodman et al., 1989; Goodman et al., 1992; Karabakhtsian et al., 1994; Lin & Lee, 1994; Wei, Goodman & Henderson, 1990). Recently, using c-myc-EMRE expression vectors linked to luciferase or CAT (chloramphenicol transferase) in HeLa cells, the presence of EMRE was associated with a response to ELF magnetic field exposure (Lin et al., 2001).

However, over the years, several replication studies have failed to confirm these findings on c-myc at the transcriptional level in HL60 and other cells at different exposure levels (Balcer-Kubiczek et al., 1998; Balcer-Kubiczek et al., 2000; Boorman et al., 2000b; Czerska et al., 1992; Desjobert et al., 1995; Greene et al., 1993; Jahreis et al., 1998; Lacy-Hulbert et al., 1995; Loberg et al., 1999; Miyakoshi et al., 1996; Morehouse & Owen, 2000a; Owen, 1998; Parker & Winters, 1992; Saffer & Thurston, 1995).

Moreover, while sparse positive findings on the expression of diverse oncogenes either at the transcriptional or protein level have been published (Campbell-Beachler et al., 1998; Lagroye & Poncy, 1998; Phillips et al., 1993; Phillips, 1993; Rao & Henderson, 1996), a number of others studies have reported an absence of effects, including effects on a number of other cancer-related genes (Balcer-Kubiczek et al., 1998; Balcer-Kubiczek et al., 2000; Loberg et al., 1999; Miller et al., 1999).

**Table 80. Genotoxic effects of magnetic fields alone or combined with genotoxic chemicals**

| Cells | Biological endpoint | Exposure conditions | Results | Reference |
|---|---|---|---|---|
| Human peripheral mononuclear cells, non proliferating 4 or 5 healthy donors | Cytogenetic assays: chromosomal aberrations (CA), micronucleus test (MN), sister chromatid exchange (SCE), alkaline comet assay (computerised analysis), cytokinesis-blocked proliferation index (CBPI) | 50 Hz 1 mT 2 h | Magnetic fields: no effects. Magnetic fields plus 1 Gy of X rays: no alterations of X-ray-induced damage. | Stronati et al., 2004 |
| Human peripheral mononuclear cells, non proliferating 4 or 5 healthy donors | Cytogenetic assays: CA, MN, SCE, comet assay (computerised analysis), CBPI | 50 Hz 1 mT 48 h | Magnetic fields: no effects. Magnetic fields plus 1 Gy of X rays: no alterations of X-ray-induced damage. | Testa et al., 2004 |
| Human diploid fibroblasts: IH-9 (28 y-old female), ES1 (6 y-old male) | Alkaline and neutral comet assay, calculation of a "comet tail factor" based on eye evaluation | 50 Hz 20–2000 µT; continuous or intermittent, 11 intermittency schedules 24 h | Continuous exposure: no effects. Intermittent exposure: induction of single strand breaks, alkali damage and double strand breaks. Highest level of damage with 5 min on / 10 min off exposure, no damage with off-time greater than 20 minutes. Threshold at 35 µT, dose-dependent increase of damages up to 2000 µT (ES1 cells). | Ivancsits et al., 2002a |
| Human diploid fibroblasts: IH-9 (28 y-old female), ES1 cells (6 y-old male), KE1 cells (43 y-old male) | Alkaline and neutral comet assay, calculation of a "comet tail factor" based on eye evaluation | 50 Hz 20–1000 µT 5 min on / 10 min off 24 h | Increase in DNA damage with exposure up to 15–19 h, then decrease in damage. When exposure was stopped at 15 h, cells recovered within the next 6 h from both single and double strand breaks. | Ivancsits et al., 2003b |

328

**Table 80. Continued**

| | | | |
|---|---|---|---|
| Human diploid fibroblasts from healthy donors: IH-9 cells (28 y-od female), ES1 cells (6 y-old male), KE1 cells (43 y-old male), AN2 cells (14 y-old female), HN3 cells (56 y-old female), WW3 cells (81 y-old male) | Alkaline and neutral comet assay, calculation of a "comet tail factor" based on eye evaluation. Statistics on duplicated experiments. | 50 Hz 1000 µT 5 min on / 10 min off 24 h | Field strength response curve in ES1 cells: see Ivancsits et al., (2002a). Cells from older donors (KE1, HN3 and WW3) exhibited higher levels of damage. Damage peaked at 15 h for youngest donors and 19 h for older ones. | Ivancsits et al., 2003a |
| *Escherichia coli* transfected with mini-Tn10 transposon | Transposition activity: count of dark clones of LacZ+ bacteria and densitometric analysis of the colour intensity. Proliferation: number, area, diameter and perimeter of clones. | 50 Hz 50, 100, 200, 500, 1000 µT 58 h | No effects on proliferation. Decreased transposition frequency. | Del Re et al., 2003 |
| *Escherichia coli* transfected with Tn10 transposon | Transposition activity: count of dark clones of LacZ+ bacteria and densitometric analysis of the colour intensity. Proliferation: number, area, diameter and perimeter of clones. Cell survival (CW and pulsed fields): colony-forming units (CFU) at the end of exposure. | 50 Hz CW and pulsed (square-wave) 50, 100, 200, 500, 1000 µT 58 h | No effects on proliferation. Increased transposition frequency at field strength above 50 µT. Pulsed field: decreased number of CFU; continuous field: increased number of CFU. | Del Re et al., 2004 |

**Table 80. Continued**

| | | | | |
|---|---|---|---|---|
| HL-60 leukemia cells and two fibroblast cell lines | Alkaline comet assay, formation of 8-OHdG adducts, cell proliferation | 50 Hz<br>0.5–1 mT<br>24, 48 or 72 h | Field strength-dependent increase in cell proliferation.<br>Increase in DNA strand breaks and 8-OHdG adducts at 24 and 72 h. Effects blocked by α-tocopherol. | Wolf et al., 2005 |
| Human peripheral blood from one healthy donor | Six replicate cultures, mitogenic stimulation with phytohemagglutinin<br>Chromosomal aberrations | 50 Hz<br>230, 470 and 700 µT<br>12 h<br>Pre-irradiation with 2 Gy of gamma rays | Magnetic field alone: no effects.<br>Gamma rays plus magnetic field: no significant effect, "borderline" significance for chromatide-type aberrations. | Hone et al., 2003<br>Lloyd et al., 2004 |
| Rat lymphocytes | Alkaline comet assay (computerised analysis) | 50 Hz<br>40 µT<br>5 or 60 min<br>± UV-A irradiation (150 J m$^{-2}$, 5 min) | Magnetic field alone or UV-A plus 5 min magnetic field: no effects.<br>UV-A plus 60 min magnetic field: enhancement of DNA damages induced by UV-A. | Zmyslony et al., 2004 |
| Human lymphocytes stimulated with phytohemagglutinin | Micronucleus assay and proliferation index<br>Sister chromatid exchange and replication index | 50 Hz<br>800 µT<br>24 h + 24 h of benzo(a)pyrene (BaP) treatment<br>± 48 h BaP treatment | 24 h co-exposure: no effects.<br>24 h co-exposure + 48 hours BaP: increase in damage induced by BaP. | Cho & Chung, 2003 |
| Transgenic rat embryo fibroblast cell line, R2 lambda LIZ | Carcinogen-induced mutation frequency | 60 Hz<br>3 mT<br>after or concurrently with MNU (N-methylnitrosurea) or menadione (2-methyl-1,4-naphthoquinone) | No enhancement of mutation frequency by magnetic field. | Suri et al., 1996 |

**Table 80. Continued**

| | | | |
|---|---|---|---|
| Human lymphocytes stimulated with phytohemagglutinin | Cytokinesis-blocked micronucleus assay | 50 Hz<br>80 or 800 µT<br>24 h ± 48 h vinblastine | Magnetic field alone: no effects.<br>No alteration of the effect of the genotoxic agent vinblastine.<br>No effect on proliferation and replication indexes. | Verheyen et al., 2003 |
| Human HL60, HL60R leukaemic cells and Raji lymphoma cells | Alkaline comet assay (SCGE, computerised analysis) 15 min after treatment | 60 Hz ± H$_2$O$_2$<br>150 µT<br>24 h | Raji cells: no effects.<br>HL60, HL60R cells: decreased in the repair of H$_2$O$_2$-induced damage. | Robison et al., 2002 |
| Human Jurkat cells | Cytokinesis-blocked micronucleus assay and proliferation index | 50 Hz<br>5 mT<br>1 and 24 h ± benzene or two genotoxic metabolites: hydroquinone (1,4-benzenediol) and 1,2,4-benzenetriol | Magnetic field alone, 1 h: no effects.<br>Magnetic field alone, 24 h: 2-fold increase in micronuclei; no effect on proliferation.<br>Co-exposures: no additional effects on chemically-induced damage. | Pasquini et al., 2003 |
| *Escherichia coli* transfected with pTN89 plasmids | Detection of mutations in the SupF gene carried by pTN89 plasmids<br>Extraction and sequencing of mutated plasmids | 60 Hz ± H$_2$O$_2$<br>5 mT<br>4 h | Magnetic field alone: no effect.<br>Magnetic field + H$_2$O$_2$: doubling in the number of mutations induced by H$_2$O$_2$; no difference in mutation spectrum and hotspots with respect to H$_2$O$_2$ alone. | Koyama et al., 2004 |

331

Recently, Loberg et al. (2000) used arrays containing cDNAs for 588 cancer related genes to investigate gene expression in normal (HME) and transformed (HBL-100) human mammary epithelial cells and human promyelocytic leukaemia (HL60) cells under a 24-hour exposure to a 60 Hz magnetic field (0.01 and 1.0 mT). Although some variations in gene expression could be seen (twofold increase or decrease), the high inter-experiment variability and the absence of a relationship between exposure intensity and differential gene expression led the authors to conclude that they could not identify a plausible genetic target for the action of magnetic fields.

Using yeast cells and the microarray and 2D Poly-Acrylamide Gel Electrophoresis (PAGE) high-throughput techniques, Nakasono et al. (2003) showed no differential expression in about 5900 genes and 1000 proteins, after a 24-h exposure to 50 Hz magnetic fields (10, 150 and 300 mT). By contrast, heat-shock, minimal culture medium, and aerobic conditions showed significant changes in expression profiles.

Yomori et al. (2002) exposed T98G human glioblastoma cells to 1, 20, 100, and 500 μT of 60 Hz elliptically polarized magnetic fields, typical of environmental magnetic fields polarization under overhead power lines. After 0.5 to 3 h of exposure, the level of c-myc, c-fos and c-jun (mRNA and protein) were found to be unaffected.

Wu et al. (2000) used the mRNA differential display technique to compare gene expression in human Daudi cells exposed for up to 24 h to a 0.8 mT, 50 Hz magnetic fields to that in sham-exposed cells. They identified one gene, the ceramide glucosyltransferase gene (GCS) whose expression was significantly decreased under magnetic field exposure. A biphasic drop was found at 20 min and then at 24 h of exposure. The product of this gene is known to be involved in cell growth and differentiation.

Using the same approach, Olivares-Banuelos et al. (2004) investigated gene expression in chromaffin cells during differentiation into neuron-like cells under treatment with nerve growth factor (NGF) or magnetic fields (60 Hz, 0.7 mT, 2 x 2 h per day over 7 days). The model of chromaffin cell differentiation was previously shown by the same group to be responsive to such magnetic field exposure (Drucker-Colin et al., 1994; Feria-Velasco et al., 1998; Verdugo-Diaz, Paromero-Rivero & Drucker-Colin, 1998). Amongst the 53 transcripts that showed a differential expression in cells exposed to magnetic field compared to cells treated with NGF cells, six genes were identified. These genes encoded phosphoglucomutase-1, thiamine pyrophosphokinase, neurofibromatosis-2 interacting protein and microtubule associated protein 2, while two other encode for unidentified proteins. Interestingly, not only all these genes, but also genes found unresponsive to ELF magnetic fields (actin, histone 2) contained CTCT sequences in their presumed regulatory regions. Although their density may be higher in the regulatory region of magnetic field responsive genes, those results show that the presence of CTCT sequences in the regulatory region of a gene is not sufficient to confer sensitivity to magnetic fields.

Santini et al. (2003) investigated the expression of cell adhesion molecules (CAMs), a class of proteins known to be involved in tumour growth and metastasis, in the MG-63 and Saos-2 osteosarcoma cell lines. Cells were exposed to a 5 mT, 50 Hz magnetic field for 7 and 14 days. Spikes and harmonics were present in the signal. The expression of two integrins (VLA-2 collagen receptor, and VLA-5 fibronectin receptor) and one protein from the CD-44 family (CD-44 hyaluronan receptor) was monitored, showing no effect in Saos-2 cells, while in MG-63 cells, the expression profile of VLA-5 and CD-44 was found to be weakly but significantly affected (14% decrease in CD-44 expression at day 7 and 10% increase in VLA-5 expression at day 14). The physiological significance of such data is unclear.

Another study looked at the expression of a protein suspected to be involved in invasiveness of brain tumours. When exposing MO54 human glioma cells to a 60 Hz, 5 mT magnetic field for 24 h, Ding, Nakahara & Miyakoshi (2002) showed that GAP-43 expression was transiently increased and followed a kinetic pattern similar to that observed after X-rays irradiation: GAP-43 levels plateaued between 5 and 10 h of exposure (twofold increase versus sham-exposed cells) and dropped to basal level at 24 h. No additive effect was noted after co-exposure to magnetic fields and X rays, suggesting that a similar mechanism might be involved in the cellular response to both types of exposure.

Cytokine receptors play an important role in immune cell homeostasis and altered expression of these proteins may be involved in carcinogenesis. For instance, tumour necrosis factor receptors (TNFR) are involved in the induction of apoptosis, and interleukin-6 receptor $\alpha$ (IL-6R$\alpha$) and transforming growth factor-$\beta$ receptor 1 (TGF$\beta$R1) exert important roles in the regulation of cell differentiation and proliferation. Zhou et al. (2002) studied the effects of a 50 Hz magnetic field (0.1 and 0.8 mT) on the expression of TNFR p55 and p75, IL-6R$\alpha$ and TGF$\beta$R1 cytokine receptors in HL60 cells exposed from 30 min to 72 h. Transcription levels of TNFR p75 and IL-6R$\alpha$ were increased only after 72 h of exposure, at either field strength. By contrast, gene expression levels of TNFR p55 and TGF$\beta$R1 were not affected under any of the exposure conditions. The biological consequences of such a differential effect of magnetic field on the different cytokine receptors are not known.

The role of the p53 tumour suppressor gene in the biological response to ELF magnetic was investigated by Czyz et al. (2004). Mouse pluripotent embryonic stem (ES) cells bearing either a wild-type or defective p53 gene, were exposed to a 50 Hz signal simulating power-line magnetic fields (at 0.1, 1.0 or 2.3 mT). A 5 min on/ 30 min off intermittent exposure was applied for 6 or 48 h during the first stages of cell differentiation. Transcript levels of regulatory genes, such as egr-1, p21, c-jun, c-myc, hsp70 and bcl-2, were analysed immediately after exposure or after a recovery time of 18 h. p53 wild-type cells were found not to be responsive to any of the exposure conditions. By contrast p53-deficient cells elicited a response under a single exposure condition: a 6-h exposure at the highest field level tested

333

resulted in a transient but significant up-regulation of c-jun, p21 and egr-1 mRNA levels. The level of egr-1 after exposure in the specified conditions was similar to the basal level found in wild-type cells. It is reported that other intermittent or continuous exposures did not induce similar effects in p53-deficient ES cells. It was suggested that that the balance between positive and negative regulators of cell cycle may be transiently altered in ES cells lacking a functional p53 gene.

The effect of ELF magnetic fields on the expression of heat shock proteins (hsps) has also been investigated. Hsps are known as chaperones, in that they assist other proteins to assemble correctly, target the appropriate cellular compartment and prevent unfolding. As a superfamily of proteins, they modulate a wide range of functions such as thermotolerance, anti-apoptosis function, immunogenicity, etc. Some of the hsps are constitutively expressed, while a number of others are inducible after the cells have been exposed to a wide range of stress signals (heat, heavy metals, etc). Some hsp proteins have also been shown to be expressed at atypical levels in tumour cells or tissue. Such observations have led to suggestions that hsps could be used as biomarkers for cellular stress in general. Their use as biomarkers for carcinogenesis is not widely validated.

In a series of papers from the Goodman group, a 60 Hz, 8 µT magnetic field was shown to increase the transcription of the heat shock genes hsp70 and SSA1 in HL60 cells and the yeast *Saccharomyces cerevisiae*, respectively (1.8-fold in 20 min) (Goodman et al., 1994). This group used the same exposure conditions — with longer exposures in some papers — and different cell lines to show that ELF magnetic fields activated heat shock factor 1 (HSF1), enhanced binding of the c-myc protein to sites within the heat shock protein promoter region and enhanced the DNA binding activity of different transcription factors such as AP1 in the hsp70 promoter region by contrast to heat shock (Lin et al., 1997; 1998a; 1998b; 1999). An increase in the hsp70 protein was also observed, with a maximum increase of 40% in normal human breast cells (HTB124) (Han et al., 1998). Moreover, an electromagnetic field response element EMRE (nCTCTn sequence) was identified in the hsp70 promoter (3 sequences) as well as in the case of c-myc (8 sequences in the promoter) (Goodman & Blank, 1998).

Pipkin et al. (1999) also showed that inducible hsp70 (hsp70B) was overexpressed after ELF magnetic field exposure (60 Hz, 1 mT), but the field strength required for the effect was higher than that reported by the Goodman group.

In a recent paper, Tokalov & Gutzeit (2004) studied the expression of a number of genes from the hsp family (hsp27, 60, 70A, 70B, 70C, 75, 78, 90, 90 and hsc70) in HL60 cells under exposure to a 50 Hz magnetic field at different strengths (10–140 µT) with or without heat shock (43 °C) for 30 minutes. Only the three hsp70 genes were overexpressed after exposure to magnetic fields alone, with a maximum induction at 80 µT and almost background levels of expression at 100 and 140 µT. Moreover, when exposure to a 100 μT magnetic field was concomitant to heat shock, the expression of the hsp70 genes was stronger than that with either treatment alone.

In contrast, other groups did not find any effects of ELF magnetic fields on hsps including hsp70 in other cell lines (Balcer-Kubiczek et al., 2000; Kang et al., 1998; Miyakoshi et al., 2000a; Parker & Winters, 1992). However, Miyakoshi et al. (2000a) showed that magnetic field exposure suppressed hsp70 expression induced by heat treatment (40–42 °C).

In a replication study of the work of the Goodman group, Morehouse & Owen (2000b) observed no significant effect on the induction of hsp70 expression and HSF-HSE binding in HL60 cells exposed to a 6.3 or 8.0 μT, 60 Hz magnetic field. Recently, Coulton et al. (2004) found no effect on the expression of hsp27, hsp70A (constitutive) and hsp70B (inducible) genes in human peripheral blood cells exposed to 50 Hz magnetic fields (20–100 μT) for 2 or 4 h. They concluded that these genes in human normal blood cells were not responsive to ELF magnetic fields

The in vitro studies on gene expression are summarized in Table 81.

### 11.4.3 Differentiation, proliferation and apoptosis

Only a few papers have dealt with differentiation, proliferation and apoptosis in recent years.

Ventura et al. (2005) exposed GTR1 embryonic stem cells to a 50 Hz, 0.8 mT magnetic field for 3 or 10 days, i.e. at the time of differentiation state for embryonic bodies and puromycin-selected cardiomyocytes, respectively. They showed that, under exposure, both embryonic bodies and cardiomyocytes overexpressed mRNA for two transcription factors known to be essential in cardiogenesis (GATA-4 and Nkx-2.5), as well as prodynorphin mRNA and the dynorphin protein, all involved in cardiac differentiation. This was correlated with the increased expression of two cardiac-specific mRNAs (a-myosin heavy chain and myosin light chain 2V) in magnetic field exposed cells and a significant increase in the number of beating cells within the 10 days of exposure.

Manni et al. (2004) exposed human oral keratinocytes to a 2 mT, 50 Hz magnetic field for up to 15 days. Exposure resulted in a number of changes with respect to sham-exposed samples that were correlated to cellular differentiation. The authors noted modifications in cells shape and morphology with a different actin distribution and an increased expression in involucrin and -catenin (markers of differentiation and adhesion) along with a decreased expression of epidermal growth factor receptors. These effects were accompanied by a diminished clonogenic capacity and a decreased cellular growth.

Table 81. Gene expression

| Cells | Biological end-point | Exposure conditions | Results | Reference |
|---|---|---|---|---|
| Hela cells | Transfected with c-myc-EMRE (nCTCTn binding sites) expression vectors linked to luciferase or chloramphenicol transferase (CAT) | 60 Hz 8 µT 30 min | Increased luciferase and CAT activities in cells transfected with c-myc-EMRE expression vector. No effect when the construct does not contain nCTCTn binding sites. | Lin et al., 2001 |
| Normal (HME) and transformed (HBL-100) human mammary epithelial cells and human promyelocytic leukaemia (HL60) cells | Gene expression using arrays containing cDNAs for 588 cancer-related genes | 60 Hz 0.01, 1.0 mT 24 h | No significant effects. High inter-experiment variability and absence of a relationship between exposure intensity and differential gene expression. | Loberg et al., 2000 |
| Yeast cells | Microarray and 2D poly-acrylamide gel electrophoresis | 50 Hz 10, 150, and 300 mT 24 h | No differential expression in about 5900 genes and 1000 proteins. | Nakasono et al., 2003 |
| T98G human glioblastoma cells | Total RNA and protein extraction ; Northern blotting | 60 Hz elliptically polarized 1, 20, 100, and 500 µT 0.5–3 h | No effects on the levels of c-myc, c-fos and c-jun (mRNA and protein). | Yomori et al., 2002 |
| Human Daudi cells | mRNA differential display technique | 50 Hz 0.8 mT 24 h | Decreased expression of the ceramide glucosyltransferase gene, involved in cell growth and differentiation. | Wu et al., 2000 |
| Chromaffin cells during differentiation in neuron-like cells | mRNA differential display technique | 60 Hz 0.7 mT 2 x 2 h d$^{-1}$, 7 d | Induction of 53 transcripts that showed a differential expression. | Olivares-Banuelos et al., 2004 |
| MG-63 and Saos-2 osteosarcoma cell lines | Expression of two integrins (VLA-2 collagen receptor, and VLA-5 fibronectin receptor) and CD-44 hyaluronan receptor | 50 Hz 5 mT 7, 14 d | No effect in Saos-2 cells. In MG-63 cell lines: 14% decrease in CD-44 expression at day 7 and 10% increase in VLA-5 expression at day 14. | Santini et al., 2003 |

336

**Table 81. Continued**

| | | | | |
|---|---|---|---|---|
| MO54 human glioma cells | Protein expression of GAP 43 using immunocytochemistry and Western blot | 60 Hz 5 mT 24 h | GAP 43 expression transiently increased; no synergy with X rays. | Ding, Nakahara & Miyakoshi, 2002 |
| HL60 human cells | Expression of TNFR p55 and p75, IL-6Rα and TGFβR1 cytokine receptors | 50 Hz 0.1, 0.8 mT 30 min – 72 h | Increase in transcription levels of TNFR p75 and IL-6Rα after 72 h of exposure only, at either field strength; no other effects. | Zhou et al., 2002 |
| Mouse pluripotent embryonic stem cells with wild-type or defective p53 gene | Transcript levels of regulatory genes analysed immediately after exposure or after a recovery time of 18 h | 50 Hz 0.1, 1.0, 2.3 mT 5 min on / 30 min off, 6 or 48 h | No effect on p53 wild-type cells. In p53-deficient cells, only a 6-h exposure at 2.3 mT resulted in a transient but significant up-regulation of c-jun, p21 and egr-1 mRNA levels. | Czyz et al., 2004 |
| HL60 human cells | Expression of hsp27, 60, 70A, 70B, 70C, 75, 78, 90α, 90β and hsc70 | 50 Hz 10–140 µT with or without heat shock (43°C) for 30 min | Overexpression of the three hsp70 genes, maximum at 80 µT; synergy with heat shock. | Tokalov & Gutzeit, 2004 |
| Human peripheral blood cells | Expression of hsp27, hsp70A (constitutive) and hsp70B (inducible) genes | 50 Hz 20–100 µT 2 or 4 h | No effects. | Coulton et al., 2004 |

A number of papers have dealt with the PC12 differentiation model (formation of neurite outgrowth) giving both positive and negative outcomes. Using the PC12D model, Takatsuki et al. (2002) found that melatonin antagonized the differentiating effect observed after the cells were exposed for 22h to a 60 Hz, 33.3 µT magnetic field combined with the geomagnetic field in the presence of the differentiation-inducer forskolin. It has to be noted that melatonin is most frequently reported to have an opposite effect on cellular differentiation.

Pirozzoli et al. (2003) exposed human neuroblastoma LAN5 cells to a 50 Hz, 1 mT magnetic field in the presence of the geomagnetic field for up to 7 days. They reported that a 24-h exposure significantly increased cell proliferation (+10%) and a 72-h exposure delayed the retinoic-acid-induced

LAN5 differentiation through increased cell proliferation and decreased expression of the B-myb protein. While exposure to a magnetic field alone did not affect apoptosis as determined using the PARP-cleavage and Hoechst assays, it counteracted camptothecin-induced apoptosis and camptothecin-repressed cellular proliferation. The effect was found to be transient (it peaked at 20 h and vanished thereafter) and dependent on the dose of camptothecin (maximum effect at 12.5 and 25 ng ml$^{-1}$).

In other studies, apoptosis and proliferation were investigated in cells exposed to ELF magnetic fields. As reported elsewhere (see 11.4.1.2), phytohemagglutinin (PHA)-stimulated human lymphocytes exposed for 24 h to a 50 Hz magnetic field at 80 or 800 µT did not undergo apoptosis, and the effect of the genotoxic agent vinblastine was not altered in the presence of the magnetic field (Verheyen et al., 2003).

The group of Miyakoshi in Japan published two papers concerning apoptosis. Apoptosis and the expression of apoptosis-related proteins (p21, bax, and bcl-2) were determined in MCF-7 human breast carcinoma cells following a 24-h or 72-h exposure to a 60 Hz magnetic field (5 mT) alone or in combination with X-rays (Ding et al., 2001). The magnetic field alone did not induce apoptosis or expression of bax and bcl-2 proteins. However, a 24-h magnetic field exposure after 12 Gy X-irradiation significantly decreased apoptosis and bax expression, but increased bcl-2 expression. In another paper, the levels of the apoptosis-related genes p21, p53, phospho-p53 (Ser15), caspase-3 and the anti-apoptosis gene bcl-2 were determined in xrs5 (KU80-deficient) and CHO-K1 (KU80-proficient) cells following exposure to a 5 mT magnetic field and X-rays (Tian et al., 2002). A significant decrease in the induction of p53, phospho-p53, caspase-3 and p21 proteins was observed in xrs5 cells when 8 Gy X-irradiation was followed by 5, 10 or 24-h magnetic field exposure. Exposure of xrs5 cells to magnetic fields for 10 h following irradiation significantly decreased X-ray-induced apoptosis from about 1.7% to 0.7%. No apoptosis was found in CHO-K1 cells within 24 h of irradiation by X-rays alone and by X-rays combined with ELF magnetic fields. The results suggested that in some cells exposure to a 5 mT ELF magnetic field may transiently suppress X-ray-induced apoptosis.

Oda & Koike (2004) examined the effect of a 5-day exposure to a 50 Hz magnetic field at 300 mT on apoptosis in primary cerebellar granule neurons, which are known to undergo apoptosis under normal conditions (5.4 mM K$^+$) in vitro. While no neuronal survival was observed in sham-exposure condition, exposure to magnetic fields prevented the apoptotic death of primary neurons. The effect was found to be dependent on the induced currents in cultured flasks (1 to 4 A m$^{-2}$) and the magnitude of the effect was comparable to that of known survival-promoters (membrane depolarization and brain-derived neurotrophic factor).

Traitcheva et al. (2003) exposed U937 and K562 human tumour cells to 50 Hz pulsed magnetic fields (10, 39 or 55mT) for 20 min to 6 h, either alone or in combination with the pro-apoptotic agent actinomycin, with or without light illumination (which generates free radicals from actinomycin). They monitored the proportion of dead cells and found that pulsed magnetic fields elicited cell death (50%) immediately after exposure (10 mT for 6 h; 55 mT for 20 min), and up to 80–90% 24 h after exposure. The effect was maximized in the presence of actinomycin or actinomycin plus light. Moreover, hyperthermia (42°C) and hyperacidity (pH = 6.5) were also found to enhance the effect of the magnetic field.

Grassi et al. (2004) investigated the effect of 50 Hz magnetic fields (5–1000 µT, 1 to 5 days of exposure) on voltage-gated $Ca^{2+}$ channels, cell proliferation and apoptosis in human neuroblastoma IMR32 and rat pituitary GH3 cells (most of the experiments being performed on IRM32 cells only). Exposure to a 50 Hz, 1 mT magnetic field significantly enhanced proliferation in both cell lines by about 40% from 24 to 72 h. In IMR32 cells, the effect was dependent on the field strength (from 0.5–1 mT). While magnetic fields did not affect apoptosis in this cell type, they were shown to inhibit puromycin- and $H_2O_2$-induced apoptosis (–22 and –33%, respectively). The effects on proliferation and apoptosis were found to be related to an increased $Ca^{2+}$ influx mainly involving voltage-gated $Ca^{2+}$ channels as determined by the use of $Ca^{2+}$-channel blockers and electrophysiological recordings (whole-cell and single-channel patch-clamp experiments).

Table 82 summarizes the in vitro studies into effects of ELF on differentiation, proliferation and apoptosis.

### 11.4.4  Gap junction intercellular communications

Gap junction intercellular communication (GJIC) operates via channels that permit the passage of ions and low molecular weight metabolites between adjacent cells, without exposure to the extracellular environment. These pathways are formed by the interaction of two hemichannels on the surface of opposing cells. These hemichannels are formed by the association of six identical subunits, named connexins (Cx), which are integral membrane proteins. GJIC is known to play an important role in cell-cell communication, cell growth and differentiation. The loss of functional GJIC or the lack of connexin expression is a common feature of cancer cells and one of the most common properties of tumour promoters, such as the phorbol ester TPA (12-0-tetradecanoylphorbol-13-acetate), is their ability to inhibit GJIC.

Three papers on the effects of ELF fields and GJIC have reported that exposure to magnetic fields (from about 0.02 to 1.6 mT, 0.5 to 24 h) modulated the effects of chemicals (TPA, chloral hydrate) and resulted in an additive loss in GJIC functionality in C3H10T1/2 mouse embryo cells (Ubeda et al., 1995), clone 9 rat liver cells (Blackman et al., 1998) and Chinese hamster lung cells (Li et al., 1999). In the later work, it was also reported that a 24-h exposure of cells to a 50 Hz, 0.8 mT magnetic field alone inhibited GJIC (while a magnetic field of 0.2 mT – but not 0.05 mT – interacted with TPA). In a attempt to reproduce the findings reported by Blackman et al. (1998), Griffin et al. (2000; 2000) did not observe any alteration in chemically-inhibited GJIC in clone 9 rat liver cells. One paper reported an increase in GJIC after exposure to a 50 Hz, 2 mT magnetic field in mouse fibroblasts (Schimmelpfeng, Stein & Dertinger, 1995).

339

**Table 82. Differentiation, proliferation and apoptosis**

| Cells | Biological endpoint | Exposure conditions | Results | Reference |
|---|---|---|---|---|
| GTR1 embryonic stem cells: embryonic bodies (undifferentiated state) and puromycin-selected cardiomyocytes (differentiated state) | Gene expression coding for tissue-restricted transcription factors and cardiomyocyte proliferation | 50 Hz 0.8 mT 3 or 10 d | Overexpression of GATA4 and Nkx-2.5 mRNA (essential in cardiogenesis) at both differentiation states. Increased expression of two cardiac-specific mRNAs. Increase in number of beating cells within 10 d of exposure. | Ventura et al., 2005 |
| Human primary oral keratinocytes (HOK cells) | Immunofluorescent staining, confocal and scanning electron microscopy Western blotting and immunofluorescent staining Clonal proliferation | 50 Hz 2 mT (field gradient: 5%) up to 15 d | Modifications in cells shape and morphology. Increased expression in two markers of differentiation and adhesion. Decreased expression of epidermal growth factor receptors. Diminished clonogenic capacity and decreased cellular growth. | Manni et al., 2004 |
| PC12D cells | Exposure in the presence of the differentiation-inducer forskolin | 60 Hz 33.3 µT combined with geomagnetic field 22 h | Melatonin antagonized the differentiating effect observed after exposure to magnetic field. | Takatsuki, Yoshikoshi & Sakanishi, 2002 |

**Table 82. Continued**

| Cells | Methods | Exposure conditions | Results | Reference |
|---|---|---|---|---|
| Human neuroblastoma LAN5 cells | Cell proliferation monitored colorimetrically. Western blotting. Apoptosis assayed by TUNEL assay, and by Hoechst staining | 50 Hz 1 mT, combined with geomagnetic field up to 7 d | Cell proliferation increased at 24 h of exposure. Delay in retinoic-acid-induced LAN5 differentiation at 72 h. No effect of field alone on apoptosis. Exposure counteracted camptothecin-induced effect on apoptosis and cellular proliferation. | Pirozzoli et al., 2003 |
| Human lymphocytes stimulated with phytohemagglutinin | Micronucleus, nuclear division index and apoptosis assays | 50 Hz 80 or 800 µT 24 h | No induction of apoptosis. No alteration of the effect of the genotoxic agent vinblastine. | Verheyen et al., 2003 |
| MCF-7 human breast carcinoma cells | Apoptosis and expression of apoptosis-related proteins (p21, bax, and bcl-2) | 60 Hz 5 mT, alone or combined with X-rays 24, 72 h | No induction of apoptosis by magnetic field alone. Transient decrease in X-ray-induced apoptosis by 24 h exposure. | Ding et al., 2001 |
| Chinese hamster ovary cells (CHO-K1) and xrs5 cells | Apoptosis and expression of apoptosis-related genes (p21, p53, phospho-p53, caspase-3 and bcl-2) | 60 Hz 5 mT, alone or combined with X-rays 5, 10, 24 h | No induction of apoptosis by magnetic field alone in both CHO-K1 and xrs5 cells. Transient decrease in X-ray-induced apoptosis by 10 h exposure in xrs5 cells. | Tian et al., 2002 |
| Rat primary cerebellar granule neurons | Neuronal survival assessed by staining with calcein-AM or propidium iodide. | 50 Hz 300 mT 5 d | Exposure prevented apoptotic death of primary neurons. Effect dependent on induced currents (1–4 A m$^{-2}$). Amplitude of effect comparable to that of known survival-promoters. | Oda & Koike, 2004 |
| U937 and K562 human tumour cells | Exposure alone or in combination with the pro-apoptotic agent actinomycin, with or without light illumination. Monitoring of the proportion of necrotic cells | 50 Hz 10, 39 or 55 mT, pulsed 20 min – 6 h | Exposure caused cell death immediately and 24 h after exposure (10 mT, 6 h; 55 mT, 20 min). Stronger effect in the presence of actinomycin or actinomycin plus light. Hyperthermia (42°C) and hyper-acidity (pH = 6.5) enhanced the effect of field exposure. | Traitcheva et al., 2003 |

**Table 82. Continued**

| | | |
|---|---|---|
| Human neuroblastoma IMR32 and rat pituitary GH3 cells | Effect on voltage-gated $Ca^{2+}$ channels, cell proliferation and apoptosis | 50 Hz<br>5–1000 µT<br>1–5 d | 1 mT exposure significantly enhanced proliferation in both cell lines.<br>In IMR32 cells, effect dependent on field strength (from 0.5 to 1 mT). No effect on apoptosis but inhibition of puromycin- and $H_2O_2$-induced apoptosis.<br>Effects on proliferation and apoptosis related to increased $Ca^{2+}$ influx. | Grassi et al., 2004 |

A series of papers from the group of Li et al. have been published recently (Chiang et al., 1999; Hu et al., 2000; Hu et al., 2001; Zeng et al., 2003). When Chinese hamster lung cells were exposed as previously described (24 h, 0.8 mT) in the presence of protein kinase C (PKC) inhibitors (staurosporine and palmitoyl carnitine) during the last hour of exposure, the effect of the magnetic field was counteracted in a dose-dependent manner and almost abolished at the highest doses of PKC inhibitors tested. According to the authors, ELF magnetic fields affected GJIC via a hyper-phosphorylation of connexins (Chiang et al., 1999). The expression and localisation of Cx43 within the cell compartments was investigated, showing that under treatment to TPA or exposure to ELF magnetic field, the phosphorylation of Cx43 was enhanced and the protein was mostly located near the nucleus, in contrast to the normal location at the plasma membrane (Zeng et al., 2003). In parallel, it was shown that ELF magnetic fields (24 h, 0.8 mT) also decreased GJIC and induced Cx43 hyperphosphorylation in mouse NIH3T3 cells but did not affect the level of the Cx43 gene transcription or the expression of Cx43 protein, which is in contradiction with the previous work on Chinese hamster lung cells. It is possible however that Cx43 is stabilised via hyperphosphorylation and that hyperphosphorylated Cx43 would be in part responsible for the observed increase in Cx43. In the NIH3T3 cells the effect of the magnetic field tested was similar to a TPA dose of 3 ng ml$^{-1}$ (Hu et al., 2000; 2001). Thus, based on this body of work, the authors conclude that ELF magnetic fields mimicked TPA in the signalling pathway leading to a decrease in GJIC, and the threshold of inhibition was 0.4 mT.

Although not related to cancer, the study of Marino, Kolomytkin & Frilot (2003) deserves to be mentioned as the effects of induced currents were investigated in HIG-82 synovial fibroblasts and 5Y neuroblastoma cells. No effects were found in nerve cells, but the authors showed a decrease in the conductance of gap junction channels under exposure to 20 mA m$^{-2}$ at 60 Hz and a significant increase in intracellular Ca$^{2+}$ at current densities of more than 10 mA m$^{-2}$. The authors hypothesised that the pain relief reported under exposure to ELF magnetic fields could be related to a drop in pro-inflammatory responses due to decreased GJIC in synovial cells. This work did not establish whether the magnetic field or the induced currents were responsible for the reported effects.

Yamaguchi et al. (2002) have also reported that pre-osteoblastic MC3T3-E1 cells elicited a decrease in GJIC after a 1-h exposure to ELF magnetic fields of up to 1.5 mT (50 % at 0.4 mT with no effect of the frequency from 30 to 120 Hz), while the well-differentiated osteoblastic ROS 17/2.8 cells did not. The effect was unrelated to Cx43 expression and distribution within the cells or intracellular Ca$^{2+}$.

The studies on gap junctions and intercellular communication are summarized in Table 83.

**Table 83. Gap junctions and intercellular communication**

| Cells | Biological endpoint | Exposure conditions | Results | Reference |
|---|---|---|---|---|
| Chinese hamster lung cells | Gap junctional inter communications; dye transfer assay: microinjection of Lucifer Yellow, determination of the number of dye-coupled cells (DCC) per injection | 50 Hz<br>0.05, 0.2, 0.4, 0.8 mT<br>24 h<br>+/- 5 ng ml$^{-1}$ TPA, 1 h<br>Field perpendicular to dishes; presence of geomagnetic field | Decrease in number of DCC at 0.8 mT only, comparable to effect of TPA. Potentiation of the effect of TPA: significant decrease versus TPA alone at and above 0.2 mT. | Li et al., 1999 |
| Chinese hamster lung cells | Gap junctional inter communications; dye transfer assay: microinjection of Lucifer Yellow, determination of the number of dye-coupled cells (DCC) per injection | 50 Hz<br>0.8 mT<br>24 h<br>Field perpendicular to dishes; presence of geomagnetic field | Magnetic fields decreased number of DCC.<br>Use of PKC inhibitors (staurosporine or palmitoyl-DL-carnitine) restored dye transfer in a dose-dependent manner. | Chiang et al., 1999 |
| Chinese hamster lung cells and NIH3T3 mouse fibroblasts | Level of connexin43 mRNA<br>Northern Blot | 50 Hz<br>0.8 mT<br>24 h<br>Field perpendicular to dishes; presence of geomagnetic field | No effect. | Hu et al., 2000 |
| NIH3T3 mouse fibroblasts | Gap junctional inter communications: fluorescence recovery after photobleaching (FRAP) analysis<br>Connexin43 expression and phosphorylation in membrane suspensions and total protein extracts<br>Western-blotting | 50 Hz<br>0.8 mT<br>24 h<br>+/- 3 ng ml$^{-1}$ TPA, 2 h<br>Field perpendicular to dishes; presence of geomagnetic field | Magnetic fields alone decreased fluorescence recovery by 50%; effect comparable to TPA.<br>Potentiation of effect of TPA, significant decrease versus TPA alone.<br>Hyperphosphorylation of connexin43, no change in level of Cx43.<br>Localisation of Cx43 in the plasma membrane. | Hu et al., 2001 |

**Table 83. Continued**

| | | | | |
|---|---|---|---|---|
| Chinese hamster lung cells | Detection of Connexin43 Western blotting, confocal microscopy, immunocytochemistry | 50 Hz 0.8 mT 24 h Field perpendicular to dishes; presence of geomagnetic field | Magnetic fields induced an internalisation of Cx43 from the membrane to the cytoplasm. Magnetic fields increased the level of Cx43 in the cytoplasm and the nucleus, effect similar to that of TPA (5 ng ml$^{-1}$; 1 h). | Zeng et al., 2003 |
| HIG-82 fibroblats (derived from rabbit synovium) and SH-SY5Y human neuroblastoma cells | Gap junctional inter communications: registration of single gap junction channel currents Calcium influx (transmembrane calcium currents) | 60 Hz currents of 2, 20 and 75 mA m$^{-2}$ | Currents of 20 mA m$^{-2}$ decreased conductance of gap junction channels. Currents of 10 mA m$^{-2}$ increased flow of current through calcium channels. | Marino, Kolomytkin & Frilot, 2003 |
| Preosteoblastic MC3T3-E1 cells and well-differentiated osteoblastic ROS 17/2.8 cells | Gap junctional inter communications; dye transfer assay: microinjection of Lucifer Yellow, determination of the number of dye-coupled cells (DCC) per injection Parachute technique: PKH26/BCECF double staining Cytosolic calcium concentration (Fura2 staining) and Connexin43 expression (Western blotting) | 30–120 Hz 0.1, 1, 3, 6 and 12.5 mT 1 and 2.5 h geomagnetic field nulled, DT< 0.6°C | No effect on ROS 17/2.8 cells. In MC3T3 cells, magnetic fields decreased the frequency of GJIC (28% of controls at 60 Hz, 1.25 mT). No effect of the frequency. No effect on intracellular Ca$^{2+}$ and Cx43 expression and localisation. | Yamaguchi et al., 2002 |

### 11.4.5    Free radicals

The effects of exposure to electric and magnetic fields on free radical species have been studied in recent years and there are three main subdivisions to this area of research: (i) the biophysical mechanisms by which magnetic fields could affect the yield and concentration of the radicals (i.e. the radical pair mechanism, see section 4.5.4); (ii) the biological and biochemical mechanisms of increased production of radicals by exposed cells, and/or their increased availability to interact with DNA; and (iii) the potential enhancement of the effect of compounds known to increase the concentration of free radicals.

The issue of free radical involvement in bioeffects has been linked closely to the role of melatonin as a free radical scavenger, as an alteration of melatonin production under exposure had been hypothesised but not proven (see Chapter 6).

Katsir & Parola (1998) reported an enhancement of the proliferation of chick embryo fibroblasts under magnetic field exposure (100 Hz, 0.7 mT, 24 h). The increase in cell proliferation was reduced in the presence of catalase, superoxide dismutase, or vitamin E, by 79, 67, and 82%, respectively. This was interpreted by the authors as an involvement of free radicals.

The synergy with free radical generating systems was investigated by two groups. Fiorani et al. (1997) studied the effect of ELF magnetic fields on rabbit erythrocytes in combination with an oxygen-radical generating system (Fe(II)/ascorbate). Exposure at 0.5 mT (50Hz) had no effect on intact erythrocytes, but increased the damage due to the presence of the iron free radical generating system, as witnessed by a 20% decay in hexokinase activity and 100% increase in methemoglobin production, compared to the effect of the oxidant system alone.

The hypothesis of the radical pair mechanism was tested by Zmyslony et al. (2004) on rat lymphocytes exposed for 1 h to 50 Hz fields at 20, 40, or 200 µT inside a pair of Helmholtz coils with its axis along or transverse to the geomagnetic field. Iron ions (from $FeCl_2$) were used as a stimulator of the oxidation processes and oxygen radical concentration was measured using a fluorescent probe. Only in the lymphocytes exposed at 40 µT along the geomagnetic field was there a decrease of fluorescence. This finding was interpreted as evidence for the radical pair mechanism, since for this configuration the magnetic field is cancelled once per period but not for other frequency and orientation configurations.

The Simko group has studied the effects of exposure on various cellular systems and have postulated recently that some of the effects that they observed could be interpreted as due to increased free radical production. In 2001, they published data on the stimulation of phagocytosis and free radical production in mouse bone marrow-derived macrophages by 50 Hz magnetic fields (0.5–1.5mT, 45 min) (Simko et al., 2001). Under exposure, an increase was observed in superoxide radical ion production and phagocytic uptake of latex beads. Stimulation with the tumour promoter TPA showed the same increased phagocytic activity as a 1 mT magnetic field. However, co-exposure with TPA led to no further increase of bead uptake, interpreted as ruling out a role for the protein kinase C signal transduction pathway.

The increased production of reactive oxygen species (ROS) was later reported by the same group (Rollwitz, Lupke & Simko, 2004) in bone marrow-derived promonocytes and macrophages exposed at 1 mT. TPA inhibited the exposure-induced production of ROS while the flavoprotein inhibitor DPI (diphenyleneiodonium chloride) did not, showing that the NADH-oxidase pathway, which produces the superoxide anion radicals, was affected, but not the NADPH pathway.

Simko and Mattsson have suggested in 2004 that EMFs might act as a stimulus to induce activated states of the cell such as phagocytosis, which then enhances the release of free radicals, leading possibly to genotoxic events. Exposure could lead to (i) direct activation of phagocytosis (or other cell specific responses) and thus of free radical production; (ii) direct stimulation of free radical production by some cells; and (iii) increase in the lifetime of free radicals leading to elevated free radical concentrations. Long-term exposure would lead to a chronically increased level of free radicals, subsequently causing an inhibition of the effects of melatonin. These speculations have not been substantiated but are of interest for further research on the role of free radicals in ELF magnetic field effects.

In Table 84 the in vitro studies into effects of ELF fields on free radicals are summarized.

### 11.4.6 *In vitro conclusions*

Generally, studies of the effects of ELF magnetic field exposure of cells have shown no induction of genotoxicity at fields below 50 mT. The notable exception is evidence from recent studies of DNA damage at field strengths as low as 35 $\mu T$; however, these studies are still being evaluated at this time and our understanding of these findings is incomplete. There is also increasing evidence that ELF magnetic fields may interact with DNA-damaging agents.

There is no clear evidence of the activation of genes associated with the control of the cell cycle. However, systematic studies analyzing the response of the whole genome have yet to be performed.

Many other cellular studies, for example on cell proliferation, apoptosis, calcium signaling, intercellular communication, heat shock protein expression and malignant transformation, have produced inconsistent or inconclusive results.

### 11.5 Overall conclusions

New human, animal and in vitro studies, published since the 2002 IARC monograph, do not change the overall classification of ELF as a possible human carcinogen.

**Table 84. Free radicals**

| Cells | Biological endpoint | Exposure conditions | Results | Reference |
|---|---|---|---|---|
| Chick embryo fibroblasts | Proliferation | 100 Hz<br>0.7 mT<br>24 h | Enhancement of proliferation under exposure; this increase was reduced in the presence of catalase, superoxide dismutase, or vitamin E. | Katsir & Parola 1998 |
| Rabbit erythrocytes (RBCs) | Exposure with oxygen-radical generating system (Fe(II)/ascorbate) | 50 Hz<br>0.2–0.5 mT<br>up to 90 min | At 0.5 mT, no effect on intact RBCs; increased damage due to the presence of the iron free radical generating system. | Fiorani et al., 1997 |
| Rat lymphocytes | Exposure with iron ions ($FeCl_2$) used as a stimulator of the oxidation processes | 50 Hz<br>20, 40 or 200 µT, field axis along or transverse to the geomagnetic field<br>1 h | Decrease of fluorescence only in lymphocytes exposed at 40 µT along geomagnetic field. | Zmyslony et al., 2004 |
| Mouse bone marrow-derived macrophages | Stimulation of phagocytosis and free radical production | 50 Hz<br>0.5–1.5 mT<br>45 min | Increase in superoxide radical ion production and phagocytic uptake of latex beads. Stimulation with TPA caused same increased phagocytic activity as 1 mT. Co-exposure with TPA led to no further increase of bead uptake. | Simko et al., 2001 |
| Mouse bone marrow-derived promonocytes and macrophages | ROS production assessed using fluorescence staining and flow cytometry; superoxide anion and nitrogen generation also assessed | 50 Hz<br>1 mT<br>45 min | Increased production of ROS. Inhibition of ROS increase by TPA, but not by the flavoprotein inhibitor DPI. | Rollwitz, Lupke & Simko, 2004 |

# 12    HEALTH RISK ASSESSMENT

## 12.1    Introduction

The control of health risks from the exposure to any physical, chemical or biological agent is informed by a scientific, ideally quantitative, assessment of potential effects at given exposure levels (risk assessment). Based upon the results of the risk assessment and taking into consideration other factors, a decision-making process aimed at eliminating or, if this is not possible, reducing to a minimum the risk from the agent (risk management) can be started. The discussion below is based on the WHO Environmental Health Criteria 210 which describes the principles for the assessment of risks to human health from exposure to chemicals (WHO, 1999). These principles are generally applicable and have been used here for ELF electric and magnetic fields.

Risk assessment is a conceptual framework that provides the mechanism for a structured review of information relevant to estimating health or the environmental effects of exposure. The risk assessment process is divided into four distinct steps: hazard identification, exposure assessment, exposure-response assessment and risk characterization.

- The purpose of *hazard identification* is to evaluate qualitatively the weight of evidence for adverse effects in humans based on the assessment of all the available data on toxicity and modes of action. Primarily two questions are addressed: (1) whether ELF fields may pose a health hazard to human beings and (2) under what circumstances an identified hazard may occur. Hazard identification is based on analyses of a variety of data that may range from observations in humans to studies conducted in laboratories, as well as possible mechanisms of action.

- *Exposure assessment* is the determination of the nature and extent of exposure to EMF under different conditions. Multiple approaches can be used to conduct exposure assessments. These include direct techniques, such as the measurement of ambient and personal exposures, and indirect methods, for example questionnaires and computational techniques.

- *Exposure-response assessment* is the process of quantitatively characterizing the relationship between the exposure received and the occurrence of an effect. For most types of possible adverse effects (i.e. neurological, behavioural, immunological, reproductive or developmental effects), it is generally considered that there is an EMF exposure level below which adverse effects will not occur (i.e. a threshold). However, for other effects such as cancer, there may not be a threshold.

- *Risk characterization* is the final step in the risk assessment process. Its purpose is to support risk managers by providing the essential scientific evidence and rationale about risk that they need

349

for decision-making. In risk characterization, estimates of the risk to human health under relevant exposure scenarios are provided. Thus, a risk characterization is an evaluation and integration of the available scientific evidence and is used to estimate the nature, importance and often the magnitude of human risk, including a recognition and characterization of uncertainty that can reasonably be estimated to result from exposure to EMF under specific circumstances.

The health risk assessment can be used as an input to risk management, which encompasses (1) all the activities needed to reach decisions on whether an exposure requires any specific action(s), (2) which actions are appropriate and (3) the undertaking of these actions. Such risk management activities are further discussed in Chapter 13.

## 12.2    Hazard identification

### 12.2.1   Biological versus adverse health effects

According to the WHO Constitution, health is a state of complete physical, mental and social well-being and not merely the absence of disease or infirmity. Before identifying any actual health hazards, it is useful to clarify the difference between a biological effect and an adverse health effect. A biological effect is any physiological response to, in this case, exposure to ELF fields. Some biological effects may have no influence on health, some may have beneficial consequences, while others may result in pathological conditions, i.e. adverse health effects. Annoyance or discomfort caused by ELF exposure may not be pathological per se but, if substantiated, can affect the physical and mental well-being of a person and the resultant effect may be considered to be an adverse health effect.

### 12.2.2   Acute effects

ELF electric and magnetic fields can affect the nervous systems of people exposed to them, resulting in adverse health consequences such as nerve stimulation, at very high exposure levels. Exposure at lower levels induces changes in the excitability of nervous tissue in the central nervous system which may affect memory, cognition and other brain functions. These acute effects on the nervous system form the basis of international guidelines. However, they are unlikely to occur at the low exposure levels in the general environment and most working environments.

Exposure to ELF electric fields also induces a surface electric charge which can lead to perceptible, but non-hazardous effects, including microshocks.

### 12.2.3   Chronic effects

Scientific evidence suggesting that everyday, chronic, low-intensity ELF magnetic field exposure poses a possible health risk is based on epidemiological studies demonstrating a consistent pattern of an increased risk of childhood leukaemia. Uncertainties in the hazard assessment include the role of control selection bias and exposure misclassification. In addition, virtually all of the laboratory evidence and the mechanistic evidence fails to support a relationship between low-level ELF magnetic field exposure and changes in biological function or disease status. Thus, on balance, the evidence is not strong enough to be considered causal and therefore ELF magnetic fields remain classified as possibly carcinogenic.

A number of other diseases have been investigated for possible association with ELF magnetic field exposure. These include other types of cancers in both children and adults, depression, suicide, reproductive dysfunction, developmental disorders, immunological modifications, neurological disease and cardiovascular disease. The scientific evidence supporting a linkage between exposure to ELF magnetic fields and any of these diseases is weaker than for childhood leukaemia and in some cases (for example, for cardiovascular disease or breast cancer) the evidence is sufficient to give confidence that magnetic fields do not cause the disease.

## 12.3    Exposure assessment

Electric and magnetic field exposures can be expressed in terms of instantaneous or temporally averaged values. Either of these can be calculated from source parameters or measured.

### 12.3.1   Residential exposures

In the case of residential exposure, data from various countries show that the geometric means of ELF magnetic field strengths across homes do not vary dramatically. Mean values of ELF electric fields in the home can be up to several tens of volts per metre. In the vicinity of some appliances, the instantaneous magnetic field values can be as much as a few hundreds of microtesla. Close to power lines, magnetic fields reach as much as approximately 20 µT and electric fields can be between several hundreds and several thousands of volts per metre.

The epidemiological studies on childhood leukaemia have focused on average residential ELF magnetic fields above 0.3 to 0.4 µT as a risk factor for cancer. Results from several extensive surveys showed that approximately 0.5–7% of children had time-averaged exposures in excess of 0.3 µT and 0.4–3.3% were exposed to in excess of 0.4 µT. Calculations based on case-control studies of ELF magnetic field exposure and childhood leukaemia resulted in approximately similar ranges.

### 12.3.2   Occupational exposures

Occupational exposure is predominantly at power frequencies and their harmonics. Magnetic field exposure in the workplace can be up to approximately 10 mT and this is invariably associated with the presence of conductors carrying high currents. In the electrical supply industry, workers may be exposed to electric fields up to 30 kV m$^{-1}$, which induce electric fields in the body and lead to increased occurrence of contact currents and microshocks.

## 12.4 Exposure-response assessment

Exposure-response assessment is the process of characterizing the relationship between the exposure received by an individual and the occurrence of an effect. There are many ways in which exposure-response relationships can be evaluated and a number of assumptions must be used to conduct such assessments.

### 12.4.1 Threshold levels

For some effects there may be a continuous relation with exposure, for others a threshold may exist. There will be a certain amount of imprecision in determining these thresholds. The degree of uncertainty is reflected partly in the value of a safety factor that is incorporated in order to derive the exposure limit.

Frequency-dependent thresholds have been identified for acute effects on electrically excitable tissues, particularly those in the central nervous system. These effects result from electric fields and currents that are induced in body tissues by ELF electric or magnetic field exposure (see Chapter 5). The ICNIRP (1998a) identified a threshold current density of 100 mA m$^{-2}$ for acute changes in functions of the central nervous system (CNS: brain and spinal cord, located in the head and trunk) and recommended basic restrictions on current density induced in these tissues of 10 mA m$^{-2}$ for workers and 2 mA m$^{-2}$ for members of the public. A general consideration of neural tissue physiology suggested that these restrictions should remain constant between 4 Hz and 1 kHz, rising above and below these frequencies. More recently, the IEEE (2002) identified a threshold induced electric field strength of 53 mV m$^{-1}$ at 20 Hz for changes in brain function in 50% of healthy adults. Effects taken into account included phosphene induction and other effects on synaptic interactions. The IEEE recommended basic restrictions on induced electric field strength in the brain of 17.7 mV m$^{-1}$ in "controlled" environments and 5.9 mV m$^{-1}$ for members of the public. The phosphene threshold rises above 20 Hz and therefore the basic restrictions recommended by the IEEE follow a frequency-proportional law up to 760 Hz, above which restrictions are based on peripheral nerve stimulation up to 100 kHz (IEEE, 2002). The net effect is that the guidance recommended by the ICNIRP (1998a) is more restrictive than that recommended by the IEEE (2002) at power frequencies (50/60 Hz) and above (see Section 12.5.1 below). The major factor responsible for this is the difference in cut-off frequency (20 Hz for the IEEE and 1 kHz for the ICNIRP) at which thresholds for electric field strength and induced current density begin to rise (Reilly, 2005).

No thresholds have not been identified for chronic effects.

### 12.4.2 Epidemiological methods

The most common means of characterizing an exposure-response relationship in epidemiology is through the derivation of estimates of relative risk or the odds ratio per unit of exposure or across exposure categories.

Most epidemiological studies have used the latter method. In summary, two recent pooled analyses of the studies on ELF magnetic fields and childhood leukaemia have presented dose-response analyses. These analyses have been conducted both on the basis of exposure categories and of continuous exposure data. All these analyses show that the risk increase becomes detectable around 0.3–0.4 µT. For exposure levels above these values, the data at present do not allow further analysis because of the small numbers of cases in the high exposure category.

## 12.5    Risk characterization

### 12.5.1    Acute effects

Exposure limits based on the acute effects on electrically excitable tissues, particularly those in the CNS, have been proposed by several international organizations. The current ICNIRP (1998a) guidelines for the general public at 50 Hz are 5 kV m$^{-1}$ for electrical fields and 100 µT for magnetic fields, and at 60 Hz are 4.2 kV m$^{-1}$ and 83 µT. For workers, the corresponding levels are 10 kV/m and 500 µT for 50 Hz and 8.3 kV m$^{-1}$ and 420 µT for 60 Hz. The IEEE (2002) exposure levels are 5 kV m$^{-1}$ and 904 µT for exposure to 60 Hz EMF for the general public. For occupational groups, the IEEE levels are 20 kV m$^{-1}$ and 2710 µT at 60 Hz. The differences in the guidelines, derived independently by the IEEE and the ICNIRP, result from the use of different adverse reaction thresholds, different safety factors and different transition frequencies, i.e. those frequencies at which the standard function changes slope (see section 12.4.1).

### 12.5.2    Chronic effects

The most common means of characterizing risks from epidemiological data for a single endpoint is to use the attributable fraction. The attributable fraction, based on an established exposure–disease relation, is the proportion of cases (of a disease) that are attributable to the exposure. The attributable fraction is based on the comparison between the number of cases in a population that occur when the population is exposed and the number that would occur in the same population if the population were not exposed, assuming that all the other population characteristics remain the same. The assumption of a causal relationship is critical to this evaluation. As noted in Chapter 11 and later in this chapter, an assumption of this kind is difficult to accept because of the numerous limitations on the epidemiological data on childhood leukaemia and ELF magnetic field exposure and a lack of supporting evidence from a large number of experimental studies. Nevertheless, a risk characterization has been performed in order to provide some insight into the possible public health impact assuming that the association is causal.

Attributable fractions for childhood leukaemia that may result from ELF magnetic field exposure have been calculated in a number of publications (Banks & Carpenter, 1988; Grandolfo, 1996; NBOSH - National Board of Occupational Safety and Health et al., 1996; NIEHS, 1999). Greenland & Kheifets (2006) have expanded on the analyses of two different sets of pooled data on childhood leukaemia and ELF magnetic field exposure (Ahlbom et al., 2000; Greenland et al., 2000) to provide an updated evaluation covering estimates for attributable fractions in a larger number of countries than were included in the pooled analyses. In global terms, most of the information on exposure comes from industrialized countries. There are a number of regions of the world, such as Africa and Latin America, where no representative information on exposure is available. Although the odds ratios from the major study regions – North America, Europe, New Zealand and parts of Asia – are similar (and therefore estimates from a pooled analysis of data obtained in these regions could be used for the present calculation), there are substantial differences in the exposure distributions between these regions. Comparable or larger differences are expected to exist with and within other regions. Therefore, the estimates of attributable fractions calculated from the data of industrialized countries cannot be confidently generalized to cover developing countries.

Greenland & Kheifets (2006) also performed an analysis of the uncertainty in the estimates of attributable fractions, by varying the assumptions made (more details on this analysis can be found in the appendix). Using the exposure distribution from case-control studies, the calculated attributable fractions are generally below 1% for the European and Japanese studies and between 1.5 and 3% for the North American studies. Based upon the exposure surveys, the attributable fraction values vary between 1 and 5% for all areas. The confidence bounds on these numbers are relatively large. Moreover, since these calculations are highly dependent on assumptions about the exposure prevalence and distribution and on the effect of exposure on the disease, they are very imprecise. Thus, assuming that the association is causal, on a worldwide scale, the best point estimates of the calculated attributable numbers (rounded to the nearest hundred) range from 100 to 2400 childhood leukaemia cases per year that might be attributable to ELF magnetic field exposure (these numbers are derived from Figures A3 and A4 in the appendix; Kheifets, Afifi & Shimkhada, 2006), representing 0.2 to 4.9% of the total annual number of leukaemia cases, which was calculated to be around 49 000 worldwide in 2000 (IARC, 2000).

### 12.5.3    Uncertainties in the risk characterization

#### 12.5.3.1 Biophysical mechanisms

The biophysical plausibility of various proposed direct and indirect interaction mechanisms for ELF electric and magnetic fields depends in particular on whether a "signal" generated in a biological process or entity by exposure to such a field can be discriminated from inherent random noise. There is considerable uncertainty as to which mechanism(s) might be relevant. Three mechanisms related to the direct interaction of fields with the human body stand out as potentially operating at lower field levels than the others: induced electric fields in networks of neural tissues, the prolongation of the lifetime of radical pairs and effects on magnetite.

## 12.5.3.2 Exposure metric

At present it is unknown which, if any, aspect of exposure might be harmful. Certain actions, while reducing one aspect of exposure, might inadvertently increase another aspect that, if it were a causal factor, would lead to increased risk. However, the assumptions are usually that less exposure is preferable and that reducing one aspect of exposure will also reduce any aspect that might be harmful. Neither of these assumptions is certain. In fact, some laboratory research has suggested that biological effects caused by EMF vary within windows of frequency and intensity of the fields. While such a complex and unusual pattern would go against some of the accepted tenets of toxicology and epidemiology, the possibility that it may be real cannot be ignored.

## 12.5.3.3 Epidemiology

The consistently observed association between average magnetic field exposure above 0.3–0.4 $\mu$T and childhood leukaemia can be due to chance, selection bias, misclassification and other factors which can potentially confound the association or a true causal relationship. Given that the pooled analyses were based on large numbers, chance as a possible explanation seems unlikely. Taking into account potential confounding factors has not changed the risk estimates and substantial confounding from factors that do not represent an aspect of the electric or magnetic fields is unlikely. Selection bias, particularly for the controls in case-control studies, may be partially responsible for the consistently observed association between ELF magnetic field exposure and childhood leukaemia. Difficulties with exposure assessment are likely to have led to substantial non-differential exposure misclassification, but this is unlikely to provide an explanation for the observed association and may in fact lead to an underestimation of the magnitude of risk. Exposure misclassification may also introduce uncertainty into the potential dose-response relation. Because the estimates of the attributable fraction are calculated from the relative risks and exposure prevalence, and since both are affected by exposure misclassification, the attributable fraction may also be affected by exposure misclassification. However, the effect on the relative risk and on the exposure misclassification tends to work in opposite directions.

## 12.6    Conclusions

Acute biological effects have been established for exposure to ELF electric and magnetic fields in the frequency range up to 100 kHz that may have adverse consequences on health. Therefore, exposure limits are needed. International guidelines exist that have addressed this issue. Compliance with these guidelines provides adequate protection.

Consistent epidemiological evidence suggests that chronic low-intensity ELF magnetic field exposure is associated with an increased risk of childhood leukaemia. However, the evidence for a causal relationship is limited, therefore exposure limits based upon epidemiological evidence are not recommended, but some precautionary measures are warranted.

# 13 PROTECTIVE MEASURES

## 13.1 Introduction

With 25 years of research into possible health risks from ELF fields, much knowledge and understanding have been gained, but important scientific uncertainties still remain. Acute effects on the nervous systems have been identified and these form the basis of international guidelines. Regarding possible long-term effects, epidemiological studies suggest that everyday, low-intensity ELF magnetic field exposure poses a possible increased risk of childhood leukaemia, but the evidence is not strong enough to be considered causal and therefore ELF magnetic fields remain classified as possibly carcinogenic. The evidence is weaker for other studied effects, including other types of cancers in both children and adults, depression, suicide, reproductive dysfunction, developmental disorders, immunological modifications, neurological disease and cardiovascular disease.

Given the lack of conclusive data on possible long-term adverse health effcts decision-makers are faced with a range of possible measures to protect public health. The chuices to be made depend not only on the assessment of the scientific data, but also on the local public health context and the level of concern and pressure from various stakeholders.

This chapter describes public health measures for the management of ELF risks. The scientific basis for current international EMF standards and guidelines is reviewed, followed by a summary of existing EMF policies. The use of precautionary-based approaches is discussed and recommendations are provided for protective measures considered to be appropriate given the degree of scientific uncertainty.

In the context of this chapter the collective term "policy-makers" refers to national and local governmental authorities, regulators and other stakeholders who are responsible for the development of policies, strategies, regulations, technical standards and operational procedures.

## 13.2 General issues in health policy

### 13.2.1 Dealing with environmental health risks

Most risk analysis approaches that deal with the impacts on health of a particular agent include three basic steps.

The first step is to identify the health risk and establish a risk profile or risk framing. This entails a brief description of the health context, the values expected to be placed at risk and the potential consequences. It also includes prioritizing the risk factor within the overall national public and occupational health context. This step would also comprise committing resources and commissioning a risk assessment.

The second step is to perform a risk assessment (hazard identification, exposure assessment, exposure-response assessment and risk characterization), involving a scientific evaluation of the effects of the risk factor as carried out in this document (see Chapter 12). Some countries have the resources to undertake their own scientific evaluation of EMF health-related effects through a formal health risk assessment process (for example, the EMF RAPID programme in the United States, NIEHS, 1999) or through an independent advisory committee (for example, the Independent Advisory Group on Non-Ionizing Radiation in the United Kingdom, AGNIR, 2001b). Other countries may go through a less formal process to develop science-based guidelines or a variation on these.

Finally, risk management strategies need to be considered, taking into account that there is more than one way of managing all health risks. Specifically, appropriate management procedures need to be devised for complex, controversial and uncertain risks. The aim in these cases is to identify ways of coping with uncertainty and inadequate information by developing sound decision-making procedures, applying appropriate levels of precaution and seeking consensus in society. The term "risk management" encompasses all of those activities required to reach decisions on whether a risk requires elimination or reduction. Risk management strategies can be broadly classified as regulatory, economic, advisory or technological, but these categories are not mutually exclusive. Thus a broad collection of elements can be factored into the final policy-making or rule-making process, such as legislative mandates (statutory guidance), political considerations, socio-economic values, costs, technical feasibility, the population at risk, the duration and magnitude of the risk, risk comparisons and the possible impact on trade between countries. Key decision-making factors such as the size of the population, resources, the costs of meeting targets, the scientific quality of the risk assessment and subsequent managerial decisions vary enormously from one decision context to another. It is also recognized that risk management is a complex multidisciplinary procedure which is seldom codified or uniform, is frequently unstructured and can respond to evolving input from a wide variety of sources. Increasingly, risk perception and risk communication are recognized as important elements that must be considered for the broadest possible public acceptance of risk management decisions.

The process of identifying, assessing and managing risks can helpfully be described in terms of distinct steps, as described in a report of the US Presidential/Congressional Commission on Risk Assessment and Risk Management (1997) which emphasizes the analysis of possible options, clarification of all stakeholders' interests and openness in the way decisions are reached. In reality, however, these steps overlap and merge into one other, and should ideally be defined as an iterative process that includes two-way feedback and stakeholder involvement at all stages (Figure 10).

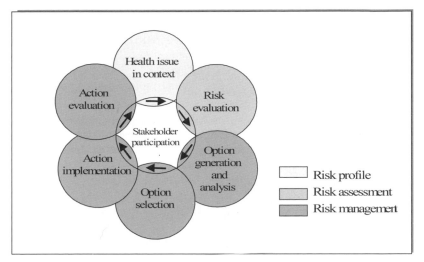

**Figure 10.** Dealing with risk: A risk analysis process that includes identifying, assessing and managing risks.

### 13.2.2 Factors affecting health policy

For policy-makers, scientific evidence carries substantial weight, but is not the exclusive criterion. Final decisions will also incorporate social values, such as the acceptability of risks, costs and benefits and cultural preferences. The question policy-makers strive to answer is "What is the best course of action to protect and promote health?"

Governmental health policies are based on a balance of "equity", i.e. the right of each citizen to an equitable level of protection and "efficiency", where cost benefit or cost-effectiveness is important. The level of risk deemed acceptable by society depends on a number of factors. Where there is an identified risk, the value that society places on the reduction of risk or disease arising from a particular agent, technology or intervention is based on the assumption that the reduction will actually occur. For involuntary exposures a notional (*de minimis*) value of lifetime mortality risk of 1 in 100 000 is accepted as a general threshold (with 1 in a million as an ideal goal) below which the risk is considered to be acceptable or impractical to improve on (WHO, 2002). For example, the risk of ionizing radiation exposure from radon is reasonably well-characterized and the exposure should be reduced so that it does not cause radiation-induced cancer in more than one per 100 000 individuals over their lifetime.

In developing policy, regulators try to maximize the benefits and minimize societal costs. The following issues are considered to be part of this process.

• *Public health/safety* – A major objective of policy is to reduce or eliminate harm to the population. Harmful effects on health are usually measured in terms of morbidity caused by the exposure and the probability that an effect would occur. They could also be measured in terms of extra cases of disease or death due to exposure, or of the number of cases avoided by reducing exposure.

- *Net cost of the policy* – The cost, referring to more than simply the monetary expense, of the policy for society as a whole, without considering any distribution of the cost, consists of several components: (a) the direct cost imposed on the entire society for any measures taken; (b) the indirect cost to society, for example, resulting from less than optimal use of the technology; and (c) cost reduction created by the policy, for example, faster implementation of a beneficial technology.

- *Public trust* – The degree of public trust in the policy and the degree of its acceptance as an effective means to adequately protect public health is an important objective in many countries. Moreover, the public's feeling of safety is important in itself, since the WHO definition of health addresses social well-being and not only the absence of disease or infirmity (WHO, 1946).

- *Stakeholder involvement* – A fair, open and transparent process is essential to good policy-making. Stakeholder involvement includes participation at each stage of policy development and opportunities to review and comment on a proposed policy prior to its implementation. Such a process may legitimately result in outcomes different from those that would be chosen by scientific experts or decision-makers alone.

- *Non-discriminatory treatment of sources* – All sources should receive the same attention when considering exposure (for example, for ELF fields, when reducing magnetic fields that result from grounding practices in the home, household appliances, power lines and transformers). The policy should focus on the most cost-effective option for reducing exposure. The policy-maker must determine whether (a) different consideration should be given to new or existing facilities and (b) there is justification for a different policy for non-voluntary and voluntary exposure. For further information, see the statement of the European Commission on the precautionary principle (EC, 2000).

- *Ethical, moral, cultural and religious constraints* – Notwithstanding stakeholder consultation, individuals and groups may differ in their views regarding whether a policy is ethical, moral and culturally acceptable or in agreement with religious beliefs. These issues can affect the implementation of a policy and need to be considered.

- *Reversibility* – The consequences of implementing a policy must be carefully considered. Policies need to be balanced and based on current information and include sufficient flexibility to be modified as new information becomes available.

## 13.3    Scientific input

Science-based evaluations of any hazards caused by EMF exposure form the basis of international guidelines on exposure limits and provide an essential input to public policy response. Criteria and procedures for determining limit values are outlined in the WHO Framework for Developing Health-based EMF Standards (WHO, 2006a).

### 13.3.1    Emission and exposure standards

Standards contain technical specifications or other precise criteria that are used consistently as rules, guidelines or definitions of characteristics to ensure that materials, products, processes and services are fit for their purpose. In the context of EMF they can be emission standards, which specify limits of emissions from a device, measurement standards, which describe how compliance with exposure or emission standards may be ensured, or exposure standards, which specify the limits of human exposure from all devices that emit EMF into a living or working environment.

Emission standards set various specifications for EMF-emitting devices and are generally based on engineering considerations, for example to minimize electromagnetic interference with other equipment and/or to optimize the efficiency of the device. Emission standards are usually developed by the International Electrotechnical Commission (IEC), the Institute of Electrical and Electronic Engineers (IEEE), the International Telecommunications Union (ITU), the Comité Européen de Normalisation Electrotechnique / European Committee for Electrotechnical Standardization (CENELEC), as well as other independent organizations and national standardization authorities.

While emission standards are aimed at ensuring, inter alia, compliance with exposure limits, they are not explicitly based on health considerations. In general, emission standards are intended to ensure that exposure to the emission from a device will be sufficiently low that its use, even in proximity to other EMF-emitting devices, will not cause exposure limits to be exceeded.

Exposure standards that limit human EMF exposure are based on studies that provide information on the health effects of EMF, as well as the physical characteristics and the sources in use, the resulting levels of exposure and the people at risk. Exposure standards generally refer to maximum levels to which whole or partial body exposure is permitted from any number of sources. This type of standard normally incorporates safety factors and provides the basic guide for limiting personal exposure. Guidelines for such standards have been issued by the International Commission on Non-Ionizing Radiation Protection (ICNIRP, 1998a), the Institute of Electrical and Electronic Engineers (IEEE, 2002) and many national authorities. These have been discussed in Chapter 12. While some countries have adopted the

ICNIRP guidelines, others use them as the de facto standard without giving them a legal basis (WHO, 2006b).

### 13.3.2 Risk in perspective

There is scientific uncertainty as to whether chronic exposure to ELF magnetic fields causes an increased risk of childhood leukaemia. In addition, given the small estimated effect resulting from such a risk, the rarity of childhood leukaemia, the rarity of average exposures higher than 0.4 µT and the uncertainty in determining the relevant exposure metric (see section 12.5.3), it is unlikely that the implementation of an exposure limit based on the childhood leukaemia data and aimed at reducing average exposure to ELF magnetic fields to below 0.4 µT, would be of overall benefit to society.

The actual exposures of the general public to ELF magnetic fields are usually considerably lower than the international exposure guidelines. However, the public's concern often focuses on the possibility of long-term effects caused by low-level environmental exposure. The classification of ELF magnetic fields as a possible carcinogen has triggered a reappraisal by some countries of whether the exposure limits for ELF provide sufficient protection. These reappraisals have led a number of countries and local governments to develop precautionary measures as discussed below.

## 13.4 Precautionary-based policy approaches

Since protecting populations is part of the political process, it is expected that different countries may choose to provide different levels of protection against environmental hazards, responding to the factors affecting health policy (see section 13.2.2). Various approaches to protection have been suggested to deal with scientific uncertainty. In recent years, increased reference has been made to precautionary policies, and in particular the Precautionary Principle.

The Precautionary Principle is a risk management tool applied in situations of scientific uncertainty where there may be need to act before there is strong proof of harm. It is intended to justify drafting provisional responses to potentially serious health threats until adequate data are available to develop more scientifically based responses. The Precautionary Principle is mentioned in international law (EU, 1992; United Nations, 1992) and is the basis for European environmental legislation (EC, 2000). It has also been referred to in some national legislation, for example in Canada (Government of Canada, 2003), and Israel (Government of Israel, 2006). The Precautionary Principle and its relationship to science and the development of standards have been discussed in several publications (Foster, Vecchia & Repacholi, 2000; Kheifets, Hester & Banerjee, 2001).

### 13.4.1 Existing precautionary ELF policies

With regard to possible effects from chronic ELF exposure, policy-makers have responded by using a wide variety of precautionary policies based on cultural, social, and legal considerations. These include the importance given to avoiding a disease that affects mostly children, the acceptability of involuntary, as opposed to voluntary, exposures and the different importance given to uncertainties in the decision-making process. Some measures are mandatory and required by law, whereas others are voluntary guidelines. Several examples are presented below.

- *Prudent avoidance* – This precautionary-based policy was developed for power-frequency EMF. It is defined as taking steps to lower human exposure to ELF fields by redirecting facilities and redesigning electrical systems and appliances at low to modest costs (Nair, Morgan & Florig, 1989). Prudent avoidance has been adopted as part of policy in several countries, including Australia, New Zealand and Sweden (see Table 85). Low-cost measures that can be taken include routing new power lines away from schools and phasing and configuring power line conductors to reduce magnetic fields near rights-of-way.

- *Passive regulatory action* – This recommendation, introduced in the USA for the ELF issue (NIEHS, 1999), advocates educating the public on ways to reduce personal exposure, rather than setting up actual measures to reduce exposure.

- *Precautionary emission control* – This policy, implemented in Switzerland, is used to reduce ELF exposure by keeping emission levels as low as "technically and operationally feasible". Measures to minimize emissions should also be "financially viable" (Swiss Federal Council, 1999). The emission levels from a device or class of devices are controlled, while the international exposure limits (ICNIRP, 1998a) are adopted as the maximum level of human exposure from all sources of EMF.

- *Precautionary exposure limits* – As a precautionary measure, some countries have reduced limits on exposure. For example, in 2003, Italy adopted ICNIRP standards but introduced two further limits for EMF exposure (Government of Italy, 2003): (a) "attention values" of one tenth of the ICNIRP reference levels for specific locations, such as children's playgrounds, residential dwellings and school premises, and (b) further restrictive "quality goals" which only apply to new sources and new homes. The chosen values for 50 Hz, 10 µT and 3 µT respectively, are arbitrary. There is no evidence of possible acute effects at that level nor evidence from epidemiological studies of leukaemia which suggests that an exposure of 3 µT is safer than an exposure of 10 or 100 µT.

Other examples of various types of precautionary policies applied to power-frequency field exposure are given in Table 86 (Kheifets et al., 2005). A complete database of EMF standards worldwide is provided on the website of the WHO International EMF Project (WHO, 2006b).

## Table 85. Examples of precautionary approaches

| Precautionary approach | Country | Measures |
|---|---|---|
| Prudent avoidance | New Zealand<br>Australia<br>Sweden | Adopt ICNIRP guidelines and add low-cost voluntary measures to reduce exposure |
| Passive regulatory action | USA | Educate the public on measures to reduce exposure |
| Precautionary emission control | Switzerland | Adopt ICNIRP guidelines and set emission limits |
| Precautionary exposure limits | Italy | Decrease exposure limits using arbitrary reduction factors |

## Table 86. Various approaches to EMF exposure limitation for the general public [a]

| Agency / country | Limits | Comments |
|---|---|---|
| *Precautionary policies based on exposure limits* | | |
| Israel, 2001 | 1 µT | Newly constructed facilities |
| Italy, 2003 | 100 µT | |
| | 10 µT | Attention value applies to exposures that occur for more than 4 hours per day |
| | 3 µT | Quality target that only applies to new lines and new homes |
| USA | 15–25 µT | Under maximum load conditions. Established by regulations in some states (e.g. Florida) and by informal guidelines in others (e.g. Minnesota) |
| | 0.2–0.4 µT | Adopted in some local ordinances (e.g. Irvine, California) |

**Table 86. Continued**

*Precautionary policies based on separation of people from sources of exposure*

| | |
|---|---|
| Ireland, 1998 | No new transmission lines or substations closer than 22 metres to an existing school or building | Local government will not grant construction permits for electrical power installations in the vicinity of schools and daycare centres |
| The Netherlands, 2005 | Increased distance between power lines and places were children can spend significant amounts of time to ensure that their mean exposure will not exceed 0.4 µT | For new buildings near existing power lines, or new power lines near existing buildings |
| USA | Restrictions on sitting new schools close to existing electric transmission lines | Adopted by the California Department of Education |
| | New lines must be buried unless technically infeasible and there must be buffer zones near residential areas, schools, day care facilities and youth camps | Adopted by the State of Connecticut |

*Precautionary policies based on costs*

| | |
|---|---|
| USA | No- or low-cost alterations to the design or routing if substantial field reduction (more than 15%) can be achieved; 4% used as benchmark of project cost | Adopted by the Public Utilities Commission for the State of California |

*Precautionary policies based on non-quantitative objectives*

| | |
|---|---|
| Australia, 2003 | Reduction of exposure where it is easily achievable | |
| Sweden, 1996 | Reduction of exposure with no recommendations regarding levels | Includes taking into account EMF when designing new transmission and distribution facilities and siting them away from sensitive areas |

[a] Source: Khalfets et al., 2005.

### 13.4.2 Cost and feasibility

The problem faced by the regulator is how to determine and evaluate the trade-off between various objectives and constraints. If zero tolerance to risk is desired, then it implies that cost is of no importance, which is problematic in a world with limited resources. On the other hand, accepting the use and introduction of technologies, provided that they have not been proven hazardous, disregards any potential health effects and may have a cost that society is not willing to pay.

From a utilitarian perspective, policy decisions cannot be made without a consideration of costs and these costs must be placed in context with the benefits. The costs and benefits of policy options should be considered at the broadest level and also presented in such a way that the costs and possible benefits to various stakeholders can be understood. All costs should be included, whether borne by industry, consumers or others. Even when allowing for the legitimate desire of society to err on the side of safety, it is likely that it will be difficult to justify more than very low-cost measures to reduce exposure to ELF fields.

Examples of approaches to considering the costs and benefits of precautionary actions on EMFs can be found in various countries. One example of an assessment of the costs of possible actions to reduce fields from power lines is in the Netherlands (Kelfkens et al., 2002). Here national geographical records were used to identify homes close to power lines, and hence to calculate the numbers of homes exposed to various levels of ELF magnetic fields. Four possible interventions were then considered: vector-sequence rearrangement, phase conductor splitting, line relocation and undergrounding, and each of these were costed for those lines where people live nearby. The effect of each of these measures on the change in distance of various field levels to the line was also calculated. Dividing the cost by the number of homes removed from exposure to the given field level provided an "average cost per dwelling gained". For 0.4 µT, this cost per dwelling for vector-sequence rearrangement, phase conductor splitting, line relocation and undergrounding was €18,000, €55,000, €128,000 and €655,000, respectively. An analysis of this kind is useful to policy-makers as it allows for the consideration and comparison of technical measures with other measures, for example, the relocation of power lines or dwellings.

Extensive "what if" policy analyses relating to EMFs from power lines and in schools were carried out in California in the late 1990s. The authors considered both a utilitarian and duty ethic approach to the question: "How certain do we need to be of the extent of the disease impact from EMFs before we would take low-cost or expensive EMF avoidance measures?" The results are summarized in a "Policy Options" document. Computer models were developed which allow users to investigate the impact of several variables, such as costs, probability of disease and extent of disease (von Winterfeldt et al., 2004). The cost–benefit analysis tended to suggest that avoidance measures at modest cost could be justified from a cost–benefit viewpoint below a "beyond a reasonable doubt" level of scientific certainty.

This approach has not been formally implemented in California, where the no- or low-cost policy has been recently reaffirmed.

Five Swedish governmental authorities published "Guidance for Decision-makers" in 1996, in which caution was recommended at reasonable expense. Examples of costing estimates were provided for several case studies. Based on their definition of the precautionary principle, measures should be considered when the fields deviate strongly from what can be deemed normal in the environment concerned (NBOSH, 1996).

When attempting to place a notional value on the benefit of preventing fatalities or cases of disease, extensive literature is available from areas other than EMFs. The two main approaches to obtaining a financial value are "human capital" and "willingness to pay". "Human capital" attempts to calculate the loss to society of a fatality, for example, by estimating the lost wages that would have been earned by that person during the rest of their life and in more sophisticated analyses including, for example, the cost to society of treating disease etc. "Willingness to pay" attempts to observe what individuals or society as a whole are willing to pay to prevent ill health or fatality, e.g. by looking at the extra salary paid to people in high-risk occupations or the amount that people are willing to pay to avoid living in an earthquake zone.

Both the "human capital" and "willingness to pay"-approaches are society-specific. For example, a WHO analysis of "The cost of diabetes in Latin America and Caribbean" (Alberto et al., 2003) used the human capital approach, calculating lost earings resulting from premature death and disability, and valued premature death in Latin America and the Caribbean at $37,000 per person. But a WHO analysis (Adams et al., 1999) of the economic value of premature death attributed to environmental tobacco smoke cites an EPA study from the USA which placed the "willingness"to pay" value of human life lost at $4.8 million per person and another study that places the value of human life lost at $5 million per person. The wage-risk trade-off method was used to determine this amount.

These examples provide an insight into how some researchers and national or local authorities have analysed several scenarios, assuming the potential health risk from ELF exposure to be important enough to implement precautionary measures. For countries without the resources to conduct such an exercise, recommendations are provided below that the Task Group considers appropriate, based on all the evidence considered.

## 13.5    Discussion and recommendations

Countries are encouraged to adopt international science-based guidelines. In the case of EMF, the international harmonization of standard-setting is a goal that countries should aim for (WHO, 2006a)

If precautionary measures are considered to complement the standards, they should be applied in such a way that they do not undermine the science-based guidelines.

Table 87. Factors relevant to the analysis of each policy option [a]

| Option | Relevant factors in considering benefits | Relevant factors in considering costs |
|---|---|---|
| Do nothing | Childhood leukaemia is a relatively rare disease, and only a small proportion of the population is exposed to levels mentioned in epidemiological studies (i.e. estimated time-weighted average above 0.3 or 0.4 µT). | No possibility of reducing burden of disease. No progress towards removal of uncertainties and better knowledge in future. |
| | There are many uncertainties regarding the effectiveness of policies, which could be reduced with scientific progres. | Undermines trust in authorities. Concerned citizens may take matters into their own hands. |
| | When the only available options are costly it may be more appropriate not to take formal action. Allows for the adaptation of policy as evidence emerges. | |
| Research | Reduces uncertainty and facilitates better decision-making. | Diversion of resources from higher priority areas. |
| | Contributes to the scientific base. | May delay actions awaiting research results. |
| | Helps in developing solutions. | |

**Table 87. Continued**

| Option | Relevant factors in considering benefits | Relevant factors in considering costs |
|---|---|---|
| Communication | A knowledgeable public<br>- can better evaluate the acceptability of different levels of ELF risks<br>- can reduce public concern due to misperceived ELF risks<br>- can increase trust in those providing the information. | Possibility of giving rise to unjustified alarm or concern.<br><br>May have limited effectiveness where the understanding of exposure is difficult or where exposure is involuntary and hard to avoid. |
| | A knowledgeable public and workers<br>- can be involved in the decision-making process regarding ELF sources<br>- can make informed decisions on what appliances to purchase or how to place them so as to minimize exposure<br>- can influence market forces to design sources in order to minimize exposure (e.g. electric blankets). | |
| Mitigation | Changes to planning of new facilities | Reassessment of the need for new facilities.<br><br>Avoid unnecessary exposure by comparing different planning scenarios so as to minimize exposure.<br><br>Use of best available technology.<br><br>Lower cost since options are dealt with in planning stage of new installations. | Requires alternative technical designs be presented for the construction of new facilities.<br><br>Costs may include sterilization of land, devaluation of property, and compensation payments.<br><br>Possibility of setting a precedent for future projects regardless of future circumstances. |

**Table 87.** Continued

| Option | | Relevant factors in considering benefits | Relevant factors in considering costs |
|---|---|---|---|
| Mitigation | Engineering changes of existing facilities | Reduction of exposure by taking protective measures such as installing shielding, changing wiring practices in houses and in distribution or transmission systems (split phasing, raising ground clearances, undergrounding etc.). | A significant part of the cost may be in identifying the instances rather than remediation. |
| | | | Changes introduced to existing installations involve a higher cost. |
| | | | Costs may include sterilization of land, devaluation of property and compensation payments. |
| | Engineering changes to appliances | Reduction of exposure to magnetic fields. | Increased cost (or increased size or weight) of appliances. |
| National standards | Exposure limits | May increase public confidence in the authority's action to protect health. | May undermine science-based guidelines. |
| | | | May give false sense of security. |
| | | | May hinder incentives for further reduction of undue exposure. |
| | | | Cost of compliance. |
| | | | Difficult to move towards less stringent standards if justified by new scientific evidence. |

a With the exception of the first option, all the options are evaluated in relation to "doing nothing" rather than adopting international guidelines.

As a result of considering the various options, policy makers will select and implement appropriate, country-specific measures for the protection of the general public and workers from exposure to ELF fields. Factors relevant to the evaluation of each policy option are given in Table 87. Precautionary measures are generally implemented through voluntary codes, encouragement and collaborative programmes rather than through mandatory enforcement, and should be seen as interim policy tools.

## Risk perception and communication

The lack of policy harmonization worldwide is one of many factors that may exacerbate public anxiety. People's perceptions of a risk depend on personal factors, external factors and the nature of the risk (Slovic, 1987). Personal factors include age, sex, and cultural or educational backgrounds, while external factors comprise the media and other forms of information dissemination, the current political and economic situation, opinion movements and the structure of the regulatory process and political decision-making in the community.

The nature of the risk can also lead to different perceptions depending on the degree of control the public has over a situation, fairness and equity aspects in locating EMF sources and fear of specific diseases (for example, cancer versus headache). The greater the number of factors that contribute to the public's perception of risk, the greater the potential for public concern. Public concern can be reduced through information and communication between the public, scientists, governments and industry. Effective risk communication is not only a presentation of the scientific calculation of risk, but also a forum for discussion on broader issues of ethical and moral concern (WHO, 2002).

## Consultation

The acceptability of the risks of ELF fields, relative to other environmental health risks, is ultimately at least as much about political and societal values and judgements as it is about scientific information. To establish public trust and confidence, stakeholders need to be involved in decision-making at the appropriate time. ELF stakeholders include government agencies, scientific and medical communities, advocacy groups, consumer protection organizations, environmental protection organizations, other affected professionals such as planners and property professionals, and industry including the electricity industry and appliance manufacturers. While there will not always be consensus on such issues, the position taken should be transparent, evidence-based and able to withstand critical scrutiny.

## Need for periodic evaluation

As new scientific information becomes available, exposure guidelines and standards should be updated. Certain studies may be more likely than others to prompt a re-evaluation of the scientific basis of the guidelines and standards because of the strength of the evidence or because of the severity of the health outcome under study. Changes to standards or policy should only be made after a proper assessment of the science base as a whole, to ensure that the conclusions of the research in a given area are consistent.

*Exposure reduction*

In recommending precautionary approaches, an overriding principle is that any actions taken should not compromise the essential health, social and economic benefits of electric power. In the light of the current scientific evidence and given the important remaining uncertainties, it is recommended that an assessment be conducted of the impact of any precautionary approach on the health, social and economic benefits of electric power. Provided that these benefits are not compromised, implementing precautionary procedures to reduce exposures is reasonable and warranted. The costs of implementing exposure reductions will vary from one country to another, making it very difficult to provide a general recommendation for balancing the costs against the risk from ELF fields. Given the weakness of the evidence for a link between exposure to ELF magnetic fields and childhood leukaemia and the limited potential impact on public health, the benefits of exposure reduction on health are unclear and thus the cost of reducing exposure should be very low.

### 13.5.1 Recommendations

In view of the above, the following recommendations are given.

- Policy-makers should establish guidelines for ELF field exposure for both the general public and workers. The best source of guidance for both exposure levels and the principles of scientific review are the international guidelines.

- Policy-makers should establish an ELF EMF protection programme that includes measurements of fields from all sources to ensure that the exposure limits are not exceeded either for the general public or workers.

- Provided that the health, social and economic benefits of electric power are not compromised, implementing very low-cost precautionary procedures to reduce exposures is reasonable and warranted.

- Policy-makers and community planners should implement very low-cost measures when constructing new facilities and designing new equipment including appliances.

- Changes to engineering practice to reduce ELF exposure from equipment or devices should be considered, provided that they yield other additional benefits, such as greater safety, or involve little or no cost.

- When changes to existing ELF sources are contemplated, ELF field reduction should be considered alongside safety, reliability and economic aspects.

- Local authorities should enforce wiring regulations to reduce unintentional ground currents when building new or rewiring existing facilities, while maintaining safety. Proactive measures to identify violations or existing problems in wiring would be expensive and unlikely to be justified.

- National authorities should implement an effective and open communication strategy to enable informed decision-making by all stakeholders; this should include information on how individuals can reduce their own exposure.

- Local authorities should improve planning of ELF EMF-emitting facilities, including better consultation between industry, local government, and citizens when siting major ELF EMF-emitting sources.

- Government and industry should promote research programmes to reduce the uncertainty of the scientific evidence on the health effects of ELF field exposure.

# APPENDIX: QUANTITATIVE RISK ASSESSMENT FOR CHILDHOOD LEUKAEMIA

Although a causal relationship between magnetic fields and childhood leukaemia has not been established, estimates of the possible public health impact which assume causality are presented below in order to provide a potentially useful input into policy analysis under different scenarios (Kheifets, Afifi & Shimkhada, 2006).

The public health impact of exposure to an agent can be based on calculations of attributable fractions. The attributable fraction, based on an established exposure-disease relation, is the proportion of the case load (of disease) that is attributable to the exposure assuming there is a causal relationship. The attributable fraction is based on the difference between the number of cases in a population that occur when the population is subject to a given exposure distribution, and the number that would occur in the same population if that distribution were changed (e.g. if exposure was reduced or eliminated by an intervention). In this calculation, it is assumed that all other population characteristics remain the same. Hence, the attributable fraction can be used to estimate the degree of incidence reduction that would be expected if exposure were reduced. Since the epidemiological literature has consistently found elevated risk of childhood leukaemia at ELF magnetic field exposure levels above 0.3 μT for the arithmetic mean and above 0.4 μT for the geometric mean, attributable-fraction estimates for these (relatively) high-level exposures allow the estimated impact on disease incidence of eliminating or reducing exposure above these levels, assuming the relation between exposure and leukaemia incidence is causal.

There are two basic pieces of information needed to make a crude estimate of the attributable fraction: (1) an estimate of the exposure effect on the disease and (2) the prevalence of exposure in the population.

## A.1    Exposure distribution

In evaluating the risks from exposure to any biologically active agent, physical, biological, or chemical, it is important to understand the distribution and magnitudes of the exposures in the general population. In order to effectively quantify the risks of childhood leukaemia, if any, from exposure to ELF magnetic fields, we must first get some estimate of the degree of exposure in children. As noted in Chapter 2, these exposures will different from country to country due to a number of factors, most notably the frequency and voltage used for power distribution.

There are two types of studies from which the exposure distribution is extracted: (1) exposure surveys to provide estimates of the exposure prevalence in children ($P_0$), and (2) case series from case-control studies to provide estimates of $P_0$ and $P_1$ where $P_1$ is the exposure prevalence in children with childhood leukaemia. Use of each of these sources provides some advantage. Case-control studies provide most relevant measurements of exposure, but may be biased, if for example, restrictions on the population (e.g. to live within a certain distance of power lines) make the case exposure prevalence in the study different from the population prevalence $P_1$; this renders unusable the case and control prevalences from studies with exposure-related restrictions. Even if the cases are representative, the controls will not be if matching has been done and the matching factors are associated with exposure; in that case the $P_0$ estimate from the study will be biased upward, toward $P_1$; fortunately, the most common matching factors were child's age and sex, which appear to be almost independent of exposure in the studies (Greenland, 2001; 2005). Exposure surveys, on the other hand, included both children and adults, as well as personal measurements throughout the day, that are thus only tangentially related to the exposure in the child's bedroom. At the very least the use of both of these sources provides a range of relevant exposures and subsequently a range of attributable fractions and numbers for consideration.

In contrast, in the case-control studies, the exposure distributions of the cases were used. For those case-control studies included in each pooled analysis, the exposure distribution reported in the pooled analysis was used. For studies not included in either pooled analysis, the exposure distribution was extracted directly from the study. (See Tables A.1 and A.2 for details of all the exposure distributions used.) It is assumed that there are no significant difference in the exposure distributions based on exposure surveys and on case-control studies. Furthermore, it is assumed that exposures obtained using personal measures are equivalent to those from household measurements, regardless of length of time of measurement.

Globally, there is disproportionately more information on exposure from industrialized countries; and among these countries, the majority of the studies have been in the USA and, to a lesser extent, in Europe. There are a number of regions of the world, such as Africa and Latin America, where no representative information on exposure is available. Furthermore, there can be substantial differences in the exposure distributions within a region; for example, exposures in Korea are probably very different from those in China and India. This poses a difficulty for a global estimation of attributable fractions and numbers since these are highly dependent on the exposure distribution, hence emphasizing the need for more data on exposure levels worldwide.

**A.2    Exposure-response  analysis  using  attributable  fraction estimates for EMF and childhood leukaemia**

If no adjustment for covariates is needed, the values of the estimates of (1) the exposure effect on the disease and (2) the prevalence of exposure in the population are simply entered into the unadjusted (crude) attributable fraction formula (Levin, 1953):

$$AF_p = P_0(RR - 1)/[P_0(RR - 1) + 1]$$

where $AF_p$ is the estimated attributable fraction and RR is the risk ratio estimate. If confounding is present, both RR and $P_0$ should be adjusted (Rothman & Greenland, 1998), but in practice only an adjusted estimate for

RR is usually available. To make this calculation for the ELF-childhood leu-kaemia relation, as leukaemia is a rare disease, the odds ratio is assumed to estimate the risk ratio. It is also assumed that the risk ratio estimates the effect in the target population, that there is no bias, and no change in the effect estimate moving from the study to the target population (Greenland, 2004). Performing analyses that incorporate uncertainty from biases and other sources of uncertainty beyond random error are highly informative and require sophisticated techniques.

The attributable number is defined as the excess number of cases attributable to exposure. For example, the attributable number associated with high exposures is interpreted as the number of cases that would be averted if these exposures were eliminated. The attributable number is obtained by multiplying the attributable fraction by the total number of cases:

$$AN = AF_p \times m_1$$

where AN is the attributable number and $m_1$ is the number of cases.

For case-control studies with adjusted odds ratios, a less biased for-mula than that given by Levin is:

$$AF_p = P_1(RR_a-1) / RR_a$$

where $RR_a$ is the adjusted rate ratio estimate (study odds ratio) and $P_1$ is the exposure prevalence among the cases in the target population (Rothman & Greenland, 1998). This formula has the advantage of requiring no adjustment of $P_1$ to be valid, and is unaffected by matching controls to cases. Further-more, assuming that exposure is independent of the adjustment factors (which appears to be approximately true in studies that did not match at all or matched on age and sex only) allows one to estimate $P_0$ from $P_1$ and $RR_a$ via the (rare-disease) formula:

$$P_0 / (1-P_0) = P_1 / (1-P_1)RR_a.$$

It is also possible to make the calculations using continuous exposure data as does Greenland et al. (2001) for 11 studies. It is not possible to do that here because such data were not available from all the sources used in this analysis, and the results in Greenland et al. (2001) indicate that results from continuous exposure would differ little from the categorical results.

Dose response functions from two pooled analyses were used for estimating the RRs. One of the differences between the two pooled analyses is in the exposure metric used: Ahlbom et al. (2000) looked at the association between the geometric mean magnetic field level and childhood leukaemia in nine epidemiologic studies, Greenland et al. (2000), however, used the arithmetic mean to examine this association in twelve studies; Greenland (2005) extended this analysis to include 14 studies using a dichotomy at

0.3 μT. The other difference in these two analyses relates to the categories used for classifying exposures. In Ahlbom et al. (2000), four categories were used relating to < 0.1 μT, 0.1–< 0.2 μT, 0.2–< 0.4 μT, and ≥ 0.4 μT. In contrast, Greenland et al. (2000) used ≤ 0.1 μT, > 0.1–≤ 0.2 μT, > 0.2 –≤ 0.3 μT, and > 0.3 μT. To address the sensitivity of attributable fraction estimates to the choice of data sets and exposure categorization, two sets of attributable fraction estimates are presented relating to these two methods for developing RRs.

In the pooled analysis by Ahlbom et al. (2000), risk for childhood leukaemia with mean residential magnetic field exposure is: OR = 1.08, (95% CI = 0.891.31) for 0.1–0.2 μT, OR = 1.11 (0.89–1.47) for 0.2–0.4 μT, OR = 2.00 (1.27–3.13) for above 0.4 μT relative to exposure below 0.1 μT. In the pooled analysis by Greenland et al. (2000) OR = 1.01 (0.84–1.21) for 0.1–0.2 μT, OR = 1.06 (0.78–1.44) for 0.2–0.3 μT, and OR = 1.68 (1.24–2.31) for exposures greater than 0.3 μT, all compared to less than 0.1 μT (both the point estimate and confidence limits remain virtually unchanged by adding 2 studies). Incorporating, in addition to the random error, all sources of bias increases the last estimate to an OR = 2.7 (0.99–32.5) (Greenland, 2005) (Note: this estimate will be used later to incorporate additional uncertainty into the attributable fraction calculations.) .

## A.3    Risk characterization

Attributable fraction (AF) estimates were made for all countries with an exposure distribution (see Figures A.1 and A.2). For the US and Germany, where there were multiple distributions, the largest of the case-control studies and the largest of the exposure surveys were used for the AF calculation used in Figure A.1. The AF estimates are divided into different exposure categories to enable a comparison of high exposures to overall exposure.

The attributable numbers (AN) of leukaemia cases were calculated for regions around the world and then added to obtain a global estimate. To compute these regional estimates, the lowest and highest exposure levels estimated in Tables A.1 and A.2 from the countries in that region were used to come up with a regional range. Where there was no information from any country in the region, the lowest and highest exposure prevalences from Tables A.1 and A.2 were used. The range of exposure prevalences for the arithmetic mean being > 0.3 μT used was 0.47% and 10.49% (Table A.1); that for the geometric mean being 0.4 μT was 0.37% and 4.78% (Table A.2). Yang's study (Yang, Ju & Myung, 2004), which is based on a larger sample and considered as more representative for non-Western regions, was used to calculate an upper range for regions with unknown levels (Latin America, Africa, Oceania). These low and high estimates were each added together to come up with a range for the entire world (Figures A.3 and A.4).

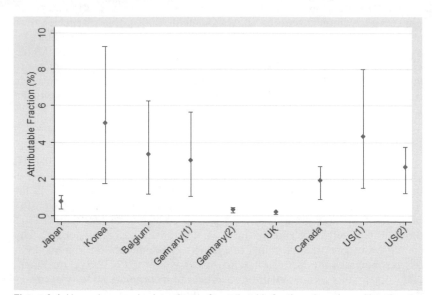

**Figure A.1.** Upper, lower and point estimates for attributable fractions, based on arithmetic mean exposure using exposure distributions for specific countries and estimate of effect from the pooled analysis by Greenland et al., 2000. (Japan: Kabuto et al., 2006; Korea: Yang, Ju & Myung, 2004; Belgium: Decat, Van den Heuvel & Mulpas, 2005; Germany(1): Brix et al., 2001; Germany(2): Schüz et al., 2001; UK: UKCCSI, 1999; Canada: McBride et al., 1999; US(1): Zaffanella & Kalton, 1998; US(2): Linet et al., 1997.)

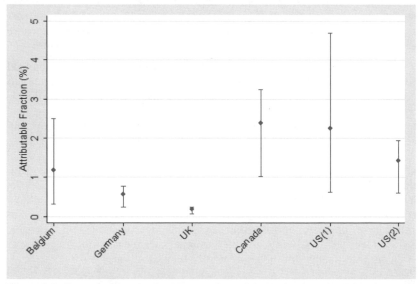

**Figure A.2.** Upper, lower and point estimates for attributable fractions, based on geometric mean exposure using exposure distributions for specific countries and estimate of effect from the pooled analysis by Ahlbom et al., 2000. (Belgium: Decat, Van den Heuvel & Mulpas, 2005; Germany: Michaelis et al., 1998; UK: UKCCSI, 1999; Canada: McBride et al., 1999; US(1): Zaffanella & Kalton, 1998; US(2): Linet et al., 1997.)

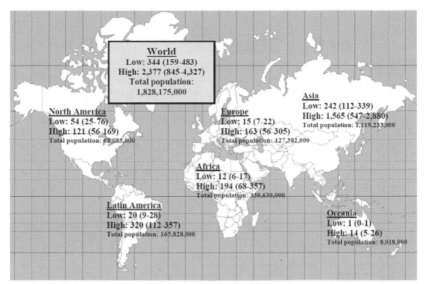

**World**
Low: 344 (159-483)
High: 2,377 (845-4,327)
Total population:
1,828,175,000

**North America**
Low: 54 (25-76)
High: 121 (56-169)
Total population: 68,083,000

**Europe**
Low: 15 (7-22)
High: 163 (56-305)
Total population: 127,382,000

**Asia**
Low: 242 (112-339)
High: 1,565 (547-2,880)
Total population: 1,119,233,000

**Africa**
Low: 12 (6-17)
High: 194 (68-357)
Total population: 339,630,000

**Latin America**
Low: 20 (9-28)
High: 320 (112-357)
Total population: 165,828,000

**Oceania**
Low: 1 (0-1)
High: 14 (5-26)
Total population: 8,018,000

**Figure A.3.** Estimated number and range of world-wide and regional cases of childhood leukaemia among children under 14 years of age that are possibly attributable to EMF arithmetic mean exposure > 0.3 µT (and the corresponding derived confidence interval). Regional range is based on the lowest level and highest exposure levels from the countries in a given region. Where there was no information from any countries in the region, the lowest and highest exposure levels overall were used.

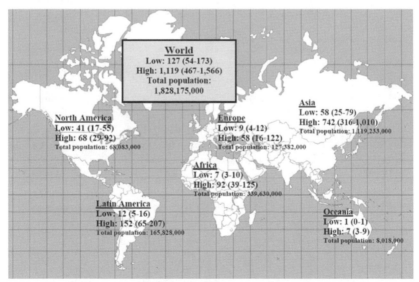

**World**
Low: 127 (54-173)
High: 1,119 (467-1,566)
Total population:
1,828,175,000

**North America**
Low: 41 (17-55)
High: 68 (29-92)
Total population: 68,083,000

**Europe**
Low: 9 (4-12)
High: 58 (16-122)
Total population: 127,382,000

**Asia**
Low: 58 (25-79)
High: 742 (316-1,010)
Total population: 1,119,233,000

**Africa**
Low: 7 (3-10)
High: 92 (39-125)
Total population: 339,630,000

**Latin America**
Low: 12 (5-16)
High: 152 (65-207)
Total population: 165,828,000

**Oceania**
Low: 1 (0-1)
High: 7 (3-9)
Total population: 8,018,000

**Figure A.4.** Estimated number and range of world-wide and regional cases of childhood leukaemia among children under 14 years of age that are possibly attributable to EMF geometric mean exposure ≥ 0.4 µT (and the corresponding derived confidence interval). Regional range is based on the lowest level and highest exposure levels from the countries in a given region. Where there was no information from any countries in the region, the lowest and highest exposure levels overall were used.

379

**Table A.1. Exposure distribution of the arithmetic mean based on exposure of cases in a case-control study or all respondents in an exposure survey**

| Country | Study | Study type | Measurement | Magnetic field category (µT) | | | | N |
|---|---|---|---|---|---|---|---|---|
| | | | | 0.1 | > 0.1–≤ 0.2 | > 0.2–≤ 0.3 | > 0.3 | |
| Belgium | Decat, Van den Heuvel & Mulpas, 2005 | Exposure survey | 24-hr personal | 81.9% | 11.5% | 1.6% | 5.1% | 251 |
| Canada | McBride et al., 1999 [a] | Case-control | 48-hr personal | 58.59% | 25.93% | 10.77% | 4.71% | 297 |
| Germany | Michaelis et al., 1998 [a] | Case-control | 24-hr bedroom | 85.23% | 9.66% | 1.70% | 3.41% | 176 |
| | Brix et al., 2001 | Exposure survey | 24-hr personal | 73.6% | 17.8% | 4.1% | 4.5% | 1952 |
| | Schüz et al., 2001 [b] | Case-control | 24-hr bedroom | 91.83% | 6.42% | 0.97% | 0.78% | 514 |
| Japan | Kabuto et al., 2006 [b] | Case-control | 7-day home | 88.46% | 5.77% | 3.85% | 1.92% | 312 |
| Korea | Yang, Ju & Myung, 2004 | Exposure survey | 24-hr personal | 64.0% | 24.2% | 4.0% | 7.8% | 409 |
| UK | UKCCSI, 1999 [b] | Case-control | 48-hr home | 92.73% | 5.31% | 1.49% | 0.47% | 1073 |
| USA | London et al., 1991 [a] | Case-control | 24-hr bedroom | 67.90% | 18.52% | 3.09% | 10.49% | 162 |
| | Linet et al., 1997 [a] | Case-control | 24-hr bedroom | 63.17% | 23.82% | 6.43% | 6.58% | 638 |
| | Zaffanella & Kalton, 1998 | Exposure survey | 24-hr personal | 64.2% | 21.1% | 7.8% | 6.6% | 995 |
| | Zaffanella, 1993 | Exposure survey | 24-hr home | 72.3% | 17.5% | 5.6% | 4.6% | 987 |

[a] Based on the distribution for pooled analysis reported by Greenland et al., 2000 .

[b] Exposure categories: < 0.1, 0.1–< 0.2, 0.2–≤ 0.4, ≥ 0.4 µT.

Table A.2. Exposure distribution of the geometric mean based on exposure of cases in a case-control study or all respondents in an exposure survey

| Country | Study | Study type | Measurement | Magnetic field category (µT) | | | | N |
|---------|-------|-----------|-------------|-------|-------------|-------------|-------|---|
| | | | | < 0.1 | 0.1–< 0.2 | 0.2–< 0.4 | ≥ 0.4 | |
| Belgium | Decat, Van den Heuvel & Mulpas, 2005 | Exposure survey | 24-hr personal | 91.9% | 4.1% | 2.8% | 1.2% | 251 |
| Canada | McBride et al., 1999 [a] | Case-control | 48-hr personal | 63.97% | 20.59% | 10.66% | 4.78% | 272 |
| Germany | Michaelis et al., 1998 [a] | Case-control | 24-hr bedroom | 89.14% | 6.86% | 2.86% | 1.14% | 175 |
| UK | UKCCSI, 1999 [a] | Case-control | 48-hr home | 94.87% | 3.54% | 1.21% | 0.37% | 1073 |
| USA | Zaffanella & Kalton, 1998 | Exposure survey | 24-hr personal | 72.6% | 17.6% | 7.5% | 2.3% | 995 |
| | Linet et al., 1997 [a] | Case-control | 24-hr bedroom | 70.25% | 18.66% | 8.24% | 2.86% | 595 |

[a] Based on the distribution for pooled analysis reported by Ahlbom et al., (2000).

381

**Table A.3. Point, low and high estimates of the proportion (AF) and number (AN) of cases in the USA for the hypothetical scenario of 50% reduction in exposure**

| Arithmetic mean | Exposures above: | | |
|---|---|---|---|
| | 0.1 µT | 0.2 µT | 0.3 µT |
| **Proportion of all cases attributable to exposure (AF):** | | | |
| Current exposure distribution[a] | 5.41% (-3.78%, 16.48%) | 5.18% (-0.05%, 11.96%) | 4.73% (1.65%, 8.73%) |
| Hypothetical distribution[b]: all exposures decreased by 50% | 1.27% (-2.02%, 5.29%) | 1.16% (-0.21%, 3.02%) | 1.01% (0.34%, 1.93%) |
| **Number of cases attributable to exposure (AN):** | | | |
| Current exposure distribution | 138 (-97, 421) | 133 (-1, 306) | 121 (42, 223) |
| Hypothetical distribution: all exposures reduced by 50% | 32 (-52, 135) | 30 (-5, 77) | 26 (9, 49) |
| Number of cases averted due to exposure reduction | 105 (-45, 286) | 103 (4, 228) | 95 (33, 174) |

| Geometric mean | 0.1 µT | 0.2 µT | 0.4 µT |
|---|---|---|---|
| **Proportion of all cases attributable to exposure (AF):** | | | |
| Current exposure distribution[a] | 3.95% (-2.83%, 12.30%) | 2.46% (-0.71%, 6.77%) | 1.67% (0.46%, 3.49%) |
| Hypothetical distribution[b]: all exposures decreased by 50% | 0.94% (-0.99%, 3.32%) | 0.37% (-0.20%, 1.17%) | 0.20% (0.05%, 0.42%) |
| **Number of cases attributable to exposure (AN):** | | | |
| Current exposure distribution | 101 (-72, 315) | 63 (-18, 173) | 43 (12, 89) |
| Hypothetical distribution: all exposures decreased by 50% | 24 (-25, 85) | 10 (-5, 30) | 5 (1, 6) |
| Number of cases averted due to exposure reduction | 77 (-47, 230) | 53 (-13, 143) | 38 (10, 83) |

[a] Calculated log-normal distribution based on Zaffanella & Kalton, 1998.

[b] Calculated log-normal distribution based on Zaffanella & Kalton, 1998, with all exposures reduced by 50%

To estimate the impact of a hypothetical scenario where the population's exposure distribution is reduced by 50%, a new exposure distribution was calculated to reflect this change. Calculating the exposure distribution shift requires knowing the mean and standard deviation of the distribution; this information was available for only one of the distributions, the USA EMF Rapid Survey, 1998 (Zaffanella & Kalton, 1998). Hence, AF and AN estimates for exposures greater than 0.1 μT, 0.2 μT, 0.3 μT or 0.4 μT were calculated for the arithmetic mean and geometric mean exposure distributions, before and after making the 50% exposure reduction in the USA (see Table A.3). The difference in the AN reflects the number of cases that would be averted due to the exposure reduction of 50%.

The conventional calculations of AF do not reflect any source of uncertainty other than random error, and informal judgments regarding the effect of possible biases. To provide additional input to policy analysis also formal Bayesian analyses are provided of the impact of high residential magnetic-field exposure (as measured by AF), accounting for uncertainties about study biases as well as uncertainties about exposure distribution. These Bayesian analyses support the idea that the public-health impact of residential fields is likely to be limited, but both no impact and a large impact remain possibilities in light of the available data (Greenland & Kheifets, 2006). The difference between the two analyses varies in both directions, but on the whole the Bayesian results make the conventional results look overoptimistic and overconfident (Table A.4).

Table A.4. Conventional estimates (with 95% confidence limits) and Bayesian (posterior) percentiles for percentage of leukaemia case load attributable to exposure > 0.3 μT versus < 0.3 μT (AF%) in 15 case-control studies of magnetic fields and childhood leukaemia and in four populations with surveys of fields [a]

| Reference | Country | Population AF% (95% limits) | |
|---|---|---|---|
| | | Conventional | Posterior |
| **Case-control:** | | | |
| Coghill, Steward & Philips, 1996 | England | 0.5 (0.2, 0.7) | 0.7 (-0.4, 18 ) |
| Dockerty et al., 1998 | N.Z. | 0.9 (0.5, 1.3) | 0.9 (-0.5, 20 ) |
| Feychting & Ahlbom, 1993 | Sweden | 3.1 (1.4, 5.2 ) | 8.6 ( 0.6, 44 ) |
| Kabuto et al., 2006 | Japan | 1.5 (0.7, 2.3 ) | 3.2 (-1.0, 24 ) |
| Linet et al., 1997 | U.S. | 2.9 (1.4, 4.2 ) | 3.5 (-1.1, 20 ) |
| London et al., 1991 | U.S. | 4.5 (2.2, 6.5 ) | 4.9 (-1.2, 27 ) |
| McBride et al., 1999 | Canada | 2.1 (1.0, 3.1 ) | 3.1 (-0.9, 23 ) |
| Michaelis et al., 1998 | Germany | 1.2 (0.6, 1.8 ) | 1.0 (-0.5, 21 ) |
| Olsen, Nielsen & Schulgen, 1993 | Denmark | 0.1 (0.1, 0.2 ) | 0.6 ( 0.0, 17 ) |
| Savitz et al., 1988 | U.S. | 2.1 (1.0, 3.5 ) | 4.7 (-1.0, 34 ) |
| Schüz et al., 2001 | Germany [b] | 0.3 (0.1, 0.5 ) | 0.7 (-0.4, 17 ) |

**Table A.4. Continued**

| Reference | Country | Population AF% (95% limits) | |
|---|---|---|---|
| | | Conventional | Posterior |
| **Case-control:** | | | |
| Tomenius, 1986 | Sweden | 0.9 (0.4, 1.4 ) | 0.7 (-0.5, 18 ) |
| Tynes & Haldorsen, 1997 | Norway | 1.0 (0.4, 1.6 ) | 0.6 ( 0.0, 15 ) |
| UKCCSI, 1999 | UK [b] | 0.2 (0.1, 0.3 ) | 0.6 (-0.4, 16 ) |
| Verkasalo et al., 1993 | Finland | 1.1 (0.5, 1.9 ) | 0.8 ( 0.0, 20 ) |
| **Surveys:** | | | |
| Brix et al., 2001 | Germany | 3.1 (1.3, 5.5) | 3.8 ( 0.0, 36 ) [c] |
| Decat, Van den Heuvel & Mulpas, 2005 | Belgium | 3.0 (1.1, 6.5) | 3.8 ( 0.0, 36 ) [c] |
| Yang, Ju & Myung, 2004 | Korea | 5.2 (2.2, 9.6) | 5.6 (-0.1, 44 ) [d] |
| Zaffanella, 1993 | U.S. | 3.2 (1.3, 5.9) | 3.9 ( 0.0, 36 ) [c] |
| Zaffanella & Kalton, 1998 | U.S. | 4.4 (1.9, 8.0) | 4.5 (-0.1, 38 ) [c] |

[a] Adopted from Greenland & Kheifets, 2006.

[b] AF for > 4 μT vs. ≤ 2 μT, excluding 2-4 μT.

[c] Adjusted using the odds-ratio model for North America (direct measurement, high prevalence) and the summary field-leukaemia odds ratio of 2.9 (CI: 0.99–8.6).

[d] Adjusted using the odds-ratio model for Kabuto (direct measurement, high prevalence).

# 14   REFERENCES

Abdeen MA, Stuchly MA (1994). Modeling of magnetic field stimulation of bent neurons. *IEEE Trans Biomed Eng*, 41(11):1092-1095.

Abramsson-Zetterberg L, Grawe J (2001). Extended exposure of adult and fetal mice to 50 Hz magnetic field does not increase the incidence of micronuclei in erythrocytes. *Bioelectromagnetics*, 22:351-357.

Adair RK (1991). Constraints on biological effects of weak extremely-low-frequency electromagnetic fields. *Phys Rev*, A 43:1039-1048.

Adair RK (1992). Criticism of Lednev's mechanism for the influence of weak magnetic fields on biological systems. *Bioelctromagnetics*, 13:231-235.

Adair RK (1994). Biological responses to weak 60 Hz electric and magnetic fields must vary as the square of the field strength. *Proc Natl Acad Sci USA*, 91:(20):9422-9425.

Adair RK (1996). Didactic discussion of stochastic resonance effects and weak signals. *Bioelectromagnetics*, 17(3):242-245.

Adair RK (1998). A physical analysis of the ion parametric resonance model. *Bioelectromagnetics*, 19(3):181-191.

Adair RK (1999). Effects of very weak magnetic fields on radical pair reformation. *Bioelectromagnetics*, 20:255-263.

Adair RK (2001). Simple neural networks for the amplification and utilization of small changes in neuron firing rates. *Proc Natl Acad Sci USA*, 98(13):7253-7258.

Adair RK, Astumian RD, Weaver JC (1998). Detection of weak electric fields by sharks, rays and skates. *Chaos*, 8(3):576-587.

Adams EK et al. *The costs of environmental tobacco smoke (ETS): An international review.* Geneva, WHO, 1999.

Adrian DJ (1977). Auditory and visual sensations stimulated by low-frequency electric currents. *Radio Sci*, 12:243-250.

Afzal SMJ, Levine GA, Liburdy RP. Environmental-level magnetic fields and estrogen-induced growth promotion in human breast and brain tumor cell lines. In: Bersani F, ed. *Electricity and Magnetism in Biology and Medicine*. Bologna, Plenum Press, 1998:473-76.

AGNIR - Advisory Group on Non-Ionising Radiation. *Health Effects related to the use of Visual Display Units.* Chilton, National Radiological Protection Board, 1994 (Documents of the NRPB, Vol. 5, No. 2).

AGNIR - Advisory Group on Non-Ionising Radiation. *ELF electromagnetic fields and neurodegenerative disease.* Chilton, National Radiological Protection Board, 2001a (Documents of the NRPB, Vol. 12, No. 4).

AGNIR - Advisory Group on Non-Ionising Radiation. *ELF electromagnetic fields and the risk of cancer.* Chilton, National Radiological Protection Board, 2001b (Documents of the NRPB, Vol. 2, No.1).

AGNIR - Advisory Group on Non-Ionising Radiation. *Magnetic fields and miscarriage.* Chilton, National Radiological Protection Board, 2002 (http://www.hpa.org.uk/radiation/publications/bulletin/e-no1/article1.htm, accessed 9-2-2007).

AGNIR - Advisory Group on Non-Ionising Radiation. *Particle deposition in the vicinity of power lines and possible effects on health.* Chilton, National Radiological Protection Board, 2004 (Documents of the NRPB, Vol. 15, No. 1).

AGNIR - Advisory Group on Non-Ionising Radiation. *Power Frequency Electromagnetic Fields, Melatonin and the Risk of Breast Cancer.* Chilton, Health Protection Agency, 2006 (Documents of the Health Protection Agency, Series B: Radiation, Chemical and Environmental Hazards, RCE-1).

Ahlbom A, Feychting M (2001). Current thinking about risks from currents. *Lancet*, 357:1143-1144.

Ahlbom A et al. (2000). A pooled analysis of magnetic fields and childhood leukaemia. *Br J Cancer*, 83(5):692-698.

Ahlbom A et al. (2004). Occupational magnetic field exposure and myocardial infarction incidence. *Epidemiology*, 15(4):403-408.

Åkerstedt T et al. (1999). A 50-Hz electromagnetic field impairs sleep. *J Sleep Res*, 8(1):77-81.

Akselrod S et al. (1981). Power spectrum analysis of heart rate fluctuation: A quantitive probe of beat-to-beat cardiovascular control. *Science*, 213(4504):220-222.

Al-Akhras MA et al. (2001). Effects of extremely low frequency magnetic field on fertility of adult male and female rats. *Bioelectromagnetics*, 22(5):340-344.

Alberto B et al. (2003). The cost of diabetes in Latin America and the Caribbean. *Bull World Health Organ*, 81:19-27.

Allan W, Pouler EM (1992). ULF waves-their relationship to the structure of the Earth's magnetosphere. *Rep Prog Phys*, 55:533-598.

Allen SG et al. *Review of occupational exposure to optical radiation and electric and magnetic fields with regard to the proposed CEC physical agents directive.* Chilton, National Radiation Protection Board, 1994 (NRPB-R265).

Anderson LE et al. (1999). Effect of 13 week magnetic fields exposures on DMBA-initiated mammary gland carcinomas in female Sprague-Dawley rats. *Carcinogenesis*, 20(8):1615-1620.

Anderson LE et al. (2000). Effects of 50- or 60-hertz, 100 microT magnetic field exposure in the DMBA mammary cancer model in Sprague-Dawley rats: possible explanations for different results from two laboratories. *Environ Health Perspect*, 108(9):797-802.

Anderson LE et al. (2001). Large granular lymphocytic (LGL) leukemia in rats exposed to intermittent 60 Hz magnetic fields. *Bioelectromagnetics*, 22(3):185-193.

Anderson RC (1990). Primary centers and secondary concentrations of tectonic activity through time in the western hemisphere of Mars. *J Geophys Res*, 95:14595-14627.

Andersson B et al. (1996). A cognitive-behavioral treatment of patients suffering from "electric hypersensitivity". Subjective effects and reactions in a double-blind provocation study. *J Occup Environ Med*, 38(8):752-758.

Anger G, Berglund A, Hansson Mild K. *[Magnetic fields in electrical locomotives] in Swedish.* Stockholm, SSI, 1997 (1997:04).

Arafa HM et al. (2003). Immunomodulatory effects of L-carnitine and q10 in mouse spleen exposed to low-frequency high-intensity magnetic field. *Toxicology*, 187(2-3):171-181.

Arnetz BB (1997). Technological stress: psychophysiological aspects of working with modern information technology. *Scand J Work Environ Health*, 23(supp 3):1997-103.

Arnetz BB, Berg M (1996). Melatonin and adrenocorticotropic hormon levels in video display unit workers during work and leisure. *J Occup Environ Med*, 38(11):1108-1110.

Asanova TP, Rakov AI (1966). [The state of health of persons working in the electric field of outdoor 400 and 500 kV switchyards]. *Gig Tr Prof Zabol*, 10:50-52.

Asanova TP, Rakov AI. *The state of health of persons working in the electric field of outdoor 400 kV and 500 kV switchyards.* Piscataway, NJ, Institute of Electrical and Electronic Engineers, 1972 (Power Engineering Society report 10).

Attwell D (2003). Interaction of low frequency electric fields with the nervous system: the retina as a model system. *Radiat Prot Dosimetry*, 106(4):341-348.

Babbitt JT et al. (2000). Hematopoietic neoplasia in C57BL/6 mice exposed to split-dose ionizing radiation and circularly polarized 60 Hz magnetic fields. *Carcinogenesis*, 21(7):1379-1389.

Bailey WH, Nyenhuis JA (2005). Thresholds for 60 Hz magnetic field stimulation of peripheral nerves in human subjects. *Bioelectromagnetics*, 26(6):462-468.

Bailey CJ, Karhu J, Ilmoniemi RJ (2001). Transcranial magnetic stimulation as a tool for cognitive studies. *Scand J Psychol*, 42(3):297-305.

Bailey WH et al. (1997). Summary and evaluation of guidelines for occupational exposure to power-frequency electric and magnetic fields. *Health Phys*, 1973(3):433-453.

Bakos J et al. (1995). Sinusodial 50 Hz, 500 µT magnetic field has no acute effect on urinary 6-sulphatoxymelatonin in Wistar rats. *Bioelectromagnetics*, 16:377-380.

Bakos J et al. (1997). Urinary 6-sulphatoxymelatonin excretion is increased in rats after 24 hours of exposure to vertical 50 Hz, 100 µT magnetic field. *Bioelectromagnetics*, 18(2):190-192.

Bakos J et al. (1999). Urinary 6-sulphatoxymelatonin excretion of rats is not changed by 24 hours of exposure to a horizontal 50-Hz, 100-µT magnetic field. *Electro Magnetobiol*, 18(1):23-31.

Balcer-Kubiczek EK et al. (1998). BIGEL analysis of gene expression in HL60 cells exposed to X-rays or 60 Hz magnetic fields. *Radiat Res*, 150:663-672.

Balcer-Kubiczek EK et al. (2000). Expression analysis of human HL60 cells exposed to 60 Hz square- or sine-wave magnetic fields. *Radiat Res*, 153(5 Pt 2):670-678.

Band PR et al. (2000). Identification of occupational cancer risks in British Columbia: A population-based case-control study of 995 incident breast cancer cases by menopausal status, controlling for confounding factors. *J Occup Environ Med*, 42:284-310.

Band PR et al. (2004). Identification of occupational cancer risks in British Columbia: a population-based case-control study of 769 cases of non-Hodgkin's lymphoma analyzed by histopathology subtypes. *J Occup Environ Med*, 46(5):479-489.

Banks RS, Carpenter DO (1988). AC electric and magnetic fields: A new health issue (article and commentary). *Health Environ Digest*, 2:1-4.

Banks RS et al. (2002). Temporal trends and misclassification in residential 60 Hz magnetic field measurements. *Bioelectromagnetics*, 23(3):196-205.

Baraton P, Hutzler B. *Magnetically induced currents in the human body*. Geneva, International Electrotechnical Commission, 1995 (Technical Report MISCT TTA1).

Baraton P, Cahouet J, Hutzler B. *Three-dimensional computation of the electric fields induced in a human body by magnetic fields*. Electricité de France, 1993 (Technical Report 93NV00013).

Baris D, Armstrong B (1990). Suicide among electric utility workers in England and Wales. *Br J Ind Med*, 47(11):788-792.

Baris D et al. (1996a). A case cohort study of suicide in relation to exposure to electric and magnetic-fields among electrical utility workers. *Occup Environ Med*, 53(1):17-24.

Baris D et al. (1996b). A mortality study of electrical utility workers in Quebec. *Occup Environ Med*, 53(1):25-31.

Barnes FS (1992). Some engineering models for interactions of electric and magnetic-fields with biological-systems. *Bioelectromagnetics*, 13(S1):67-85.

Baroncelli P et al. (1986). A health examination of railway high-voltage substation workers exposed to ELF electromagnetic fields. *Am J Ind Med*, 10(1):45-55.

Basser PJ, Roth BJ (1991). Stimulation of a myelinated nerve axon by electromagnetic induction. *Med & Biol Eng & Comput*, 29:261-268.

Baum A et al. (1995). A histopathological study on alterations in DMBA-induced mammary carcinogenesis is rats with 50 Hz, 100 µT magnetic field exposure. *Carcinogenesis*, 16:119-125.

Baumgardt-Elms C et al. (2002). Testicular cancer and electromagnetic fields (EMF) in the workplace: results of a population-based case-control study in Germany. *Cancer Causes Control*, 13(10):895-902.

Bawin SM, Adey WR (1976). Sensitivity of calcium binding in cerebral tissue to weak environmental electric fields oscillating at low frequency. *Proc Natl Acad Sci USA*, 78(6):1999-2003.

Begenisich T, Melvin JE (1998). Regulation of chloride channels in secretory epithelia. *J Membr Biol*, 163(2):77-85.

Belanger K et al. (1998). Spontaneous abortion and exposure to electric blankets and heated water beds. *Epidemiology*, 9(1):36-42.

Bell G et al. (1992). Electrical states in the rabbit brain can be altered by light and electromagnetic-fields. *Brain Res*, 570(1-2):307-315.

Bell GB, Marino AA, Chesson AL (1994a). Frequency-specific blocking in the human brain caused by electromagnetic fields. *Neuroreport*, 5(4):510-512.

Bell GB, Marino AA, Chesson AL (1994b). Frequency-specific responses in the human brain caused by electromagnetic fields. *J Neurol Sci*, 123(1-2):26-32.

Bell GB et al. (1991). Human sensitivity to weak magnetic-fields. *Lancet*, 338(8781):1521-1522.

Bellossi A (1991). Effect of pulsed magnetic fields on leukemia-prone AKR mice. No-effect on mortality through five generations. *Leuk Res*, 15(10):899-902.

Beniashvili DS, Bilanishvili VG, Menabde MZ (1991). Low-frequency electromagnetic-radiation enhances the induction of rat mammary-tumors by nitrosomethyl urea. *Cancer Lett*, 61(1):75-79.

Beraldi R et al. (2003). Mouse early embryos obtained by natural breeding or in vitro fertilization display a differential sensitivity to extremely low-frequency electromagnetic fields. *Mutat Res*, 538(1-2):163-170.

Berman E et al. (1990). Development of chicken embryos in a pulsed magnetic field. *Bioelectromagnetics*, 11:169-187.

Bergqvist U, Vogel E, eds. *Possible health implications of subjective symptoms and electromagnetic fields. A report prepared by a European group of experts for the European Commission, DG V.* Stockholm, National Institute for Working Life, 1997 (Arbete och hälsa, 19).

Bernhardt J, Pauly H (1973). On the generation of potential differences across the membranes of ellipsoidal cells in an alternating electrical field. *Biophysik*, 10:89-98.

Bethwaite P et al. (2001). Acute leukemia in electrical workers: A New Zealand case-control study. *Cancer Causes Control*, 12:683-689.

Bhatia S et al. Epidemiology and etiology.In: *Childhood leukemias*. Cambridge, University Press, 1999:38-49.

Bjork J et al. (2001). Are occupational, hobby, or lifestyle exposures associated with Philadelphia chromosome positive chronic myeloid leukaemia? *Occup Environ Med*, 58(11):722-727.

Blackman CF, Benane SG, House DE (1993). Evidence for direct effect of magnetic-fields on neurite outgrowth. *FASEB J*, 7(9):801-806.

Blackman CF, Benane SG, House DE (2001). The influence of 1.2 microT, 60 Hz magnetic fields on melatonin- and tamoxifen-induced inhibition of MCF-7 cell growth. *Bioelectromagnetics*, 22(2):122-128.

Blackman CF et al. (1982). Effects of ELF fields on calcium-ion efflux from brain tissue in vitro. *Radiat Res*, 92:510-520.

Blackman CF et al. (1985). Effects of ELF (1-120 Hz) and modulated (50 Hz) RF fields on the efflux of calcium ions from brain tissue in vitro. *Bioelectromagnetics*, 6(1):1-11.

Blackman CF et al. (1998). Double blind test of magnetic field effects on neurite outgrowth. *Bioelectromagnetics*, 19(4):204-209.

Blackwell RP (1986). Effects of extremely-low-frequency electric fields on neuronal activity in rat brain. *Bioelectromagnetics*, 7:425-434.

Blackwell RP, Reed AL (1985). Effects of electric field exposure on some indices of CNS arousal in the mouse. *Bioelectromagnetics*, 6:105-107.

Blakemore LJ, Trombley PQ (2003). Kinetic variability of AMPA receptors among olfactory bulb neurons in culture. *Neuroreport*, 14(7):965-970.

Blanchard JP, Blackman CF (1994). Clarification and application of an ion parametric resonance model for magnetic field interactions with biological systems. *Bioelectromagnetics*, 15(3):217-238.

Bliokh PV, Nickolaenko AP, Filippov F. *Schumann resonances in the earth-ionosphere cavity.* Stevenage, Herts., Peter Peregrinus, 1980 (IEE Electromagnetic Waves Series, 9 [translation]).

Bogdanov MB et al. (1998). Elevated "hydroxyl radical" generation in vivo in an animal model of amyotrophic lateral sclerosis. *J Neurochem*, 71(3):1321-1324.

Bonhomme-Faivre L et al. (1998). Study of human neurovegetative and hematologic effects of environmental low-frequency (50-Hz) electromagnetic fields produced by transformers. *Arch Environ Health*, 53(2):87-92.

Boorman GA et al. (1997). Eight-week toxicity study of 60 Hz magnetic field in F344 rats and B6C3F1 mice. *Fundamental and applied toxicology*, 35:55-63.

Boorman GA et al. (1999a). Effect of 26 week magnetic field exposures in a DMBA initiation-promotion mammary gland model in Sprague-Dawley rats. *Carcinogenesis*, 20(5):899-904.

Boorman GA et al. (1999b). Chronic toxicity/oncogenicity evaluation of 60 Hz (power frequency) magnetic fields in F344/N rats. *Toxicol Pathol*, 27(3):267-278.

Boorman GA et al. (2000a). Magnetic fields and mammary cancer in rodents: a critical review and evaluation of published literature. *Radiat Res*, 153(5 Pt 2):617-626.

Boorman GA et al. (2000b). Evaluation of in vitro effects of 50 and 60 Hz magnetic fields in regional EMF exposure facilities. *Radiat Res*, 153(5 Pt2):648-657.

Boorman GA et al. (2000c). Leukemia and lymphoma incidence in rodents exposed to low-frequency magnetic fields. *Radiat Res*, 153(5 Pt 2):627-636.

Bourland JD, Nyenhuis JA, Schaefer DJ (1999). Physiologic effects of intense MR imaging gradient fields. *Neuroimaging Clin N Am*, 9(2):363-377.

Bowman JD et al. (1988). Exposures to extremely low frequency (ELF) electromagnetic fields in occupations with elevated leukemia rates. *Appl Ind Hyg*, 3:189-194.

Bracken MB et al. (1995). Exposure to electromagnetic-fields during pregnancy with emphasis on electrically heated beds - Association with birth-weight and intrauterine growth-retardation. *Epidemiology*, 6(3):263-270.

Bracken TD, Senior RS, Bailey WH (2005). DC electric fields from corona-generated space charge near AC transmission lines. *IEEE Trans Power Delivery*, 20(2):1692-1702.

Bracken T, Senior R, Dudman J (2005). 60-Hertz electric-field exposures in transmission line towers. *J Occup Environ Hyg*, 2(9):444-455.

Bracken TD, Senior R, Tuominen M (2004). Evaluating occupational 60-hertz electric-field exposures for guideline compliance. *J Occup Environ Hyg*, 1(10):672-679.

Bracken TD et al. *The EMDEX Project: residential study, final report.* Palo Alto, CA, Electric Power Research Institute, 1994.

Brendel H, Niehaus M, Lerchl A (2000). Direct suppressive effects of weak magnetic fields (50 Hz and 16 2/3 Hz) on melatonin synthesis in the pineal gland of Djungarian hamsters (*Phodopus sungorus*). *J Pineal Res*, 29(4):228-233.

Brent RL (1999). Reproductive and teratologic effects of low-frequency electromagnetic fields: A review of in vivo and in vitro studies using animal models. *Teratology*, 59(4):261-286.

Brent RL et al. (1993). Reproductive and teratologic effects of electromagnetic-fields. *Reprod Toxicol*, 7(6):535-580.

Brix J et al. (2001). Measurement of the individual exposure to 50 and 16 2/3 Hz magnetic fields within the Bavarian population. *Bioelectromagnetics*, 22(5):323-332.

Brocklehurst B, McLauchlan KA (1996). Free radical mechanism for the effects of environmental electromagnetic fields on biological systems. *Int J Radiat Biol*, 69(1):3-24.

Brown RH (1997). Amyotrophic lateral sclerosis. Insights from genetics. *Arch Neurol*, 54(10):1246-1250.

Buiatti E et al. (1984). Risk factors in male infertility: A case-control study. *Archiv Environ Helath*, 39(4):266-270.

Bullard EC (1948). The magnetic field within the earth. *Mon Not R Astron Soc Geophys*, Suppl. 5:248-258.

Burch JB, Reif JS, Yost MG (1999). Geomagnetic disturbances are associated with reduced nocturnal excretion of a melatonin metabolite in humans. *Neurosci Lett*, 266:209-212.

Burch JB et al. (1998). Nocturnal excretion of a urinary melatonin metabolite among electric utility workers. *Scand J Work Environ Health*, 24(3):183-189.

Burch JB et al. (1999). Reduced excretion of a melatonin metabolite in workers exposed to 60 Hz magnetic fields. *Am J Epidemiol*, 150(1):27-36.

Burch JB et al. (2000). Melatonin metabolite levels in workers exposed to 60-Hz magnetic fields: work in substations and with 3-phase conductors. *J Occup Environ Med*, 42(2):136-142.

Burch JB et al. (2002). Melatonin metabolite excretion among cellular telephone users. *Int J Radiat Biol*, 78(11):1029-1036.

Burchard JF et al. (1996). Biological effects of electric and magnetic fields on productivity of dairy cows. *J Dairy Sci*, 79(9):1549-1554.

Burchard JF et al. (2004). Lack of effect of 10 kV/m 60 Hz electric field exposure on pregnant dairy heifer hormones. *Bioelectromagnetics*, 25(4):308-312.

Burgess P, Clark M (1994). Cosmic radiation and powerlines. *Radiol Prot Bull*, 151:17-19.

Cahalan MD, Wulff H, Chandy KG (2001). Molecular properties and physiological roles of ion channels in the immune system. *J Clin Immunol*, 21(4):235-252.

Cameron IL, Hunter KE, Winters WD (1985). Retardation of embroyogenesis by extremely low frequency 60 Hz electromagnetic fields. *Physiol Chem Phys Med NMR*, 17(1):135-138.

Campbell-Beachler M et al. (1998). Effect of 60 Hz magnetic field exposure on c-*fos* expression in stimulated PC12 cells. *Mol Cell Biochem*, 189:107-111.

Cancer Research UK. 2004 (http://www.cancerresearchuk.org/, accessed 20-2-2007).

Canedo L, Cantu RG, Hernandez R (2003). Magnetic field exposure during gestation: pineal and cerebral cortex serotonin in the rat. *Int J Dev Neurosci*, 21(5):263-266.

Cano MI, Pollan M (2001). Non-Hodgkin's lymphomas and occupation in Sweden. *Int Arch Occup Environ Health*, 74(6):443-449.

Cantoni O et al. (1995). The effect of 50 Hz sinusoidal electric and/or magnetic fields on the rate of repair of DNA single/double strand breaks in oxidatively injured cells. *Biochem Molecul Biol Int*, 37(4):681-689.

Cantoni O et al. (1996). Effect of 50 Hz sinusoidal electric and/or magnetic-fields on the rate of repair of DNA single-strand breaks in cultured-mammalian-cells exposed to 3 different carcinogens - Methylmethane sulfonate, chromate and 254 nm UV-radiation. *Biochem Molecul Biol Int*, 38(3):527-533.

Caputa K et al. (2002). Modelling fields induced in humans by 50/60 Hz magnetic fields: reliability of the results and effects of model variations. *Phys Med Biol*, 47(8):1391-1398.

Carpenter RHS (1972). Electrical stimulation of the human eye in different adaptational states. *J Physiol*, 221:137-148.

Carron C et al. (2000). TEL-JAK2 transgenic mice develop T-cell leukemia. *Blood*, 95(12):3891-3899.

Carstensen EL (1985). Sensitivity of the human eye to power frequency electric fields. *IEEE Trans Biomed Eng*, 32(8):561-565.

Cartwright RA, Staines A (1992). Acute leukaemias. *Baillieres Clin Haematol*, 5(1):1-26.

Catterall WA (1995). Structure and function of voltage-gated ion channels. *Annu Rev Biochem*, 64:493-531.

Catterall WA (2000). From ionic currents to molecular mechanisms: the structure and function of voltage-gated sodium channels. *Neuron*, 26(1):13-25.

Chacon L (2000). 50-Hz sinusoidal magnetic field effect on in vitro pineal N-acetyltransferase activity. *Electro Magnetobiol*, 19:339-343.

Chadwick P, Lowes F (1998). Magnetic fields on British trains. *Ann Occup Hyg*, 42(5):331-335.

Chang RC et al. (2001). Neurons reduce glial responses to lipopolysaccharide (LPS) and prevent injury of microglial cells from over-activation by LPS. *J Neurochem*, 76(4):1042-1049.

Charles LE et al. (2003). Electromagnetic fields, polychlorinated biphenyls, and prostate cancer mortality in electric utility workers. *Am J Epidemiol*, 157(8):683-691.

Checcucci A. An epidemiological investigation of HV substation workers: study design and preliminary results. In: Grandolfo M, Michaelson SM, Rindi A, eds. *Biological effects and dosimetry of static and ELF electromagnetic fields*. New York, Springer, 1985:557-569.

Chen KM, Chuang HR, Lin CJ (1986). Quantification of interaction between ELF-LF electric fields and human bodies. *IEEE Trans Biomed Eng*, 33(8):746-756.

Chernoff N, Rogers JM, Kavet R (1992). A review of the literature on potential reproductive and developmental toxicity of electric and magnetic fields. *Toxicology*, 74(2-3):91-126.

Chiang H et al. (1995). Pulsed magnetic field from video display terminals enhances teratogenic effects of cytosine arabinoside in mice. *Bioelectromagnetics*, 16(1):70-74.

Chiang H et al. (1999). The mechanism of suppression of gap junctional intercellular communication by 50 Hz magnetic fields. *Electro Magnetobiol*, 18(3):243-247.

Chiba A et al. (1984). Application of finite element method to analysis of induced current densities inside human model exposed to 60-Hz electric field. *IEEE Trans Power Apparatus Systems*, 103:1895-1902.

Chiu RS, Stuchly MA (2005). Electric fields in bone marrow substructures at power-line frequencies. *IEEE Trans Biomed Eng*, 52(6):1103-1109.

Cho YH, Chung HW (2003). The effect of extremely low frequency electromagnetic fields (ELF-EMF) on the frequency of micronuclei and sister chromatid exchange in human lymphocytes induced by benzo(a)pyrene. *Toxicol Lett*, 143(1):37-44.

Chokroverty S et al. (1995). Magnetic brain stimulation: safety studies. *Electroencephalogr Clin Neurophysiol*, 97(1):36-42.

Chung MK, Kim JC, Myung SH (2004). Lack of adverse effects in pregnant/lactating female rats and their offspring following pre- and postnatal exposure to ELF magnetic fields. *Bioelectromagnetics*, 25(4):236-244.

Chung MK et al. (2003). Developmental toxicity evaluation of ELF magnetic fields in Sprague-Dawley rats. *Bioelectromagnetics*, 24(4):231-40.

Cintolesi F et al. (2003). Anisotropic recombination of an immobilized photoinduced radical pair in a 50 microT magnetic fields: a model avian photomagnetoreceptor. *Chem Phys*, 182:1-18.

Coelho AM, Easley SP, Rogers WR (1991). Effects of exposure to 30 kV/m, 60-Hz electric fields on the social behaviour of baboons. *Bioelectromagnetics*, 12(2):117-135.

Coelho AM, Rogers WR, Easley SP (1995). Effects of concurrent ecposure to 60 Hz electric and magnetic fields on the social behavior of baboons. *Bioelectromagnetics*, 16(Suppl 3):71-92.

Coghill RW, Steward J, Philips A (1996). Extra low frequency electric and magnetic fields in the bedplace of children diagnosed with leukaemia: a case-control study. *Eur J Cancer Prev*, 5(3):153 158.

Conti P et al. (1999). Effect of electromagnetic fields on several CD markers and transcription and expression of CD4. *Immunobiology*, 201(1):36-48.

Cook CM, Thomas AW, Prato FS (2002). Human electrophysiological and cognitive effects of exposure to ELF magnetic and ELF modulated RF and microwave fields: a review of recent studies. *Bioelectromagnetics*, 23(2):144-157.

Cook MR et al. (1992). A replication study of human exposure to 60-Hz fields - Effects on neurobehavioral measures. *Bioelectromagnetics*, 13(4):261-285.

Cooper MS (1984). Gap junctions increase the sensitivity of tissue cells to exogenous electric fields. *J Theor Biol*, 111(1):123-130.

Cooper PJ, Garny A, Kohl P (2003). Cardiac electrophysiology: theoretical considerations of a potential target for weak electromagnetic field effects. *Radiat Prot Dosimetry*, 106(4):363-368.

Cooper TJ. Occupational exposure to electric and magnetic fields in the context of the ICNIRP guidelines. Chilton, Didcot, National Radiological Protection Board, 2002 (NRPB-W24).

Coulton LA et al. (2004). Effect of 50 Hz electromagnetic fields on the induction of heat-shock protein gene exprcssion in human leukocytes. *Radiat Res*, 161(4):430-434.

Cox CF et al. (1993). A test for teratological effects of power frequency magnetic fields on chick embryos. *IEEE Trans Biomed Eng*, 40(7):605-610.

Coyle JT, Puttfarcken P (1993). Oxidative stress, glutamate, and neurodegenerative disorders. *Science*, 262(5134):689-695.

Crasson M (2003). 50-60 Hz electric and magnetic field effects on cognitive function in humans: a review. *Radiat Prot Dosimetry*, 106(4):333-340.

Crasson M, Legros JJ (2005). Absence of daytime 50 Hz, 100 microT(rms) magnetic field or bright light exposure effect on human performance and psychophysiological parameters. *Bioelectromagnetics*, 26(3):225-233.

Crasson M et al. (1999). 50 Hz magnetic field exposure influence on human performance and psychophysiological parameters: two double-blind experimental studies. *Bioelectromagnetics*, 20(8):474-486.

Crasson M et al. (2001). Daytime 50 Hz magnetic field exposure and plasma melatonin and urinary 6 sulfatoxymelatonin concentration profiles in humans. *J Pineal Res*, 31(3):234-241.

Creim JA et al. (1984). Attempts to produce taste-aversion learning in rats exposed to 60-Hz electric fields. *Bioelectromagnetics*, 5:271-282.

Crumpton MJ, Collins AR (2004). Are environmental electromagnetic fields genotoxic? *DNA Repair (Amst)*, 3(10):1385-1387.

Cruz DC et al. (1999). Physical trauma and family history of neurodegenerative diseases in amyotrophic lateral sclerosis: a population-based case-control study. *Neuroepidemiology*, 18(2):101-110.

Czerska E et al. (1992). Comparison of the effect of ELF on c-myc oncogene expression in normal and transformed human cells. *Ann N Y Acad Sci*, 649:340-342.

Czyz J et al. (2004). Non-thermal effects of power-line magnetic fields (50 Hz) on gene expression levels of pluripotent embryonic stem cells-the role of tumour suppressor p53. *Mutat Res*, 557(1):63-74.

Danish National Board of Health. *[The activity in the hospital care system] (in Danish)*. Copenhagen, Danish National Board of Health, 1981.

Dasdag S et al. (2002). Effects of extremely low frequency electromagnetic fields on hematologic and immunologic parameters in welders. *Arch Med Res*, 33(1):29-32.

Davanipour Z et al. (1997). Amyotrophic-lateral-sclerosis and occupational exposure to electromagnetic-fields. *Bioelectromagnetics*, 18(1):28-35.

Davis S et al. (2001). Residential magnetic fields, light-at-night, and nocturnal urinary 6-sulfatoxymelatonin concentration in women. *Am J Epidemiol*, 154(7):591-600.

Davis S, Mirick DK, Stevens RG (2002). Residential magnetic fields and the risk of breast cancer. *Am J Epidemiol*, 155(5):446-454.

Dawson BV et al. (1998). Evaluation of potentail health effects of 10 kHz magnetic fields: a rodent reproductive study. *Bioelectromagnetics*, 19(3):162-171.

Dawson TW (1997). An analytic solution for verification of computer models for low-frequency magnetic induction. *Radio Science*, 32(2):343-367.

Dawson TW, Stuchly M (1996). Analytic validation of a three-dimensional scalar-potential finite-difference code for low-frequency magnetic induction. *Appl Comput Eletromag Soc (ACES) J*, 11(3):72-81.

Dawson TW, Stuchly MA (1998). High resolution organ dosimetry for human exposure to low frequency magnetic fields. *IEEE Trans Magn*, 34(3):708-718.

Dawson TW, Caputa K, Stuchly MA (1997a). A comparison of 60 Hz uniform magnetic and electric induction in the human body. *Phys Med Biol*, 42:2319-2329.

Dawson TW, Caputa K, Stuchly MA (1997b). Influence of human model resolution on computed currents induced in organs by 60-Hz magnetic fields. *Bioelectromagnetics*, 18(7):478-490.

Dawson TW, Caputa K, Stuchly MA (1998). High-resolution organ dosimetry to human exposure to low-frequency electric fields. *IEEE Trans Power Delivery*, 13:366-376.

Dawson TW, Caputa K, Stuchly MA (1999a). High-resolution magnetic field numerical dosimetry for live-line workers. *IEEE Trans Magn*, 35:1131-1138.

Dawson TW, Caputa K, Stuchly MA (1999b). Magnetic induction at 60 Hz in the human heart: a comparison between the in situ and isolated scenarios. *Bioelectromagnetics*, 20(4):233-243.

Dawson TW, Caputa K, Stuchly MA (1999c). Numerical evaluation of 60 Hz magnetic induction in the human body in complex occupational environments. *Phys Med Biol*, 44(4):1025-1040.

Dawson TW, Caputa K, Stuchly MA (1999d). Organ dosimetry for human exposure to non-uniform 60-Hz magnetic fields. *IEEE Transactions on Power Delivery*, 14(4):1234-1239.

Dawson TW, Moerloose JD, Stuchly M (1996). Comparison of magnetically induced ELF fields in humans computed by FDTD and scalar potential FD codes. *Applied Computational Electromagnetics Society (ACES) J*, 11(3):63-71.

Dawson TW, Potter ME, Stuchly MA (2001). Accuracy evaluation of modelling of low frequency field interactions with the human body. *Appl Comput Eletromag Soc (ACES) J*, 16(2):162-172.

Dawson TW et al. (2001). Induced electric fields in the human body associated with 60 Hz contact currents. *IEEE Trans Biomed Eng*, 48(9):1020-1026.

de Bruyn L, de Jager L (1994). Electric Field Exposure and Evidence of Stress in Mice. *Environ Res*, 65:149-160.

De Roos AJ et al. (2003). Occupation and the risk of adult glioma in the United States. *Cancer Causes Control*, 14(2):139-150.

de Seze R et al. (1993). Effects of time-varying uniform magnetic fields on natural killer cell activity and antibody response in mice. *Bioelectromagnetics*, 14(5):405-412.

De Vita R et al. (1995). Effects of 50 Hz magnetic fields on mouse spermatogenesis monitored by flow cyctometric analysis. *Bioelectromagnetics*, 16:330-334.

Deapen DM, Henderson BE (1986). A case-control study of amyotrophic lateral sclerosis. *Am J Epidemiol*, 123(5):790-799.

Decat G, Van den Heuvel I, Mulpas L. *Monitoring survey of the 50 Hz magnetic field for the estimation of the proportion of Belgian children exposed to the epidemiological cut-off points of 0.2, 0.3, and 0.4 micro Tesla*. Erembodegem, Flemish Environmental Agency, 2005 (Final Report of the BBEMG Research Contract).

Dekker JM et al. (1997). Heart rate variability from short electrocardiographic recordings predicts mortality from all causes in middle aged and elderly men. The Zutphen study. *Am J Epidemiol*, 145(10):899-908.

Del Re B et al. (2003). Extremely low frequency magnetic fields affect transposition activity in Escherichia coli. *Radiat Environ Biophys*, 42(2):113-118.

Del Re B et al. (2004). Various effects on transposition activity and survival of Escherichia coli cells due to different ELF-MF signals. *Radiat Environ Biophys*, 43(4):265-270.

Delgado JMR et al. (1982). Embryological changes induced by weak, extremely low frequency electromagnetic fields. *J Anat*, 134(4):533-551.

Delpizzo V (1990). A model to assess personal exposure to ELF magnetic fields from common household sources. *Bioelectromagnetics*, 11:139-147.

Delpizzo V (1994). Epidemiological studies of work with video display terminals and adverse pregnancy outcomes (1984-1992). *Am J Ind Med*, 26:465-480.

Deno DW (1977). Currents induced in the human body by high voltage transmission line electric field - measurement and calculation of distribution and dose. *IEEE Trans Power Apparatus Systems*, 96:1517-1527.

Deno D, Zaffanella LE. Field effects of overhead transmission lines and stations.In: *Transmission Line Reference Book: 345 kV and above*. Palo Alto, CA, EPRI, 1982:329-419.

Desjobert H et al. (1995). Effects of 50 Hz magnetic-fields on c-myc transcript levels in nonsynchronized and synchronized human-cells. *Bioelectromagnetics*, 16(5):277-283.

Devevey L et al. (2000). Absence of the effects of 50 Hz magnetic fields on the progression of acute myeloid leukaemia in rats. *Int J Radiat Biol*, 76(6):853-862.

Dicarlo AL et al. (1999). Short-term magnetic field exposures (60 Hz) induce protection against ultraviolet radiation damage. *Int J Radiat Biol*, 75(12):1541-1549.

Dickinson HO, Parker L (1999). Quantifying the effect of population mixing on childhood leukaemia risk: the Seascale cluster. *Br J Cancer*, 81(1):144-151.

Dietrich FM, Jacobs WL. *Survey and assessment of electric and magnetic field public exposure in the transportation environment*. US Department of Transportation, Federal Railroad Administration, 1999 (Report No PB99-130908).

DiGiovanni J et al. (1999). Lack of effect of 60 Hz magnetic field on biomarkers of tumor promotion in the skin of SENCAR mice. *Carcinogenesis*, 20(4):685-689.

Dimbylow PJ (1987). Finite difference calculations of current densities in a homogeneous model of a man exposed to extremely low frequency electric fields. *Bioelectromagnetics*, 8:355-375.

Dimbylow PJ (1997). FDTD calculations of the whole-body averaged SAR in an anatomically realistic voxel model of the human body from 1 MHz to 1 GHz. *Phys Med Biol*, 42(3):479-490.

Dimbylow PJ (1998). Induced current densities from low-frequency magnetic fields in a 2 mm resolution, anatomically realistic model of the body. *Phys Med Biol*, 42:221-230.

Dimbylow PJ (2000). Current densities in a 2 mm resolution anatomically realistic model of the body induced by low frequency electric fields. *Phys Med Biol*, 45:1013-1022.

Dimbylow PJ (2005). Development of the female voxel phantom, NAOMI, and its application to calculations of induced current densities and electric fields from applied low frequency magnetic and electric fields. *Phys Med Biol*, 50(6):1047-1070.

Ding GR, Nakahara T, Miyakoshi J (2002). Exposure to power frequency magnetic fields and X-rays induces GAP-43 gene expression in human glioma MO54 cells. *Bioelectromagnetics*, 23(8):586-591.

Ding GR et al. (2001). Increase in hypoxanthine–guanine phosphoribosyl transferase gene mutations by exposure to electric field. *Life Sci*, 68:1041-1046.

Dlugosz L et al. (1992). Congenital defects and electric bed heating in New York State: a register-based case-control study. *Am J Epidemiol*, 135(9):1000-1011.

Dockerty JD et al. (1998). Electromagnetic field exposures and childhood cancers in New Zealand. *Cancer Causes Control*, 9(3):299-309.

Dockerty JD et al. (1999). Electromagnetic field exposures and childhood leukemia in New Zealand. *Lancet*, 354(9194):1918-1919.

Dolezalek H. Atmospheric electricity. In: Weast RC, ed. *Handbook of Chemistry and Physics*. Boca Raton, FL, CRC Press Inc., 1979.

Donnelly KE, Agnew D. *Exposure assesment methods for a childhood epidemiology study*. Pickering, Ontario Hydro Health and Safety Division, 1991 (HSD-ST-9).

Dovan T, Kaune WT, Savitz DA (1993). Repeatability of measurements of residential magnetic fields and wire codes. *Bioelectromagnetics*, 14(2):145-159.

Dowman R et al. (1989). Chronic exposure of primates to 60-Hz electric and magnetic fields: III. Neurophysiologic effects. *Bioelectromagnetics*, 10(3):303-317.

Dowson DI et al. (1988). Overhead high-voltage cables and recurrent headache and depressions. *Practitioner*, 232(1447):435-436.

Draper GJ, Kroll ME, Stiller CA (1994). Childhood cancer. *Cancer Surv*, 19-20:493-517.

Draper G et al. (2005). Childhood cancer in relation to distance from high voltage power lines in England and Wales: a case-control study. *Br Med J*, 330(7503):1290.

Drucker-Colin R et al. (1994). Comparison between low frequency magnetic field stimulation and nerve growth factor treatment of cultured chromaffin cells, on neurite growth, noradrenaline release, excitable properties, and grafting in nigrostriatal lesioned rats. *Mol Cell Neurosci*, 5(6):485-498.

Easley SP, Coelho AM, Rogers WR (1991). Effects of exposure to a 60-kV/m, 60-Hz electric field on the social behavior of baboons. *Bioelectromagnetics*, 12:361-375.

EC - Commission of the European Communities. *Non-ionizing radiation. Sources, exposure and health effects*. Luxembourg, Office for Official Publications of the European Communities, 1996.

EC - Commission of the European Communities. *Communication on the Precautionary Principle*. 2000 (http://europa.eu.int/comm/off/com/health_consumer/precaution.htm, accessed 16-2-2007).

Edmonds DT (1993). Larmor precession as a mechanism for the detection of static and alternating magnetic fields. *Bioelectrochem Bioenerg*, 30:3-12.

Ekström T, Mild KH, Holmberg B (1998). Mammary tumours in Sprague-Dawley rats after initiation with DMBA followed by exposure to 50 Hz electromagnetic fields in a promotional scheme. *Cancer Lett*, 123(1):107-111.

Elbetieha A, Al-Akhras MA, Darmani H (2002). Long-term exposure of male and female mice to 50 Hz magnetic field: effects on fertility. *Bioelectromagnetics*, 23(2):168-172.

Engelborghs S, D'Hooge R, De Deyn PP (2000). Pathophysiology of epilepsy. *Acta Neurol Belg*, 100(4):201-213.

EPA - US Environmental Protection Agency. *EMF in your environment: magnetic field measurements of everyday electrical devices*. Washington, DC, US Environmental Protection Agency, 1992.

Eriksson A et al. *50 Hz magnetic fields in dwellings*. Stockholm, National Board of Occupational Safety and Health, 1987 (1987:6).

Eskelinen T et al. (2002). Use of spot measurements for assessing residential ELF magnetic field exposure: a validity study. *Bioelectromagnetics*, 23(2):173-176.

EU - European Union (1992). Treaty on European Union. *Official Journal of the European Communities*, C 191.

Eveson RW et al. (2000). The effects of weak magnetic fields on radical recombination reactions in micelles. *Int J Radiat Biol*, 76(11):1509-1522.

Fabbro-Peray P, Daures JP, Rossi JF (2001). Environmental risk factors for non-Hodgkin's lymphoma: a population-based case-control study in Languedoc-Roussillon, France. *Cancer Causes Control*, 12(3):201-212.

Fairbairn DW, O'Neill KL (1994). The effects of electromagnetic fields exposure on the formation of DNA sinlge strand breaks in human cells. *Cell Mol Biol*, 40(4):561-567.

Fam WZ, Mikhail EL (1993). A system for the exposure of small laboratory animals to a 25-mT 60-Hz alternating or traveling magnetic field. *IEEE Trans Biomed Eng*, 40(7):708-711.

Fam WZ, Mikhail EL (1996). Lymphoma induced in mice chronically exposed to very strong low-frequency electromagnetic-field. *Cancer Lett*, 105(2):257-269.

Farrell JM et al. (1997). The effect of pulsed and sinusoidal magnetic fields on the morphology of developing chick embryos. *Bioelectromagnetics*, 18(431):431-438.

Fear EC, Stuchly MA (1998a). A novel equivalent circuit model for gap-connected cells. *Phys Med Biol*, 43(6):1439-1448.

Fear EC, Stuchly MA (1998b). Biological cells with gap junctions in low-frequency electric fields. *IEEE Trans Biomed Eng*, 45(7):856-866.

Fear EC, Stuchly MA (1998c). Modeling assemblies of biological cells exposed to electric fields. *IEEE Trans Biomed Eng*, 45(10):1259-1271.

Fedrowitz M, Kamino K, Löscher W (2004). Significant differences in the effects of magnetic field exposure on 7,12-dimethylbenz(a)anthracene-induced mammary carcinogenesis in two substrains of Sprague-Dawley rats. *Cancer Res*, 64(1):243-251.

Fedrowitz M, Westermann J, Löscher W (2002). Magnetic field exposure increases cell proliferation but does not affect melatonin levels in the mammary gland of female Sprague Dawley rats. *Cancer Res*, 62(5):1356-1363.

Felaco M et al. (1999). Impact of extremely low frequency electromagnetic fields on CD4 expression in peripheral blood mononuclear cells. *Mol Cell Biochem*, 201(1-2):49-55.

Felician O, Sandson TA (1999). The neurobiology and pharmacotherapy of Alzheimer's disease. *J Neuropsychiatry Clin Neurosci*, 11(1):19-31.

Feria-Velasco A et al. (1998). Neuronal differentiation of chromaffin cells in vitro, induced by extremely low frequency magnetic fields or nerve growth factor: a histological and ultrastructural comparative study. *J Neurosci Res*, 53(5):569-582.

Fews AP et al. (1999a). Increased exposure to pollutant aerosols under high voltage power lines. *Int J Radiat Biol*, 75(12):1505-1521.

Fews AP et al. (1999b). Corona ions from powerlines and increased exposure to pollutant aerosols. *Int J Radiat Biol*, 75(12):1523-1531.

Fews AP et al. (2002). Modification of atmospheric DC fields by space charge from high-voltage power lines. *Atmosph Res*, 63:271-289.

Feychting M, Ahlbom A (1993). Magnetic fields and cancer in children residing near Swedish high-voltage power lines. *Am J Epidemiol*, 138(7):467-481.

Feychting M, Ahlbom A (1994). Magnetic fields, leukemia, and central nervous system tumors in Swedish adults residing near high-voltage power lines. *Epidemology*, 5(5):501-509.

Feychting M, Ahlbom A (2000). With regard to the relative merits of contemporary measurements and historical calculated fields in the Swedish childhood cancer study. *Epidemiology*, 11:357-358.

Feychting M, Forssen U, Floderus B (1997). Occupational and residential magnetic field exposure and leukemia and central nervous system tumors. *Epidemiology*, 8(4):384-389.

Feychting M et al. (1998). Dementia and occupational exposure to magnetic fields. *Scand J Work Environ Health*, 24(1):46-53.

Feychting M et al. (2003). Occupational magnetic field exposure and neurodegenerative disease. *Epidemiology*, 14(4):413-419.

Fincham SM et al. (2000). Is occupation a risk factor for thyroid cancer? *J Occup Environ Med*, 42(3):318-322.

Finkelstein MM (1999). Re: magnetic field exposure and cardiovascular disease mortality among electric utility workers - letter to editor. *Am J Epidemiol*, 150(11):1258.

Fiorani M et al. (1992). Electric and or magnetic field effects on DNA structure and function in cultured human cells. *Mutat Res*, 282(1):25-29.

Fiorani M et al. (1997). In vitro effects of 50 Hz magnetic fields on oxidatively damaged rabbit red blood cells. *Bioelectromagnetics*, 18(2):125-131.

Fitzpatrick SM, Rothman DL (2000). Meeting report: transcranial magnetic stimulation and studies of human cognition. *J Cogn Neurosci*, 12(4):704-709.

Floderus B (1996). Is job title an adequate surrogate to measure magnetic field exposure. *Epidemiology*, 7(2):115-116.

Floderus B, Persson T, Stenlund C (1996). Magnetic field exposures in the workplace: reference distribution and exposures in occupational groups. *Int J Occup Environ Helath*, 2:226-238.

Floderus B, Stenlund C, Persson T (1999). Occupational magnetic field exposure and site-specific cancer incidence: a Swedish cohort study. *Cancer Causes Control*, 10(5):323-332.

Floderus B et al. (1993). Occupational exposure to electromagnetic fields in relation to leukemia and brain tumors: a case-control study in Sweden. *Cancer Causes Control*, 4(5):465-476.

Flodin U, Seneby A, Tegenfeldt C (2000). Provocation of electric hypersensitivity under everyday conditions. *Scand J Environ Health*, 26(2):93-98.

Florig HK, Hoburg JF (1990). Power-frequency magnetic fields from electric blankets. *Health Phys*, 58(4):493-502.

Forssén UM et al. (2000). Occupational and residential magnetic field exposure and breast cancer in females. *Epidemiology*, 11(1):24-29.

Forssén UM et al. (2004). Occupational magnetic field exposure among women in Stockholm County, Sweden. *Occup Environ Med*, 61(7):594-602.

Forssén UM et al. (2005). Occupational magnetic fields and female breast cancer: a case-control study using Swedish population registers and new exposure data. *Am J Epidemiol*, 161(3):250-259.

Foster KR (1992). Health-effects of low-level electromagnetic fields: Phantom or not-so-phantom risk? *Health Phys*, 62(5):429-435.

Foster KR, Schwan HP (1989). Dielectric properties of tissues and biological materials: a critical review. *Crit Rev Biomed Eng*, 17(1):25-104.

Foster KR, Schwan HP. Dielectric properties of tissue.In: Polk C, Postow E, eds. *Handbook in biological effects of electromagnetic fields*. New York, CRC Publishers, 1996.

Foster KR, Vecchia P, Repacholi MH (2000). Science and the precautionary principle. *Science*, 288(12 May, 5468):979-981.

Francis JT, Gluckman BJ, Schiff SJ (2003). Sensitivity of neurons to weak electric fields. *J Neurosci*, 23(19):7255-7261.

Frankenhaeuser B, Huxley AF (1964). The action potential in the myelinated nerve fibre of Xenopus laevis as computed on the basis of voltage clamp data. *J Physiol*, 171:302-315.

Free MJ et al. (1981). Endocrinological effects of strong 60-Hz electric fields on rats. *Bioelectromagnetics*, 2:105-121.

Friedman DR et al. (1996). Childhood exposure to magnetic fields: residential area measurements compared to personal dosimetry. *Epidemiology*, 7(2):151-155.

Frolen H, Svedenstal BM, Paulsson LE (1993). Effects of pulsed magnetic-fields on the developing mouse embryo. *Bioelectromagnetics*, 14(3):197-204.

Fry RJM, Carnes BA. Age, sex and other factors in radiation carcinogenesis. In: Baverstock KF, Stather JW, eds. *Low dose radiation: biological basis of risk assessment*. London, Taylor & Francis, 1989:196-206.

Furse CM, Gandhi OP (1998). Calculation of electric fields and currents induced in a millimeter-resolution human model at 60 Hz using the FDTD method. *Bioelectromagnetics*, 19:293-299.

Gabriel C, Gabriel S, Corthout E (1996). The dielectric properties of biological tissues: I. Literature survey. *Phys Med Biol*, 41(11):2231-2249.

Gallagher JP, Sanders M (1987). Trauma and amyotrophic lateral sclerosis: a report of 78 patients. *Acta Neurol Scand*, 75(2):145-150.

Gamberale F et al. (1989). Acute effects of ELF electromagnetic fields: a field study of linesmen working with 400 kV power lines. *Br J Ind Med*, 46:729-737.

Gandhi OP (1995). Some numerical methods for dosimetry: extremely low frequencies to microwave frequencies. *Radio Science*, 30(1):161-177.

Gandhi OP, Chen JY (1992). Numerical dosimetry at power-line frequencies using anatomically based models. *Bioelectromagnetics*, 13(Suppl 1):43-60.

Gandhi OP, DeFord JF (1988). Calculation of EM power deposition for operator exposure to RF introduction heaters. *IEEE Trans Electromag Compat*, 30:63-68.

Gandhi OP et al. (2001). Currents induced in anatomic models of the human for uniform and nonuniform power frequency magnetic fields. *Bioelectromagnetics*, 22(2):112-121.

Gangi S, Johansson O (2000). A theoretical model based upon mast cells and histamine to explain the recently proclaimed sensitivity to electric and/or magnetic fields in humans. *Med Hypoth*, 54:663-671.

Gardner KM et al. (2002). Occupations and breast cancer risk among Chinese women in urban Shanghai. *Am J Ind Med*, 42(4):296-308.

Garland GD. *Introduction to geography: mantle, core and crust*. Toronto, W.B. Saunders Company, 1979.

Gauger JR. *Household appliance magnetic field survey*. Arlington, VA, Naval Electronic Systems Command, 1984 (ITT Research Institute Report EO 6549-3).

Gawel M, Zaiwalla Z, Rose FC (1983). Antecedent events in motor neuron disease. *J Neurol Neurosurg Psychiatry*, 46(11):1041-1043.

Gibbons DL et al. (1999). An E mu-BCL-2 transgene facilitates leukaemogenesis by ionizing radiation. *Oncogene*, 18(26):3870-3877.

Gilham C et al. (2005). Day care in infancy and risk of childhood acute lymphoblastic leukaemia: findings from UK case-control study. *Br Med J*, 330(7503):1294.

Gluckman BJ et al. (2001). Adaptive electric field control of epileptic seizures. *J Neurosci*, 21(2):590-600.

Gona AG et al. (1993). Effects of 60 Hz electric and magnetic-fields on the development of the rat cerebellum. *Bioelectromagnetics*, 14(5):433-447.

Goodman R, Blank M (1998). Magnetic field stress induces expression of hsp70. *Cell Stress Chaperones*, 3(2):79-88.

Goodman R et al. (1989). Exposure of human cells to low-frequency electromagnetic fields results in quantitative changes in transcripts. *Biochim Biophys Acta*, 1009(3):216-220.

Goodman R et al. (1992). Exposure to electric and magnetic (EM) fields increases transcripts in HL-60 cells - does adaptation to EM fields occur? *Bioelectrochem Bioenerg*, 29(2):185-192.

Goodman R et al. (1994). Increased levels of hsp 70 transcript induced when cells are exposed to low frequency electromagnetic fields. *Bioelectrochem Bioenerg*, 33:115-120.

Gothe CJ, Odoni CM, Nilsson CG (1995). The environmental somatization syndrome. *Psychosomatics*, 36:1-11.

Gourdon CG. Efforts of French railroads to reduce traction of electromagnetic fields. In: Blank M, ed. *Electricity and magnetism in biology and medicine*. San Francisco, San Francisco Press, 1993:259-263.

Government of Canada (2003). *Framework for the application of precaution in science-based decision making about risk*. (http://www.pco-bcp.gc.ca/docs/Publications/precaution/precaution_e.pdf, accessed 15-2-2007).

Government of Israel (2006). *Non-Ionizing Radiation Law, 2006 (No. 5766)*. (http:// www.sviva.gov.il/Enviroment/Static/Binaries/Articals/non-ionizing_radiation_law_1.pdf, accessed 15-2-2007).

Government of Italy (2003). Decree of the president of the council of ministers 8 July 2003. Establishment of exposure limits, attention values, and quality goals to protect the population against power frequency (50 Hz) electric and magnetic fields generated by power lines (in Italian). *Official Gazette of the Italian Republic*, Serie Generale 200:11-12.

Graham C, Cook MR (1999). Human sleep in 60 Hz magnetic fields. *Bioelectromagnetics*, 20(5):277-283.

Graham C, Cook MR, Riffle DW (1997). Human melatonin during continuous magnetic field exposure. *Bioelectromagnetics*, 18(2):166-171.

Graham C et al. (1994). Dose response study of human exposure to 60 Hz electric and magnetic fields. *Bioelectromagnetic*, 15:447-463.

Graham C et al. (1996). Nocturnal melatonin levels in human volunteers exposed to intermittent 60 Hz magnetic-fields. *Bioelectromagnetics*, 17(4):263-273.

Graham C et al. (1998). Prediction of nocturnal plasma melatonin from morning urinary measures. *J Pineal Res*, 24(4):230-238.

Graham C et al. (1999). Human exposure to 60-Hz magnetic fields: neurophysiological effects. *Int J Psychophysiol*, 33:169-175.

Graham C et al. (2000a). Cardiac autonomic control mechanisms in power-frequency magnetic fields: a multistudy analysis. *Environ Health Perspect*, 108(8):737-742.

Graham C et al. (2000b). Multi-night exposure to 60 Hz magnetic fields: effects on melatonin and its enzymatic metabolite. *J Pineal Res*, 28:1-8.

Graham C et al. (2000c). Nocturnal magnetic exposure: Gender-specific effects on heart rate variability and sleep. *Clinical Neurophysiol*, 111(11):1936-1941.

Graham C et al. (2000d). Heart rate variability and physiological arousal in men exposed to 60 Hz magnetic fields. *Bioelectromagnetics*, 21(3):480-482.

Graham C et al. (2000e). Exposure to strong ELF magnetic fields does not alter cardiac autonomic control mechanisms. *Bioelectromagnetics*, 21(3):413-421.

Graham C et al. (2001a). Examination of the melatonin hypothesis in women exposed at night to EMF or bright light. *Environ Health Perspect*, 109(5):501-507.

Graham C et al. (2001b). Melatonin and 6-OHMS in high-intensity magnetic fields. *J Pineal Res*, 31(1):85-88.

Graham C et al. (2001c). All-night exposure to EMF does not alter urinary melatonin, 6-OHMS or immune measures in older men and women. *J Pineal Res*, 13:109-113.

Grandolfo M (1996). Extremely low frequency magnetic fields and cancer. *Eur J Cancer Prev*, 5(5):379-381.

Grassi C et al. (2004). Effects of 50 Hz electromagnetic fields on voltage-gated Ca2+ channels and their role in modulation of neuroendocrine cell proliferation and death. *Cell Calcium*, 35(4):307-315.

Greaves MF (2002). Childhood leukaemia. *Br Med J*, 324(7322):283-287.

Greaves MF, Alexander FE (1993). An infectious etiology for common acute lymphoblastic leukemia in childhood? *Leukemia*, 7(3):349-360.

Green LM et al. (1999a). Childhood leukaemia and personal monitoring of residential exposures to electric and magnetic fields in Ontario, Canada. *Cancer Causes Control*, 10:233-243.

Green LM et al. (1999b). A case-control study of childhood leukemia in southern Ontario, Canada, and exposure to magnetic fields in residences. *Int J Cancer*, 82:161-170.

Greenberg RS, Shuster JL (1985). Epidemiology of cancer in children. *Epidemiol Rev*, 7:22-48.

Greene JJ et al. (1993). Gene-specific modulation of RNA synthesis and degradation by extremely low frequency electromagnetic fields. *Cell Mol Biol*, 39(3):261-268.

Greenland S (2001). Estimation of population attributable fractions from fitted incidence ratios and exposure survey data, with an application to electromagnetic fields and childhood leukemia. *Biometrics*, 57(1):182-188.

Greenland S (2004). Model-based estimation of relative risks and other epidemiologic measures in studies of common outcomes and in case-control studies. *Am J Epidemiol*, 160(4):301-305.

Greenland S (2005). Multiple-bias modelling for analysis of observational data. *J Royal Statist Soc*, 168(2):267-308.

Greenland S, Kheifets L (2006). Leukemia attributable to residential magnetic fields: results from analyses allowing for study biases. *Risk Anal*, 26(2):471-482.

Greenland S et al. (2000). A pooled analysis of magnetic fields, wire codes, and childhood leukemia. *Epidemiology*, 11(6):624-634.

Griefahn B et al. (2001). Experiments on the effects of a continuous 16.7 Hz magnetic field on melatonin secretion, core body temperature, and heart rates in humans. *Bioelectromagnetics*, 22(8):581-588.

Griefahn B et al. (2002). Experiments on effects of an intermittent 16.7-Hz magnetic field on salivary melatonin concentrations, rectal temperature, and heart rate in humans. *Int Arch Occup Environ Health*, 75(3):171-178.

Griffin GD, Williams MW, Gailey PC (2000). Cellular communication in clone 9 cells exposed to magnetic fields. *Radiat Res*, 153:690-698.

Griffin GD et al. (2000). Power frequency magnetic field exposure and gap junctional communication in Clone 9 cells. *Bioelectrochem*, 51(2):117-123.

Griffiths SD et al. (1992). Clonal characteristics of acute lymphoblastic cells derived from BCR/ABL p190 transgenic mice. *Oncogene*, 7(7):1391-1399.

Grissom CB (1995). Magnetic field effects in biology: A survey of possible mechanisms with emphasis on radical-pair recombination. *Chem Rev*, 95:3-24.

Grota LJ et al. (1994). Electric-field exposure alters serum melatonin but not pineal melatonin synthesis in male-rats. *Bioelectromagnetics*, 15(5):427-437.

Guenel P et al. (1993). Design of a job exposure matrix on electric and magnetic fields: selection of an efficient job classification for workers in thermoelectric power production plants. *Int J Epidemiol*, 22(Suppl 2):S16-S21.

Gunnarsson LG et al. (1992). A case-control study of motor neurone disease: its relation to heritability, and occupational exposures, particularly to solvents. *Br J Ind Med*, 49:791-798.

Gunnarsson LG et al. (1991). Amyotrophic lateral sclerosis in Sweden in relation to occupation. *Acta Neurol Scand*, 83(6):394-398.

Gurney JG et al. (1995). Childhood cancer occurrence in relation to power-line configurations: a study of potential selection bias in case-control studies. *Epidemiology*, 6(1):31-35.

Gurvich EB et al. Occupational and nonoccupational exposed to extremely low frequency electromagnetic fields as a risk factor. In: Repacholi M, Rubtsova NB, Muc AM, eds. *Electromagnetic fields: biological effects and hygienic standardization. Proceedings of an international meeting, Moscow, 18-22 May, 1998*. Geneva, WHO, 1999:275-278.

Hackman RM, Graves HB (1981). Corticosterone levels in mice exposed to high-intensity electric fields. *Behav Neural Biol*, 32(2):201-213.

Hahn H, Wojnowski L, Miller G (1999). The patched signalling pathway in tumourigenesis and development: lessons from animal models. *J Mol Med*, 77:459-468.

Håkansson N et al. (2002). Cancer incidence and magnetic field exposure in industries using resistance welding in Sweden. *Occup Environ Med*, 59(7):481-486.

Håkansson N et al. (2003). Neurodegenerative diseases in welders and other workers exposed to high levels of magnetic fields. *Epidemiology*, 14(4):420-426.

Hamalainen AM et al. Exposure to magnetic fields at work and public areas at the Finnish railways. In: *Proceedings of the Second World Congress for Electricity and Magnetism in Medicine and Biology, Bologna, Italy*, 1999, 785-787.

Han L et al. (1998). Application of magnetic field-induced heat shock protein 70 for presurgical cytoprotection. *J Cell Biochem*, 71(4):577-583.

Hansen NH et al. (2000). EMF exposure assessment in the Finnish garment industry: evaluation of proposed EMF exposure metrics. *Bioelectromagnetics*, 21(1):57-67.

Harland JD, Liburdy RP (1997). Environmental magnetic fields inhibit the antiproliferative action of tamoxifen and melatonin in a human breast cancer cell line. *Bioelectromagnetics*, 18(8):555-562.

Harland JD, Levine GA, Liburdy RP. Differential inhibition of tamoxifen's oncostatic functions in a human breast cancer cell line by a 12 mG (1.2 mT) magnetic field. In: Bersani F, ed. *Electricity and Magnetism in Biology and Medicine*. Bologna, Plenum Press, 1998:465-468.

Harrington JM et al. (2001). Leukaemia mortality in relation to magnetic field exposure: findings from a study of United Kingdom electricity generation and transmission workers, 1973-97. *Occup Environ Med*, 58:307-314.

Harris AW et al. (1998). A test of lymphoma induction by long-term exposure of E mu-Pim1 transgenic mice to 50 Hz magnetic fields. *Radiat Res*, 149(3):300-307.

Hart FX (1992). Numerical and analytical methods to determine the current density distributions produced in human and rat models by electric and magnetic fields. *Bioelectromagtnetics*, 13(Suppl. 1):27-42.

Hatch EE et al. (2000). Do confounding or selection factors of residential wiring codes and magnetic fields distort finding of electromagnetic fields studies? *Epidemiology*, 11(2):189-198.

Hatch M (1992). The epidemiology of electric and magnetic field exposures in the power frequency range and reproductive outcomes. *Paediatr Perinat Epidemiol*, 6(2):198-214.

Hauf R. Electric and magnetic fields at power frequencies with particular reference to 50 and 60 Hz. In: Suess MJ, ed. *Non-ionizing radiation protection*. Copenhagen, WHO, 1982:175-197.

Hauf R (1989). Biological effect of low frequency electromagnetic fields. *Oesterreichische Zeitschrift fur Elektrizitaetswirtschaft*, 42:298-300.

Häussler M et al. (1999). Exposure of rats to a 50-Hz, 100 µT magnetic field does not affect the ex vivo production of interleukins by activated T or B lymphocytes. *Bioelectromagnetics*, 20(5):295-305.

Haynal A, Regli F (1964). [Amyotrophic lateral sclerosis associated with accumulated electric injury]. *Confin Neurol*, 24:189-198.

HCN - Health Council of the Netherlands - ELF Electromagnetic Fields Committee. *Electromagnetic fields: annual update 2003*. The Hague, Health Council of the Netherlands, 2004 (Publication no. 2004/01).

Hefeneider SH et al. (2001). Long-term effects of 60-Hz electric vs. magnetic fields on IL-1 and IL-2 activity in sheep. *Bioelectromagnetics*, 22(3):170-177.

Heikkinen P et al. (2001). Effects of 50 Hz magnetic fields on cancer induced by ionizing radiation in mice. *Int J Radiat Biol*, 77(4):483-495.

Henshaw DL, Reiter RJ (2005). Do magnetic fields cause increased risk of childhood leukemia via melatonin disruption? *Bioelectromagnetics*, 26(Suppl. 7):S86-S97.

Henshaw DL et al. (1996a). Author's reply to letter to the editor. *Int J Radiat Biol*, 69(5):653-657.

Henshaw DL et al. (1996b). Enhanced deposition of radon daughter nuclei in the vicinity of power frequency electromagnetic fields. *Int J Radiat Biol*, 69(1):25-38.

Heusser K, Tellschaft D, Thoss F (1997). Influence of an alternating 3 Hz magnetic field with an induction of 0.1 millitesla on chosen parameters of the human occipital EEG. *Neurosci Lett*, 239(2-3):57-60.

Hille B. *Ionic channels of excitable membranes*, 3rd ed. Sunderland, MA, Sinauer Associates, 2001.

Hille R, Anderson RF (2001). Coupled electron/proton transfer in complex flavoproteins: solvent kinetic isotope effect studies of electron transfer in xanthine oxidase and trimethylamine dehydrogenase. *J Biol Chem*, 276(33):31193-31201.

Hillert L et al. (2002). Prevalence of self-reported hypersensitivity to electric or magnetic fields in a population-based questionnaire survey. *Scand J Work Environ Health*, 28(1):33-41.

Hintenlang DE (1993). Synergistic effects of ionizing-radiation and 60 Hz magnetic-fields. *Bioelectromagnetics*, 14(6):545-551.

Hirata A et al. (2001). Dosimetry in models of child and adult for low-frequency electric field. *IEEE Trans Biomed Eng*, 48(9):1007-1012.

Hjeresen DL et al. (1980). Effects of 60-Hz electricfields on avoidance behavior and activity of rats. *Bioelectromagnetics*, 1:299-312.

Hjeresen DL et al. (1982). A behavioral response of swine to a 60-Hz electric field. *Bioelectromagnetics*, 3:443-451.

Hocking B (1994). Non ionising electromagnetic radiation. *Aust Fam Physician*, 23(7):1388-1389.

Hodgkin AL, Huxley AF (1952). A quantitative description of membrane current and its application to conduction and excitation in nerve. *J Physiol*, 117(4):500-544.

Holder JW, Elmore E, Barrett JC (1993). Gap junction function and cancer. *Cancer Res*, 53(15):3475-3485.

Hone P et al. (2003). Possible associations between ELF electromagnetic fields, DNA damage response processes and childhood leukaemia. *Br J Cancer*, 88(12):1939-1941.

Hong SC et al. (2001). Chronic exposure to ELF magnetic fields during night sleep with electric sheets: effects on diurnal melatonin rhythms in men. *Bioelectromagnetics*, 22(2):138-143.

Hopwood A (1992). Natural radiation focused by power lines: new evidence. *Electronics World & Wireless World*, (November):912-915.

Hore PJ (2005). Rapporteur's report: Sources and interaction mechanisms. *Prog Biophys Mol Biol*, 87(2-3):205-212.

House RV, McCormick DL (2000). Modulation of natural killer cell function after exposure to 60 Hz magnetic fields: confirmation of the effect in mature B6C3F1 mice. *Radiat Res*, 153(5 Pt 2).722-724.

House RV et al. (1996). Immune function and host defense in rodents exposed to 60-Hz magnetic fields. *Fundam Appl Toxicol*, 34(2):228-239.

Hoyes KP, Hendry JH, Lord BI (2000). Modification of murine adult haemopoiesis and response to methyl nitrosourea following exposure to radiation at different developmental stages. *Int J Radiat Biol*, 76(1):77-85.

Hu GL et al. (2000). Absence of ELF magnetic field effects on transcription of the connexin43 gene. *Electro Magnetobiol*, 19:345-350.

Hu GL et al. (2001). ELF magnetic field inhibits gap junctional intercellular communication and induces hyperphosphorylation of connexin43 in NIH3T3 cells. *Bioelectromagnetics*, 22:568-573.

Hutzler B et al. Exposure to 50 Hz magnetic fields during live work. In: *CIGRE (International Conference on Large High Voltage Electric Systems) Session 1994*. Paris, CIGRE, 1994:1-9.

Huuskonen H, Juutilainen J, Komulainen H (1993). Effects of low-frequency magnetic fields on fetal development in rats. *Bioelectromagnetics*, 14(3):205-213.

Huuskonen H, Juutilainen J, Komulainen H (2001). Development of preimplantation mouse embryos after exposure to a 50 Hz magnetic field in vitro. *Toxicol Lett*, 122(2):149-155.

Huuskonen H, Lindbohm ML, Juutilainen J (1998). Teratogenic and reproductive effects of low-frequency magnetic fields. *Mutat Res*, 410(2):167-183.

Huuskonen H et al. (1998a). Effects of gestational exposure to a video display terminal-like magnetic field (20-kHz) on CBA/S mice. *Teratology*, 58(5):190-196.

Huuskonen H et al. (1998b). Effects of low-frequency magnetic fields on fetal development in CBA/Ca mice. *Bioelectromagnetics*, 19(8):477-485.

IARC - International Agency for Research on Cancer (1992). Mechanisms of carcinogenesis in risk identification. *IARC Scientific Publications*, No. 116.

IARC - International Agency for Research on Cancer (2000). *International Association of Cancer Registries - Globocan 2000 Database Version 1.0*. (http://www-dep.iarc.fr/globocan/globocan.html, accessed 1-3-2005).

IARC Working Group on the Evaluation of Carcinogenic Risks to Humans. *Non-ionizing radiation, Part 1. Static and extremely low-frequency (ELF) electric and magnetic fields*. Lyon, IARC, 2002 (Monographs on the Evaluation of Carcinogenic Risks to Humans, 80).

Ichinose TY et al. (2004). Immune markers and ornithine decarboxylase activity among electric utility workers. *J Occup Environ Med*, 46(2):104-112.

401

ICNIRP - International Commission on Non-ionizing Radiation Protection (1998a). Guidelines for limiting exposure to time-varying electric, magnetic, and electromagnetic fields (up to 300 GHz). *Health Phys*, 74(4):494-522.

ICNIRP - International Commission on Non-ionizing Radiation Protection (1998b). Response to questions and comments on the guidelines for limiting exposure to time-varying electric, magnetic and electromagnetic fields (up to 300 GHz). *Health Phys*, 75(4):438-439.

ICNIRP - International Commission on Non-ionizing Radiation Protection. *Possible health risk to the general public from the use of security and similar devices. Report of a concerted action within the project: "Environment and Health, Health impact of electromagnetic fields" of the 5th Framework Programme of the European Commission.* Bernhardt JH, McKinlay A, Matthes R, eds. Munich, International Commission on Non-ionizing Radiation Protection, 2002 (ICNIRP 12/2002).

ICNIRP - International Commission on Non-ionizing Radiation Protection. *Exposure to static and low frequency electromagnetic fields, biological effects and health consequences (0 - 100 kHz).* Bernhardt JH et al., eds. Oberschleissheim, International Commission on Non-ionizing Radiation Protection, 2003 (ICNIRP 13/2003).

ICNIRP - International Commission on Non-Ionizing Radiation Protection (2004). ICNIRP statement related to the use of security and similar devices utilizing electromagnetic fields. *Health Phys*, 87(2):187-196.

IEC - International Electrotechnical Commission. *Safety of household and similar electric appliances, part 1: general requirements.* Geneva, International Electrotechnical Commission, 1994 (IEC 60335-1).

IEC - International Electrotechnical Commission. *Committee draft. Measurement and evaluation of high frequency (9 kHz to 300 GHz) electromagnetic fields with regard to human exposure.* Geneva, International Electrotechnical Commission, 2000 (85/214/CD).

IEEE Standards Coordinating Committee 28. *IEEE standard for safety levels with respect to human exposure to electromagnetic fields, 0-3 kHz.* New York, NY, IEEE - The Institute of Electrical and Electronics Engineers, 2002 (IEEE Std C95.6-2002).

Ikeda K et al. (2003). No effects of extremely low frequency magnetic fields found on cytotoxic activities and cytokine production of human peripheral blood mononuclear cells in vitro. *Bioelectromagnetics*, 24(1):21-31.

Irgens A et al. (1997). Male proportion in offspring of parents exposed to strong static and extremely low-frequency electromagnetic fields in Norway. *Am J Ind Med*, 32(5):557-561.

Ishido M (2001). Magnetic fields (MF) of 50 Hz at 1.2 µT as well as 100 µT cause uncoupling of inhibitory pathways of adenylyl cyclase mediated by melatonin a1 receptor in MF-sensitive MCF-7 cells. *Carcinogenesis*, 22(7):1043-1048.

Ivancsits S et al. (2002a). Induction of DNA strand breaks by intermittent exposure to extremely-low-frequency electromagnetic fields in human diploid fibroblasts. *Mutat Res*, 519(1-2):1-13.

Ivancsits S et al. (2002b). Vanadate induces DNA strand breaks in cultured human fibroblasts at doses relevant to occupational exposure. *Mutat Res*, 519(1-2):25-35.

Ivancsits S et al. (2003a). Age-related effects on induction of DNA strand breaks by intermittent exposure to electromagnetic fields. *Mech Ageing Dev*, 124(7):847-850.

Ivancsits S et al. (2003b). Intermittent extremely low frequency electromagnetic fields cause DNA damage in a dose-dependent way. *Int Arch Occup Environ Health*, 76(6):431-436.

Jackson JD (1992). Are the stray 60-Hz electromagnetic fields associated with the distribution and use of electric power a significant cause of cancer? *Proc Natl Acad Sci USA*, 89:3508-3510.

Jacobson GA et al. (2005). Subthreshold voltage noise of rat neocortical pyramidal neurones. *J Physiol*, 564(Pt 1):145-160.

Jaffa K (2001). Pooled analysis of magnetic fields, wire codes, and childhood leukemia. *Epidemiology*, 12(4):472-474.

Jaffa K, Kim H, Aldrich TE (2000). The relative merits of contemporary measurements and historical calculated fields in the Swedish childhood cancer study. *Epidemiology*, 11(3):353-356.

Jahreis GP et al. (1998). Absence of 60-Hz, 0.1-mT magnetic field-induced changes in oncogene transcription rates or levels in CEM-CM3 cells. *Biochim Biophys Acta*, 1443(3):334-342.

Jan LY, Jan YN (1989). Voltage-sensitive ion channels. *Cell*, 56(1):13-25.

Jandova A et al. (1999). Effects of sinusoidal magnetic field on adherence inhibition of leucocytes: preliminary results. *Bioelectrochem Bioenerg*, 48(2):317-319.

Jandova A et al. (2001). Effects of sinusoidal magnetic field on adherence inhibition of leukocytes. *Electromag Biol Med*, 20(3):397-413.

Järvholm B, Stenberg A (2002). Suicide mortality among electricians in the Swedish construction industry. *Occup Environ Med*, 59(3):199-200.

Jefferys JG (1994). Experimental neurobiology of epilepsies. *Curr Opin Neurol*, 7(2):113-122.

Jefferys JG (1995). Nonsynaptic modulation of neuronal activity in the brain: electric currents and extracellular ions. *Physiol Rev*, 75(4):689-723.

Jefferys JG et al. (2003). Effects of weak electric fields on the activity of neurons and neuronal networks. *Radiat Prot Dosimetry*, 106(4):321-323.

Jerry RA, Popel AS, Brownell WE (1996). Potential distribution for a sperioidal cell having a conductive membrane in an electric field. *IEEE Trans Biomed Eng*, 43:970-972.

Johansen C (2000). Exposure to electromagnetic fields and risk of central nervous system disease in utility workers. *Epidemiology*, 11(5):539-543.

Johansen C, Olsen JH (1998a). Mortality from amyotrophic lateral sclerosis, other chronic disorders, and electric shocks among utility workers. *Am J Epidemiol*, 148(4):362-368.

Johansen C, Olsen JH (1998b). Risk of cancer among Danish utility workers: a nationwide cohort study. *Am J Epidemiol*, 147(6):548-555.

Johansen C et al. (1999). Multiple sclerosis among utility workers. *Neurology*, 52(6):1279-1282.

Johansen C et al. (2002). Risk of severe cardiac arrhythmia in male utility workers: a nationwide Danish cohort study. *Am J Epidemiol*, 156(9):857-861.

Johansson O, Hilliges M, Han SW (1996). A screening of skin changes, with special emphasis on neurochemical marker antibody evaluation, in patients claiming to suffer from "screen dermatitis" as compared to normal healthy controls. *Exp Dermatol*, 5(5):279-285.

Johansson O et al. (1994). Skin changes in patients claiming to suffer from "screen dermatitis": a two-case open-field provocation study. *Exp Dermatol*, 3(5):234-238.

Johansson O et al. (2001). Cutaneous mast cells are altered in normal healthy volunteers sitting in front of ordinary TVs/PCs - results from open-field provocation experiments. *J Cutan Pathol*, 28(10):513-519.

John TM, Liu G-Y, Brown GM (1998). 60 Hz magnetic field exposure and urinary 6-sulphatoxymelatonin levels in rats. *Bioelectromagnetics*, 19(3):172-180.

Jokela K, Puranen L, Sihvonen AP (2004). Assessment of the magnetic field exposure due to the battery current of digital mobile phones. *Health Phys*, 86(1):56-66.

Jones TL et al. (1993). Selection bias from differential residential-mobility as an explanation for associations of wire codes with childhood cancer. *J Clin Epidemiol*, 46(6):545-548.

Juutilainen J (1986). Effects of low frequency magnetic fields on chick embryos. Dependence on incubation temperature and storage of the eggs. *Z Naturforsch [C ]*, 41(11-12):1111-1115.

Juutilainen J. *Measurements of 50 Hz magnetic fields in Finnish homes*. Helsinki, Imatran Voima Oy, 1989 (Imatran Voima Oy Research Reports IVO-A-02/89).

Juutilainen J (1991). Effects of low-frequency magnetic fields on embryonic development and pregnancy. *Scand J Work Environ Health*, 17(3):149-58.

Juutilainen J (2003). Developmental effects of extremely low frequency electric and magnetic fields. *Radiat Prot Dosimetry*, 106(4):385-390.

Juutilainen J, Läära E, Saali K (1987). Relationship between field strength and abnormal development in chick embryos exposed to 50 Hz magnetic fields. *Int J Radiat Biol*, 52(5):787-793.

Juutilainen J, Lang S (1997). Genotoxic, carcinogenic and teratogenic effects of electromagnetic fields: introduction and overview. *Mutat Res*, 387(3):165-171.

Juutilainen J, Saali K (1986). Development of chick embryos in 1 Hz to 100 kHz magnetic fields. *Radiat Environ Biophys*, 25:135-140.

Juutilainen J et al. (1993). Early-pregnancy loss and exposure to 50-Hz magnetic-fields. *Bioelectromagnetics*, 14(3):229-236.

Juutilainen J et al. (2000). Nocturnal 6-hydroxymelatonin sulfate excretion in female workers exposed to magnetic fields. *J Pineal Res*, 28(2):97-104.

Kabat GC et al. (2003). Electric blanket use and breast cancer on Long Island. *Epidemiology*, 14(5):514-520.

Kabuto M et al. (2006). Childhood leukemia and magnetic fields in Japan: a case-control study of childhood leukemia and residential power-frequency magnetic fields in Japan. *Int J Cancer*, 119(3):643-650.

Kandel ER, Schwartz JH, Jessell TM. *Principles of neural science*, Vol. 65. Norwalk, CT, Appleton & Lange, 1991:1009.

Kang K-I et al. (1998). Luciferase activity and synthesis of HSP70 and HSP90 are insensitive to 50Hz electromagnetic fields. *Life Sci*, 63(6):489-497.

Karabakhtsian R et al. (1994). Calcium is necessary in the cell response to EM fields. *FEBS Lett*, 349:1-6.

Karasek M, Lerchl A (2002). Melatonin and magnetic fields. *Neuro Endocrinol Lett*, 23(Suppl 1):84-87.

Kato M, Shigemitsu T. Effects of 50 Hz magnetic fields on pineal function in the rat. In: Stevens RG, Wilson BW, Anderson LE, eds. *The melatonin hypothesis, breast cancer and use of electric power*. Columbus, OH, Battelle Press, 1997:337-376.

Kato M et al. (1993). Effects of exposure to a circularly polarized 50-Hz magnetic field on plasma and pineal melatonin levels in rats. *Bioelectromagnetics*, 14:1997-106.

Kato M et al. (1994a). Circularly polarized 50-Hz magnetic field exposure reduces pineal gland and blood melatonin concentrations of Long-Evans rats. *Neurosci Lett*, 166:59-62.

Kato M et al. (1994b). Circularly polarized, sinusoidal, 50 Hz magnetic field exposure does not influence plasma testosterone levels of rats. *Bioelectromagnetics*, 15:513-518.

Kato M et al. (1994c). Horizontal or vertical 50-Hz, 1-micro T magnetic fields have no effect on pineal gland or plasma melatonin concentration of albino rats. *Neurosci Lett*, 168:205-208.

Kato M et al. (1994d). Recovery of nocturnal melatonin concentration takes place within one week following cessation of 50 Hz circulary polarized magnetic field exposure for six weeks. *Bioelectromagnetics*, 15:489-492.

Katsir G, Parola AH (1998). Enhanced proliferation caused by a low frequency weak magnetic field in chick embryo fibroblasts is suppressed by radical scavengers. *Biochem Biophys Res Commun*, 252(3):753-756.

Kaune WT, McCreary FA (1985). Numerical calculation and measurement of 60-Hz current densities induced in an upright grounded cylinder. *Bioelectromagnetics*, 6(3):209-220.

Kaune WT, Forsythe WC (1985). Current densities measured in human models exposed to 60-Hz electric fields. *Bioelectromagnetics*, 6:13-32.

Kaune WT, Zafanella LE (1992). Analysis of magnetic field produced far from electric power lines. *IEEE Trans Power Delivery*, 7(4):2082-2091.

Kaune WT, Zaffanella LE (1994). Assessing historical exposures of children to power-frequency magnetic fields. *J Expo Anal Environ Epidemiol*, 4:149-170.

Kaune WT, Kistler LM, Miller MC. Comparison of the coupling of grounded and ungrounded humans to vertical 60 Hz electric fields. In: Anderson LE, Kelman BJ, Weige RJ, eds. *Interaction of biological systems with static and ELF electric and magnetic fields*. Richland, WA, Pacific Northwest Laboratory, 1987:185-195.

Kaune WT et al. (1978). A method for the exposure of miniature swine to vertical 60 Hz electric fields. *IEEE Trans Biomed Eng*, 25(3):276-283.

Kaune WT et al. (1987). Residential magnetic and electric fields. *Bioelectromagnetics*, 8(4):315-335.

Kaune WT et al. (1994). Development of a protocol for assessing time-weighted-average exposures of young children to power-frequency magnetic fields. *Bioelectromagnetics*, 15(1):33-51.

Kaune WT et al. (1998). Temporal characteristics of transmission-line loadings in the Swedish childhood cancer study. *Bioelectromagnetics*, 19(6):354-365.

Kavaliers M, Ossenkopp KP (1986a). Magnetic field inhibition of morphine-induced analgesia and behavioral activity in mice: evidence for involvement of calcium ions. *Brain Res*, 379(1):30-38.

Kavaliers M, Ossenkopp KP (1986b). Stress-induced opioid analgesia and activity in mice: inhibitory influences of exposure to magnetic fields. *Psychopharmacology (Berl)*, 89(4):440-443.

Kavaliers M, Ossenkopp KP (1991). Opioid system and magnetic field effects in the land snail, Cepaea nemoralis. *Biol Bull*, 180:301-309.

Kavaliers M, Ossenkopp KP (1993). Repeated naloxone treatments and exposures to weak 60-Hz magnetic fields have 'analgesic' effects in snails. *Brain Res*, 620(1):159-162.

Kavaliers M, Ossenkopp KP, Hirst M (1984). Magnetic fields abolish the enhanced nocturnal analgesic response to morphine in mice. *Physiol Behav*, 32(2):261-264.

Kavaliers M, Ossenkopp KP, Tysdale DM (1991). Evidence for the involvement of protein kinase C in the modulation of morphine-induced 'analgesia' and the inhibitory effects of exposure to 60-Hz magnetic fields in the snail, Cepaea nemoralis. *Brain Res*, 554(1-2):65-71.

Kavaliers M, Wiebe JP, Ossenkopp KP (1998). Brief exposure of mice to 60 Hz magnetic fields reduces the analgesic effects of the neuroactive steroid, 3 alpha-hydroxy-4-pregnen-20-one. *Neurosci Lett*, 257:155-158.

Kavaliers M et al. Opioid systems and the biological effects of magnetic fields. In: Frey AH, ed. *On the nature of electromagnetic field interactions with biological systems*. Austin, TX, RG Landes Co, 1994:181-194.

Kavaliers M et al. (1996). Spatial learning in deer mice: sex differences and the effects of endogenous opioids and 60 Hz magnetic fields. *J Comp Physio A*, 179:715-724.

Kavaliers M et al. (1998). Evidence for the involvement of nitric oxide and nitric oxide synthase in the modulation of opioid-induced antinociception and the inhibitory effects of exposure to 60-Hz magnetic fields in the land snail. *Brain Res*, 809(1):50-57.

Kavet R (2005). Contact current hypothesis: summary of results to date. *Bioelectromagnetics*, 26(Suppl 7):S75-S85.

Kavet R, Zaffanella LE (2002). Contact voltage measured in residences: implications to the association between magnetic fields and childhood leukemia. *Bioelectromagnetics*, 23(6):464-474.

Kavet R, Silva JM, Thornton D (1992). Magnetic field exposure assessment for adult residents of maine who live near and far away from overhead transmission lines. *Bioelctromagnetics*, 13:35-55.

Kavet R et al. (2000). The possible role of contact current in cancer risk associated with residential magnetic fields. *Bioelectromagnetics*, 21(7):538-553.

Kavet R et al. (2001). Evaluation of biological effects, dosimetric models, and exposure assessment related to ELF electric- and magnetic-field guidelines. *Appl Occup Environ Hyg*, 16(12):1118-1138.

Kavet R et al. (2004). Association of residential magnetic fields with contact voltage. *Bioelectromagnetics*, 25(7):530-536.

Kazantzis N, Podd J, Whittington C (1998). Acute effects of 50 Hz, 100 microT magnetic field exposure on visual duration discrimination at two different times of the day. *Bioelectromagnetics*, 19(5):310-317.

Keetley V et al. (2001). Neuropsychological sequelae of 50 Hz magnetic fields. *Int J Radiat Biol*, 77(6):735-742.

Keisu L (1996). [Successful treatment of "electricity hypersensitivity". The patient was assisted in curing himself]. *Lakartidningen*, 93(18):1753-1755.

Kelfkens G et al. Costs and benefits of the reduction of magnetic fields due to overhead power lines. In: *Proceedings of the 2nd International Workshop on Biological Effects of EMFs, 7-11 October 2002, Rhodes, Greece*, 2002, 309-317.

Kelsh MA, Sahl JD (1997). Mortality among a cohort of electric utility workers, 1960-1991. *Am J Ind Med*, 31:534-544.

Kelsh MA, Kheifets L, Smith R (2000). The impact of work environment, utility, and sampling design on occupational magnetic field exposure summaries. *AIHA J*, 61(2):174-182.

Kelsh MA et al. (2003). Occupational magnetic field exposures of garment workers: results of personal and survey measurements. *Bioelectromagnetics*, 24(5):316-326.

Kharazi AI, Babbitt JT, Hahn TJ (1999). Primary brain tumor incidence in mice exposed to split-dose ionizing radiation and circularly polarized 60 Hz magnetic fields. *Cancer Lett*, 147(1-2):149-156.

Kheifets L, Shimkhada R (2005). Childhood leukemia and EMF: review of the epidemiologic evidence. *Bioelectromagnetics*, 26(Suppl 7):S51-S59.

Kheifets L, Afifi AA, Shimkhada R (2006). Public health impact of extremely low-frequency electromagnetic fields. *Environ Health Perspect*, 114(10):1532-1537.

Kheifets L, Hester GL, Banerjee GL (2001). The precautionary principle and EMF: implementation and evaluation. *J Risk Res*, 4(2):113-125.

Kheifets LI, Kavet R, Sussman SS (1997). Wire codes, magnetic fields, and childhood cancer. *Bioelectromagnetics*, 18(2):99-110.

Kheifets L, Swanson J, Greenland S (2006). Childhood leukemia, electric and magnetic fields, and temporal trends. *Bioelectromagnetics*, 27(7):545-552.

Kheifets LI et al. (1995). Occupational electric and magnetic field exposure and brain cancer. a meta-analysis. *J Occup Environ Med*, 37(12):1237-1241.

Kheifets LI et al. (1997). Occupational electric and magnetic field exposure and leukemia. A meta-analysis. *J Occup Environ Med*, 39(11):1074-1091.

Kheifets L et al. (2005). Developing policy in the face of scientific uncertainty: interpreting 0.3 microT or 0.4 microT cutpoints from EMF epidemiologic studies. *Risk Anal*, 25(4):927-935.

Kim J et al. (2004). Extremely low frequency magnetic field effects on premorbid behaviors produced by cocaine in the mouse. *Bioelectromagnetics*, 25(4):245-250.

Kinlen LF (1994). Leukemia. *Cancer Surv*, 19–20:475-491.

Kirschvink JL (1997). Homing in on vertebrates. *Nature*, 390:339-340.

Kirschvink JL, Kirschvink AK (1991). Is geomagnetic sensitivity real? Replication of the Walker-Bitterman magnetic conditioning experiment in honey bees. *Am Zool*, 31:169-185.

Kirschvink JL et al. (1992). Magnetite in human tissues a mechanism for the biological effects of weak elf magnetic fields. *Bioelectromagnetics*, 13(Suppl 1):101-113.

Kleiger RE et al. (1987). Decreased heart rate variability and its association with increased mortality after acute myocardial infarction. *Am J Cardiol*, 59(4):256-262.

Kleinerman RA et al. (2005). Self-reported electrical appliance use and risk of adult brain tumors. *Am J Epidemiol*, 161(2):136-146.

Kliukiene J, Tynes T, Andersen A (2003). Follow-up of radio and telegraph operators with exposure to electromagnetic fields and risk of breast cancer. *Eur J Cancer Prev*, 12(4):301-307.

Kliukiene J, Tynes T, Andersen A (2004). Residential and occupational exposures to 50-Hz magnetic fields and breast cancer in women: a population-based study. *Am J Epidemiol*, 159(9):852-861.

Knave B et al. (1979). Long-term exposure to electric fields. A cross-sectional epidemiologic investigation on occupationally exposed high voltage substation workers. *Scand J Environ Health*, 5:115-125.

Koc M, Polat P (2001). Epidemiology and aetiological factors of male breast cancer: a ten years retrospective study in eastern Turkey. *Eur J Cancer Prev*, 10(6):531-534.

Koch WE et al. (1993). Examination of the development of chicken embryos following exposure to magnetic-fields. *Comp Biochem Physiol*, 105(4):617-624.

Kondo K, Tsubaki T (1981). Case-control studies of motor neuron disease: association with mechanical injuries. *Arch Neurol*, 38(4):220-226.

König HL et al. *Biological effects of environmental electromagnetism*. New York, Springer-Verlag, 1981.

Kornberg H, Sagan L. *Biological effects of high-voltage fields - an update, Vol.1*. Palo Alto, CA, Electric Power Research Institute, 1979.

Korneva HA et al. (1999). Effects of low-level 50 Hz magnetic fields on the level of host defense and on spleen colony formation. *Bioelectromagnetics*, 20(1):57-63.

Korpinen L, Partanen J (1994a). Influence of 50 Hz electric and magnetic fields on the pulse rate of human heart. *Bioelectromagnetics*, 15(6):503-512.

Korpinen L, Partanen J (1994b). The influence of 50 Hz electric and magnetic fields on the extrasystoles of human heart. *Rev Environ Health*, 10(2):105-112.

Korpinen L, Partanen J (1995). The influence of 50-Hz electric and magnetic fields on human cardiovascular autonomic function tests. *Electro Magnetobiol*, 14:135-147.

Korpinen L, Partanen J (1996). Influences of 50-Hz electric and magnetic fields on human blood pressure. *Radiat Environ Biophys*, 35:199-204.

Korpinen L, Partanen J, Uusitalo A (1993). Influence of 50 Hz electric and magnetic fields on the human heart. *Bioelectromagnetics*, 14:329-340.

Kotnik T, Miklavcic D (2000). Theoretical evaluation of the distributed power dissipation in biological cells exposed to electric fields. *Bioelectromagnetics*, 21(5):385-394.

Kowalczuk CI et al. (1994). Effects of prenatal exposure to 50 Hz magnetic fields on development in mice: I. Implantation rate and fetal development. *Bioelectromagnetics*, 15(4):349-361.

Kowalczuk CI et al. (1995). Dominant lethal studies in male mice after exposure to a 50 Hz magnetic field. *Mutat Res*, 328:229-237.

Koyama S et al. (2004). ELF electromagnetic fields increase hydrogen peroxide ($H_2O_2$)-induced mutations in pTN89 plasmids. *Mutat Res*, 560(1):27-32.

Kraut A, Tate R, Tran N (1994). Residential electric consumption and childhood cancer in Canada (1971-1986). *Arch Environ Health*, 49(3):156-159.

Krishnan G et al. (2003). Occupation and adult gliomas in the San Francisco Bay Area. *J Occup Environ Med*, 45:639-647.

Kroese ED et al. (1997). Use of E mu-PIM-1 transgenic mice short-term in vivo carcinogenicity testing: lymphoma induction by benzo[a]pyrene, but not by TPA. *Carcinogenesis*, 18(5):975-980.

Kumlin T et al. (1998a). Epidermal ornithine decarboxylase and polyamines in mice exposed to 50 Hz magnetic fields and UV radiation. *Bioelectromagnetics*, 19(6):388-391.

Kumlin T et al. (1998b). Effects of 50 Hz magnetic fields on UV-induced skin tumourigenesis in ODC-transgenic and non-transgenic mice. *Int J Radiat Biol*, 1973(1):113-121.

Kumlin T et al. (2002). p53-independent apoptosis in UV-irradiated mouse skin: possible inhibition by 50 Hz magnetic fields. *Radiat Environ Biophys*, 41(2):155-158.

Kurokawa Y et al. (2003a). Acute exposure to 50 Hz magnetic fields with harmonics and transient components: lack of effects on nighttime hormonal secretion in men. *Bioelectromagnetics*, 24(1):12-20.

Kurokawa Y et al. (2003b). No influence of short-term exposure to 50-Hz magnetic fields on cognitive performance function in human. *Int Arch Occup Environ Health*, 76(6):437-442 (2003a).

Labreche F et al. (2003). Occupational exposures to extremely low frequency magnetic fields and postmenopausal breast cancer. *Am J Ind Med*, 44(6):643-652.

Lacy-Hulbert A, Metcalfe JC, Hesketh R (1998). Biological responses to electromagnetic fields. *FASEB J*, 12(6):395-420.

Lacy-Hulbert A et al. (1995). No effect of 60 Hz electromagnetic fields on MYC or ß-Actin expression in human leukemic cells. *Radiat Res*, 144:9-17.

Lagroye I, Poncy JL (1997). The effect of 50 Hz electromagnetic fields on the formation of micronuclei in rodent cell lines exposed to gamma radiation. *Int J Radiat Biol*, 72(2):249-254.

Lagroye I, Poncy JL (1998). Influence of 50-Hz magnetic fields and ionizing radiation on *c-jun* and *c-fos* oncoproteins. *Bioelectromagnetics*, 19(2):112-116.

Lai H (1996). Spatial learning deficit in the rat after exposure to a 60 Hz magnetic field. *Bioelectromagnetics*, 17(6):494-496.

Lai H, Carino M (1999). 60 Hz magnetic fields and central cholinergic activity: effects of exposure intensity and duration. *Bioelectromagnetics*, 20(5):284-289.

Lai H, Singh NP (1997a). Acute exposure to a 60 Hz magnetic field increases DNA strand breaks in rat brain cells. *Bioelectromagnetics*, 18(2):156-165.

Lai H, Singh NP (1997b). Melatonin and N-tert-butyl-alpha-phenylnitrone block 60-Hz magnetic field-induced DNA single and double strand breaks in rat brain cells. *J Pineal Res*, 22(3):152-162.

Lai H, Singh NP (2004). Magnetic-field-induced DNA strand breaks in brain cells of the rat. *Environ Health Perspect*, 112(6):687-694.

Lai H, Carino MA, Ushijima I (1998). Acute exposure to a 60 Hz magnetic field affects rats' water-maze performance. *Bioelectromagnetics*, 19(2):117-122.

Lai H et al. (1993). Effects of a 60 Hz magnetic field on central cholinergic systems of the rat. *Bioelectromagnetics*, 14(1):5-15.

Leal J et al. (1989). Embryonic development and weak changes of the geomagnetic field. *J Bioelectr*, 7:141-153.

LeBien TW (2000). Fates of human B-cell precursors. *Blood*, 96(1):9-23.

Lednev VV (1991). Possible mechanism for the influence of weak magnetic fields on biological systems. *Bioelectromagnetics*, 12:71-75.

Lednev VV. Possible mechanism for the effect of weak magnetic fields on biological systems. Correction of the basic expression and its consequences. In: Blank M, ed. *Electricity and magnetism in biology and medicine*. San Francisco, San Francisco Press, 1993:550-552.

Lednev VV. Interference with vibrational energy sublevels of ions bound in calcium-binding proteins as the basis for the interaction of weak magnetic fields with biological systems. In: Frey AH, ed. *On the nature of electromagnetic field interactions with biological systems*. Austin, TX, RG Landes Co, 1994:59-72.

Lee GM et al. (2000). The use of electric bed heaters and the risk of clinically recognized spontaneous abortion. *Epidemiology*, 11(4):406-415.

Lee GM et al. (2002). A nested case-control study of residential and personal magnetic field measures and miscarriages. *Epidemiology*, 13(1):21-31.

Lee JM et al. (1993). Melatonin secretion and puberty in female lambs exposed to environmental electric and magnetic fields. *Biol Reprod*, 49(4):857-864.

Lee JM et al. (1995). Melatonin and puberty in female lambs exposed to EMF: a replicate study. *Bioelectromagnetics*, 16(2):119-123.

Leeper E et al. (1991). Modification of the 1979 "Denver wire code" for different wire or plumbing types. *Bioelectromagnetics*, 12(5):315-318.

Leitgeb N, Schroettner J (2002). Electric current perception study challenges electric safety limits. *J Med Eng Technol*, 26(4):168-172.

Leitgeb N, Schroettner J, Cech R (2005). Electric current perception of the general population including children and the elderly. *J Med Eng Technol*, 29(5):215-218.

Leman ES et al. (2001). Studies of the interactions between melatonin and 2 Hz, 0.3 mT PEMF on the proliferation and invasion of human breast cancer cells. *Bioelectromagnetics*, 22(3):178-184.

Lerchl A et al. (1991). Evidence that extremely low-frequency $Ca^{2+}$ cyclotron resonance depresses pineal melatonin synthesis in vitro. *Neurosci Lett*, 124(2):213-215.

Leuchtag HR . Do sodium channels in biological membranes undergo ferroelectric-superionic transitions? In: *Applications of Ferroelectrics, IEEE 7th International Symposium*, 1990, 279-283.

Levallois P et al. (1995). Electric and magnetic-field exposures for people living near a 735-kilovolt power-line. *Environ Health Perspect*, 103(9):832-837.

Levallois P et al. (2001). Effects of electric and magnetic fields from high-power lines on female urinary excretion of 6-sulfatoxymelatonin. *Am J Epidemiol*, 154(7):601-609.

Levallois P et al. (2002). Study of self-reported hypersensitivity to electromagnetic fields in California. *Environ Health Perspect*, 110(Suppl 4):619-623.

Levin ML (1953). The occurrence of lung cancer in man. *Acta Unio Int Contra Cancrum*, 9:531-541.

Lewy H, Massot O, Touitou Y (2003). Magnetic field (50 Hz) increases N-acetyltransferase, hydroxy-indole-O-methyltransferase activity and melatonin release through an indirect pathway. *Int J Radiat Biol*, 79(6):431-435.

Li CM et al. (1999). Effects of 50 Hz magnetic fields on gap junctional intercellular communication. *Bioelectromagnetics*, 20(5):290-294.

Li CY, Sung FC, Wu SC (2002). Risk of cognitive impairment in relation to elevated exposure to electromagnetic fields. *J Occup Environ Med*, 44(1):66-72.

Li DK, Neutra RR (2002). Magnetic fields and miscarriage. *Epidemiology*, 13(2):237-238.

Li DK, Checkoway H, Mueller BA (1995). Electric blanket use during pregnancy in relation to the risk of congenital urinary tract anomalies among women with a history of subfertility. *Epidemiology*, 6(5):485-489.

Li DK et al. (2001). A population-based prospective cohort study of personal exposure to magnetic fields during pregnancy and the risk of miscarriage. *Epidemiology*, 13(1):9-20.

Liao D et al. (1997). Cardiac autonomic function and incident coronary heart disease: A population-base case-cohort study. The ARIC study. *Am J Epidemiol*, 145(8):696-706.

Liboff AR, McLeod BR, Smith SD (1989). Rotating magnetic fields and ion cyclotron resonance. *J Bioelect*, 8(1):119-125.

Liburdy RP et al. (1993). ELF magnetic fields, breast cancer, and melatonin: 60 Hz fields block melatonin's oncostatic action on ER+ breast cancer cell proliferation. *J Pineal Res*, 14:89-1997.

Lightfoot T (2005). Aetiology of childhood leukemia. *Bioelectromagnetics*, 13(Suppl 7):S5-S11.

Lin H, Blank M, Goodman R (1999). A magnetic field-responsive domain in the human HSP70 promoter. *J Cell Biochem*, 75(1):170-176.

Lin H et al. (1997). Electromagnetic field exposure induces rapid, transitory heat shock factor activation in humans cells. *J Cell Biochem*, 66:402-488.

Lin H et al. (1998a). Magnetic field activation of protein-DNA binding. *J Cell Biochem*, 70(3):297-303.

Lin H et al. (1998b). Myc-mediated transactivation of HSP70 expression following exposure to magnetic fields. *J Cell Biochem*, 69(2):181-188.

Lin H et al. (2001). Regulating genes with electromagnetic response elements. *J Cell Biochem*, 81(1):143-148.

Lin RS, Lee WC (1994). Risk of childhood leukemia in areas passed by high power lines. *Rev Environ Health*, 10(2):97-103.

Lindbohm ML et al. (1992). Magnetic fields of video display terminals and spontaneous abortion. *Am J Epidemiol*, 136(9):1041-1051.

Linet MS, Devesa SS (1991). Descriptive epidemiology of childhood leukaemia. *Br J Cancer*, 63(3):424-429.

Linet MS et al. (1997). Residential exposure to magnetic fields and acute lymphoblastic leukemia in children. *New Engl J Med*, 337:1-7.

Linet MS et al. (1999). Cancer surveillance series: recent trends in childhood cancer incidence and mortality in the United States. *J Natl Cancer Inst*, 91(12):1051-1058.

Litvak E, Foster KR, Repacholi MH (2002). Health and safety implications of exposure to electromagnetic fields in the frequency range 300 Hz to 10 MHz. *Bioelectromagnetics*, 23(1):68-82.

Liu DL, Nazaroff WW (2003). Particle penetration through building cracks. *Aerosol Sci Tech*, 37:565-573.

Liu D et al. (1994). Hydroxyl radicals generated in vivo kill neurons in the rat spinal cord: electrophysiological, histological, and neurochemical results. *J Neurochem*, 62(1):37-44.

Liu Y et al. (2005). Magnetic field effect on singlet oxygen production in a biochemical system. *Chem Commun (Camb )*, (2):174-176.

Livingston GK et al. (1991). Reproductive integrity of mammalian cells exposed to power frequency electromagnetic fields. *Environ Mol Mutagen*, 17:49-58.

Lloyd D et al. (2004). The repair of gamma-ray-induced chromosomal damage in human lymphocytes after exposure to extremely low frequency electromagnetic fields. *Cytogenet Genome Res*, 104(1-4):188-192.

Loberg LI et al. (1999). Gene expression in human breast epithelial cells exposed to 60 Hz magnetic fields. *Carcinogenesis*, 20(8):1633-1636.

Loberg LI et al. (2000). Expression of cancer-related genes in human cells exposed to 60 Hz magnetic fields. *Radiat Res*, 153(5 Pt 2):679-684.

Lombardi F et al. (1987). Heart rate variability as an index of sympathovagal interaction after acute myocardial infarction. *Am J Cardiol*, 60(16):1239-1245.

London SJ et al. (1991). Exposure to residential electric and magnetic-fields and risk of childhood leukemia. *Am J Epidemiol*, 134(9):923-937.

London SJ et al. (1994). Exposure to magnetic fields among electrical workers in relation to leukemia risk in Los Angeles county. *Am J Ind Med*, 26:47-60.

London SJ et al. (2003). Residential magnetic field exposure and breast cancer risk: a nested case-control study from a multiethnic cohort in Los Angeles County. *Am J Epidemiol*, 158:969-980.

Lonne-Rahm S et al. (2000). Provocation with stress and electricity of patients with "sensitivity to electricity". *J Occup Environ Med*, 42(5):512-516.

Loomis DP, Savitz DA (1990). Mortality from brain cancer and leukaemia among electrical workers. *Br J Ind Med*, 47(9):633-638.

Loomis DP et al. (1994). Organization and classification of work history data in industry-wide studies: an application to the electric power industry. *Am J Ind Med*, 26(3):413-425.

Lorimore SA et al. (1990). Lack of acute effects of 20 mT, 50 Hz magnetic fields on murine haemopoiesis. *Int J Radiat Biol*, 58:713-723.

Löscher W (2001). Do cocarcinogenic effects of ELF electromagnetic fields require repeated long-term interaction with carcinogens? Characteristics of positive studies using the DMBA breast cancer model in rats. *Bioelectromagnetics*, 22(8):603-614.

Löscher W, Mevissen M (1995). Linear relationship between flux-density and tumor co-promoting effect of prolonged magnetic-field exposure in a breast-cancer model. *Cancer Lett*, 96(2):175-180.

Löscher W, Mevissen M, Häußler M (1997). Seasonal influence on 7,12-Dimethylbenz[a]anthracene-indu mammary carcinogenesis in Sprague-Dawley rats under controlled laboratory conditions. *Pharmacology & Toxicology, 81:265-27.*

Löscher W, Mevissen M, Lerchl A (1998). Exposure of female rats to a 100-microT 50 Hz magnetic field does not induce consistent changes in nocturnal levels of melatonin. *Radiat Res*, 150(5):557-567.

Löscher W et al. (1993). Tumor promotion in a breast-cancer model by exposure to a weak alternating magnetic-field. *Cancer Lett*, 71(1-3):75-81.

Löscher W et al. (1994). Effects of weak alternating magnetic-fields on nocturnal melatonin production and mammary carcinogenesis in rats. *Oncology*, 51(3):288-295.

Lotan M, Schwartz M (1994). Cross talk between the immune system and the nervous system in response to injury: implications for regeneration. *FASEB J*, 8(13):1026-1033.

Lovely RH et al. (1992). Rats are not aversive when exposed to 60-Hz magnetic fields at 3.03 mT. *Bioelectromagnetics*, 13:351-362.

Lövsund F, Öberg PA, Nilsson SEG (1982). ELF magnetic fields in electro-steel and welding industries.

Lövsund P et al. (1980). Magnetophosphenes: a quantitative analysis of thresholds. *Med Biol Eng Comput*, 18(3):326-334.

Luben RA, Morgan AP . Independent replication of 60 Hz, 1.2 µT EMF effects on melatonin and tamoxifen responses of MCF-7 breast cancer cells in vitro. In: *BioElectroMagnetics Society, 20th Annual Meeting*, 1998, A3.

Lundsberg LS, Bracken MB, Belanger K (1995). Occupationally related magnetic field exposure and male subfertility. *Fertil Steril*, 63(2):384-391.

Lupke M, Rollwitz J, Simko M (2004). Cell activating capacity of 50 Hz magnetic fields to release reactive oxygen intermediates in human umbilical cord blood-derived monocytes and in Mono Mac 6 cells. *Free Radic Res*, 38(9):985-993.

Lyskov E, Sandström M, Hansson Mild K (2001a). Neurophysiological study of patients with perceived 'electrical hypersensitivity'. *Int J Psychophysiol*, 42(3):233-241.

Lyskov E, Sandström M, Hansson Mild K (2001b). Provocation study of persons with perceived electrical hypersensitivity and controls using magnetic field exposure and recording of electrophysiological characteristics. *Bioelectromagnetics*, 22(7):457-462.

Lyskov E et al. (1993a). Influence of short-term exposure of magnetic field on the bioelectrical processes of the brain and performance. *Int J Psychophysiol*, 14:227-231.

Lyskov E et al. (1993b). Effects of 45-Hz magnetic fields on the functional state of the human brain. *Bioelectromagnetics*, 14(2):87-95.

Lyskov EB et al. (1993c). Effects of 45-Hz magnetic fields on cortical EEG in rats. *Electro Magnetobiol*, 12:179-185.

Maddock BJ (1992). Overhead line design in relation to electric and magnetic field limits. *Power Engineer J*, 6(5):217-224.

Mader DL, Peralta SB (1992). Residential exposure to 60-Hz magnetic-fields from appliances. *Bioelectromagnetics*, 13(4):287-301.

Mader DL et al. (1990). A simple model for calculating residential 60-Hz magnetic fields. *Bioelectromagnetics*, 11(4):283-296.

Maffeo S, Miller MW, Carstensen EL (1984). Lack of effect of weak low frequency electromagnetic fields on chick embryogenesis. *J Anat*, 139:613-618.

Makar TK et al. (1994). Vitamin E, ascorbate, glutathione, glutathione disulfide, and enzymes of glutathione metabolism in cultures of chick astrocytes and neurons: evidence that astrocytes play an important role in antioxidative processes in the brain. *J Neurochem*, 62(1):45-53.

Malik M, Farrell T, Camm AJ (1990). Circadian rhythm of heart rate variability after acute myocardial infarction and its influence on the prognostic value of heart rate variability. *Am J Cardiol*, 66(15):1049-1054.

Malmivuo J, Plonsey R. *Bioelectromagnetism*. New York, Oxford Press, 1995.

Mandeville R et al. (1997). Evaluation of the potential carcinogenicity of 60 Hz linear sinusoidal continuous-wave magnetic fields in Fisher F344 rats. *FASEB-J*, 11:1127-1136.

Mandeville R et al. (2000). Evaluation of the potential promoting effect of 60 Hz magnetic fields on N-ethyl-N-nitrosourea induced neurogenic tumors in female F344 rats. *Bioelectromagnetics*, 21(2):84-93.

Manni V et al. (2004). Low electromagnetic field (50 Hz) induces differentiation on primary human oral keratinocytes (HOK). *Bioelectromagnetics*, 25(2):118-126.

Mant J et al. (2006). Clinicians didn't reliably distinguish between different causes of cardiac death using case histories. *J Clin Epidemiol*, 59(8):862-867.

Maresh CM et al. (1988). Exercise testing in the evaluation of human responses to powerline frequency fields. *Aviat Space Environ Med*, 59(12):1139-1145.

Margonato V et al. (1993). Biologic effects of prolonged exposure to ELF electromagnetic-fields in rats. I. 50 Hz electric fields. *Bioelectromagnetics*, 14(5):479-493.

Margonato V et al. (1995). Biological effects of prolonged exposure to ELF electromagnetic fields in rats: II. 50 Hz magnetic fields. *Bioelectromagnetics*, 16(6):343-355.

Marino AA, Bell GB, Chesson A (1996). Low-level EMFs are transduced like other stimuli. *J Neurol Sci*, 144:99-106.

Marino AA, Kolomytkin OV, Frilot C (2003). Extracellular currents alter gap junction intercellular communication in synovial fibroblasts. *Bioelectromagnetics*, 24(3):199-205.

Martin GJ et al. (1987). Heart rate variability and sudden death secondary to coronary artery disease during ambulatory electrocardiographic monitoring. *Am J Cardiol*, 60(1):86-89.

Martinez SF et al. (1992). Pineal 'synaptic ribbons' and serum melatonin levels in the rat following the pulse action of 52-Gs (50-Hz) magnetic fields: an evolutive analysis over 21 days. *Acta Anat (Basel)*, 143(4):289-293.

Maslanyj MP. *Power-frequency electromagnetic fields associated with local area electricity substations*. Chilton, Didcot, National Radiological Protection Board, 1996 (NRPB-M751).

Maslanyj MP et al. (2007). Investigation of the sources of residential power frequency magnetic field exposure in the UK Childhood Cancer Study. *J Radiol Prot*, 27(1):41-58.

Mathie A, Kennard LE, Veale EL (2003). Neuronal ion channels and their sensitivity to extremely low frequency weak electric field effects. *Radiat Prot Dosimetry*, 106(4):311-316.

McBride M (1998). Childhood cancer and environmental contaminants. *Can J Pub Health*, 89(suppl 1):S53-S62.

McBride ML et al. (1999). Power-frequency electric and magnetic fields and risk of childhood leukemia in Canada. *Am J Epidemiol*, 149(9):831-842.

McCann J, Kavet R, Rafferty CN (2000). Assessing the potential carcinogenic activity of magnetic fields using animal models. *Environ Health Perspect*, 108(Suppl 1):79-100.

McCann J, Kheifets L, Rafferty CN (1998). Cancer risk assessment of extremely low frequency electric and magnetic fields: a critical review of methodology. *Environ Health Perspect*, 106:701-717.

McCormick DA. Membrane properties and neurotransmitter actions. In: Shepherd GM, ed. *The synaptic organisation of the brain*. Oxford, Oxford University Press, 1998:37-76.

McCormick DL et al. (1998). Exposure to 60-Hz magnetic fields and risk of lymphoma in PIM transgenic and TSG-*p53*(*p53* knockout) mice. *Carcinogenesis*, 19(9):1649-1653.

McCormick DL et al. (1999). Chronic toxicity/oncogenicity evaluation of 60 Hz (power frequency) magnetic fields in B6C3F1 mice. *Toxicol Pathol*, 27(3):279-285.

McDowall ME (1986). Mortality of persons resident in the vicinity of electricity transmission facilities. *Br J Cancer*, 53:271-279.

McElroy JA et al. (2001). Electric blanket or mattress cover use and breast cancer incidence in women 50-79 years of age. *Epidemiology*, 12(6):613-617.

McElroy JA et al. (2002). Endometrial cancer incidence in relation to electric blanket use. *Am J Epidemiol*, 156(3):262-267.

McGivern RF, Sokol RZ, Adey WR (1990). Prenatal exposure to a low-frequency electromagnetic field demasculinizes adult scent marking behavior and increases accessory sex organ weights in rats. *Teratology*, 411:1-8.

McKay BE, Persinger MA (2000). Application timing of complex magnetic fields delineates windows of posttraining-pretesting vulnerability for spatial and motivational behaviors in rats. *Int J Neurosci*, 103(1-4):69-77.

McKinlay A, Repacholi M (2003). International workshop on weak electric field effects in the body. *Radiat Protect Dosimetry*, 106(4):295-296.

McKinlay AF et al. *Review of the scientific evidence for limiting exposure to electromagnetic fields (0-300 GHz)*. Chilton, Didcot, National Radiological Protection Board, 2004 (Documents of the NRPB, Vol. 15, No. 3).

McLauchlan K (1992). Are environmental magnetic fields dangerous? *Physics World*, 5:41-45.

McLean JRN et al. (1991). Cancer promotion in a mouse-skin model by a 60 Hz magnetic-field .2. Tumor-development and immune-response. *Bioelectromagnetics*, 12(5):273-287.

McLean J et al. (1995). A 60-Hz magnetic field increases the incidence of squamous cells carcinomas in mice previously exposed to chemical carcinogens. *Cancer Lett*, 92(2):121-125.

McLean JRN et al. (1997). The effect of 60-Hz magnetic fields on co-promotion of chemically induced skin tumours on SENCAR mice: a discussion of three studies. *Environ Health Persp*, 105:94-96.

McMahan S, Ericson J, Meyer J (1994). Depressive symptomatology in women and residential proximity to high-voltage transmission lines. *Am J Epidemiol*, 139(1):58-63.

Merchant CJ, Renew DC, Swanson J (1994a). Exposures to power-frequency magnetic fields in the home. *J Radiol Prot*, 14(1):77-87.

Merchant CJ, Renew DC, Swanson J (1994b). Occupational exposures to power-frequency magnetic fields in the electricity supply industry. *J Radiol Prot*, 14(2):155-164.

Merchant CJ, Renew DC, Swanson J. Origins and magnitudes of exposure to power-frequency magnetic fields in the UK. In: *CIGRE (International Conference on Large High Voltage Electric Systems) Session 1994, vol. 2.* Paris, CIGRE, 1994c:36-105.

Mevissen M, Häußler M (1998). Acceleration of mammary tumorigenesis by exposure of 7,12-dimethylbenz[a]anthracene - treated female rats in a 50Hz 100-µT magnetic-field: replication study. *J Toxicol Environ Health A*, 53(5):401-418.

Mevissen M, Buntenkotter S, Löscher W (1994). Effects of static and time-varying (50-Hz) magnetic-fields on reproduction and fetal development in rats. *Teratology*, 50(3):229-237.

Mevissen M, Häußler M, Löscher W (1999). Alterations in ornithine decarboxylase activity in the rat mammary gland after different periods of 50 Hz magnetic field exposure. *Bioelectromagnetics*, 20(6):338-346.

Mevissen M, Kietzmann M, Löscher W (1995). In-vivo exposure of rats to a weak alternating magnetic-field increases ornithine decarboxylase activity in the mammary-gland by a similar extent as the carcinogen dmba. *Cancer Lett*, 90(2):207-214.

Mevissen M, Lerchl A, Löscher W (1996). Study on pineal function and DMBA-induced breast-cancer formation in rats during exposure to a 100-mg, 50-Hz magnetic-field. *J Toxicol Environ Health*, 48(2):169-185.

Mevissen M et al. Effects of AC magnetic field on DMBA-induced mammary carcinogenesis in Sprague-Dawley rats. In: Blank M, ed. *Electricity and magnetism in biology and medicine*. San Francisco, San Francisco Press, 1993a:413-415.

Mevissen M et al. (1993b). Effects of magnetic-fields on mammary tumor development induced by 7,12-dimethylbenz(a)anthracene in rats. *Bioelectromagnetrics*, 14:131-143.

Mevissen M et al. (1996). Exposure of DMBA-treated female rats in a 50-Hz, 50-µT magnetic-field: effects on mammary-tumor growth, melatonin levels, and T-lymphocyte activation. *Carcinogenesis*, 17(5):903-910.

Mevissen M et al. (1998). Complex effects of long-term 50 Hz magnetic field exposure in vivo on immune functions in female Sprague-Dawley rats depend on duration of exposure. *Bioelectromagnetics*, 19(4):259-270.

Mezei G, Kheifets L (2001). Is there any evidence for differential misclassification or for bias away from the null in the Swedish childhood cancer study? *Epidemiology*, 12:750-752.

Mezei G, Kheifets LI (2002). Clues to the possible viral etiology of childhood leukaemia. *Technology*, 9:3-14.

Mezei G, Kheifets L (2006). Selection bias and its implications for case-control studies: a case study of magnetic field exposure and childhood leukaemia. *Int J Epidemiol*, 35(2):397-406.

Mezei G et al. (2001). Household appliance use and residential exposure to 60 Hz magnetic fields. *J Expo Anal Environ Epidemiol*, 11(1):41-49.

Mezei G et al. (2006). Analyses of magnetic-field peak-exposure summary measures. *J Expo Sci Environ Epidemiol*, 16(6):477-485.

Michaelis J et al. (1997). Childhood leukemia and electromagnetic fields: results of a population-based case-control study in Germany. *Cancer Causes Control*, 8(2):167-174.

Michaelis J et al. (1998). Combined risk estimates for two German population-based case-control studies on residential magnetic fields and childhood acute leukemia. *Epidemiology*, 9:92-94.

Milham S (1982). Mortality from leukemia in workers exposed to electrical and magnetic fields. *N Engl J Med*, 307(4):249.

Milham S (1985a). Mortality in workers exposed to electromagnetic fields. *Environ Health Perspect*, 62:297-300.

Milham S (1985b). Silent keys: leukaemia mortality in amateur radio operators. *Lancet*, (April 6):812.

Milham S, Hatfield J, Tell R (1999). Magnetic fields from steel-belted radial tires: implications for epidemiologic studies. *Bioelectromagnetics*, 20:440-445.

Milham S, Ossiander EM (2001). Historical evidence that residential electrification caused the emergence of the childhood leukemia peak. *Med Hypotheses*, 56(3):290-295.

Miller SC et al. (1999). NF-kappaB or AP-1-dependent reporter gene expression is not altered in human U937 cells exposed to power-line frequency magnetic fields. *Radiat Res*, 151(3):310-318.

Mills KM et al. (2000). Reliability of proxy-reported and self-reported household appliance use. *Epidemiology*, 11(5):581-588.

Milunsky A et al. (1992). Maternal zinc and fetal neural tube defects. *Teratology*, 46(4):341-348.

413

Mirabolghasemi G, Azarnia M (2002). Developmental changes in *Drosophila melanogaster* following exposure to alternating electromagnetic fields. *Bioelectromagnetics*, 23(6):416-420.

Miyakoshi J et al. (1999). Long-term exposure to a magnetic field (5 mT at 60 Hz) increases X-ray -induced mutations. *J Radiat Res*, 40:13-21.

Miyakoshi J et al. (1996). Exposure to magnetic field (5 mt at 60 Hz) does not affect cell growth and c-myc gene expression. *J Radiat Res (Tokyo)*, 37(3):185-191.

Miyakoshi J et al. (2000a). Suppression of heat-induced HSP-70 by simultaneous exposure to 50 mT magnetic field. *Life Sci*, 66:1187-1196.

Miyakoshi J et al. (2000b). Exposure to strong magnetic fields at power frequency potentiates X-ray-induced DNA strand breaks. *J Radiat Res (Tokyo)*, 41(3):293-302.

Miyakoshi J et al. (2000c). Exposure to extremely low frequency magnetic fields suppresses X-ray-induced transformation in mouse C3H10T1/2 cells. *Biochem Biophys Res Commun*, 271(2):323-327.

Moorman PG et al. (1999). Participation rates in a case-control study: the impact of age, race, and race of interviewer. *Ann Epidemiol*, 9(3):188-195.

Morehouse CA, Owen RD (2000a). Exposure of Daudi cells to low-frequency magnetic fields does not elevate MYC steady-state mRNA levels. *Radiat Res*, 153(5 Pt 2):663-669.

Morehouse CA, Owen RD (2000b). Exposure to low-frequency electromagnetic fields does not alter HSP70 expression or HSF-HSE binding in HL60 cells. *Radiat Res*, 153(5 Pt2):658-662.

Morris JE, Phillips RD (1982). Effects of 60-Hz electric fields on specific humoral and cellular components of the immune system. *Bioelectromagnetics*, 3:341-347.

Morris JE et al. In vitro exposure of MCF-7 human mammary cells to 60 Hz magnetic fields. In: *BioElectroMagnetics Society, 20th Annual Meeting*, 1998, 125A.

Morris JE et al. (1999). Clinical progression of transplanted large granular lymphocytic leukemia in Fischer 344 rats exposed to 60 Hz magnetic fields. *Bioelectromagnetics*, 20(1):48-56.

Mostafa RM, Mostafa YM, Ennaceur A (2002). Effects of exposure to extremely low-frequency magnetic field of 2 G intensity on memory and corticosterone level in rats. *Physiol Behav*, 76(4-5):589-595.

Mubarak AA (1996). Does high voltage electricity have an effect on the sex distribution of offspring? *Hum Reprod*, 11(1):230-231.

Muc AM. *Electromagnetic fields associated with transportation systems*. Toronto, Ontario, Health Canada, 2001.

Mueller CH, Krueger H, Schierz C (2002). Project NEMESIS: Perception of a 50 Hz electric and magnetic field at low intensities (laboratory experiment). *Bioelectromagnetics*, 23(1):26-36.

Murphy JC et al. (1993). Power frequency electric and magnetic fields: A review of genetic toxicology. *Mut Res*, 296(3):221-240.

Murthy KK, Rogers WR, Smith HD (1995). Initial studies on the effects of combined 60 Hz electric and magnetic field exposure on the human system of nonhuman primates. *Bioelectromagnetics*, 16(Suppl 3):93-102.

Nagano A et al. (1991). Ventilatory effects of percutaneous magnetophrenic stimulation. *Front Med Biol Eng*, 3(2):97-112.

Nair I, Morgan MG, Florig HK. *Biological effects of power frequency electric and magnetic fields: background paper*. Washington, DC, Office of Technology Assessment, Congress of the United States, 1989 (OTA-BP-E-53).

Nakasono S et al. (2003). Effect of power-frequency magnetic fields on genome-scale gene expression in Saccharomyces cerevisiae. *Radiat Res*, 160(1):25-37.

National Grid (2007a). *Transmission - Table of calculated magnetic fields produced by underground cables in operation in the UK*. (http://www.emfs.info/Source_underground_mag_fld_table.asp, accessed 22-2-2007).

National Grid (2007b). *What is the average field from a transmission line?* (http://www.emfs.info/Source_overhead_avrgfield.asp, accessed 22-2-2007).

Navas-Acien A et al. (2002). Interactive effect of chemical substances and occupational electromagnetic field exposure on the risk of gliomas and meningiomas in Swedish men. *Cancer Epidemiol Biomarkers Prev*, 11(12):1678-1683.

414

NBOSH - National Board of Occupational Safety and Health et al. *Low-frequency electric and magnetic fields: the precautionary principle for national authorities. Guidance for decision-makers.* Stockholm, National Board of Occupational Safety and Health, 1996.

Negishi T et al. (2002). Studies of 50 Hz circularly polarized magnetic fields of up to 350 microT on reproduction and embryo-fetal development in rats: exposure during organogenesis or during preimplantation. *Bioelectromagnetics*, 23(5):369-389.

Neutra RR, Del Pizzo V (1996). When "Wire Codes" predict cancer better than spot measurements of magnetic fields. *Epidemiology*, 7(3):217-218.

Niehaus M et al. (1997). Growth retardation, testicular stimulation, and increased melatonin synthesis by weak magnetic fields (50Hz) in Djhungarian hamsters, *Phodopus sungorus. Biochem Biophysi Res Commun*, 234:707-711.

NIEHS - National Institute of Environmental Health Sciences. *Questions and answers about EMF electric and magnetic fields associated with the use of electric power.* Washington, DC, National Institute of Environmental Health Sciences, 1995 (DOE/EE-0040).

NIEHS - National Institute of Environmental Health Sciences. *Assessment of health effects from exposure to power-line frequency electric and magnetic fields. National Institute of Environmental Health Sciences Working Group Report.* Portier CJ, Wolfe MS, eds. Research Triangle Park, NC, National Institute of Health, 1998 (NIH Publication No 98-3981).

NIEHS - National Institute of Environmental Health Sciences. *Report on health effects from exposure to power-line frequency electric and magnetic fields. report to Congress.* Research Triangle Park, NC, National Institute of Health, 1999 (NIH Publication No 99-4493).

Nilius B, Droogmans G (2001). Ion channels and their functional role in vascular endothelium. *Physiol Rev*, 81(4):1415-1459.

NIOSH - National Institute for Occupational Safety and Health, National Institute of Environmental Health Sciences, US Department of Energy. *Questions and answers - EMF in the workplace. Electric and magnetic fields associated with the use of electric power.* Washinton, DC, National Institute of Environmental Health Sciences, 1996.

Noonan CW et al. (2002). Occupational exposure to magnetic fields in case-referent studies of neurodegenerative diseases. *Scand J Work Environ Health*, 28(1):42-48.

Nordenson I et al. Effect of low-frequency magnetic fields on the chromosomal level in human amniotic cells. In: Norden B, Ramel C, eds. *Interaction mechanisms of low-level electromagnetic fields in living systems - Resonant phenomena.* Oxford, University Press, 1992:240-250.

Nordenson I et al. (2001). Chromosomal aberrations in peripheral lymphocytes of train engine drivers. *Bioelectromagnetics*, 22(5):306-315.

Nordström S, Birk E, Gustavsson L (1983). Reproductive hazards among workers at high voltage substations. *Bioelectromagnetic*, 4:91-101.

NRC - National Research Council. *Possible health effects of exposure to residential electric and magnetic fields.* Washington, DC, National Academy Press, 1997.

Nyenhuis JA et al. Health effects and safety of intense gradient fields. In: Shellock FG, ed. *Magnetic resonance procedures: health effects and safety.* Boca Raton, London, New York, Washington, DC, CRC Press, 2001:31-54.

Oda T, Koike T (2004). Magnetic field exposure saves rat cerebellar granule neurons from apoptosis in vitro. *Neurosci Lett*, 365(2):83-86.

Ohnishi Y et al. (2002). Effects of power frequency alternating magnetic fields on reproduction and pre-natal development of mice. *J Toxicol Sci*, 27(3):131-138.

Olivares-Banuelos T et al. (2004). Differentiation of chromaffin cells elicited by ELF MF modifies gene expression pattern. *Cell Biol Int*, 28(4):273-279.

Olsen JH, Nielsen A, Schulgen G (1993). Residence near high-voltage facilities and risk of cancer in children. *Br Med J*, 307(6909):891-895.

Olsen RG (1994). Power-transmission electromagnetics. *IEEE Antennas Propagation Mag*, 36:7-16.

Oppenheimer M, Preston-Martin S (2002). Adult onset acute myelogenous leukemia and electromagnetic fields in Los Angeles County: bed-heating and occupational exposures. *Bioelectromagnetics*, 23(6):411-415.

Orr JL, Rogers WR, Smith HD (1995a). Detection threshold for 60 Hz electric fields by nonhuman primates. *Bioelectromagnetics*, 16(Suppl 3):23-34.

Orr JL, Rogers WR, Smith HD (1995b). Exposure of baboons to combined 60 Hz electric and magnetic fields does not produce work stoppage or affect operant performance on a match-to-sample task. *Bioelectromagnetics*, 16(Suppl 3):61-70.

Ossenkopp K-P, Kavaliers M (1987). Morphine-induced analgesia and exposure to low-intensity 60-Hz magnetic fields: inhibition of nocturnal analgesia in mice is a function of magnetic field intensity. *Brain Res*, 418(2):356-360.

Otaka Y et al. (2002). Carcinogenicity test in B6C3F1 mice after parental and prenatal exposure to 50 Hz magnetic fields. *Bioelectromagnetics*, 23(3):206-213.

Owen RD (1998). MYC mRNA abundance is unchanged in subcultures of HL60 cells exposed to power-frequency magnetic fields. *Radiat Res*, 150:23-30.

Pafkova H, Jerabek J (1994). Interaction of MF 50 Hz, 10 mT with high dose of X-rays: evaluation of embryotoxicity in chick embryos. *Rev Environ Health*, 10(3-4):235-241.

Pafkova H et al. (1996). Developmental effects of magnetic field (50 Hz) in combination with ionizing radiation and chemical teratogens. *Toxicol Lett*, 88(1-3):313-316.

Parazzini F et al. (1993). Video display terminal use during pregnancy and reproductive outcome a meta-analysis. *J Epidemiol Community Health*, 47(4):265-268.

Parker JE, Winters W (1992). Expression of gene-specific rna in cultured-cells exposed to rotating 60 Hz magnetic-fields. *Biochem Cell Biol*, 70(3-4):237-241.

Parpura V et al. (1994). Glutamate-mediated astrocyte-neuron signalling. *Nature*, 369(6483):744-747.

Pasquini R et al. (2003). Micronucleus induction in cells co-exposed in vitro to 50 Hz magnetic field and benzene, 1,4-benzenediol (hydroquinone) or 1,2,4-benzenetriol. *Toxicol In Vitro*, 17(5-6):581-586.

Pattengale PK. Classification of mouse lymphoid cell neoplasms.In: Jones TC et al., eds. *Hemopoietic system*. Springer-Verlag Telos, 1990:137-143.

Pattengale PK (1994). Tumours of the lymphohaematopoietic system. *IARC Sci Publ*, (111):651-670.

Pattengale PK, Taylor CR (1983). Experimental models of lymphoproliferative disease. The mouse as a model for human non-Hodgkin's lymphomas and related leukemias. *Am J Pathol*, 113(2):237-265.

Perry FS et al. (1981). Environmental power-frequency magnetic fields and suicide. *Health Phys*, 41(2):267-277.

Perry S, Pearl L, Binns R (1989). Power frequency magnetic field: depressive illness and myocardial infarction. *Public Health*, 103(3):177-180.

Perry VH, Brown MC, Gordon S (1987). The macrophage response to central and peripheral nerve injury. A possible role for macrophages in regeneration. *J Exp Med*, 165(4):1218-1223.

Petridou E et al. (1993). Suggestions of concomitant changes of electric power consumption and childhood leukemia in Greece. *Scand J Soc Med*, 21:(4):281-285.

Pfluger DH, Minder CE (1996). Effects of exposure to 16.7 hz magnetic fields on urinary 6-hydroxymelatonin sulfate excretion of Swiss railway workers. *J Pineal Res*, 21(2):91-100.

Phillips JL (1993). Effects of electromagnetic field exposure on gene transcription. *J Cell Biochem*, 51(4):381-386.

Phillips JL, McChesney L (1991). Effect of 72 Hz pulsed magnetic field exposure on macromolecular synthesis in CCRF-CEM cells. *Cancer Biochem Biophys*, 12(1):1-7.

Phillips JL et al. (1993). Effect of 72 Hz pulsed magnetic field exposure on ras p21 expression in CCRF-CEM cells. *Cancer Biochem Biophys*, 13(3):187-193.

Picazo ML et al. (1995). Long-term effects of elf magnetic fields on the mouse testis and serum testosterone levels. *Electro Magnetobiol*, 14(2):127-134.

Picazo ML et al. (1996). Changes in mouse adrenal gland functionality under second-generation chronic exposure to ELF magnetic fields: I. Males. *Electro Magnetobiol*, 15(2):85-98.

Picazo ML et al. (1998). Inhibition of melatonin in the plasma of third-generation male mice under the action of elf magnetic fields. *Electro Magnetobiol*, 17(1):75-85.

Pipkin JL et al. (1999). Induction of stress proteins by electromagnetic fields in cultured HL-60 cells. *Bioelectromagnetics*, 20(6):347-357.

Pirozzoli MC et al. (2003). Effects of 50 Hz electromagnetic field exposure on apoptosis and differentiation in a neuroblastoma cell line. *Bioelectromagnetics*, 24(7):510-516.

Plonsey R, Barr RC. *Bioelectricity, a quantitative approach*. New York, Plenum Press, 1988.

Podd JV et al. (1995). Do ELF magnetic fields affect human reaction time? *Bioelectromagnetics*, 16:317-323.

Podd J et al. (2002). Brief exposure to a 50 Hz, 100 microT magnetic field: effects on reaction time, accuracy, and recognition memory. *Bioelectromagnetics*, 23(3):189-195.

Polk C. Sources, propagation, amplitude, and temporal variation of extremely low frequency (0-100 Hz) electromagnetic fields. In: Llaurado JG, Sances A, Battoclettie JH, eds. *Biological and clinical effects of low frequency magnetic and electric fields*. Springfield, IL, Charles C. Thomas, 1974:21-48.

Polk C (1992). Dosimetry of extremely-low-frequency magnetic-fields. *Bioelectroamgetics*, 13(Suppl. 1):209-235.

Pollan M, Gustavsson P, Floderus B (2001). Breast cancer, occupation, and exposure to electromagnetic fields among Swedish men. *Am J Ind Med*, 39(3):276-285.

Poole C et al. (1993). Depressive symptoms and headaches in relation to proximity of residence to an alternating-current transmission line right-of-way. *Am J Epidemiol*, 137(3):318-330.

Portet R, Cabanes J (1988). Development of young rats and rabbits exposed to a strong electric field. *Bioelectromagnetics*, 9:95-104.

Potter ME, Okoniewski M, Stuchly MA (2000). Low frequency finite difference time domain (FDTD) for modeling of induced fields in humans close to line sources. *J Comput Physics*, 162:82-103.

Prato FS, Kavaliers M, Carson JJL (1996). Behaviuoral responses to magnetic fields by land snails are dependent on both magnetic field direction and light. *Proc R Soc Lond B*, 263:1437-1442.

Prato FS, Kavaliers M, Thomas AW (2000). Extremely low frequency magnetic fields can either increase or decrease analgaesia in the land snail depending on field and light conditions. *Bioelectromagnetics*, 21(4):287-301.

Prato FS et al. (1995). Possible mechanisms by which extremely-low-frequency magnetic fields affect opioid function. *FASEB J*, 9(9):807-814.

Prato FS et al. (1997). Light-dependent and -independent behavioural effects of extremely low frequency magnetic fields in a land snail are consistent with a parametric resonance mechanism. *Bioelectromagnetics*, 18(3):284-291.

Preece AW, Wesnes KA, Iwi GR (1998). The effect of a 50-Hz magnetic field on cognitive function in humans. *Int J Radiat Biol*, 74(4):463-470.

Preece AW et al. (1996). Domestic magnetic field exposures in Avon. *Phys Med Biol*, 41(1):71-81.

Preece AW et al. (1997). Magnetic fields from domestic appliances in the UK. *Phys Med Biol*, 42:67-76.

Putinas J, Michaelson SM (1990). Humoral responsiveness of mice exposed to a 500 μT, 60 Hz magnetic field. *Bioelectrochem Bioenerg*, 24(371-374):371-374.

Qiu C et al. (2004). Occupational exposure to electromagnetic fields and risk of Alzheimer's disease. *Epidemiology*, 15(6):687-694.

Quaglino D et al. (2004). The effect on rat thymocytes of the simultaneous in vivo exposure to 50-Hz electric and magnetic field and to continuous light. *Scientific World Journal*, 4(Suppl 2):91-99.

Quinlan WJ et al. (1985). Neuroendocrine parameters in the rat exposed to 60-Hz electric fields. *Bioelectromagnetics*, 6:381-389.

Ragan HA et al. (1983). Hematologic and serum chemistry studies in rats exposed to 60-Hz electric fields. *Bioelectromagnetics*, 4(1):79-90.

Rankin RF et al. (2002). Results of a multisite study of U.S. residential magnetic fields. *J Expo Anal Environ Epidemiol*, 12(1):9-20.

Rannug A, Holmberg B, Mild KH (1993). A rat liver foci promotion study with 50-Hz magnetic fields. *Environ Res*, 62(2):223-229.

Rannug A et al. (1993a). A study on skin tumour formation in mice with 50 Hz magnetic field exposure. *Carcinogenesis*, 14(4):573-578.

Rannug A et al. (1993b). Rat-liver foci study on coexposure with 50 Hz magnetic-fields and known carcinogens. *Bioelectromagnetics*, 14(1):17-27.

Rannug A et al. (1994). Intermittent 50 Hz magnetic field and skin tumour promotion in SEN-CAR mice. *Carcinogenesis*, 15(2):153-157.

Rao S, Henderson AS (1996). Regulation of c-fos is affected by electromagnetic-fields. *J Cell Biochem*, 63(3):358-365.

Rauch GB et al. (1992). A comparison of international residential grounding practices and associated magnetic fields. *IEEE Trans Power Delivery*, 7(2):743-748.

Rea WJ et al. (1991). Electromagnetic-field sensitivity. *J Bioelect*, 10(1-2):241-256.

Rechavi G, Ramot B, Ben-Bassat I (1992). The role of infection in childhood leukemia: what can be learned from the male predominance? *Acta Haematol*, 88:58-60.

Reese JA, Jostes RF, Frazier ME (1988). Exposure of mammalian cells to 60-Hz magnetic or electric fields: analysis for DNA singles-strand breaks. *Bioelectromagnetics*, 9(3):237-247.

Reichmanis M et al. (1979). Relation between suicide and the electromagnetic field of overhead power lines. *Physiol Chem & Physics*, 11.

Reilly JP. *Electrical stimulation and electropathology*. Cambridge, University Press, 1992.

Reilly JP. *Applied bioelectricity: from electrical stimulation to electropathology*. New York, Springer Verlag, 1998a.

Reilly JP. Cardiac sensitivity to stimulation. In: Reilly JP, ed. *Applied bioelectricity: from electrical stimulation to electropathology*. New York, Springer Verlag, 1998b:194-239.

Reilly JP (1999). Comments concerning "Guidelines for limiting exposure to time-varying electric, magnetic and electromagnetic fields (up to 300 GHz). *Health Phys*, 76(3):314-315.

Reilly JP (2002). Neuroelectric mechanisms applied to low frequency electric and magnetic field exposure guidelines - part I: sinusoidal waveforms. *Health Phys*, 83(3):341-355.

Reilly JP (2005). An analysis of differences in the low-frequency electric and magnetic field exposure standards of ICES and ICNIRP. *Health Phys*, 89(1):71-80.

Reilly JP, Freeman VT, Larkin WD (1985). Sensory effect of transient electrical stimulation - evaluation with a neuroelectric model. *IEEE Trans Biomed Eng*, 32(12):1001-1011.

Reilly KM et al. (2000). Nf1;Trp53 mutant mice develop glioblastoma with evidence of strain-specific effects. *Nat Genet*, 26(1):109-113.

Reipert BM et al. (1997). Apoptosis in haemopoietic progenitor cells exposed to extremely low-frequency magnetic fields. *Life Sci*, 61(16):1571-1582.

Reiter RJ. Melatonin biosynthesis, regulation, and effects. In: Stevens RG, Wilson BW, Anderson LE, eds. *The melatonin hypothesis: breast cancer and the use of electric power*. Columbus, OH, Battelle Press, 1997:25-48.

Reiter RJ et al. (1988). Reduction of the nocturnal rise in pineal melatonin levels in rats exposed to 60-Hz electric fields in utero and for 23 days after birth. *Life Sci*, 42(22):2203-2206.

Renew DC, Male JC, Maddock BJ. Power frequency magnetic fields: measurement and exposure assessment. In: *CIGRE (International Conference on Large High Voltage Electric Systems) Session 1990*. Paris, CIGRE, 1990.

Ries LAG et al. *SEER cancer statistics review, 1973–1998*. Bethesda, MD, National Cancer Institute, 2001.

Ritz T, Adem S, Schulten K (2000). A model for photoreceptor-based magnetoreception in birds. *Biophys J*, 78(2):707-718.

Ritz T et al. (2004). Resonance effects indicate a radical-pair mechanism for avian magnetic compass. *Nature*, 429:177-180.

Robert E et al. (1996). Case-control study on maternal residential proximity to high voltage power lines and congenital anomalies in France. *Paediatr Perinat Epidemiol*, 10(1):32-38.

Robison JG et al. (2002). Decreased DNA repair rates and protection from heat induced apoptosis mediated by electromagnetic field exposure. *Bioelectromagnetics*, 23(2):106-112.

Rogers WR, Orr JL, Smith HD (1995). Nonhuman primates will not respond to turn off strong 60 Hz electric fields. *Bioelectromagnetics*, 16(Suppl 3):46-60.

Rogers WR et al. (1995a). Regularly scheduled, day-time, slow-onset 60 Hz electric and magnetic field exposure does not depress serum melatonin concentration in nonhuman primates. *Bioelectromagnetics*, 16(Suppl 3):111-118.

Rogers WR et al. (1995b). Rapid-onset/offset, variably scheduled 60 Hz electric and magnetic field exposure reduces nocturnal serum melatonin concentration in nonhuman primates. *Bioelectromagnetics*, 16(Suppl 3):119-122.

Rollwitz J, Lupke M, Simko M (2004). Fifty-hertz magnetic fields induce free radical formation in mouse bone marrow-derived promonocytes and macrophages. *Biochim Biophys Acta*, 1674(3):231-238.

Rommereim DN et al. (1987). Reproduction and development in rats chronically exposed to 60-Hz electric fields. *Bioelectromagnetics*, 8:243-258.

Rommereim DN et al. (1990). Reproduction, growth, and development of rats during chronic exposure to multiple field strengths of 60-Hz electric fields. *Fundam Appl Toxicol*, 14(3):608-621.

Rommereim DN et al. (1996). Development toxicology evaluation of 60-Hz horizontal magnetic fields in rats. *Appl Occup Environ Hyg*, 11(4).

Rosen LA, Barber I, Lyle DB (1998). A 0.5 G, 60 Hz magnetic field suppresses melatonin production in pinealocytes. *Bioelectromagnetics*, 19(2):123-127.

Rosenberg RS, Duffy PH, Sacher GA (1981). Effects of intermittent 60-Hz voltage electric fields on metabolism, activity, and temperature in mice. *Bioelectromagnetics*, 2:291-303.

Rosenberg RS et al. (1983). Relationship between field strength and arousal response in mice exposed to 60-Hz electric fields. *Bioelectromagnetics*, 4:181-191.

Rothman KJ, Greenland S. *Modern epidemiology*, 2nd ed. Philadelphia, Lippincott, 1998.

Rothwell NJ (1997). Neuroimmune interactions: The role of cytokines. Sixteenth Gaddum memorial lecture December 1996. *Br J Pharmacol*, 121(5):841-847.

Roy S et al. (1995). The phorbol 12-myristate 13-acetate (PMA)-induced oxidative burst in rat peritoneal neutrophils in increased by 0.1 mT (60 Hz) magnetic field. *FEBS Lett*, 376:164-166.

Rubin GJ, Das MJ, Wessely S (2005). Electromagnetic hypersensitivity: a systematic review of provocation studies. *Psychosom Med*, 67(2):224-232.

Rubtsova NB, Tikhonova GI, Gurvich EB. Study of commercial frequency electromagnetic field effects on human health and their hygienic rating criteria. In: Repacholi M, Rubtsova NB, Muc AM, eds. *Electromagnetic fields: biological effects and hygienic standardization. Proceedings of an international meeting, Moscow, 18-22 May, 1998*. Geneva, World Health Organization, 1999:445-455.

Rudolph K et al. (1985). Weak 50-Hz electromagnetic fields activate rat open field behavior. *Physiol Behav*, 35(4):505-508.

Russo IH, Russo J (1996). Mammary gland neoplasia in long-term rodent studies. *Environ Health Perspect*, 104(9):938-967.

Ryan BM et al. (1996). Developmental toxicity study of 60 Hz (power frequency) magnetic fields in rats. *Teratology*, 54(2):73-83.

Ryan BM et al. (1999). Multigeneration reproduction toxicity assessment of 60-Hz magnetic fields using a continuous breeding protocol in rats. *Teratology*, 59(3):156-162.

Ryan K et al. (2000). Radio frequency radiation of millimeter wave length: potential occupational safety issues relating to surface heating. *Health Phys*, 78(2).170-181.

Saffer JD, Thurston SJ (1995). Short exposures to 60 Hz magnetic-fields do not alter MYC expression in HL-60 or Daudi cells. *Radiat Res*, 144(1):18-25.

Sagan PM et al. (1987). Detection of 60-hertz vertical electric fields by rats. *Bioelectromagnetics*, 8(3):303-313.

Sahl J et al. (2002). Occupational magnetic field exposure and cardiovascular mortality in a cohort of electric utility workers. *Am J Epidemiol*, 156(10):913-918.

Sait ML, Wood AW, Sadafi HA (1999). A study of heart rate and heart rate variability in human subjects exposed to occupational levels of 50 Hz circularly polarised magnetic fields. *Med Engin Phys*, 21:361-369.

Salzinger K et al. (1990). Altered operant behavior of adult rats after perinatal exposure to a 60-Hz electromagnetic field. *Bioelectromagnetics*, 11:105-116.

Sandström M et al. (1993). A survey of electric and magnetic fields among VDT operators in offices. *IEEE Trans EMC*, 35:394-397.

Sandström M et al. (1997). Neurophysiological effects of flickering light in patients with perceived electrical hypersensitivity. *J Occup Environ Med*, 39(1):15-22.

Santini MT et al. (2003). Effects of a 50 Hz sinusoidal magnetic field on cell adhesion molecule expression in two human osteosarcoma cell lines (MG-63 and Saos-2). *Bioelectromagnetics*, 24(5):327-338.

Sasser LB et al. Effect of 60 Hz electric fields on pineal melatonin during various times of the dark period. In: *Project Resumes, DOE Annual Review of Research on Biological Effects of 50 and 60 Hz Electric and Magnetic Fields*. Milwaukee, WI, US Department of Energy, 1991:A-24.

Sasser LB et al. (1996). Exposure to 60 Hz magnetic fields does not alter clinical progression of LGL leukemia in Fischer rats. *Carcinogenesis*, 17(12):2681-2687.

Sasser LB et al. (1998). Lack of a co-promoting effect of a 60 Hz magnetic field on skin tumorigenesis in SENCAR mice. *Carcinogenesis*, 19(9):1617-1621.

Sastre A, Cook MR, Graham C (1998). Nocturnal exposure to intermittent 60 Hz magnetic fields alters human cardiac rhythm. *Bioelectromagnetics*, 19(2):98-106.

Saunders RD (2003). Rapporteur report: Weak field interactions in the CNS. *Rad Prot Dos*, 106(4):357-361.

Saunders RD, Jefferys JG (2002). Weak electric field interactions in the central nervous system. *Health Phys*, 83(3):366-375.

Savitz DA (2002). Magnetic fields and miscarriage. *Epidemiology*, 13(1):1-4.

Savitz DA, Ananth CV (1994). Residential magnetic fields, wire codes, and pregnancy outcome. *Bioelectromagnetics*, 15(3):271-273.

Savitz DA, Loomis DP (1995). Magnetic field exposure in relation to leukemia and brain cancer mortality among electric utility workers. *Am J Epidemiol*, 141(2):123-134.

Savitz DA, Checkoway H, Loomis D.P. (1998). Magnetic field exposure and neurodegenerative disease mortality among electric utility workers. *Epidemiology*, 9(4 July):398-404.

Savitz DA, Loomis DP, Tse CK (1998). Electrical occupations and neurodegenerative diseases: analysis of US mortality data. *Arch Environ Health*, 53(1):71-74.

Savitz DA et al. (1988). Case-control study of childhood cancer and exposure to 60-Hz magnetic fields. *Am J Epidemiol*, 128(1):21-38.

Savitz DA et al. (1997). Lung cancer in relation to employment in the electrical utility industry and exposure to magnetic fields. *Occup Environ Med*, 54:396-402.

Savitz DA et al. (1999). Magnetic field exposure and cardiovascular disease mortality among electric utility workers. *Am J Epidemiol*, 149(2):135-142.

Scaiano JC, Monahan S, Renaud J (2006). Dramatic effect of magnetite particles on the dynamics of photogenerated free radicals. *Photochem Photobiol*, 65:759-762.

Scaiano JC et al. (1994). Application of the radical pair mechanism to free radicals in organized systems. *Bioelectromagnetics*, 15:549-554.

Scarfi MR et al. (2005). Evaluation of genotoxic effects in human fibroblasts after intermittent exposure to 50 Hz electromagnetic fields: a confirmatory study. *Radiat Res*, 164(3):270-276.

Schienle A et al. (1996). Atmospheric electromagnetism: individual differences in brain electrical response to simulated sferics. *Int J Psychophysiol*, 21(2-3):177-188.

Schimmelpfeng J, Stein J-C, Dertinger H (1995). Action of 50 Hz magnetic fields on cyclic AMP and intercellular communications in monolayers and speroids of mammalian cells. *Bioelectromagnetics*, 16:361-386.

Schlehofer B et al. (2005). Occupational risk factors for low grade and high grade glioma: results from an international case control study of adult brain tumours. *Int J Cancer*, 113(1):116-125.

Schnitzer PG, A.F.Olshan, J.D.Erickson (1995). Paternal occupation and risk of birth defects in offspring. *Epidemiology*, 6(6):577-583.

Schnorr TM et al. (1991). Video Display Terminals and the risk of spontaneous abortion. *N Engl J Med*, 324(11):727-733.

Schoenfeld ER et al. (2003). Electromagnetic fields and breast cancer on Long Island: a case-control study. *Am J Epidemiol*, 158(1):47-58.

Schulten K. Magnetic field effects in chemistry and biology. In: Aachen PG, ed. *Festkorperprobleme XXII: Advances in Solid State Physics*. Braunschweig, Vieweg, 1982:61-83.

Schumann WO (1952). Uber die strahlungslosen Eigenschwingungen einer leitenden Kugel, die von einer Luftschicht und einer Ionospharenhulle umgeben ist. *Zeitschrift fur Naturforschung*, 7a:149-152.

Schüz J et al. (2000). Extremely low-frequency magnetic fields in residences in Germany. Distribution of measurements, comparison of two methods for assessing exposure, and predictors for the occurrence of magnetic fields above background level. *Radiat Environ Biophys*, 39(4):233-240.

Schüz J et al. (2001). Residential magnetic fields as a risk factor for childhood acute leukaemia: Results from a German population-based case-control study. *Int J Cancer*, 91(5):728-735 (2001a).

Selmaoui B, Touitou Y (1995). Sinusoidal 50-Hz magnetic fields depress rat pineal NAT activity and serum melatonin. Role of duration and intensity of exposure. *Life Sci*, 57(14):1351-1358.

Selmaoui B, Touitou Y (1999). Age-related differences in serum melatonin and pineal NAT activity and in the response of rat pineal to a 50-Hz magnetic field. *Life Sci*, 64(24):2291-2297.

Selmaoui B, Lambrozo J, Touitou Y (1996). Magnetic-fields and pineal function in humans: evaluation of nocturnal acute exposure to extremely-low-frequency magnetic-fields on serum melatonin and urinary 6-sulfatoxymelatonin circadian-rhythms. *Life Sci*, 58(18):1539-1549.

Selmaoui B, Lambrozo J, Touitou Y (1997). Endocrine function in young men exposed for one night to a 50-Hz magnetic field. A circadian study of pituitary, thyroid and adrenocortical hormones. *Life Sci*, 61(5):473-486.

Selmaoui B et al. (1996). Acute exposure to 50 Hz magnetic field does not effect hematologic or immunologic functions in healthy young men: a circadian study. *Bioelectromagnetics*, 17(5):364-372.

Sentman DD (1987). Magnetic elliptical polarization of Schumann resonances. *Radio Sci*, 22:595-605.

Shah PN, Mhatre MC, Kothari LS (1984). Effect of melatonin on mammary carcinogenesis in intact and pinealectomized rats in varying photoperiods. *Cancer Res*, 44(8):3403-3407.

Shaw GM (2001). Adverse human reproductive outcomes and electromagnetic fields: A brief summary of the epidemiologic literature. *Bioelectromagnetics*, 22(Suppl 5):5-18.

Shaw GM, Croen LA (1993). Human adverse reproductive outcomes and electromagnetic field exposures: review of epidemiologic studies. *Environ Health Perspect*, 101(Suppl. 4):107-119.

Shaw GM et al. (1999). Maternal periconceptional use of electric bed-heating devices and risk for neural tube defects and orofacial clefts. *Teratology*, 60(3):124-129.

Shellock FG. *Magnetic resonance procedures: Health effects and safety*. Boca Raton London New York Washington, DC, CRC Press., 2001.

Shen YH et al. (1997). The effects of 50 Hz magnetic field exposure on DMBA induced thymic lymphoma leukemia in mice. *Bioelectromagnetics*, 18(5):360-364.

Shepherd GM, Koch C. Introduction to synaptic circuits.In: Shepherd GM, ed. *The synaptic organisation of the brain*. Oxford, Oxford University Press, 1998:1-36.

Sheppard AR, Kavet R, Renew DC (2002). Exposure guidelines for low-frequency electric and magnetic fields: report from the Brussels workshop. *Health Phys*, 83(3):324-332.

Shiau Y, Valentino AR (1981). ELF electric field coupling to dielectric spheroidal models of biological objects. *IEEE Trans Biomed Eng*, 28(6):429-437.

Sienkiewicz Z (2003). Rapporteur report: Other tissues. *Radiat Prot Dosimetry*, 106(4):391-396.

Sienkiewicz ZJ, Haylock RGE, Saunders RD (1996). Acute exposure to power-frequency magnetic fields has no effect on the acquisition of a spatial learning task by adult male mice. *Bioelectromagnetics*, 17(3):180-186 (1996a).

Sienkiewicz ZJ, Haylock RG, Saunders RD (1998). Deficits in spatial learning after exposure of mice to a 50 Hz magnetic field. *Bioelectromagnetics*, 19(2):79-84 (1998b).

Sienkiewicz ZJ, Larder S, Saunders RD (1996). Prenatal exposure to a 50 Hz magnetic field has no effect on spatial learning in adult mice. *Bioelectromagnetics*, 17(3):249-252 (1996b).

Sienkiewicz ZJ, Saunders RD, Kowalczuk CI. *Biological effects of exposure to non-ionising electromagnetic fields and radiation: II. Extremely low frequency electric and magnetic fields.* Chilton, National Radiological Protection Board, 1991 (NRPB-R239).

Sienkiewicz ZJ et al. Biological effects of electromagnetic fields and radiation.In: Stone WR, ed. *The review of radio science 1990-1992.* New York, Oxford University Press, 1993:737-770.

Sienkiewicz ZJ et al. (1994). Effects of prenatal exposure to 50 Hz magnetic fields on development in mice: II. Postnatal development and behavior. *Bioelectromagnetics*, 15(4):363-375.

Sienkiewicz ZJ et al. (1998). 50 Hz magnetic field effects on the performance of a spatial learning task by mice. *Bioelectromagnetics*, 19(8):486-493 (1998a).

Sienkiewicz ZJ et al. (2001). Single, brief exposure to a 50 Hz magnetic field does not affect the performance of an object recognition task in adult mice. *Bioelectromagnetics*, 22(1):19-26.

Sikov MR et al. (1987). Developmental studies of Hanford miniature swine exposed to 60 Hz electric fields. *Bioelectromagnetics*, 8:229-242.

Silny J . Influence of low-frequency magnetic field (LMF) on the organism. In: *Proceedings of the 4th Symposium on Electromagnetic Compatibility.* Zurich, 1981, 175-180.

Silny J. Changes in VEP caused by strong magnetic fields.In: Nodar RH, Barber C, eds. *Evoked potentials II.* Boston, Butterworth Publishers, 1984:272-279.

Silny J . Effects of low-frequency, high intensity magnetic field on the organism. In: *Proceedings of the IEEE International Conference on Electric and Magnetic Fields in Medicine and Biology.* London, 1985, 104.

Silny J. The influence thresholds of the time-varying magnetic field in the human organism. In: Bernhardt JH, ed. *Biological effects of static and extremely low frequency magnetic fields.* Munich, MMV Medizin Verlag München, 1986.

Silny J (1999). Electrical hypersensitivity in humans - fact or fiction? *Zbl Hyg Umweltmed*, 202:219-233.

Silva M et al. (1989). Power-frequency magnetic fields in the home. *IEEE Trans Power Delivery*, 4:465-478.

Simko M, Kriehuber R, Lange S (1998). Micronucleus formation in human amnion cells after exposure to 50Hz magnetic fields applied horizontally and vertically. *Mut Res*, 418(2-3):101-111.

Simko M, Mattsson MO (2004). Extremely low frequency electromagnetic fields as effectors of cellular responses in vitro: possible immune cell activation. *J Cell Biochem*, 93(1):83-92.

Simko M et al. (1998). Effects of 50 Hz EMF exposure on micronucleus formation and apoptosis in transformed and nontransformed human cell lines. *Bioelectromagnetics*, 19(2):85-91.

Simko M et al. (2001). Micronucleus induction in Syrian hamster embryo cells following exposure to 50 Hz magnetic fields, benzo(a)pyrene, and TPA in vitro. *Mut Res*, 495(1-2):43-50.

Skauli KS, Reitan JB, Walther BT (2000). Hatching in zebrafish (*Danio rerio*) embryos exposed to a 50 Hz magnetic field. *Bioelectromagnetics*, 21(5):407-410.

Skedsmo A, Vistnes AI (2000). Deflection of cosmic radiation near power lines - a theoretical approach. *Health Phys*, 78(6):679-686.

Skinner J et al. (2002). Exposure to power frequency electric fields and the risk of childhood cancer in the UK. *Br J Cancer*, 87(11):1257-1266.

Skotte JH (1994). Exposure to power-frequency electromagnetic fields in Denmark. *Scand J Work Environ Health*, 20:132-138.

Sloane JA et al. (1999). Increased microglial activation and protein nitration in white matter of the aging monkey. *Neurobiol Aging*, 20(4):395-405.

Slovic P (1987). Perception of risk. *Science*, 236:280-285.

Smith RF, Clarke RL, Justesen DR (1994). Behavioral sensitivity of rats to extremely-low-frequency magnetic fields. *Bioelectromagnetics*, 15(5):411-426.

Sobel E et al. (1995). Occupations with exposure to electromagnetic-fields: a possible risk factor for Alzheimers-disease. *Am J Epidemiol*, 142(5):515-524.

Sobel E et al. (1996). Elevated risk of Alzheimers-disease among workers with likely electromagnetic-field exposure. *Neurology*, 47(6):1477-1481.

Sokejima S, Kagamimori S, Tatsumura T (1996). Electric power consumption and leukaemia death rate in Japan. *Lancet*, 348(9030):821-822.

Sommer AM, Lerchl A (2004). The risk of lymphoma in AKR/J mice does not rise with chronic exposure to 50 Hz magnetic fields (1 microT and 100 microT). *Radiat Res*, 162(2):194-200.

Sorahan T, Nichols L (2004). Mortality from cardiovascular disease in relation to magnetic field exposure: findings from a study of UK electricity generation and transmission workers, 1973-1997. *Am J Ind Med*, 45(1):93-102.

Speciale SG et al. (1998). The neurotoxin 1-methyl-4-phenylpyridinium is sequestered within neurons that contain the vesicular monoamine transporter. *Neuroscience*, 84(4):1177-1185.

Spiegel RJ (1977). High-voltage electric field coupling to humans using moment method techniques. *IEEE Trans Biomed Eng*, BME-24:466-472.

Spiegel RJ (1981). Numerical determination of induced currents in humans and baboons exposed to 60 Hz electric fields. *IEEE Trans Electromag Compat*, 23:382-390.

Spinelli JJ et al. (2001). Assessing response bias as an explanation for the observation of low socioeconomic status (SES) as a risk factor for childhood leukemia (Abstract). *Am J Epidemiol*, 153:S254 (948).

Sritara P et al. (2003). Twelve-year changes in vascular risk factors and their associations with mortality in a cohort of 3499 Thais: the Electricity Generating Authority of Thailand Study. *Int J Epidemiol*, 32(3):461-468.

Stather JW et al. (1996). Comment on the paper: enhanced deposition of radon daughter nuclei in the vicinity of power frequency electromagnetic fields. *Int J Radiat Biol*, 69(5):645-649.

Steiner UE, Ulrich T (1989). Magnetic field effects in chemical kinetics and related phenomena. *Chem Rev*, 89(1):51-147.

Stell M, Sheppard AR, Adey WR (1993). The effect of moving air on detection of a 60-Hz electric field. *Bioelectromagnetics*, 14(1):67-78.

Stering P. Retina.In: Shepherd GM, ed. *The synaptic oarganization of the brain*. Oxford, Oxford University Press, 1998:205-254.

Stern S (1995). Do rats show a behavioral sensitivity to low-level magnetic fields? *Bioelectromagnetics*, 16(5):335-336.

Stern S, Laties VG (1985). 60-Hz electric fields: detection by female rats. *Bioelectromagnetics*, 6(1):99-103.

Stern S, Laties VG (1989). Comparison of 60-Hz electric fields and incandescent light as aversive stimuli controlling the behavior of rats. *Bioelectromagnetics*, 10(1):99-109.

Stern S et al. (1983). Behavioral detection of 60-Hz electric fields by rats. *Bioelectromagnetics*, 4(3):215-247.

Stern S et al. (1996). Exposure to combined static and 60 Hz magnetic fields: failure to replicate a reported behavioral effect. *Bioelectromagnetics*, 17(4):279-292.

Stevens RG (1987). Electric power use and breast cancer: a hypothesis. *Am J Epidemiol*, 125(4).

Stevens RG (2001). Light in the built environment: potential role of circadian disruption in endocrine disruption and breast cancer. *Cancer Causes Control*, 12:279-287.

Stollery BT (1986). Effects of 50 Hz electric currents on mood and verbal reasoning skills. *Br J Ind Med*, 43:339-349.

Stollery BT (1987). Effects of 50 Hz electric currents on vigilance and concentration. *Br J Ind Med*, 44(2):111-118.

Stopps GJ, Janischewskyj W, Alcock VMD. *Epidemiological study of workers maintaining HV equipment and lines in Ontario*. Montreal, Canadian Electrical Association, 1979.

Stronati L et al. (2004). Absence of genotoxicity in human blood cells exposed to 50 Hz magnetic fields as assessed by comet assay, chromosome aberration, micronucleus, and sister chromatid exchange analyses. *Bioelectromagnetics*, 25(1):41-48.

Stuchly MA, Dawson TW (2000). Interaction of low-frequency electric and magnetic fields with the human body. *Proceedings of the IEEE*, 88(5):643-664.

Stuchly MA, Dawson TW (2002). Human body exposure to power lines: relation of induced quantities to external magnetic fields. *Health Phys*, 83(3):330-340.

Stuchly MA, Gandhi OP (2000). Inter-laboratory comparison of numerical dosimetry for human exposure to 60 Hz electric and magnetic fields. *Bioelectromagnetics*, 21(3):167-174.

Stuchly MA, Lecuyer DW (1989). Exposure to electromagnetic fields in arc welding. *Health Phys*, 56:297-302.

Stuchly MA, Lecuyer DW, McLean J (1991). Cancer promotion in a mouse-skin model by a 60-Hz magnetic-field .1. Experimental design and exposure system. *Bioelectromagnetics*, 12(5):261-271.

Stuchly MA, Zhao S (1996). Magnetic field-induced currents in the human body in proximity of power lines. *IEEE Trans Power Delivery*, 11(1):102-108.

Stuchly MA et al. *Validation of computational methods for evaluation of electric fields and currents induced in humans exposed to electric and magnetic fields*. Palo Alto, CA, Electric Power Research Institute, 1998 (EPRI TR-111768).

Stuchly MA et al. (1988). Teratological assessment of exposure to time-varying magnetic field. *Teratology*, 38:461-466.

Stuchly MA et al. (1992). Modification of tumor promotion in the mouse skin by exposure to an alternating magnetic-field. *Cancer Lett*, 65(1):1-7.

Sukkar MY, El-Munshid HA, Ardawi MSM. *Concise human physiology*. Oxford, Blackwell Science Ltd, 2000.

Sun WQ et al. (1995). Characterization of the 60-Hz magnetic fields in schools of the Carleton Board of Education. *AIHA J*, 56:12-15.

Suri A et al. (1996). A 3 milliTesla 60 Hz magnetic field is neither mutagenic nor co-mutagenic in the presence of menadione and MNU in a transgenic rat cell line. *Mut Res*, 372:23-31.

Svedenstål B-M, Holmberg B (1993). Lymphoma development among mice exposed to X-rays and pulsed magnetic fields. *Int J Radiat Biol*, 64(1):119-125.

Svedenstål B-M, Johanson K-J (1995). Fetal loss in mice exposed to magnetic fields during early pregnancy. *Bioelectromagnetics*, 16:284-289.

Svedenstål B-M, Johanson K-J, Hansson Mild K (1999). DNA damage induced in brain cells of CBA mice exposed to magnetic fields. *In Vivo*, 13:551-552.

Svedenstål B-M et al. (1999). DNA damage, cell kinetics and ODC activities studied in CBA mice exposed to electromagnetic fields generated by transmission lines. *In Vivo*, 13:507-514.

Swanbeck G, Bleeker T (1989). Skin problems from visual display units. Provocation of skin symptoms under experimental conditions. *Acta Derm Venereol (Stockh)*, 69(1):46-51.

Swanson J (1996). Long-term variations in the exposure of the population of England and Wales to power-frequency magnetic fields. *J Radiol Prot*, 16(4):287-301.

Swanson J, Jeffers D (1999). Possible mechanisms by which electric fields from power lines might affect airborne particles harmful to health. *J Radiol Prot*, 19(3):213-229.

Swanson J, Kaune WT (1999). Comparison of residential power-frequency magnetic fields away from appliances in different countries. *Bioelectromagnetics*, 20(4):244-254.

Swanson J, Kheifets L (2006). Biophysical mechanisms: a component in the weight of evidence for health effects of power-frequency electric and magnetic fields. *Radiat Res*, 165(4):470-478.

Swiss Federal Council (1999). *Ordinance relating to protection from non-ionizing radiation (ONIR)*. (http://www.bafu.admin.ch/elektrosmog/01079/index.html?lang=en, accessed 20-2-2007).

Tabor Z, Michalski J, Rokita E (2004). Influence of 50 Hz magnetic field on human heart rate variability: linear and nonlinear analysis. *Bioelectromagnetics*, 25(6):474-480.

Takagi T (2000). Roles of ion channels in EPSP integration at neuronal dendrites. *Neurosci Res*, 37:167-171.

Takatsuki H, Yoshikoshi A, Sakanishi A (2002). Stimulation of neurite outgrowth in PC12D cells by ELF magnetic field and suppression by melatonin. *Colloids Surf B Biointerfaces*, 26:379-386.

Taki M, Suzuki Y, Wake K (2003). Dosimetry considerations in the head and retina for extremely low frequency electric fields. *Radiat Prot Dosimetry*, 106(4):349-356.

Tamarkin L et al. (1981). Melatonin inhibition and pinealectomy enhancement of 7,12-dimethlbanz(a)anthracene-induced mammary tumors in the rat. *Cancer Res*, 41:4432-4436.

Tarone RE et al. (1998). Residential wire codes: reproducibility and relation with measured magnetic fields. *Occup Environ Med*, 55:333-339.

Taylor WR, Smith RG (2004). Transmission of scotopic signals from the rod to rod-bipolar cell in the mammalian retina. *Vision Res*, 44(28):3269-3276.

Teitelbaum SL et al. (2003). Occupation and breast cancer in women 20-44 years of age (United States). *Cancer Causes Control*, 14(7):627-637.

Tenforde TS, Kaune WT (1987). Interaction of extremely low frequency electric and magnetic fields with humans. *Health Phys*, 53(6):585-606.

Terol FF, Panchon A (1995). Exposure of domestic quail embryos to extremely-low-frequency magnetic-fields. *Int J Radiat Biol*, 68(3):321-330.

Testa A et al. (2004). Evaluation of genotoxic effect of low level 50 Hz magnetic fields on human blood cells using different cytogenetic assays. *Bioelectromagnetics*, 25(8):613-619.

Theriault G et al. (1994). Cancer risks associated with occupational exposure to magnetic fields among electric utility workers in Ontario and Quebec, Canada, and France - 1970-1989. *Am J Epidemiol*, 139(6):550-572.

Thomas AW, Persinger MA (1997). Daily post-training exposure to pulsed magnetic fields that evoke mophine-like analgesia affects consequent motivation but not proficiency in maze learnings in rats. *Electro Magnetobiol*, 16(1):33-41.

Thomas RL, Schrot J, Liboff AR (1986). Low intensity magnetic fields alter operant behaviour in rats. *Bioelectromagnetics*, 7:349-357.

Thompson JM et al. (1995). Cortisol secretion and growth in ewe lambs chronically exposed to electric and magnetic fields of a 60-Hertz 500-kV AC transmission line. *J Anim Sci*, 73(11):3274-3280.

Thomson RA, Michaelson SM, Nguyen QA (1988). Influence of 60-Hertz magnetic fields on leukemia. *Bioelectromagnetics*, 9(2):149-158.

Thun-Battersby S, Mevissen M, Löscher W (1999). Exposure of Sprague-Dawley rats to a 50 Hz, 100 microTesla magnetic field for 27 weeks facilitates mammary tumorigenesis in the 7,12-dimethylbenz[a]-anthracene model of breast cancer. *Cancer Res*, 59(15):3627-3633 (1999b).

Thun-Battersby S, Westermann J, Löscher W (1999). Lymphocyte subset analyses in blood, spleen and lymph nodes of female Sprague-Dawley rats after short or prolonged exposure to a 50 Hz 100-microT magnetic field. *Radiat Res*, 152(4):436-443 (1999a).

Tian F et al. (2002). Exposure to power frequency magnetic fields suppresses X-ray-induced apoptosis transiently in Ku80-deficient xrs5 cells. *Biochem Biophys Res Commun*, 292(2):355-361.

Timmel CR et al. (1998). Effects of weak magnetic fields on free radical recombination reactions. *Mol Phys*, 95(1):71-89.

Tokalov SV, Gutzeit HO (2004). Weak electromagnetic fields (50 Hz) elicit a stress response in human cells. *Environ Res*, 94(2):145-151.

Tomenius L (1986). 50-Hz electromagnetic environment and the incidence of childhood tumors in Stockholm County. *Bioelectromagnetics*, 7(2):191-207.

425

Toomingas A (1996). Provocation of the electromagnetic distress syndrome. *Scand J Work Environ Health*, 22:457-459.

Tornqvist S (1998). Paternal work in the power industry: effects on children at delivery. *J Occup Environ Med*, 40(2):111-117.

Touitou Y et al. (2003). Magnetic fields and the melatonin hypothesis: a study of workers chronically exposed to 50-Hz magnetic fields. *Am J Physiol Regul Integr Comp Physiol*, 284(6):R1529-R1535.

Traitcheva N et al. (2003). ELF fields and photooxidation yielding lethal effects on cancer cells. *Bioelectromagnetics*, 24(2):148-150.

Tranchina D, Nicholson C (1986). A model for the polarization of neurons by extrinsically applied electric fields. *Biophys J*, 50(6):1139-1156.

Tremblay L et al. (1996). Differential modulation of natural and adaptive immunity in fischer rats exposed for 6 weeks to 60 Hz linear sinusoidal continuous-wave magnetic fields. *Bioelectromagnetics*, 17(5):373-383.

Trimmel M, Schweiger E (1998). Effects of an ELF (50-Hz, 1mT) electromagnetic field (EMF) on concentration in visual attention, perception and memory including effects of EMF sensitivity. *Toxicol Lett*, 96-97:377-382.

Tripp HM, Warman GR, Arendt J (2003). Circularly polarised MF (500 microT 50 Hz) does not acutely suppress melatonin secretion from cultured Wistar rat pineal glands. *Bioelectromagnetics*, 24(2):118-124.

Truong H, Smith C, Yellon SM (1996). Photoperiod control of the melatonin rhythm and reproductive maturation in the juvenile Djungarian hamster: 60-Hz magnetic field exposure effects. *Biol Reprod*, 55(2):455-460.

Truong H, Yellon SM (1997). Effect of varous acute 60 Hz magnetic field exposure on the nocturnal malatonin rise in the adult Djungarian hamster. *J Pineal Res*, 72:177-183.

Trzeciak HI et al. (1993). Behavioral effects of long-term exposure to magnetic fields in rats. *Bioelectromagnetics*, 14:287-297.

Tsuji H et al. (1996). Impact of reduced heart rate variability on risk for cardiac events. The Framingham Heart Study. *Circulation*, 94(Suppl 11):2850-2855.

Tuschl H et al. (2000). Occupational exposure to static, ELF, VF and VLF magnetic fields and immune parameters. *Int J Occup Med Environ Health*, 13(1):39-50.

Tynes T, Haldorsen T (1997). Electromagnetic fields and cancer in children residing near Norwegian high-voltage power lines. *Am J Epidemiol*, 145(3):219-226.

Tynes T, Haldorsen T (2003). Residential and occupational exposure to 50 Hz magnetic fields and hematological cancers in Norway. *Cancer Causes Control*, 14(8):715-720.

Tynes T, Klaeboe L, Haldorsen T (2003). Residential and occupational exposure to 50 Hz magnetic fields and malignant melanoma: a population based study. *Occup Environ Med*, 60(5):343-347.

Tynes T et al. (1996). Incidence of breast cancer in norwegian female radio and telegraph operators. *Cancer Causes Control*, 7(2):197-204.

Ubeda A, Trillo MA, Leal J (1987). Magnetic field effects on embryonic development: influence of the organism orientation. *Med Sci Res*, 15:531-532.

Ubeda A et al. (1983). Pulse shape of magnetic fields influences chick embryogenesis. *J Anat*, 137(3):513-536.

Ubeda A et al. (1994). Chick embryo development can be irreversibly altered by early exposure to weak extremely-low-frequency magnetic fields. *Bioelectromagnetics*, 15(5):385-398.

Ubeda A et al. (1995). A 50 Hz magnetic field blocks melatonin-induced enhancement of junctional transfer in normal C3H/10T1/2 cells. *Carcinogenesis*, 16(12):2945-2949.

Ueno S (1999). Biomagnetic approaches to studying the brain. *IEEE Eng Med Biol Mag*, 18(3):108-120.

Uhl GR (1998). Hypothesis: the role of dopaminergic transporters in selective vulnerability of cells in Parkinson's disease. *Ann Neurol*, 43(5):555-560.

UKCCSI - UK Childhood Cancer Study Investigators (1999). Exposure to power-frequency magnetic fields and the risk of childhood cancer. *Lancet*, 353(9194):1925-1931.

UKCCSI - UK Childhood Cancer Study Investigators (2000). Childhood cancer and residential proximity to power lines. *Br J Cancer*, 83(11):1573-1580.

UN - United Nations (2002). *The 2002 Revision Population Database*. (http://esa.un.org/unpp/index.asp?panel=2, accessed 1-3-2005).

UNCED - United Nations Conference on Environment and Development (1992). *Rio Declaration on Environment and Development*. (http://www.un.org/esa/documents/ga/conf151/aconf15126-1.htm, accessed 20-2-2007).

UNSCEAR - United Nations Scientific Committee on the Effects of Atomic Radiation. *Sources and effects of ionizing radiation. Report to the General Assembly, with scientific annexes*. New York, NY, United Nations, 1993.

Ushiyama A, Ohkubo C (2004). Acute effects of low-frequency electromagnetic fields on leukocyte-endothelial interactions in vivo. *In Vivo*, 18(2):125-132 (2004a).

Ushiyama A et al. (2004). Subchronic effects on leukocyte-endothelial interactions in mice by whole body exposure to extremely low frequency electromagnetic fields. *In Vivo*, 18(4):425-432 (2004b).

US Presidential/Congressional Commission on Risk Assessment and Risk Management (1997). Framework for environmental health risk management. (http://www.riskworld.com/nreports/1997/risk-rpt/pdf/epajan.pfd, accessed 20-2-2007)

Vaishnav S et al. (1994). Relation between heart rate variability early after acute myocardial infarction and long-term mortality. *Am J Cardiol*, 73(9):653-657.

Valberg PA, Kavet R, Rafferty CN (1997). Can low-level 50/60 Hz electric and magnetic fields cause biological effects? *Radiat Res*, 148.2-21.

Van Den Heuvel R et al. (2001). Haemopoietic cell proliferation in murine bone marrow cells exposed to extreme low frequency (ELF) electromagnetic fields. *Toxicology In Vitro*, 15:351-355.

van Wijngaarden E (2003). An exploratory investigation of suicide and occupational exposure. *J Occup Environ Med*, 45(1):96-101.

van Wijngaarden E et al. (2000). Exposure to electromagnetic fields and suicide among electric utility workers: a nested case-control study. *West J Med*, 173(2):94-100.

van Wijngaarden E et al. (2001a). Population-based case-control study of occupational exposure to electromagnetic fields and breast cancer. *Ann Epidemiol*, 11(5):297-303.

van Wijngaarden E et al. (2001b). Mortality patterns by occupation in a cohort of electric utility workers. *Am J Ind Med*, 40(6):667-673.

Vasquez BJ et al. (1988). Diurnal patterns in brain biogenic amines of rats exposed to 60-Hz electric fields. *Bioelectromagnetics*, 9:229-236.

Ventura C et al. (2005). Turning on stem cell cardiogenesis with extremely low frequency magnetic fields. *FASEB J*, 19(1):155-157.

Verbeek S et al. (1991). Mice bearing the Em-myc and Em-pim-1 transgenes develop pre-B-cell leukaemia prenatally. *Mol Cell Biol*, 11(2):1176-1179.

Verdugo-Diaz L, Paromero-Rivero M, Drucker-Colin R (1998). Differntiation of chromaffin cells by extremely low frequency magnetic fields changes ratios of catecholamine type messenger. *Biochem Bioenerg*, 46:297-300.

Verheyen GR et al. (2003). Effect of coexposure to 50 Hz magnetic fields and an aneugen on human lymphocytes, determined by the cytokinesis block micronucleus assay. *Bioelectromagnetics*, 24(3):160-164.

Verkasalo PK et al. (1993). Risk of cancer in Finnish children living close to power lines. *Br Med J*, 307(6909):895-899.

Verkasalo PK et al. (1996). Magnetic fields of high voltage power lines and risk of cancer in Finnish adults: nationwide cohort study. *Br Med J*, 313(7064):1047-1051.

Verkasalo PK et al. (1997). Magnetic fields of transmission lines and depression. *Am J Epidemiol*, 146(12):1037-1045.

Veyrot D (2003). Rapporteur report: interaction mechanisms. *Radiat Prot Dosimetry*, 106(4):317-319.

Villeneuve PJ et al.(2002).Brain cancer and occupational exposure to magnetic fields among men: results from a Canadian population-based case-control study. *Int J Epidemiol*, 31(1):210-217.

Vistnes AI, Gjoetterud K (2001). Why arguments based on photon energy may be highly misleading for power line frequency electromagnetic fields. *Bioelectromagnetics*, 22(3):200-204.

Vistnes AI et al. (1997a). Exposure of children to residential magnetic fields in Norway. *Bioelectromagnetics*, 18:47-57.

Vistnes AI et al. (1997b). Exposure of children to residential magnetic-fields in Norway - Is proximity to power-lines an adequate predictor of exposure? *Bioelectromagnetics*, 18(1):47-57.

von Winterfeldt D et al. (2004). Managing potential health risks from electric powerlines: a decision analysis caught in controversy. *Risk Anal*, 24(6):1487-1502.

Wake K et al. (1998). Induced current density distribution in a human related to magnetophosphenes. *Trans IEE Japan*, 118-A:806-811.

Walker MM, Bitterman ME (1985). Conditioned responding to magnetic fields by honeybees. *J Comp Physiol*, A157:67-71.

Walleczek J, Shiu EC, Hahn GA (1999). Increase in radiation-induced HPRT gene mutation frequency after nonthermal exposure to nonionizing 60 Hz electromagnetic fields. *Radiat Res*, 151(4):489-497.

Walsh V, Ashbridge E, Cowey A (1998). Cortical plasticity in perceptual learning demonstrated by transcranial magnetic stimulation. *Neuropsychologia*, 36(1):45-49.

Warman GR et al. (2003a). Acute exposure to circularly polarized 50-Hz magnetic fields of 200-300 microT does not affect the pattern of melatonin secretion in young men. *J Clin Endocrinol Metab*, 88(12):5668-5673.

Warman GR et al. (2003b). Circadian neuroendocrine physiology and electromagnetic field studies: precautions and complexities. *Radiat Prot Dosimetry*, 106(4):369-373.

Wassermann EM (1998). Risk and safety of repetitive transcranial magnetic stimulation: report and suggested guidelines from the International Workshop on the Safety of Repetitive Transcranial Magnetic Stimulation, June 5-7, 1996. *Electroencephalogr Clin Neurophysiol*, 108(1):1-16.

Weaver JC, Vaughan TE (1998). Theoretical limits on the threshold for the response of long cells to weak extremely low frequency electric fields due to ionic and molecular flux rectification. *Biophys J*, 75(5):2251-2254.

Wechsler LS et al. (1991). A pilot study of occupational and environmental risk factors for Parkinson's disease. *Neurotoxicology*, 12(3):387-392.

Wei LX, Goodman R, Henderson A (1990). Changes in levels of c-myc and histone H2B following exposure of cells to low-frequency sinusoidal electromagnetic fields: evidence for a window effect. *Bioelectromagnetics*, 11(4):269-272.

Weigel RJ, Lundstrom DL (1987). Effect of relative humidity on the movement of rat vibrissae in a 60-Hz electric field. *Bioelectromagnetics*, 8:107-110.

Wenzl TB (1997). Estimating magnetic field exposures of rail maintenance workers. *AIHA J*, 58:667-671.

Wertheimer N, Leeper E (1979). Electrical wiring configurations and childhood cancer. *Am J Epidemiol*, 109(3):273-284.

Wertheimer N, Leeper E (1982). Adult cancer related to electrical wires near the home. *Int J Epidemiol*, 11(4):345-355.

Wertheimer N, Leeper E (1986). Possible effects of electric blankets and heated waterbeds on fetal development. *Bioelectromagnetics*, 7(1):13-22.

Wertheimer N, Leeper E (1989). Fetal loss associated with two seasonal sources of electromagnetic field exposure. *Am J Epidemiol*, 129:220-224.

Wesseling C et al. (2002). Cancer of the brain and nervous system and occupational exposures in Finnish women. *J Occup Environ Med*, 44(7):663-668.

Whittington CJ, Podd JV, Rapley BR (1996). Acute effects of 50 Hz magnetic field exposure on human visual task and cardiovascular performance. *Bioelectromagnetics*, 17(2):131-137.

WHO - World Health Organization (1946). *Preamble to the Constitution of the World Health Organization as adopted by the International Health Conference, New York, 19-22 June, 1946.* (http://www.searo.who.int/aboutsearo/pdf/const.pdf, accessed 16-2-2007).

WHO - World Health Organization. *Extremely low frequency (ELF) fields.* Environmental Health Criteria, Vol. 35. Geneva, World Health Organization, 1984.

WHO - World Health Organization. *Magnetic fields.* Environmental Health Criteria, Vol. 69. Geneva, World Health Organization, 1987.

WHO - World Health Organization. *Revised guidelines for the preparation of Environmental Health Criteria monographs.* Geneva, World Health Organization, 1990 (PCS/90.69).

WHO - World Health Organization. *Electromagnetic fields (300 Hz to 300 GHz).* Environmental Health Criteria, Vol. 137. Geneva, World Health Organization, 1993.

WHO - World Health Organization. *Principles for the assessment of risks to human health from exposure to chemicals.* Environmental Health Criteria, Vol. 210. Geneva, World Health Organization, 1999.

WHO - World Health Organization. *World Health Report, Reducing risks, promoting healthy life.* Geneva, World Health Organization, 2002.

WHO - World Health Organization (2005). *WHO International Seminar and Working Group meeting on EMF hypersensitivity.* (http://www.who.int/peh-emf/meetings/hypersensitivity_prague2004/en/index.html, accessed 6-3-2007).

WHO - World Health Organization. *Framework for developing health-based EMF standards.* Geneva, World Health Organization, 2006a.

WHO - World Health Organization (2006b). *WHO EMF standards world wide database.* (http://www.who.int/docstore/peh-emf/EMFStandards/who-0102/Worldmap5.htm, accessed 18-2-2007).

Wiley MJ et al. (1992). The effects of continuous exposure to 20-kHz sawtooth magnetic fields on the litters of CD-1 mice. *Teratology,* 46(4):391-398.

Willett EV et al. (2003). Occupational exposure to electromagnetic fields and acute leukaemia: analysis of a case-control study. *Occup Environ Med,* 60(8):577-583.

Willich SN et al. (1993). Sudden cardiac death. Support for a role of triggering in causation. *Circulation,* 87(5):1442-1450.

Wilson BW, Chess EK, Anderson LE (1986). 60-Hz electric-field effects on pineal melatonin rhythms: time course for onset and recovery. *Bioelectromagnetics,* 7(2):239-242.

Wilson BW et al. (1981). Chronic exposure to 60 Hz electric fields: effects on pineal function in the rat. *Bioelectromagnetics,* 2(4):371-380.

Wilson BW et al. (1983). Erratum. Chronic exposure to 60 Hz electric fields: Effects on pineal function in the rat. *Bioelectromagnetics,* 4:293.

Wilson BW et al. (1990). Evidence for an effect of ELF electromagnetic fields on human pineal gland function. *J Pineal Res,* 9:259-269.

Wilson BW et al. (1996). Magnetic-field characteristics of electric bed-heating devices. *Bioelectromagnetics,* 17(3):174-179.

Wilson BW et al. (1999). Effects of 60 Hz magnetic field exposure on the pineal and hypothalamic-pituitary-gonadal axis in the Siberian hamster (*Phodopus sungorus*). *Bioelectromagnetics,* 20(4):224-232.

Winker R et al. (2005). Chromosomal damage in human diploid fibroblasts by intermittent exposure to extremely low-frequency electromagnetic fields. *Mutat Res,* 585(1-2):43-49.

WMA - World Medical Association (2004). *Declaration of Helsinki: Ethical Principles for Medical Research Involving Human Subjects.* (http://www.wma.net/e/ethicsunit/helsinki.htm, accessed 12-2-2007).

Wolf FI et al. (2005). 50-Hz extremely low frequency electromagnetic fields enhance cell proliferation and DNA damage: possible involvement of a redox mechanism. *Biochim Biophys Acta,* 1743(1-2):120-129.

Wood AW et al. (1998). Changes in human plasma melatonin profiles in response to 50 Hz magnetic field exposure. *J Pineal Res,* 25(2):116-127.

Wu RY et al. (2000). The effect of 50 Hz magnetic field on GCSmRNA expression in lymphoma B cell by mRNA differential display. *J Cell Biochem,* 79(3):460-470.

Wu SC et al. (1957). Experimental test of parity conservation in beta decay. *Phys Rev,* 105:1413-1415.

Yamaguchi DT et al. (2002). Inhibition of gap junction intercellular communication by extremely low-frequency electromagnetic fields in osteoblast-like models is dependent on cell differentiation. *J Cell Physiol*, 190(2):180-188.

Yang KH, Ju MN, Myung SH . Sample of Korean's occupational and residential exposures to ELF magnetic field over a 24-hour period. In: *Abstracts of the 26th Annual Meeting of the Bioelectromagnetics Society*. Washington, DC, Bioelectromagnetics Society, 2004, 188-189.

Yasui M et al. (1997). Carcinogenicity test of 50 Hz sinusoidal magnetic fields in rats. *Bioelectromagnetics*, 18:531-540.

Yellon SM (1994). Acute 60 Hz magnetic field exposure effects on the melatonin rhytm in the pineal gland and circulation of the Djungarian hamster. *J Pineal Res*, 16(3):136-144.

Yellon SM (1996). 60-Hz magnetic field exposure effects on the melatonin fhythm and photoperiod control of reproduction. *Am J Physiol*, 270(5 Pt 1):E816-E821.

Yellon SM, Truong HN (1998). Melatonin rhythm onset in the adult Siberian hamster: influence of photoperiod but not 60-Hz magnetic field exposure on melatonin content in the Pineal gland and in circulation. *J Biol Rhythms*, 13(1):52-59.

Yomori H et al. (2002). Elliptically polarized magnetic fields do not alter immediate early response genes expression levels in human glioblastoma cells. *Bioelectromagnetics*, 23(2):89-96.

Youngstedt SD et al. (2002). No association of 6-sulfatoxymelatonin with in-bed 60-Hz magnetic field exposure or illumination level among older adults. *Environ Res*, 89(3):201-209.

Yu MC et al. (1993). Effects of 60 Hz electric and magnetic-fields on maturation of the rat neopallium. *Bioelectromagnetics*, 14(5):449-458.

Zaffanella L. *Survey of residential magnetic field source. Volume 1: Goals, results and conclusions. Volume 2: Protocol, data analysis and management.* Palo Alto, CA, Electric Power Research Institute, 1993 (EPRI TR-102759-V1 and TR-102759-V2).

Zaffanella L, Kalton GW. *Survey of personal magnetic field exposure. Phase II: 1000-person survey. EMF RAPID Program Engineering Project No.6.* Oak Ridge, TN, Lockheed Martin Energy Systems, 1998.

Zahm SH, Devesa SS (1995). Childhood cancer: overview of incidence trends and environmental carcinogens. *Environ Health Perspect*, 103(6):177-184.

Zecca L et al. (1991). Neurotransmitter amino acid variations in striatum of rats exposed to 50 Hz electric fields. *Biochim Biophys Acta*, 1075:1-5.

Zecca L et al. (1998). Biological effects of prolonged exposure to ELF electromagnetic fields in rats: III. 50 Hz electromagnetic fields. *Bioelectromagnetics*, 19(1):57-66.

Zeng QL et al. (2003). ELF magnetic fields induce internalization of gap junction protein connexin 43 in Chinese hamster lung cells. *Bioelectromagnetics*, 24(2):134-138.

Zhadin MN, Deryugina ON, Pisachenko TM (1999). Influence of combined DC and AC magnetic fields on rat behaviour. *Bioelectromagnetics*, 20(6):378-386.

Zhou J et al. (2002). Gene expression of cytokine receptors in HL60 cells exposed to a 50 Hz magnetic field. *Bioelectromagnetics*, 23(5):339-346.

Zhu K et al. (2003). Use of electric bedding devices and risk of breast cancer in African-American women. *Am J Epidemiol*, 158(8):798-806.

Zhu S, Way Q, Zhu L (2001). [The effects of electromagnetic fields of extremely low frequency on the immune system in electric rail way workers] in Chinese. *J Labour Medicine*, 18(5):291-293.

Zhu S et al. (2002). [The effects of the electromagnetic fields of extremely low frequency on the health in electric railway workers] in Chinese. *Chin J Environ Occup Med*, 19(2):79-99.

Zimmerman S et al. (1990). Influence of 60-Hz magnetic fields on sea urchin development. *Bioelectromagnetics*, 11:37-45.

Zmyslony M et al. (2004). Effects of in vitro exposure to power frequency magnetic fields on UV-induced DNA damage of rat lymphocytes. *Bioelectromagnetics*, 25(7):560.

Zubal G (1994). Computerised three-dimensional segmented human anatomy. *Med Phys*, 21(2):299-303.

430

**AC**
Alternating current. An electrical current whose magnitude and direction vary cyclically, as opposed to direct current, whose direction remains constant.

**Action potential (nerve impulse or "spike")**
A sudden brief reversal of the local membrane electrical potential that occurs once a threshold depolarisation has been exceeded and which quickly propagates down a nerve axon conveying "digitally" encoded information.

**Acute effect**
Effect of short duration and occurring rapidly (usually in the first 24 h or up to 14 d) following a single dose or short exposure to a substance or radiation.

**Adverse health effect**
A biological effect which has a detrimental effect on mental, physical and/or general well being of exposed people, either in the short term or long term.

**Antibody**
A class of proteins produced by (B) lymphocytes that recognises and binds to a specific antigen, thereby aiding its elimination, or elimination of the agent, such as a bacterium, expressing it.

**Antigen**
Any substance, usually (but not always) foreign, that provokes an antigen-specific immune response, such as antibody-binding.

**Apoptosis**
A specific form of cell death during which cells degrade their own DNA. Apoptosis can occur normally during organ formation, or as a result of DNA or cellular damage.

**Autonomic nervous system**
A part of the peripheral nervous system that regulates the visceral or "housekeeping" functions of the body, such as heart-rate and blood pressure. It's cell bodies lie either in the central nervous system, or in ganglia in other parts of the body.

**Background levels**
The amounts of EMF found (that are not due to an obviously specific source) in a typical environment of an industrialized society.

**Basic restrictions**
Restrictions on exposure to time-varying electric, magnetic, and electromagnetic fields that are based directly on established health effects. Depending upon the frequency of the field, the physical quantities used to specify these restrictions are induced electric field (E), current density (J), specific energy absorption rate (SAR), and power density (S). Only power density in air, outside the body, can be readily measured in exposed individuals.

**Bias**
A systematic tendency to error as a consequence of the design or conduct of a study.

**Biological effect**
A measurable change in a biological system in response (for example) to an electromagnetic field.

**Biophysical mechanisms**
Physical and/or chemical interactions of electric and magnetic fields with biological systems.

**Blind study**
A study in which the subject or, in the case of studies using animals, tissues or cell cultures, the experimenter, is unaware of whether exposure is to the agent under test or to a neutral or comparison agent until completion of the experiment, in order to avoid unconscious subjective bias affecting the study outcome.

**Blood-brain barrier**
A physiological "barrier" comprising endothelial and epithelial cells that regulates the composition of cerebrospinal fluid of the central nervous system.

**Calcium efflux**
The release of calcium ions from a sample into a surrounding solution.

**Cancer**
An uncontrolled and abnormal proliferation of cells that causes disease.

**Carcinogen**
An agent that can induce cancer.

**Carcinoma**
A tumour arising from epithelial tissue (e.g. glands; breast; skin; linings of the urogenital, intestinal and respiratory systems).

**Case-control study**
An investigation into the extent to which a group of persons with a specific disease (the cases) and comparable persons who do not have the disease (the controls) differ with respect to exposure to putative risk factors.

**Causal relationship**
A causal relationship occurs between two agents when one causes the other. For example, researchers are studying whether there is a causal relationship between EMF and cancer, meaning that they are studying to see if EMF causes, or affects the progress of, cancer.

**Cell signalling (pathways)**
A sequence of intracellular changes linking a "signalling event", such as activation of membrane-bound ion channels or ligand-receptors, and a "response", such as a change in gene expression, for example, leading to increased proliferation.

**Central nervous system (CNS)**
Usually taken to mean the cells, such as neurons and glial cells, of the brain and spinal cord. It also includes the retina, which is formed as an outgrowth of the forebrain.

**Chromosome**
A single molecule of DNA, comprising a large number of genes and other DNA, together with associated protein molecules that condense during cell division to form a deeply staining, rod-shaped body.

**Chronic effect**
Consequence which develops slowly and has a long-lasting course (often but not always irreversible).

**Circulary polarized**
If the electric field is viewed as a point in space, the locus of the end point of the vector will rotate and trace out an ellipse, once each cycle.

**Cognition**
Information processing by the brain, including processes such as attention, perception, learning, reasoning, comprehending and memory.

**Cohort study**
An investigation involving the identification of a group of individuals (the cohort) about whom certain exposure information is collected, and the ascertainment of occurrence of diseases at later times. For each individual, information on prior exposure can be related to subsequent disease experience. Cohort studies may be conducted prospectively or retrospectively.

**Combined analysis**
Analysis of data pertaining to the same topic that have been collected in several different studies. Usually based on individual level data from each of the available studies, rather than on the published findings (see Meta analysis).

**Comet assay**
A single cell electrophoresis assay in which DNA is caused to migrate away from the nucleus by an applied electric field. The extent of migration gives a measure of DNA damage.

**Conductance**
The reciprocal of resistance. Symbol: G. Unit: siemens (S).

**Conductivity, electrical**
The scalar or vector quantity which, when multiplied by the electric field strength, yields the conduction current density; it is the reciprocal of resistivity. Expressed in siemens per meter ($S\ m^{-1}$).

**Confidence interval (CI)**
An interval calculated from data when making inferences about an unknown parameter. In hypothetical repetitions of the study, the interval will include the parameter in question on a specified percentage of occasions (e.g. 90% for a 90% confidence interval).

**Confounding**
Spurious findings due to the effect of a variable that is correlated with both the exposure and disease under study.

**Contact current**
Current flowing between an energized, isolated, conductive (metal) object and ground through an electrical circuit representing the equivalent impedance of the human body.

**Continuous exposure**
Exposure for durations exceeding the corresponding averaging time. Exposure for less than the averaging time is called short-term exposure.

**Continuous wave (CW)**
A wave whose successive oscillations are identical under steady-state conditions.

**Coronary thrombosis**
A blood clot which blocks one of the coronary arteries, leading to a heart attack.

**Current density**
A vector of which the integral over a given surface is equal to the current flowing through the surface; the mean density in a linear conductor is equal to the current divided by the cross-sectional area of the conductor. Unit: ampere per square meter $(A\ m^{-2})$.

**Diastole**
The period of relaxation of heart muscle, following contraction (systole).

**Dielectric constant**
See Permittivity.

**Dielectric material**
A class of materials that act as electric insulators. For this class, the conductivity is presumed to be zero, or very small. The positive and negative charges in dielectrics are tightly bound together so that there is no actual transport of charge under the influence of a field. Such material alters electromagnetic fields because of induced charges formed by the interaction of the dielectric with the incident field.

**Differentiation (cellular)**
The development of a specialised cellular structure and function from less specialised "precursor" cells such as stem cells which is generally accompanied by a loss of proliferative capacity.

**Dipole**
A centre-fed open antenna excited in such a way that the standing wave of current is symmetrical about the mid point of the antenna.

**Dose**
A term for the amount of a chemical or physical agent delivered to a target organ. Since neither the target organ nor the mechanism of delivery are well understood for most biological effects of EMF fields, an EMF dose can sel-

dom be defined, and the concept of exposure metric (see below) is used instead.

**Dose-response relationship**
Mathematical description of the relationship between the dose and occurrence of the disease.

**Dosimetry**
Measurement or determination by calculation of the internal electric field strength or induced current density, or of the specific absorption (SA) or specific absorption rate (SAR) distribution in humans or animals exposed to electromagnetic fields.

**Double blind study**
A volunteer study in which the subject and the experimenter until completion are unaware of whether exposure is to the agent under test or to a neutral or comparison agent, in order to avoid unconscious subjective bias affecting the study outcome.

**Duty factor**
The ratio of the sum of pulse durations to a stated averaging time. For repetitive phenomena, the averaging time is the pulse repetition period.

**Electric and magnetic fields or electromagnetic fields (EMF)**
The combination of time-varying electric and magnetic fields.

**Electric field**
A vector field $E$ measured in volts per metre (V m$^{-1}$).

**Electric field strength ($E$)**
Force exerted by an electric field on an electric point charge, divided by the electric charge. Expressed in newtons per coulomb or volts per metre (N C$^{-1}$ = V m$^{-1}$).

**Electrical ground**
The earth or a metal surface placed in contact with the earth, or connected to the earth with a conductor.

**Electrocardiogram (ECG)**
A recording of the electrical activity of the heart from electrodes placed on the body.

**Electroencephalogram (EEG)**
A recording of the electrical activity of the brain from electrodes placed on the head.

**Electromagnetic energy**
The energy stored in an electromagnetic field. Expressed in joule (J).

**Electromagnetic interference (EMI)**
Degradation of the performance of a device, a piece of equipment, or a system caused by an electromagnetic disturbance.

**Electroretinogram (ERG)**
A recording of the electrical activity of the retina from electrodes placed on the surface of the eye and the head.

**Embryo**
The stage of prenatal development between the fertilised ovum and the completion of major organ development. In humans, this occurs in the first trimester.

**Enteric nervous system**
Comprises the intrinsic neurons of the gut, about the same in number (approximately 100 million) as those of the spinal cord, and which exhibit a high degree of independence from the central nervous system.

**Epidemiology**
The study of the distribution of disease in populations and of the factors that influence this distribution.

**Epilepsy**
Epileptic seizures arise from an excessively synchronous and sustained discharge of a group of neurons; a persistent increase in neuronal excitability is a key feature.

**Event-related (or evoked) potential (ERP or EP)**
A recording of the electrical activity of the brain after a stimulus event, such as a visual or auditory stimulus (resulting in VEPs and AEPs respectively). Late components are associated with cognitive processing.

**Exposure**
The subjection of a person to electric, magnetic, or electromagnetic fields or to contact currents other than those originating from physiological processes in the body and other natural phenomena.

**Exposure standard**
A standard that limits EMF exposure to humans. See Standard.

**Exposure, intermittent**
This term refers to alternating periods of exposure and absence of exposure varying from a few seconds to several hours. If exposure lasting a few minutes to a few hours alternates with periods of absence of exposure lasting 18-24 hours (exposure repeated on successive days), "repeated exposure" might be a more appropriate term.

**Exposure, long term**
This term indicates exposure during a major part of the lifetime of the biological system involved; it may, therefore, vary from a few weeks to many years in duration.

**Exposure metric**
A single number that summarizes an electric and/or magnetic field exposure over a period of time. An exposure metric is usually determined by a combination of the instrument's signal processing and the data analysis performed after the measurement.

**Exposure, partial-body**
Exposure that results when EMF are substantially non-uniform over the body. Fields that are non-uniform over volumes comparable to the human body may occur due to highly directional sources, standing waves, re-radiating sources, or in the near field region of a radiating structure.

**Exposure, short term**
Exposure for durations less than the corresponding averaging time.

**Exposure, whole-body**
Pertains to the case in which the entire body is exposed to the incident electromagnetic energy or the case in which the cross section (physical area) of the body is smaller than the cross section of the incident radiation beam.

**Extremities**
Limbs of the body.

**Fetus (foetus)**
The stage of prenatal development between the embryo and birth.

**Fibrillation (ventricular)**
The loss of organised ventricular contractions of the heart.

**Field strength**
The magnitude of the electric or magnetic field, normally the root-mean-square value.

**Free radicals**
Highly reactive chemical species (part of a molecule) with an unpaired electron.

**Free space**
An ideal perfectly homogeneous medium possessing a relative dielectric constant of unity, in which there is nothing to reflect, refract, or absorb energy. A perfect vacuum possesses these qualities.

**Frequency**
The number of cycles completed by electromagnetic waves in 1 s; usually expressed in hertz (Hz).

**Frequency response**
An instrument's output as a function of frequency relative to the magnitude of the input signal. Specification of an instrument's frequency response includes the type of filter and its bandwidth.

**Gene expression**
The production of a functional protein or an RNA molecule from genetic information (genes) encoded by DNA.

**Genotoxin**
An agent which damages DNA and RNA

**Geomagnetic fields**
Magnetic fields originating from the earth (including the atmosphere). Predominantly a static magnetic field, but includes some oscillating components and transients.

**Guideline**
A recommended limit for a substance or an agent intended to protect human health or the environment.

**Haematology**
The study of blood; its formation, normal composition, function and pathology.

**Harmonic**
A frequency which is a multiple of the frequency under consideration.

**Health**
A state of complete physical, mental and social well-being and not merely the absence of disease or infirmity.

**Health hazard**
A biological effect that is detrimental to health or well-being.

**Immune system**
The body's primary defence against abnormal growth of cells (i.e. tumours) and infectious agents such as bacteria, viruses, and parasites.

**Impedance, wave**
The ratio of the complex number (vector) representing the transverse electric field at a point, to that representing the transverse magnetic field at that point. Expressed in ohm ($\Omega$).

**Implantation**
The attachment of the early embryo to the uterine wall.

**In vitro**
Experimental studies of cells or tissues, usually in a sustaining oxygenated, fluid medium. Literally means "in glass", isolated from the living organism and artificially maintained, as in a test tube or culture dish.

**In vivo**
Occurring within the whole living body. 'In life'; experimental studies of processes in living organisms.

**Latency**
The time between exposure to an injurious agent and the manifestation of a response.

**Leukocyte**
A white blood cell.

**Lymphocyte**
White blood cells produced in lymphoid tissue that initiate adaptive, antigen-specific immune responses. Some T-lymphocytes are cytotoxic; B-lymphocytes secrete antibodies.

**Macrophage**
A phagocytic cell derived from myeloid progenitor cells found in various tissues.

**Magnetic field strength (*H*)**
A field vector, $H$, that is equal to the magnetic flux density divided by the permeability of the medium. Expressed in units of amperes per meter (A m$^{-1}$).

**Magnetic flux density (*B*)**
The force on a moving unit positive charge at a point in a magnetic field per unit velocity. A vector field quantity, $B$, expressed in tesla (T).

**Malignant**
Neoplasms or tumours that have become invasive.

**Meta-analysis**
Analysis of data pertaining to the same topic that have been collected in several different studies. Usually refers to an analysis based on published findings from individual studies, rather than on the original data sets (see Combined analysis).

**Metabolic rate**
See Resting metabolic rate.

**Metabolism**
The biochemical reactions by which energy is made available for the use of an organism from the time a nutrient substance enters, until it has been utilized and the waste products eliminated.

**Metastasis**
Tumour cells that leave their site of origin and migrate to other sites in the body.

**Micronucleus**
Chromosome fragments that have not been lost on cell division.

**Mutation**
A stable heritable change in the DNA at a specific site in the in the genome of a cell by an agent (mutagen) such as ionising radiation.

**Natural killer (NK) cells**
Lymphocytes that are not antigen-specific but nevertheless bind to and kill certain tumour and virus-infected cells.

**Neonate, neonatal**
Newly born.

**Neoplasm**
New growth of abnormal tissue.

**Neural network**
Group of interacting neurons.

**Neural tube defect**
A defect of the newly formed precursor of the central nervous system, commonly anencephaly (failure of brain to develop), encephalocele (cyst of the brain), and spina bifida (defects in the closure of the neural tube).

**Neuron**
Nerve cell, specialised for the transmission of neural information.

**Neurotransmitter**
A substance released by a neuron that causes a post-synaptic response that is relatively quick in onset (< 1 ms) and short (< 10's ms) in duration, as distinct from the more prolonged action of neuromodulators.

**Neutrophil**
Phagocytic white blood cells derived from myeloid progenitor cells.

**Non-differential measurement errors**
Errors in exposure assessment that do not depend on whether or not someone develops the disease under study.

**Occupational exposure**
Exposure experienced by adults who are generally exposed under known conditions and are trained to be aware of potential risk and to take appropriate precautions.

**Odds ratio**
The ratio of the odds of disease occurrence in a group with exposure to a factor to that in an unexposed group; within each group, the odds are the ratio of the numbers of diseased and non-diseased individuals.

**Oncogene**
A gene which contributes to cancer in a dominant fashion through the mutation and/or abnormal expression of a gene (proto-oncogene) involved in regulating cell proliferation.

**Operant behaviour**
Behaviour, such as pressing a lever, which is "shaped" by rewards (such as food pellets) or punishment (such as a mild electric shock).

**Organogenesis**
The process of organ formation in developing organisms.

**Peripheral nervous system (somatic)**
The part of the nervous system that mainly deals with the voluntary and conscious aspects of neural control such as voluntary muscle (motor) contraction and sensations such as those of warmth or pressure. The cell bodies lie within the spinal cord, but the peripheral nerves (axons) terminate on muscle fibres or in specialised sensory receptors throughout the body.

**Permeability**
The scalar or tensor quantity whose product by the magnetic field strength is the magnetic flux density. Note: For isotropic media, the permeability is a scalar; for anisotropic media, a matrix.
Synonym: absolute permeability. If the permeability of a material or medium

440

is divided by the permeability of vacuum (magnetic constant) $\mu_0$, the result is termed relative permeability ($\mu$). Unit: henry per metre (H m$^{-1}$).

**Permittivity; dielectric constant**
A constant defining the influence of an isotropic medium on the forces of attraction or repulsion between electrified bodies. Symbol: $\varepsilon$. Unit: farad per metre (F m$^{-1}$).

**Permittivity, relative**
The ratio of the permittivity of a dielectric to that of a vacuum. Symbol: $\varepsilon_r$.

**Phase**
Of a periodic phenomenon, the fraction of a period through which the time has advanced relative to an arbitrary time origin.

**Phosphene**
The perception of flickering light in the periphery of the visual field induced by non-visual means such as a trans-retinal electric current.

**Prospective study**
An epidemiological study in which data on exposures and disease outcome are collected as the events occur, unlike a retrospective study (see below). Some cohort studies are conducted prospectively.

**Public exposure**
All exposure to EMF experienced by members of the general public, excluding occupational exposure and exposure during medical procedures.

**Recall bias**
Bias resulting from the tendency of a class of subjects to recall relevant events better than other subjects.

**Reference level**
EMF exposure level provided for practical exposure assessment purposes to determine whether the basic restrictions are likely to be exceeded. Some reference levels are derived from relevant basic restrictions using measurement and/or computational techniques and some address perception and adverse indirect effects of exposure to EMF.

**Reinforcement (behavioural)**
An action such as reward or punishment that increases the likelihood of a certain behaviour.

**Relative risk**
The ratio of the disease rate in the group under study to that in a comparison group, with adjustment for confounding factors such as age, if necessary.

**Reproductive effects**
Effects on reproduction which may include, but not be limited to, alterations in sexual behaviour, onset of puberty, fertility, gestation, parturition, lactation, pregnancy outcomes, premature reproductive senescence, or modifications in other functions that are dependent on the integrity of the reproductive system.

**Resonance**
The change in amplitude occurring as the frequency of the wave approaches or coincides with a natural frequency of the medium.

**Retrospective study**
An epidemiological study in which data on exposures and disease outcome are collected some time after the event, unlike a prospective study (see above). Examples include case-control studies and some cohort studies.

**Root-mean-square (RMS)**
Certain electrical effects are proportional to the square root of the mean value of the square of a periodic function (over one period). This value is known as the effective value or the root-mean-square (RMS) value, since it is derived by first squaring the function, determining the mean value of the squares obtained, and extracting the square root of the mean value to determine the end result.

**Safety factor**
A reduction factor incorporated into limits in standards or guidelines that allows for uncertainties in the determination of a threshold level of exposure, above which established health effects begin to appear.

**Selection bias**
Bias resulting from a faulty way to select subjects for a study. Epidemiological studies depend on a reliable comparison between subjects with a disease and a reference population as to their exposure. If the subjects chosen for a study are not representative of the corresponding population, the comparison becomes flawed and the association between disease and exposure becomes biased.

**Shield**
A mechanical barrier or enclosure provided for protection. The term is modified in accordance with the type of protection afforded; e.g., a magnetic shield is a shield designed to afford protection against magnetic fields.

**Short term exposure**
See exposure, short term

**Significance level**
The probability of obtaining a result at least as extreme as that observed in the absence of a raised risk. A result that would arise less than 1 in 20 times in the absence of an underlying effect is often referred to as being "statistically significant".

**Sinus arrhythmia**
The normal variation of heart rate during the breathing cycle.

**Spatial average**
The root mean square of the field over an area equivalent to the vertical cross section of the adult human body, as applied to the measurement of electric or magnetic fields in the assessment of whole-body exposure.

**Spot measurements**
Magnetic field measurements taken at various individual locations throughout a room or area.

**Standard**
1) A documented agreement containing technical specifications or other precise criteria to be used consistently as rules, guidelines or definitions of characteristics to ensure that materials, products, processes and services are fit for their purpose.
2) A legally enforceable limit for a substance or an agent intended to protect human health or the environment. Exceeding the standard could result in unacceptable harm.

**Static field**
A field vector that does not vary with time.

**Statistical power**
The probability that, with a specified degree of confidence, an underlying effect of a given magnitude will be detected in a study.

**Synapse**
A junction between two neurons, or between a neuron and a muscle fibre, that allows the transmission of electrical information, usually by means of a chemical transmitter (neurotransmitter) released from the presynaptic terminal of one neuron onto the closely juxtaposed post-synaptic terminal of the other.

**Systole**
The period of contraction of heart muscle following relaxation (diastole).

**Teratogen**
An agent that can cause birth defects.

**Threshold**
The lowest dose of an agent at which a specified measurable effect is observed and below which it is not observed.

**Thrombosis**
Blocking of an artery or vein by a blood clot.

**Time-weighted average (TWA)**
The average of various measurements, each of which is given more or less weight according to how much time a person is likely to spend in the spot where that measurement was taken. The term is used more generally to indicate the average of field levels over a specific amount of time. This is one method used to summarize exposure to exposure to magnetic fields.

**Transcription factor**
A protein that binds to a DNA sequence with a "regulatory" function thereby, directly or indirectly, affecting the initiation of transcription.

**Transformation**
Conversion of cells to a state of unrestrained growth in culture, resembling or identical with a tumour-forming (tumorigenic) state.

443

**Transgenic organism**
A genetically modified organism, which has foreign DNA such as a gene stably integrated into its genome.

**Transients**
Brief bursts of high frequency fields, usually resulting from mechanical switching of AC electricity.

**Transmission lines**
High voltage power lines that carry large quantities of power over large distances.

**Tumour**
A growth of tissue resulting from abnormal cell proliferation.

**Tumour initiator**
An agent that can produce an initial carcinogenic event such as a mutation.

**Tumour progression**
The process by which initiated and promoted cells become increasingly malignant.

**Tumour promoter**
An agent that can stimulate the proliferation (clonal expansion) of initiated cells.

**Tumour suppressor gene**
A normal cellular gene involved in regulating cell proliferation whose mutation and/or abnormal expression can contribute to cancer in a recessive manner.

**Vasoconstriction**
The contraction of blood vessels, making them narrower.

**Vasodilatation (or vasodilation)**
The relaxation of blood vessels, making them wider.

**Vigilance tasks**
Responding to unusual and infrequent stimuli (signals) occurring against a background of usual and frequent stimuli (events). Vigilance can be either visual or auditory.

**Voltage-gated ion channel**
Cell membrane proteins that allow the passage of particular ion species across the cell membrane in response to the opening of a molecular "gate" which is steeply sensitive to the transmembrane voltage. They are associated with electrical excitability.

**Wavelength ($\lambda$)**
The distance between two successive points of a periodic wave in the direction of propagation, in which the oscillation has the same phase. Symbol: $\lambda$. Unit: metre (m).

**Wild type (gene)**
The gene that is found in nature or in the standard laboratory stock for a given organism.

**Working memory**
An active system for temporarily storing and manipulating information needed in the execution of complex cognitive tasks.

# 16 RESUME ET RECOMMANDATIONS RELATIVES AUX ETUDES A MENER

La présente monographie des critères d'hygiène de l'environnement porte sur les effets éventuels sur la santé d'une exposition à des champs électriques et magnétiques d'extrêmement basse fréquence (EBF). On y examine les caractéristiques physiques des champs EBF ainsi que les sources d'exposition et le mesurage des champs. Toutefois, ses principaux objectifs sont d'examiner la littérature scientifique sur les effets biologiques d'une exposition aux champs EBF afin de pouvoir évaluer les risques pour la santé associés à l'exposition à ces champs et d'utiliser cette évaluation du risque sanitaire pour formuler des recommandations relatives aux programmes de protection sanitaire à l'intention des autorités nationales.

Les fréquences qui nous occupent sont situées au-dessus de 0 Hz et jusqu'à 100 kHz. La majorité des études a porté sur les effets des champs magnétiques à la fréquence des réseaux (50 ou 60 Hz), quelques études seulement portant sur les champs électriques à ces mêmes fréquences. En outre, un certain nombre d'études a été réalisé sur les champs magnétiques de très basse fréquence (VLF, 3–30 kHz), liés aux champs magnétiques à gradient commuté utilisés dans l'imagerie par résonance magnétique et aux champs VLF plus faibles, émis par les terminaux à écran cathodique et les postes de télévision.

Ce document récapitule les principales conclusions et recommandations de chaque section ainsi que les conclusions générales du processus d'évaluation des risques sanitaires. Les termes utilisés dans cette monographie pour indiquer le "poids de la preuve" en faveur d'un effet donné sur la santé sont les suivants. Les éléments d'appréciation sont "limités" lorsqu'ils ne se rapportent qu'à une seule étude ou lorsqu'il reste des questions sans réponse concernant la conception, la conduite ou l'interprétation d'un certain nombre d'études. On dit que les éléments d'appréciation sont "insuffisants" lorsque les études ne peuvent être interprétées comme montrant la présence ou l'absence d'un effet du fait d'insuffisances importantes sur le plan qualitatif ou quantitatif, ou lorsqu'aucune donnée n'est disponible.

On a également recensé des lacunes importantes dans les connaissances et on a résumé dans la section intitulée "Recommandations de recherche" les études nécessaires pour les combler.

## 16.1 Résumé

### 16.1.1 Sources, mesurage et expositions

Les champs électriques et magnétiques existent partout où de l'électricité est produite, transmise ou distribuée dans des lignes ou des câbles électriques, ou utilisée dans des appareils électriques. Depuis que l'électricité fait partie intégrante de notre mode de vie moderne, ces champs sont omniprésents dans notre environnement.

L'intensité du champ électrique se mesure en volts par mètre ($V\ m^{-1}$) ou en kilovolts par mètre ($kV\ m^{-1}$) et l'induction magnétique en teslas (T), ou plus communément en millitéslas (mT) ou en microteslas ($\mu T$).

Dans les habitations, l'exposition aux champs magnétiques à la fréquence du réseau ne montre pas de variations spectaculaires dans le monde. La moyenne géométrique du champ magnétique dans les habitations se situe entre 0,025 et 0,07 $\mu T$ en Europe et entre 0,055 et 0,11 $\mu T$ aux Etats-Unis. Les valeurs moyennes du champ électrique dans les habitations sont de l'ordre de plusieurs dizaines de volts par mètre. Au voisinage de certains appareils domestiques, les valeurs instantanées du champ magnétique peuvent atteindre quelques centaines de microteslas. A proximité des lignes électriques à haute tension, les champs magnétiques atteignent près de 20 $\mu T$ et les champs électriques jusqu'à plusieurs milliers de volts par mètre.

Peu d'enfants subissent, là où ils habitent, des expositions à des champs magnétiques de 50 ou 60 Hz dont la moyenne dans le temps est supérieure aux niveaux associés avec une incidence accrue de leucémie infantile (voir section 16.1.10). Près de 1 à 4% d'entre eux ont des expositions moyennes supérieures à 0,3 $\mu T$ et seuls 1 à 2% des expositions médianes supérieures à 0,4 $\mu T$.

L'exposition professionnelle, bien qu'elle soit principalement due à des champs à la fréquence du réseau, peut également comporter l'exposition à d'autres fréquences. Les expositions moyennes au champ magnétique sur les lieux de travail se sont avérées plus élevées au sein des "professions liées à l'électricité" que dans les autres, telles que par exemple le travail de bureau. Elles sont comprises entre 0,4 et 0,6 $\mu T$ pour les électriciens et les ingénieurs en électricité et autour de 1,0 $\mu T$ pour les agents travaillant sur les lignes électriques, les expositions les plus élevées concernant les soudeurs, les conducteurs de trains et les opérateurs de machines à coudre (plus de 3 $\mu T$). Les expositions maximales aux champs magnétiques sur les lieux de travail peuvent atteindre près de 10 mT et sont invariablement associées à la présence de conducteurs transportant des courants forts. Dans le secteur de l'alimentation électrique, les agents peuvent être exposés à des champs électriques atteignant 30 $kV\ m^{-1}$.

### 16.1.2   Champs électriques et magnétiques dans l'organisme

L'exposition à des champs électriques et magnétiques EBF externes induit des champs et des courants électriques dans l'organisme. La dosimétrie décrit le rapport entre le champ externe et les champ électriques et la densité de courant induits dans l'organisme, ou d'autres paramètres associés à l'exposition à ces champs. Le champ électrique et la densité de courant induits localement présentent un intérêt particulier parce qu'ils sont en rapport avec la stimulation des tissus excitables tels que nerfs et muscles.

Le corps de l'homme et des animaux perturbe sensiblement la distribution spatiale d'un champ électrique EBF. Aux fréquences basses, le corps est un bon conducteur et les lignes du champ perturbé à l'extérieur de l'organisme sont presque perpendiculaires à la surface du corps. Des charges oscillantes sont induites à la surface de l'organisme exposé et ce sont elles qui produisent des courants dans l'organisme. Les principales caractéristiques de la dosimétrie concernant l'exposition de l'homme aux champs électriques EBF sont les suivantes:

- Le champ électrique à l'intérieur de l'organisme est normalement cinq ou six fois plus faible que le champ électrique externe.

- Lorsque le champ vertical est la cause principale de l'exposition, la direction dominante des champs induits est également verticale.

- Pour un champ électrique externe donné, les champs induits les plus forts le sont dans le corps humain en contact parfait avec le sol par l'intermédiaire des pieds (mise à la terre électrique) et les champs les plus faibles dans le corps isolé du sol ("espace libre").

- Le courant total circulant dans un organisme en contact parfait avec le sol est déterminé par la taille et la forme de l'organisme (notamment la posture), plutôt que par la conductivité des tissus.

- La distribution des courants induits dans les divers organes et tissus est déterminée par la conductivité de ces tissus et organes.

- La distribution d'un champ électrique induit est également fonction des conductivités, mais moins que celle du courant induit.

- Il existe également un phénomène indépendant dans lequel le courant est produit dans l'organisme du fait d'un contact avec un objet conducteur situé dans un champ électrique.

Concernant les champs magnétiques, la perméabilité des tissus est la même que celle de l'air, de sorte que le champ dans les tissus est le même que le champ extérieur. Le corps de l'homme et des animaux ne perturbe pas sensiblement ce champ. La principale interaction des champs magnétiques est l'induction, suivant la loi de Faraday, de champs électriques et des densités de courant associées dans les tissus conducteurs. Les principales caractéristiques de la dosimétrie concernant l'exposition de l'homme aux champs magnétiques EBF sont les suivantes:

- Le champ et le courant électrique induit dépendent de l'orientation du champ extérieur. Les champs induits dans l'organisme dans son ensemble sont plus grands lorsque le champ est aligné de l'avant vers l'arrière du corps, mais, pour certains organes, les valeurs les plus élevées s'observent lorsque le champ est appliqué de côté.

- Les champs électriques les plus faibles sont induits par un champ magnétique orienté le long de l'axe vertical du corps.

- Pour une intensité et une orientation donnée du champ magnétique, l'intensité des champs électriques induits dans un organisme augmentent avec sa taille.

- La distribution du champ électrique induit est modifiée par la conductivité des divers organes et tissus. Ceux-ci ont un effet limité sur la distribution de la densité du courant induit.

### 16.1.3 Mécanismes biophysiques

Il faut évaluer la plausibilité des divers mécanismes proposés d'interaction directe et indirecte des champs électriques et magnétiques EBF. En particulier, on veut savoir si on peut distinguer un "signal" produit dans un processus biologique par l'exposition à un champ, d'un bruit aléatoire intrinsèque, et si le mécanisme remet en question les principes et connaissances scientifiques actuels. De nombreux mécanismes ne deviennent plausibles qu'à des intensités de champs supérieures à un certain niveau. Néanmoins, l'absence de mécanismes plausibles répertoriés n'exclut pas la possibilité d'effets sur la santé même avec des champs très faibles, pour autant qu'on respecte les principes scientifiques fondamentaux.

Parmi les nombreux mécanismes proposés concernant l'interaction directe des champs avec le corps humain, il en est trois qui pourraient opérer à des intensités de champs plus faibles que les autres: les champs électriques induits dans les réseaux de neurones, les paires de radicaux libres et la présence de magnétite.

Les champs électriques induits dans les tissus par l'exposition à des champs électriques ou magnétiques EBF vont directement stimuler les fibres nerveuses simples myélinisées, et il s'agit d'un mécanisme plausible sur le plan biophysique, lorsque l'intensité du champ interne dépasse quelques $V\ m^{-1}$. Des champs beaucoup plus faibles peuvent modifier la transmission synaptique dans les réseaux neuronaux, au contraire des cellules isolées. Ce traitement du signal par les systèmes nerveux est communément employé par les organismes multicellulaires pour détecter les signaux environnementaux faibles. On a proposé une limite inférieure pour la discrimination par les réseaux nerveux de 1 mV/m, mais, d'après les données actuelles, des valeurs seuils situées autour de 10 à 100 $mV\ m^{-1}$ semblent plus probables.

Le mécanisme des paires de radicaux libres est une modalité acceptée par laquelle les champs magnétiques peuvent modifier des types particuliers de réactions chimiques. On décrit généralement une augmentation de la concentration de radicaux libres sous exposition à des champs faibles et une diminution dans des champs intenses. On a observé ces augmentations dans des champs magnétiques de moins de 1 mT. Il semblerait qu'il y ait un lien entre ce mécanisme et le système de navigation des oiseaux au cours de leur migration. Pour des raisons théoriques et parce que les modifications produites par les champs magnétiques EBF et statiques sont analogues, on pense que des champs à la fréquence du réseau, bien moins intenses que le champ géomagnétique d'environ 50 µT, sont peu susceptibles d'être biologiquement importants.

Les cristaux de magnétite, qui sont de petits cristaux ferromagnétiques d'oxyde de fer de diverses formes, se retrouvent dans les tissus animaux et humains, même si c'est à l'état de traces. Comme les radicaux libres,

449

ils ont été reliés au système d'orientation et de navigation des animaux migrateurs, bien que la présence de quantités de magnétite à l'état de traces dans le cerveau humain ne lui confère pas d'aptitude à détecter le champ géomagnétique faible. Les calculs basés sur des hypothèses extrêmes laissent à penser que le seuil des effets des champs EBF sur les cristaux de magnétite se situe autour de 5 µT.

Les autres interactions biophysiques directes des champs, comme la cassure des liaisons chimiques, les forces exercées sur les particules chargées et les divers mécanismes de "résonance" en bande étroite ne sont pas considérées comme apportant des explications plausibles aux interactions avec les champs rencontrés dans les environnements publics et professionnels.

Concernant les effets indirects, la charge électrique de surface induite par les champs électriques peut être perçue et entraîner des microchocs douloureux lorsque l'on touche un objet conducteur. Des courants de contact peuvent se produire lorsque, par exemple, de jeunes enfants touchent un robinet de baignoire dans certaines habitations. Cela produit de petits champs électriques, peut-être au-dessus du niveau de bruit de fond, dans la moelle osseuse. Toutefois, on ignore s'ils présentent un risque pour la santé.

Les lignes à haute tension produisent des nuages d'ions chargés électriquement par suite de la décharge par effet couronne. Il semble qu'elles pourraient accroître le dépôt des polluants de l'air sur la peau et dans les voies aériennes, avec d'éventuelles conséquences indésirables pour la santé. Toutefois, il semble peu probable que les ions de la couronne aient plus qu'un effet minime, si ce n'est nul, sur les risques sanitaires à long terme même chez les sujets les plus exposés.

Aucun des trois mécanismes directs évoqués ci-dessus ne semble constituer une cause plausible d'incidence accrue des maladies aux niveaux d'exposition généralement rencontrés. En réalité, ils ne deviendraient plausibles qu'à des intensités bien plus élevées, et les mécanismes indirects n'ont pour l'instant pas été suffisamment étudiés. Cette absence de mécanisme répertorié plausible n'exclut pas la possibilité d'effets indésirables pour la santé, mais crée véritablement un besoin de preuves plus solides venant de la biologie et de l'épidémiologie.

### 16.1.4 Neurocomportement

L'exposition à des champs électriques à la fréquence du réseau provoque des réponses biologiques bien définies, allant de la perception simple à la gêne, par biais des effets de la charge électrique de surface. Ces réponses dépendent de l'intensité du champ, des conditions environnementales ambiantes et de la sensibilité individuelle. Les seuils de perception directe chez 10% des volontaires se situent entre 2 et 20 kV m$^{-1}$, tandis que 5% trouvent que des valeurs de 15 à 20 kV m$^{-1}$ sont gênantes. La décharge d'étincelles qu'émet une personne avec le sol est douloureuse pour 7% des volontaires dans un champ de 5 kV m$^{-1}$. Les seuils pour une décharge à partir d'un objet chargé à travers une personne ayant les pieds au sol dépend de la taille de l'objet et exigent par conséquent une évaluation précise.

Les champs magnétiques de forte intensité et pulsés peuvent stimuler les tissus nerveux périphériques ou centraux; de tels effets peuvent se produire au cours des examens d'imagerie par résonance magnétique (IRM) et sont utilisés dans la stimulation magnétique transcrânienne. Le seuil de champ électrique nécessaire pour provoquer une stimulation nerveuse directe pourrait ne pas dépasser quelques volts par mètre (V/m). Ce seuil est probablement constant sur une gamme de fréquences située entre quelques hertz (Hz) et quelques kilohertz (kHz). Les personnes souffrant d'épilepsie ou prédisposées à cette maladie risquent d'être plus sensibles aux champs électriques EBF induits dans le système nerveux central (SNC). En outre, la sensibilité à la stimulation électrique du SNC semble très probablement être associée à des antécédents familiaux de crises convulsives et à l'utilisation d'antidépresseurs tricycliques, de neuroleptiques et autres médicaments qui abaissent le seuil convulsivogène.

La fonction de la rétine, qui fait partie du SNC, peut être modifiée par l'exposition à des champs magnétiques EBF beaucoup plus faibles que ceux qui provoquent une stimulation nerveuse directe. Une sensation d'éclairs lumineux, appelés phosphènes magnétiques ou magnéto-phosphènes, résulte de l'interaction du champ électrique induit avec les cellules de la rétine électriquement excitables. La valeur seuil du champ électrique induit dans le liquide extracellulaire de la rétine a été estimée entre 10 et 100 mV m$^{-1}$ à 20 Hz. Cependant, une incertitude considérable est attachée à ces valeurs.

Les données relatives à d'autres effets neuro-comportementaux observés dans les études sur des volontaires, par exemple les effets sur l'activité électrique du cerveau, la cognition, le sommeil, l'hypersensibilité et l'humeur sont moins nettes. En général, ces études ont été effectuées à des niveaux d'exposition situés au-dessous de ceux nécessaires pour provoquer les effets décrits ci-dessus et n'ont produit que des effets au mieux subtils et transitoires. Les conditions nécessaires pour déclencher ces réponses ne sont aujourd'hui pas bien connues. Il semblerait qu'il existe des effets sur le temps de réaction et sur une moindre précision observée dans l'exécution de certaines tâches cognitives, ce que viennent conforter les résultats d'études sur l'activité électrique générale du cerveau. Les études cherchant à déterminer si les champs magnétiques modifient la qualité du sommeil ont donné des résultats variables. Il est possible que cette variabilité puisse être attribuée en partie aux différences observées dans la conception de ces études.

Certaines personnes affirment être hypersensibles aux champs électromagnétiques en général. Toutefois, les données des études de provocation en double aveugle laissent à penser que les symptômes rapportés ne sont pas liés à l'exposition aux champs magnétiques EBF.

Il n'y a que des données contradictoires et peu concluantes indiquant que l'exposition aux champs électriques et magnétiques EBF puissent provoquer des symptômes dépressifs ou des suicides. Ainsi, ces données sont considérées comme insuffisantes.

Chez les animaux, la possibilité qu'une exposition aux champs EBF puisse modifier les fonctions neuro-comportementales a été explorée sous divers angles et pour toute une série de conditions d'exposition. Peu d'effets ont été établis avec certitude. Il y a des preuves convaincantes que les champs électriques à la fréquence du secteur peuvent être détectés par les animaux, très probablement par suite d'effets de charge de surface, et puissent provoquer une stimulation ou un stress bénin transitoire. Chez le rat, le seuil de détection se situe entre 3 et 13 kV m$^{-1}$. On a montré que des champs supérieurs à 50 kV m$^{-1}$ provoquaient une réaction d'aversion chez les rongeurs. Les autres modifications éventuelles dues aux champs sont moins bien définies; les études en laboratoire n'ont permis d'obtenir que des effets subtils et transitoires. Il semblerait que l'exposition aux champs magnétiques puisse moduler les fonctions des systèmes de neurotransmetteurs opioïdes et cholinergiques dans le cerveau, ce qui est conforté par les résultats d'études s'intéressant aux effets sur l'analgésie et sur l'acquisition et l'exécution de tâches liées à la mémoire spatiale.

### 16.1.5  Système neuroendocrinien

Les résultats des études effectuées chez des volontaires, ainsi que des études épidémiologiques en milieu résidentiel et professionnel, laissent à penser que le système neuroendocrinien n'est pas affecté par l'exposition à des champs électriques ou magnétiques à la fréquence du réseau. Cela vaut particulièrement pour les concentrations circulantes d'hormones spécifiques du système neuroendocrinien, notamment la mélatonine, libérée par l'épiphyse, et pour un certain nombre d'hormones impliquées dans le contrôle du métabolisme et de la physiologie de l'organisme libérées par l'hypophyse. On a parfois observé des différences infimes dans la chronologie de la libération de la mélatonine associées à certaines caractéristiques de l'exposition, mais ces résultats n'ont pas été uniformes. Il est très difficile d'éliminer certains facteurs de confusion dus à toutes sortes d'éléments environnementaux et du mode de vie qui pourraient également modifier les concentrations d'hormones. La plupart des études en laboratoire sur les effets de l'exposition aux EBF sur les concentrations nocturnes de mélatonine chez des volontaires ont montré qu'elle n'avait aucun effet lorsqu'on avait pris soin de neutraliser les éventuels facteurs de confusion.

Parmi les nombreuses études réalisées chez l'animal pour analyser les effets des champs électriques et magnétiques à la fréquence du réseau sur les concentrations pinéales et sériques de mélatonine chez le rat, certaines ont rapporté que l'exposition entraînait une suppression nocturne de la mélatonine. Les changements de concentration de mélatonine observés dans des études antérieures portant sur des expositions à des champs électriques allant jusqu'à 100 kV m$^{-1}$ n'ont pas pu être reproduits. Les résultats d'une série d'études plus récentes, qui ont montré que les champs magnétiques polarisés circulairement supprimaient les concentrations nocturnes de mélatonine, ont perdu du poids du fait de comparaisons inappropriées entre animaux exposés et témoins historiques. Les données d'autres expériences réalisées chez les rongeurs, couvrant des degrés d'intensité allant de quelques microteslas à

5 mT, ont été ambiguës, certains résultats montrant une dépression de la mélatonine et d'autres aucune modification. Chez les animaux se reproduisant à une saison déterminée, la preuve d'un effet de l'exposition à des champs à la fréquence du réseau sur les concentrations de mélatonine et sur l'état reproductif dépendant de la mélatonine est principalement négative. Aucun effet convaincant sur les concentrations de mélatonine n'a été observé dans une étude réalisée chez des primates non humains chroniquement exposés à des champs à la fréquence du réseau, bien qu'une étude préliminaire effectuée sur deux animaux ait rapporté une suppression de la mélatonine en réponse à une exposition irrégulière et intermittente.

Les effets de l'exposition à des champs EBF sur la production de mélatonine ou sa libération dans des épiphyses isolées ont été variables, bien que relativement peu d'études in vitro aient été effectuées. Les éléments de preuve indiquant que l'exposition aux EBF interfère avec l'action de la mélatonine sur les cellules de cancer du sein in vitro sont particulièrement intéressants. Toutefois, ce système souffre de l'inconvénient que les lignées cellulaires montrent fréquemment en culture une dérive génotypique et phénotypique qui peut empêcher leur transfert entre laboratoires.

Aucun effet réplicable n'a été observé sur les hormones liées au stress de l'axe hypophyso-surrénalien de toutes sortes d'espèces de mammifères, à l'exception possible d'un stress de courte durée faisant suite au début d'une exposition à un champ électrique EBF suffisamment intense pour être perçu. De la même façon, alors que peu d'études ont été effectuées, on a observé des effets principalement négatifs ou irréguliers au niveau des concentrations d'hormones de croissance et d'hormones participant au contrôle de l'activité métabolique, ou associées au contrôle de la reproduction et du développement sexuel.

Dans l'ensemble, ces données n'indiquent pas que les champs électriques et/ou magnétiques EBF modifient le système neuroendocrinien et ont des répercussions indésirables sur la santé humaine, et les éléments de preuve sont donc considérés comme insuffisants.

### 16.1.6 Troubles neurodégénératifs

L'hypothèse a été émise suivant laquelle l'exposition aux champs EBF serait associée à plusieurs maladies neurodégénératives. Concernant la maladie de Parkinson et la sclérose en plaques, le nombre d'études est faible et rien ne permet de penser qu'il y ait une association avec ces maladies.

Pour la maladie d'Alzheimer et la sclérose latérale amyotrophique (SLA), davantage d'études ont été publiées. Certains de ces rapports laissent à penser que les personnes ayant des professions dans le secteur de l'électricité pourraient avoir un risque accru de SLA. Jusqu'ici, aucun mécanisme biologique n'a été établi qui pourrait expliquer une telle association, la maladie ayant pu apparaître à cause de facteurs de confusion liés à ce type de professions, par exemple les chocs électriques. Dans l'ensemble, les éléments en faveur d'une association entre exposition aux EBF et SLA sont considérés comme insuffisants. Les quelques études portant sur l'association entre exposition aux EBF et maladie d'Alzheimer ont donné des résultats variables. Toutefois, la meilleure qualité des études axées sur la morbidité par Alzheimer, plutôt que sur la mortalité, n'indique aucune association. Dans l'ensemble, les éléments en faveur d'une association entre l'exposition aux EBF et la maladie d'Alzheimer sont insuffisants.

### 16.1.7 Troubles cardio-vasculaires

Les études expérimentales sur l'exposition à court et long terme indiquent que si le choc électrique constitue un risque manifeste pour la santé, les autres effets cardio-vasculaires dangereux associés aux champs EBF ont peu de chances de se produire aux niveaux d'exposition communément rencontrés dans l'environnement naturel ou professionnel. Bien qu'on ait signalé dans la littérature diverses modifications cardio-vasculaires, la majorité des effets sont mineurs et les études n'ont pas donné de résultats homogènes. Aucune des études de la morbidité et de la mortalité des maladies cardio-vasculaires n'a montré d'association avec l'exposition, sauf une. Le fait de savoir s'il existe une association entre l'exposition et l'altération du contrôle autonome du coeur donne lieu à bien des conjectures. Dans l'ensemble, les éléments dont on dispose ne sont pas en faveur d'une association entre exposition aux EBF et maladie cardio-vasculaire.

### 16.1.8 Immunologie et hématologie

Les données concernant les effets des champs électriques ou magnétiques EBF sur des constituants du système immunitaire sont généralement peu homogènes. La plupart des populations cellulaires et marqueurs fonctionnels ne sont pas perturbés par l'exposition. Cependant, dans certaines études humaines réalisées avec des champs allant de 10 µT à 2 mT, on a observé des modifications des cellules Natural Killer (NK), qui ont montré à la fois une augmentation et une diminution de leur nombre, et dans la numération leucocytaire totale qui a montré soit une absence de modification, soit une diminution du nombre de leucocytes. Dans des études réalisées chez l'animal, on a observé une diminution de l'activité des cellules NK chez la souris femelle, mais pas chez les mâles ni chez les rats des deux sexes. Les numérations leucocytaires ont également montré une certaine variabilité, avec des diminutions ou une absence de modification, rapportées dans différentes études. Les expositions auxquelles étaient soumis les animaux allaient de 2 µT à 30 mT. La difficulté qu'il y a à interpréter les effets potentiels de ces données sur la santé est due aux grandes variations enregistrées dans les conditions d'exposition et environnementales, ainsi qu'au nombre relativement faible de sujets testés et à la vaste gamme des paramètres biologiques étudiés.

Il y a eu peu d'études sur les effets des champs magnétiques EBF sur le système hématologique. Dans les expériences évaluant les numérations leucocytaires différentielles, les expositions allaient de 2 µT à 2 mT. Aucun effet constant de l'exposition aiguë aux champs magnétiques EBF ou aux champs magnétiques et électriques EBF combinés n'a été trouvé dans les études réalisées chez l'homme ou chez l'animal.

Par conséquent, d'une manière générale, les éléments en faveur d'effets des champs électriques ou magnétiques EBF sur les systèmes immunitaire et hématologique sont considérés comme insuffisants.

### 16.1.9   Reproduction et développement

Dans l'ensemble, les études épidémiologiques n'ont pas montré d'association entre leurs résultats dans le domaine de la reproduction de l'homme et l'exposition maternelle ou paternelle à des champs EBF. Il existe des éléments en faveur d'un risque accru de fausse-couche associé à l'exposition maternelle au champ magnétique, mais ils sont insuffisants.

Les effets d'expositions aux champs électriques EBF jusqu'à 150 kV m$^{-1}$ ont été évalués chez plusieurs espèces de mammifères, notamment dans des études sur l'exposition de grands groupes et sur plusieurs générations. Les résultats montrent systématiquement qu'il n'y a aucun effet indésirable sur le développement.

L'exposition de mammifères aux champs magnétiques EBF jusqu'à 20 mT n'entraîne pas de malformations externes, squelettiques ou viscérales grossières. Certaines études montrent une augmentation des anomalies mineures du squelette chez le rat et la souris. Ces variations sont relativement courantes dans les études de tératologie et sont souvent considérées comme sans signification biologique. Toutefois, des effets subtils des champs magnétiques sur le développement squelettique ne peuvent être écartés. Très peu d'études ont été publiées sur les effets sur la reproduction et il est impossible d'en tirer des conclusions.

Plusieurs études sur des modèles expérimentaux autres que mammifères (embryons de poulets, poissons, oursins et insectes) ont donné des résultats indiquant que les champs magnétiques EBF de l'ordre du microtesla peuvent perturber le début du développement. Mais les résultats de ces modèles expérimentaux ont moins de poids dans l'évaluation générale de la toxicité sur le développement que ceux des études correspondantes réalisées chez les mammifères.

Dans l'ensemble, les éléments en faveur d'effets sur le développement et la reproduction sont insuffisants.

### 16.1.10  Cancer

La classification du Centre International de Recherche sur le Caner (CIRC, IARC) des champs magnétiques EBF comme étant "peut-être cancérogènes pour l'homme" (IARC, 2002) est basée sur l'ensemble des données disponibles en 2001. L'examen de la littérature dans la présente monographie des critères d'hygiène de l'environnement est principalement axé sur des études publiées après l'analyse du CIRC.

*Epidémiologie*

La classification du CIRC a été fortement influencée par les associations observées dans les études épidémiologiques sur la leucémie infantile.

455

Le fait de classer ces éléments comme étant limités n'est pas modifié avec l'adjonction de deux études sur la leucémie infantile publiées après 2002. Depuis la publication de la monographie du CIRC, les éléments relatifs à d'autres cancers chez l'enfant restent insuffisants.

Un certain nombre de rapports a été publié à la suite de la monographie du CIRC concernant le risque de cancer du sein chez la femme adulte associé à l'exposition à des champs magnétiques EBF. Ces études sont de taille plus importante que les précédentes et moins susceptibles de présenter des biais et sont dans l'ensemble négatives. Elles ont donc considérablement affaibli les éléments en faveur d'une association entre exposition à des champs magnétiques EBF et risque de cancer du sein chez la femme et ne vont plus du tout dans le sens d'une telle association.

Dans le cas des tumeurs cérébrales et des leucémies chez l'adulte, les nouvelles études publiées après la monographie du CIRC ne modifient pas la conclusion selon laquelle les éléments en faveur d'une association entre champs magnétiques EBF et ces maladies restent insuffisants.

Pour les autres maladies et tous les autres cancers, les éléments restent insuffisants.

*Etudes sur les animaux de laboratoire*

Il n'existe actuellement aucun modèle animal approprié de la forme de leucémie infantile la plus commune, la leucémie aiguë lymphoblastique. Trois études indépendantes à grande échelle effectuées chez le rat n'ont fourni aucune preuve d'un effet des champs magnétiques EBF sur l'incidence des tumeurs mammaires spontanées. La plupart des études rapportent l'absence d'effets des champs magnétiques EBF sur la leucémie ou le lymphome dans les modèles murins. Plusieurs études à grande échelle et à long terme effectuées chez des rongeurs n'ont montré aucune augmentation systématique d'aucun type de cancer, notamment des tumeurs hématopoïétiques, mammaires, cérébrales et cutanées.

Un nombre non négligeable d'études a examiné les effets des champs magnétiques EBF sur les tumeurs mammaires induites chimiquement chez le rat. Elles ont obtenu des résultats variables qui peuvent être dus entièrement ou partiellement à des différences dans les protocoles expérimentaux, par exemple à l'utilisation de sous-souches particulières. La plupart des études sur les effets de l'exposition à des champs magnétiques EBF sur des modèles de leucémie/lymphome chimiquement induits ou induits par le rayonnement n'ont pas montré d'effets. Les études sur les lésions hépatiques précancéreuses, les tumeurs cutanées et cérébrales chimiquement induites ont en majorité rapporté l'absence d'effets. Une étude a signalé une accélération de la genèse tumorale cutanée induite par les UV après exposition à des champs magnétiques EBF.

Deux groupes ont signalé des niveaux accrus de lésions des brins d'ADN dans le tissu cérébral suite à une exposition *in vivo* à des champs magnétiques EBF. Toutefois, d'autres groupes, en utilisant toutes sortes de modèles murins de génotoxicité, n'ont trouvé aucun signe d'effets génotoxiques. Les résultats des études s'intéressant aux effets non génotoxiques en rapport avec le cancer ne permettent pas de tirer des conclusions.

Dans l'ensemble, rien ne permet de penser que l'exposition à des champs magnétiques EBF seule puisse provoquer des tumeurs. Les éléments indiquant que l'exposition à un champ magnétique EBF peut favoriser le développement d'une tumeur lorsqu'elle est associée à des facteurs cancérogènes sont insuffisants.

*Etudes in vitro*

En général, les études sur les effets de l'exposition de cellules à un champ EBF ont montré qu'il n'y avait pas d'effets génotoxiques pour des intensités de champ inférieures à 50 mT. Il existe cependant une exception notable, à savoir les données d'études récentes signalant une altération de l'ADN à des champs aussi faibles que 35 µT; cependant, ces études sont encore en cours d'évaluation et notre compréhension de ces résultats reste incomplète. Tout porte également à croire que les champs magnétiques EBF peuvent interagir avec des agents altérant d'ADN.

Il n'y a pas de preuve nette d'une activation des gènes associés au contrôle du cycle cellulaire par des champs magnétiques EBF. Cependant, il faut encore mener des études systématiques analysant la réponse de l'ensemble du génome.

De nombreuses autres études à l'échelle cellulaire, par exemple sur la prolifération cellulaire, le phénomène d'apoptose, le signal calcique et la transformation maligne, ont donné des résultats non homogènes ou ne permettant pas de tirer de conclusions.

*Conclusion générale*

Les nouvelles études réalisées chez l'homme, chez l'animal et in vitro et publiées depuis la monographie du CIRC en 2002 ne modifient en rien la classification générale des champs magnétiques EBF, considérés comme cancérogènes possibles pour l'homme.

### 16.1.11 Evaluation du risque pour la santé

D'après la Constitution de l'OMS, la santé est un état de bien-être physique, mental et social complet et pas simplement l'absence de maladie ou d'infirmité. Une évaluation du risque est un cadre conceptuel pour un examen structuré des informations utiles à l'estimation des résultats sur la santé ou l'environnement. L'évaluation du risque sanitaire peut être utilisée comme un élément de la gestion du risque qui englobe toutes les activités nécessaires pour parvenir à des décisions relatives au fait qu'une exposition exige ou non des mesures particulières et la mise en oeuvre de celles-ci.

Dans l'évaluation des risques pour la santé de l'homme, de solides données concernant l'homme, chaque fois qu'elles sont disponibles, sont généralement plus instructives que celles recueillies chez l'animal. Les études chez l'animal et les études in vitro peuvent étayer les données des études chez l'homme, combler les lacunes laissées par les études chez l'homme, ou être utilisées pour prendre une décision relative aux risques lorsque les études chez l'homme sont insuffisantes ou absentes.

Toutes les études, qu'elles aient des résultats positifs ou négatifs (présence ou absence d'effets), doivent être évaluées et jugées pour elles-mêmes puis toutes ensembles à partir des données disponibles. Il est important de déterminer dans quelle mesure une série d'éléments modifie la probabilité pour qu'une exposition provoque un résultat. Les éléments de preuve de l'existence d'un effet sont généralement renforcés si les résultats de différents types d'études (épidémiologiques et expérimentales) laissent entrevoir la même conclusion et/ou lorsque de multiples études du même type donnent le même résultat.

*Effets aigus*

Des effets biologiques aigus ont été établis pour une exposition aux champs électriques et magnétiques EBF dans la gamme de fréquences allant jusqu'à 100 kHz, effets qui peuvent avoir des conséquences indésirables sur la santé. Par conséquent, des limites d'exposition sont nécessaires. Il existe des directives internationales qui traitent de cette question. L'observance de ces directives assure une protection suffisante contre les effets aigus.

*Effets chroniques*

Les données scientifiques laissant à penser que l'exposition quotidienne chronique à des champs magnétiques à la fréquence du réseau, de faible intensité (au-dessus de 0,3–0,4 µT), constitue un risque pour la santé sont basées sur des études épidémiologiques mettant en évidence un profil homogène de risque de leucémie infantile accru. Les incertitudes de cette évaluation du risque incluent le biais de sélection des témoins et les erreurs de classification de l'exposition sur la relation entre champs magnétiques et leucémie infantile. En outre, pratiquement toutes les données de laboratoire et toutes les données mécanistiques ne vont pas dans le sens d'une association entre champs magnétiques EBF de faible intensité et modifications de fonctions biologiques ou de l'état sanitaire. Ainsi, tout bien considéré, les éléments de preuve ne sont pas suffisamment solides pour être considérés comme établissant un lien de causalité, mais le sont suffisamment pour rester préoccupants.

Bien que l'on n'ait pas pu établir une relation de cause à effet entre l'exposition à un champ magnétique EBF et la leucémie infantile, son effet possible sur la santé publique a été calculé en partant du principe de causalité de façon à fournir un élément potentiellement utile à la politique de santé. Toutefois, ces calculs dépendent fortement de la distribution de l'exposition et d'autres hypothèses et sont par conséquent très imprécis. En partant du principe que l'association est causale, le nombre de cas de leucémie infantile dans le monde qui pourrait être attribué à l'exposition peut, selon les estimations, se situer entre 100 et 2400 cas par an. Toutefois, cela ne représente que

0,2 à 4,9% de l'incidence annuelle totale des cas de leucémie, estimée à 49 000 dans le monde en 2000. Ainsi, dans le contexte mondial, l'impact sur la santé publique, pour autant qu'il y en ait, serait limité et incertain.

On a étudié un certain nombre d'autres maladies à la recherche d'une association éventuelle avec une exposition aux champs magnétiques EBF. Parmi elles figurent des cancers de l'enfant et de l'adulte, la dépression, le suicide, des dysfonctionnements de l'appareil reproducteur, des troubles du développement, des modifications immunologiques et des maladies neurologiques. Les données scientifiques en faveur d'un lien entre champs magnétiques EBF et l'une quelconque de ces maladies sont beaucoup plus ténues que pour la leucémie infantile et, dans certains cas (par exemple, s'agissant des maladies cardio-vasculaires ou du cancer du sein), elles sont suffisantes pour que l'on soit assuré que les champs magnétiques EBF ne provoquent pas ces maladies.

### 16.1.12 Mesures de protection

Il est essentiel de mettre en application des limites d'exposition de façon à se protéger des effets indésirables établis de l'exposition aux champs électriques et magnétiques EBF. Ces limites d'exposition doivent être basées sur un examen rigoureux de toutes les données scientifiques pertinentes.

Seuls des effets aigus ont été établis et il existe deux directives internationales relatives aux limites d'exposition (ICNIRP, 1998a; IEEE, 2002) destinées à protéger contre ces effets.

En même temps que ces effets aigus attestés, il existe des incertitudes concernant l'existence d'effets chroniques, à cause des éléments limités qui existent en faveur d'un lien entre exposition aux champs magnétiques EBF et leucémie infantile. Par conséquent, il est justifié de faire appel à des stratégies prudentes. Toutefois, il n'est pas recommandé de réduire les valeurs limites figurant dans les normes relatives à l'exposition jusqu'à un niveau arbitraire au nom du principe de précaution. De telles pratiques sapent les fondements scientifiques sur lesquels les limites sont basées et risquent de constituer une approche coûteuse, mais pas nécessairement efficace, d'assurer la protection.

La mise en œuvre d'autres types de mesures de précaution adaptées pour réduire l'exposition est raisonnable et justifiée. Toutefois, l'énergie électrique apporte des bienfaits évidents sur le plan sanitaire, social et économique et il ne faut pas que ces mesures les mettent en péril. Qui plus est, étant donné la faiblesse des éléments en faveur d'un lien entre exposition aux champs magnétiques EBF et leucémie infantile et les effets limités sur la santé publique si un tel lien existe, il est malaisé de déterminer les bienfaits qu'apporterait pour la santé une réduction de l'exposition. Ainsi, le coût des mesures de précaution doit être très bas. Le coût de la mise en oeuvre des réductions d'exposition variera d'un pays à l'autre, ce qui fait qu'il est très difficile de formuler une recommandation générale visant à équilibrer les coûts face à un risque potentiel imputable aux champs EBF.

Compte tenu de ce qui précède, les recommandations qui suivent ont été formulées.

- Les responsables de l'élaboration des politiques sanitaires doivent établir des lignes directives concernant l'exposition aux champs EBF à l'intention du grand public et des entreprises. Les directives internationales constituent la meilleure source d'orientation, aussi bien pour les niveaux d'exposition que pour les principes de l'évaluation scientifique des risques.

- Les responsables de l'élaboration des politiques doivent mettre en place un programme de protection contre les champs EBF comportant la mesure des champs de toutes origines pour veiller à ce que les limites d'exposition ne soient pas dépassées pour le grand public et lors d'expositions professionnelles.

- A condition de ne pas mettre en péril les bienfaits apportés sur le plan sanitaire, social et économique par l'énergie électrique, la mise en œuvre de mesures de précaution à très bas coût afin de réduire l'exposition est raisonnable et justifiée.

- Les responsables de l'élaboration des politiques sanitaires, les autorités locales et les fabricants doivent mettre en œuvre des mesures à très bas coût lorsqu'ils construisent de nouvelles installations et conçoivent un nouvel équipement, notamment de nouveaux appareils.

- Il faut envisager d'apporter des modifications aux pratiques de l'ingénierie afin de réduire l'exposition aux EBF des appareils ou dispositifs, à condition qu'elles se conjuguent avec d'autres avantages, par exemple une meilleure sécurité ou un coût faible ou nul.

- Lorsque l'on envisage d'apporter des changements aux sources EBF existantes, il faut étudier les possibilités de réduction du champ EBF en même temps que les aspects liés à la sécurité, à la fiabilité et au volet économique du projet.

- Les autorités locales doivent faire appliquer les réglementations relatives aux installations électriques afin de réduire les courants de terre non intentionnels lorsque l'on construit de nouvelles installations ou que l'on refait les installations existantes, tout en conservant la sécurité. Des mesures proactives visant à recenser les violations de ces règles ou les problèmes existants dans les installations électriques seraient coûteuses et peu susceptibles d'être justifiées.

- Les autorités nationales doivent mettre en œuvre une stratégie de communication efficace et ouverte pour permettre une prise de décision éclairée par toutes les parties prenantes ; celle-ci doit comprendre des informations sur la façon dont les personnes peuvent réduire leur propre exposition.

- Les autorités locales doivent améliorer la planification des installations émettrices de champs EBF, notamment en procédant à des consultations plus larges entre l'industrie, les pouvoirs publics locaux et les citoyens lorsqu'il s'agit d'implanter d'importantes sources EBF.

- Les pouvoirs publics et l'industrie doivent promouvoir des programmes de recherche visant à réduire l'incertitude des données scientifiques concernant les effets sanitaires de l'exposition aux champs EBF.

## 16.2    Recommandations en matière de recherche

La détermination des lacunes dans les connaissances relatives aux effets sanitaires possibles d'une exposition aux champs EBF constitue une part essentielle de cette évaluation du risque sanitaire. Il en a résulté les recommandations qui suivent relatives à la recherche à venir (résumées au Tableau 1).

La priorité des priorités pour la recherche est de s'intéresser aux fréquences intermédiaires, se situant communément entre 300 Hz et 100 kHz, étant donné l'actuel manque de données les concernant. Une très faible partie du corpus de connaissances nécessaires pour une évaluation du risque a été rassemblée et la plupart des études existantes ont donné des résultats variables, qui doivent être mieux étayés. Les normes générales de constitution d'une base de données sur les fréquences intermédiaires, qui soit suffisante pour l'évaluation du risque sanitaire, comprennent l'évaluation de l'exposition, des études épidémiologiques, des études sur l'homme en laboratoire et des études sur l'animal et sur les cellules (in vitro) (ICNIRP, 2003; ICNIRP, 2004; Litvak et al., 2002).

Pour toutes les études sur des volontaires, il est obligatoire que la recherche sur les sujets humains soit effectuée en conformité totale avec les principes éthiques, y compris les dispositions de la déclaration d'Helsinki (WMA, 2004).

Pour les études de laboratoire, on accordera la priorité aux réponses notifiées (i) pour lesquelles il y a au moins quelques éléments de réplication ou de confirmation, (ii) qui sont potentiellement en rapport avec la cancérogenèse (par exemple, la génotoxicité), (iii) qui sont suffisamment solides pour permettre une analyse mécanistique et (iv) qui se produisent dans des modèles mammifères ou humains.

### 16.2.1    Sources, mesurage et expositions

La caractérisation plus précise des habitations ayant une exposition élevée aux EBF dans différents pays, afin de déterminer la contribution relative des sources internes et externes, ainsi que l'influence des pratiques en matière d'installation électrique/de mise à la terre et autres caractéristiques des habitations, pourraient fournir des indications concernant une méthode pertinente de mesure de l'exposition pour les évaluations épidémiologiques. Mieux connaître l'exposition fœtale et infantile aux champs EBF en est une composante importante, surtout s'agissant de l'exposition à un chauffage électrique par le sol ou aux transformateurs dans les immeubles.

On soupçonne que, dans certains cas d'exposition professionnelle, les limites d'exposition aux champs EBF des directives actuelles sont dépassées. Davantage d'informations sont nécessaires sur l'exposition professionnelle (y compris aux fréquences qui ne sont pas celles du réseau) liée par exemple à l'entretien des lignes sous tension, au travail à l'intérieur ou à proximité de l'entrefer des aimants d'IRM (et donc des champs EBF à gradient commuté) et aux réseaux de transport de l'électricité. De la même façon, des connaissances supplémentaires sont nécessaires concernant l'exposition du grand public qui pourrait approcher les limites des directives, notamment s'agissant de sources telles que les systèmes de sécurité, les systèmes de démagnétisation des bibliothèques, les appareils de cuisson par induction et de chauffage de l'eau.

L'exposition à des courants de contact a été proposée comme explication possible de l'association entre champs magnétiques EBF et leucémie infantile. Des recherches sont nécessaires dans des pays autres que les Etats-Unis d'Amérique afin d'évaluer la possibilité que les pratiques de mise à la terre et de plomberie utilisées dans les habitations donnent naissance à des courants de contact. Ces études auront la priorité dans les pays dans lesquels les résultats épidémiologiques concernant les EBF et la leucémie infantile sont significatifs.

### 16.2.2 Dosimétrie

Dans le passé, la plupart des recherches en laboratoire était fondée sur les courants électriques induits dans l'organisme, et la dosimétrie était ainsi axée sur cette quantité. Ce n'est que récemment que les travaux ont commencé à explorer les rapports entre exposition externe et champs électriques induits. Pour mieux comprendre les effets biologiques, on a besoin de davantage de données sur les champs électriques internes dans différentes conditions d'exposition.

Il faudrait procéder à une estimation des champs électriques internes dus à l'influence combinée des champs électriques et magnétiques externes dans différentes configurations. L'addition vectorielle des champs électriques et magnétiques qui sont sans relation de phase et variables dans l'espace est nécessaire pour déterminer les restrictions de base à respecter.

Très peu d'évaluations ont été effectuées sur des modèles précis de femme enceinte et de fœtus comportant une modélisation anatomique appropriée. Il est important d'estimer l'éventuelle induction de champs électriques chez le fœtus en relation avec le problème de la leucémie infantile car les expositions tant professionnelles que résidentielles de la mère sont importantes.

Il faut affiner encore les modèles micro-dosimétriques pour pouvoir tenir compte de l'architecture cellulaire des réseaux nerveux et autres systèmes infra-organiques complexes dont on sait qu'ils sont plus sensibles aux effets induits par le champ électrique. Ce processus de modélisation doit également se pencher sur les influences s'exerçant sur les potentiels électriques de la membrane cellulaire et sur la libération des neurotransmetteurs.

### 16.2.3 Mécanismes biophysiques

Il y a trois sujets principaux pour lesquels il y a des limites évidentes à la compréhension que l'on a des mécanismes: les paires de radicaux libres, les particules magnétiques présentes dans l'organisme et le rapport signal/bruit dans les systèmes multicellulaires, tels que les réseaux neuronaux.

Le mécanisme des paires de radicaux libres est l'un des mécanismes d'interaction de faible intensité les plus plausibles, mais il reste à montrer qu'il est capable d'assurer la médiation d'effets importants dans le métabolisme et le fonctionnement cellulaire. Il est particulièrement important de comprendre quelle est la limite inférieure d'exposition à laquelle il agit, de façon à pouvoir estimer s'il pourrait ou non constituer un mécanisme pertinent de cancérogenèse. Etant donné les études récentes dans lesquelles les espèces oxygénées radicalaires ont été augmentées dans les cellules immunitaires exposées aux champs EBF, il est recommandé d'utiliser comme modèle cellulaire, pour l'analyse du potentiel de ce mécanisme des paires de radicaux libres, des cellules du système immunitaire qui produisent des espèces oxygénées radicalaires dans le cadre de leur réponse immunitaire.

Bien que la présence de particules magnétiques (cristaux de magnétite) dans le cerveau humain ne semble pas, d'après ce que l'on sait actuellement, conférer une sensibilité aux champs magnétiques EBF environnementaux, les approches théoriques et expérimentales à venir devraient déterminer si une telle sensibilité pourrait exister dans certaines conditions. En outre, toute modification du mécanisme des paires de radicaux libres évoqué ci-dessus, engendrée par la présence de magnétite, devrait être recherchée.

Il convient d'analyser de façon approfondie la mesure dans laquelle des mécanismes multicellulaires opèrent dans le cerveau pour augmenter le rapport signal/bruit, afin d'élaborer un cadre théorique permettant de quantifier le phénomène ou de déterminer ses limites. L'étude complémentaire du seuil et de la fréquence de réponse dans les réseaux neuronaux de l'hippocampe et d'autres parties du cerveau devrait être effectuée in vitro.

### 16.2.4 Neuro-comportement

Il est recommandé d'effectuer des études sur des volontaires en laboratoire sur les effets possibles sur le sommeil et sur la réalisation de tâches mentalement éprouvantes, au moyen d'approches méthodologiques harmonisées. Il faut préciser les réponses dose-réponse à des densités de flux magnétique supérieures à celles utilisées auparavant, et pour une gamme élargie de fréquences (c'est-à-dire dans la gamme des kilohertz).

Les études sur des adultes volontaires et sur les animaux laissent à penser que des effets cognitifs aigus peuvent se produire avec les expositions à court terme à des champs électriques ou magnétiques intenses. La caractérisation de ces effets est très importante pour l'élaboration de limites relatives à l'exposition, mais on manque de données précises concernant les effets dépendant du champ chez l'enfant. La mise en oeuvre d'études en laboratoire de la cognition et des modifications de l'électroencéphalogramme (ECG) enregistrées chez les personnes exposées aux champs EBF est recommandée, notamment chez les adultes régulièrement soumis à une exposition professionnelle et chez les enfants.

Les études comportementales sur des animaux immatures offrent un indicateur utile des effets cognitifs éventuels chez l'enfant. Les effets possibles d'une exposition pré- et postnatale aux champs magnétiques EBF sur le développement du système nerveux et la fonction cognitive devraient être étudiés. Ces études pourraient être utilement complétées par l'analyse des effets de l'exposition aux champs magnétiques EBF et aux champs électriques induits sur la croissance des cellules nerveuses au moyen de coupes de cerveaux ou de neurones en culture.

Il est nécessaire de s'intéresser plus avant aux conséquences sanitaires potentielles que laissent entrevoir les données expérimentales montrant des réponses opioïdes et cholinergiques chez l'animal. Les études portant sur la modulation des réponses opioïdes et cholinergiques chez l'animal doivent être étendues et il convient de définir des paramètres d'exposition et le fondement biologique de ces réponses comportementales.

### 16.2.5  Système neuroendocrinien

La base de données existante relative à la réponse neuroendocrinienne n'indique pas que l'exposition aux champs EBF pourrait avoir des effets indésirables sur la santé humaine. Par conséquent, aucune recommandation relative à des recherches supplémentaires n'est formulée.

### 16.2.6  Troubles neurodégénératifs

Plusieurs études ont montré un risque accru de sclérose latérale amyotrophique dans les "professions liées à l'électricité". On considère qu'il est important d'étudier cette association plus avant, de façon à découvrir si les champs magnétiques EBF font partie des causes de cette maladie neurodégénérative rare. Cette recherche demande de grandes études de cohortes prospectives comportant des informations sur l'exposition aux champs magnétiques EBF, aux chocs électriques et à d'autres facteurs de risque.

Il n'est pas certain que les champs magnétiques EBF constituent un facteur de risque de la maladie d'Alzheimer. Les données actuellement disponibles ne sont pas suffisantes et cette association doit être analysée de façon approfondie. L'utilisation des données de morbidité plutôt que de mortalité revêt une importance particulière.

### 16.2.7 Troubles cardio-vasculaires

Des recherches plus approfondies sur l'association entre champs magnétiques EBF et risque de maladie cardiovasculaire ne sont pas considérées comme une priorité.

### 16.2.8 Immunologie et hématologie

Les modifications observées dans les paramètres immunitaires et hématologiques d'adultes exposés aux champs magnétiques EBF ont montré des variations et il n'y a pratiquement aucune donnée issue de la recherche qui soit disponible sur les enfants. Par conséquent, la recommandation est de mener des études sur les effets de l'exposition aux EBF sur le développement des systèmes immunitaires et hématopoïétiques chez le jeune animal.

### 16.2.9 Reproduction et développement

Il semblerait qu'il y ait un risque accru de fausse couche associé à l'exposition aux champs magnétiques EBF. Etant donné l'effet potentiellement important pour la santé publique d'une telle association, une recherche épidémiologique approfondie est recommandée.

### 16.2.10 Cancer

La priorité des priorités pour la recherche dans ce domaine consiste à résoudre le conflit entre les données épidémiologiques (qui montrent une association entre l'exposition aux champs magnétiques EBF et un risque accru de leucémie infantile) et les données expérimentales et mécanistiques (qui ne sont pas en faveur d'une telle association). Il est recommandé que les épidémiologistes et les spécialistes des sciences expérimentales collaborent dans ce domaine. Pour que les nouvelles études épidémiologiques soient instructives, elles doivent être axées sur de nouveaux aspects de l'exposition, sur l'interaction potentielle avec d'autres facteurs ou sur les groupes fortement exposés, ou doivent être novatrices à un autre titre dans ce domaine de recherche. De plus, il est également recommandé de mettre à jour les analyses existantes groupées, en ajoutant les données des études récentes et en donnant un nouvel éclairage à ces analyses.

Les études sur les tumeurs cérébrales chez l'enfant ont donné des résultats variables. Comme pour la leucémie infantile, une analyse groupée des études sur ces tumeurs serait très instructive et elle est donc recommandée. Une telle analyse globale peut, à peu de frais, donner un aperçu plus vaste et meilleur des données existantes, notamment sur l'existence d'un biais de sélection et, si les études sont suffisamment homogènes, peut offrir une meilleure estimation du risque.

Concernant le cancer du sein chez l'adulte, des études plus récentes ont montré de façon convaincante qu'il n'y avait aucune association avec l'exposition aux champs magnétiques EBF. Par conséquent, d'autres recherches sur une telle association devraient se voir accorder une très faible priorité à l'avenir.

Concernant la leucémie et le cancer du cerveau chez l'adulte, la recommandation est de mettre en œuvre de grandes cohortes de sujets exposés professionnellement qui existent. Les études sur l'exposition professionnelle, les analyses et les méta-analyses groupées relatives à la leucémie et au cancer du cerveau ont donné des résultats variables et peu concluants. Toutefois, de nouvelles données ont été publiées par la suite qui devraient être utilisées pour actualiser ces analyses.

La priorité est d'examiner les données épidémiologiques en établissant des modèles animaux et in vitro appropriés pour les réponses aux champs magnétiques EBF de faible intensité, modèles qui soient largement transférables d'un laboratoire à l'autre.

Les modèles de rongeurs transgéniques utilisés pour l'étude de la leucémie infantile doivent être développés de façon à fournir des modèles animaux expérimentaux permettant d'étudier les effets de l'exposition aux champs magnétiques EBF. Par ailleurs, pour les études existantes sur l'animal, la majorité des données disponibles indiquent qu'il n'y a pas d'effets cancérogènes dus aux seuls champs magnétiques EBF. Il faut par conséquent accorder un rang de priorité élevé aux études in vitro et chez l'animal dans lesquelles les champs magnétiques EBF sont rigoureusement évalués en tant que cofacteurs de la cancérogenèse.

Concernant les autres études in vitro, les expériences faisant état d'effets génotoxiques de l'exposition à un champ magnétique EBF intermittent doivent être reproduites.

### 16.2.11 Mesures de protection

Il est recommandé d'effectuer des recherches sur l'élaboration de politiques de protection sanitaire et sur la mise en oeuvre de celles-ci dans les secteurs où il n'y a pas de certitude scientifique, plus précisément sur le recours au principe de précaution, l'interprétation de ce dernier et l'évaluation des effets des mesures de précaution prises contre les champs magnétiques EBF et autres agents rangés dans les "cancérogènes possibles pour l'homme". Lorsqu'il y a incertitude quant au risque sanitaire potentiel qu'un agent représente pour la société, des mesures de précaution peuvent être justifiées pour garantir la protection appropriée du grand public et des travailleurs. Seules des recherches limitées ont été effectuées dans ce domaine pour les champs magnétiques EBF et, parce qu'elles sont importantes, des recherches complémentaires sont nécessaires. Elles permettront peut-être aux pays d'intégrer le principe de précaution dans leurs politiques de protection de la santé.

Il est conseillé de procéder à une recherche approfondie sur la perception du risque et la communication sur les risques spécifiquement axée sur les champs électromagnétiques. Les facteurs psychologiques et sociologiques qui influent sur la perception du risque en général ont été largement étudiés. Toutefois, une recherche limitée a été menée pour analyser l'importance relative de ces facteurs dans le cas des champs électromagnétiques ou pour répertorier d'autres facteurs qui seraient spécifiques aux champs électromagnétiques. Les études récentes laissent à penser que les mesures de précaution qui véhiculent implicitement des messages de risque peuvent modifier la perception du risque en augmentant ou en réduisant l'inquiétude. Des études approfondies dans ce domaine sont par conséquent justifiées.

Il convient de mener à bien une recherche sur l'élaboration d'une analyse coût-bénéfice/coût-efficacité afin d'atténuer l'exposition aux champs magnétiques EBF. Le recours à des analyses coût/bénéfice et coût/efficacité, afin d'évaluer si une orientation politique est bénéfique pour la société, a fait l'objet de recherches dans de nombreux secteurs de l'action des pouvoirs publics. L'élaboration d'un cadre qui recensera les paramètres nécessaires pour pouvoir effectuer cette analyse s'agissant des champs magnétiques EBF est nécessaire. Vu les incertitudes de l'évaluation, il faudra incorporer des paramètres quantifiables et non quantifiables.

## Tableau 1. Recommandations de recherche

| Sources, mesures et expositions | Priorité |
|---|---|
| Caractérisation approfondie des habitations soumises à une forte exposition au champ magnétique EBF dans différents pays | Moyenne |
| Recensement des lacunes dans les connaissances concernant l'exposition professionnelle aux EBF, par exemple s'agissant de l'IRM | Elevée |
| Evaluation de la capacité des installations électriques domestiques, en dehors des Etats-Unis d'Amérique, à induire des courants de contact chez l'enfant | Moyenne |
| **Dosimétrie** | |
| Dosimétrie numérique complémentaire reliant les champs électriques et magnétiques externes aux champs électriques internes, en particulier s'agissant de l'exposition à des champs électriques et magnétiques combinés dans diverses orientations | Moyenne |
| Calcul des champs et courants électriques induits chez la femme enceinte et chez le fœtus | Moyenne |
| Affinement des modèles micro-dosimétriques prenant en compte l'architecture cellulaire des réseaux nerveux et autres systèmes tissulaires complexes | Moyenne |
| **Mécanismes biophysiques** | |
| Etude approfondie des mécanismes des paires de radicaux dans les cellules immunitaires qui génèrent des espèces radicalaires de l'oxygène dans le cadre de leur fonction phénotypique | Moyenne |
| Etude théorique et expérimentale approfondie du rôle possible de la magnétite dans la sensibilité au champ magnétique EBF | Faible |

| | |
|---|---|
| Détermination des seuils de réponse aux champs électriques internes induits par les EBF sur les systèmes multicellulaires, comme les réseaux nerveux, à l'aide de méthodes théoriques et in vitro | Elevée |

**Neurocomportement**

| | |
|---|---|
| Etudes cognitives, sur le sommeil et l'EEG de volontaires, notamment des enfants et des sujets exposés professionnellement, dans un large éventail de fréquences EBF à des densités de flux élevées | Moyenne |
| Etudes de la fonction cognitive chez l'animal après exposition pré- et postnatale | Moyenne |
| Etude approfondie des réponses opioïdes et cholinergiques chez l'animal | Faible |

**Troubles neurodégénératifs**

| | |
|---|---|
| Etudes complémentaires sur le risque de sclérose latérale amyotrophique dans les professions liées à l'électricité et en rapport avec une exposition à un champ magnétique EBF et de maladie d'Alzheimer en rapport avec l'exposition à un champ magnétique EBF | Elevée |

**Immunologie et hématologie**

| | |
|---|---|
| Etudes sur les conséquences de l'exposition à un champ magnétique EBF sur le développement des systèmes immunitaires et hématopoïétiques chez le jeune animal | Faible |

**Reproduction et développement**

| | |
|---|---|
| Etude complémentaire sur le lien éventuel qui existerait entre fausses couches et exposition à un champ magnétique EBF | Faible |

**Cancer**

| | |
|---|---|
| Actualisation des analyses groupées existantes sur la leucémie infantile à l'aide des nouvelles données | Elevée |
| Analyses groupées des études existantes sur les tumeurs cérébrales chez l'enfant | Elevée |
| Mise à jour des méta-analyses existantes relatives à la leucémie et aux tumeurs cérébrales chez l'adulte et aux cohortes de sujets exposés professionnellement | Moyenne |
| Mise au point de modèles murins transgéniques de leucémie infantile utilisables dans les études sur les EBF | Elevée |
| Evaluation des effets co-cancérogènes au moyen d'études in vitro chez l'animal | Elevée |
| Tentative de reproduction des études de génotoxicité in vitro | Moyenne |

**Mesures de protection**

| | |
|---|---|
| Recherche sur l'élaboration de politiques de protection de la santé et sur leur mise en oeuvre dans les secteurs où il n'y a pas de certitude scientifique | Moyenne |

| | |
|---|---|
| Recherche complémentaire sur la perception du risque et la communication sur les risques axée sur les champs électromagnétiques | Moyenne |
| Elaboration d'une analyse coût-bénéfice/coût-efficacité pour l'atténuation des champs EBF | Moyenne |

# 17 РЕЗЮМЕ И РЕКОМЕНДАЦИИ Дlц ДАЛЬНЕЙШИХ ИССЛЕДОВАНИЙ

В настоящей монографии, посвященной медицинским критериям окружающей среды (МКОС), рассматриваются возможное влияние на здоровье воздействия электрического и магнитного полей сверхнизкой частоты (СНЧ). В монографии рассматриваются физические характеристики полей СНЧ, а также источники излучения и измерения. Однако главная цель состоит в обзоре научной литературы, касающейся биологических эффектов воздействия полей СНЧ для того, чтобы оценить риск для здоровья, возникающий в связи с воздействием этого поля, и использовать эту оценку риска для здоровья для составления рекомендаций, предназначенных для национальных органов, занимающихся программами защиты здоровья.

Рассматриваемые частоты находятся в диапазоне от 0 Гц до 100 кГц. Значительное большинство исследований проводилось в отношении магнитных полей промышленной частоты (50 или 60 Гц) и лишь немногие исследования касались электрических полей промышленной частоты. Кроме того, было проведено несколько исследований, касающихся полей очень низких частот (ОНЧ, 3–30 кГц), магнитных полей переменного градиента, применяющихся в магнитно-резонансной томографии, и более слабых полей ОНЧ, создаваемых видеодисплейными терминалами и телевизорами.

В данной главе обобщаются основные выводы и рекомендации по каждому разделу, а также общие выводы в отношении процесса оценки риска для здоровья. В монографии для выражения убедительности данных по отношению к определенному медицинскому результату используются следующие термины. Данные именуются «ограниченными», когда они являются результатом лишь одного исследования или когда имеются нерешенные вопросы, касающиеся постановки, проведения или интерпретации ряда исследований. Термин «неадекватные» данные используется в тех случаях, когда исследования нельзя истолковать таким образом, чтобы показать наличие либо отсутствие какого-либо эффекта вследствие существенных качественных или количественных ограничений или в тех случаях, когда данные отсутствуют.

Были также выявлены основные пробелы в информации и исследования, которые необходимо провести для ликвидации этих пробелов, они были обобщены в разделе, озаглавленном «Рекомендации в отношении научных исследований».

## 17.1 Резюме

### 17.1.1 *Источники, измерения и воздействия на организм человека*

Электрические и магнитные поля существуют повсюду, где генерируется, транспортируется или распределяется электроэнергия по линиям или кабелям электропередачи или используется в электрических приборах. Поскольку использование электричества является неотъемлемой частью нашего современного образа жизни, эти поля повсеместно существуют в нашем окружении.

Напряженность электрического поля измеряется в вольтах на метр (В/м) или в киловольтах на метр (кВ/м), а в отношении магнитных полей индукция изменяется в теслах (Тл) или чаще в миллитеслах (мТл) или в микротеслах (мкТл).

Воздействие магнитных полей промышленной частоты в местах проживания людей в различных странах мира отличается незначительно. Среднее геометрическое значение интенсивности магнитного поля в домашних условиях колеблется от 0,025 и 0,07 мкТл в Европе и 0,055 и 0,11 мкТл в США. Среднее значение напряженности электрического поля в домашних условиях находится в пределах нескольких десятков вольт на метр. В непосредственной близости от некоторых приборов мгновенные значения магнитной индукции могут составлять несколько сотен микротесла. Вблизи линий электропередачи магнитные поля достигают приблизительно 20 мкТл, а напряженность электрических полей может составлять несколько тысяч вольт на метр.

Лишь незначительное количество детей подвержены воздействию магнитных полей частотой 50 или 60 Гц в домашних условиях ,с уровнями, усредненными по времени воздействия, превышающими уровни, которые обусловливают повышенную заболеваемость детей лейкемией (см. Раздел 17.1.10). Приблизительно 1%-4% подвергаются воздействию магнитной индукции, превышающей 0,3 мкТл и лишь 1%–2% подвергаются усредненному воздействию, превышающему 0,4 мкТл.

Производственное воздействие, хотя и обусловленное, главным образом, полями промышленной частоты, может также включать в себя воздействие других частот. Средняя экспозиция к магнитному полю на рабочем месте оказалась выше у работников «электрических профессий», нежели у лиц с другими занятиями, такими как работа в офисе, и составляла от 0,4–0,6 мкТл для электриков и электроинженеров до приблизительно 1,0 мкТл для рабочих, обслуживающих линии электропередачи, при наиболее высоких уровнях воздействия для таких профессий, как сварщики, водители электровозов и операторы швейных машин (свыше 3 мкТл). Максимальная интенсивность магнитного поля на рабочем месте может достигать приблизительно 10 мТл, и это неизменно связано с высокими значениями пропускаемого в проводах электротока. В секторе электроснабжения работающие могут подвергаться воздействию электрических полей, значение которых составляет до 30 кВ/м.

## 17.1.2 Электрические и магнитные поля в организме

При воздействии внешних электрических и магнитных полей сверхнизких частот в организме наводятся электрические поля и токи. При помощи измерений выявлена взаимосвязь между внешними полями и наведенным электрическим полем и плотностью тока в организме или другими параметрами, обусловленными воздействием этих полей. Локально индуцированное электрическое поле и плотность тока представляют особый интерес, поскольку они могут стимулировать возбудимые ткани, такие как нервные и мышечные волокна.

Организм человека и животных в значительной степени видоизменяет пространственное распределение электрического поля СНЧ. На низких частотах тело является хорошим проводником, и искаженные линии поля вне организма практически перпендикулярны поверхности тела. На поверхности подвергающегося воздействию организма возникают колеблющиеся заряды, которые индуцируют токи внутри организма. Основные результаты дозиметрии, касающиеся воздействия электрических полей СНЧ на организм человека, выглядят следующим образом:

- Электрическое поле, имеющееся внутри организма, обычно обладает напряженностью на пять или шесть порядков меньшей, чем внешнее электрическое поле.

- При действии на организм поля преимущественно вертикальной направленности, преобладающая направленность наведенных полей также вертикальна.

- При данном внешнем электрическом поле наиболее сильные поля наводятся в теле человека, ноги которого плотно контактируют с землей (электрически заземлены ), и наиболее слабые поля наводятся в теле, изолированном от земли (в "свободном пространстве").

- Общий ток, протекающий в теле, находящемся в тесном контакте с землей, определяется преимущественно габаритами и формой тела (включая позу), а не проводимостью тканей.

- Распределение наведенных токов по различным органам и тканям определяется проводимостью этих тканей.

- Распределение наведенного электрического поля также обусловлено проводимостью, однако в меньшей степени, нежели наведенный ток.

- Имеет место также явление, состоящее в том, что в теле возникает ток при наличии контакта с проводящим предметом, находящимся в электрическом поле.

Что касается магнитных полей, то для них проницаемость тканей та же, что и проницаемость воздуха, поэтому магнитное поле в тканях такое же, как и внешнее поле. Организмы человека и животных не вносят существенного возмущения в поле. Основным результатом воздействия магнитных полей является индукция электрических полей, открытая Фарадеем и обусловленная плотностью тока в проводящих тканях. Основные результаты измерения воздействия магнитных полей СНЧ на организм человека состоят в следующем:

- Наведенное электрическое поле и ток зависят от ориентации внешнего поля. Наведенные поля в организме в целом достигают наибольшего значения в тех случаях, когда линии поля идут в направлении от фронтальной к задней части тела, однако в отношении отдельных органов наивысшие значения достигаются в тех случаях, когда линии поля имеют боковую направленность (от края до края).

- Наиболее слабые электрические поля индуцируются магнитным полем, ориентированным вдоль вертикальной оси тела.

- При определенной напряженности и ориентации магнитного поля более сильные электрические поля наводятся в более массивном теле.

- Распределение наведенного электрического поля обусловлено проводимостью различных органов и тканей. Они оказывают ограниченное влияние на распределение плотности наведенного тока.

### 17.1.3 Биофизические механизмы

Различные предлагаемые механизмы прямого и косвенного взаимодействия электрических и магнитных полей СНЧ изучаются на предмет обоснованности, в частности, в какой степени "сигнал", индуцированный в биологическом процессе в результате воздействия какого-либо поля, может быть выделен из флуктуационного шума, и противоречит ли этот механизм научным принципам и нынешним научным знаниям. Действие многих механизмов становится очевидным лишь при значениях поля, превышающих определенный уровень. Тем не менее, отсутствие выявленных очевидных механизмов не исключает возможности воздействия на здоровье даже при весьма низких уровнях поля при условии того, что это не противоречит основным научным принципам.

Из многочисленных предлагаемых механизмов прямого взаимодействия полей с организмом человека выделяются три механизма в качестве вероятно действующих при более низких интенсивностях поля, нежели другие: индуцированные электрические поля в нейронных сетях радикальные пары и магнетиты.

Электрические поля, наведенные в тканях электрическими или магнитными полями СНЧ, непосредственно стимулируют одиночные миелиновые нервные волокна биофизически понятным образом в тех случаях, когда напряженность внутреннего поля превышает несколько вольт на метр. В отличие от отдельных клеток значительно более слабые поля могут оказывать влияние на синаптическую передачу в нейронных сетях . Подобная обработка сигналов нервными системами обычно используется многоклеточными организмами для выявления слабых сигналов окружающей среды. Было высказано предположение, что нижним пределом интенсивности сигнала, различаемого нейронной сетью, является 1 мВ/м, однако, учитывая современные данные, более вероятными представляются пороговые значения в диапазоне 10–100 мВ/м.

Механизм действия радикальных пар является общепринятым пониманием того, каким образом магнитные поля могут оказывать влияние на специфические типы химических реакций, обычно путем увеличения концентрации реактивных свободных радикалов в слабых полях и снижения концентраций в сильных полях. Эти увеличения проявлялись в магнитных полях с индукцией менее 1 мТл. Имеются определенные данные, увязывающие этот механизм со способностью перелетных птиц определять направление перелета. Также, исходя из теоретических предпосылок, и в силу того, что изменения, вызываемые СНЧ и постоянными магнитными полями сходны, предполагается, что поля промышленной частоты с интенсивностью значительно меньшей, чем геомагнитное поле с индукцией около 50 мкТл, вряд ли могут иметь существенное биологическое значение.

Магнетитовые кристаллы, мелкие ферромагнитные кристаллы оксидов железа различной формы, присутствуют в тканях животных и человека, хотя и в незначительных количествах. Подобно свободным радикалам их присутствие связывают со способностью мигрирующих животных к ориентированию и навигации, хотя присутствие чрезвычайно малых количеств магнетита в мозге человека не наделяет его способностью выявлять наличие слабого геомагнитного поля. Расчеты, основанные на крайних предположениях, позволяют сделать вывод о том, что нижний предел эффектов воздействия полей СНЧ на магнетитовые кристаллы составляет 5 мкТл.

Другие виды прямого биофизического воздействия полей, такие как нарушение химических связей, воздействие на заряженные частицы и различные механизмы узкополосного "резонанса" не рассматриваются, что продиктовано желанием дать достоверное объяснение воздействию полей, которое имеет место в повседневной жизни и

Что касается непрямых эффектов, поверхностные электрические заряды, индуцируемые электрическими полями могут ощущаться, они могут приводить к болезненным микроударам при соприкасании с проводящим предметом. Контактные токи могут возникать, когда, например, дети касаются водопроводного крана в ванной. При этом возникают незначительные электрические поля в костном мозге, значение которых, возможно, превышает фоновый уровень. Однако, представляет ли это риск для здоровья, неизвестно.

Высоковольтные линии электропередач продуцируют большое количество электрически заряженных ионов при коронном разряде. Предполагается, что они способствуют отложению переносимых воздухом загрязняющих веществ на коже и в дыхательных путях, что, возможно, отрицательно сказывается на здоровье. Однако представляется маловероятным, чтобы ионы, появляющиеся в результате коронного разряда, обладали более чем незначительным или вообще каким-либо влиянием на долгосрочный риск для здоровья даже у тех лиц, которые экспонированы в наибольшей степени.

Ни один из трех прямых механизмов не представляет собой достоверную причину увеличения заболеваемости при тех уровнях воздействия, которым обычно подвергаются люди. Фактически они становятся достоверными при более значительных уровнях, а косвенные механизмы изучены в недостаточной степени. Подобное отсутствие установленного достоверного механизма не исключает возможности неблагоприятного влияния на здоровье, но порождает необходимость располагать более прочными фактическими данными из области биологии и эпидемиологии.

### 17.1.4 Нейроповедение

Воздействие электрических полей промышленной частоты вызывает вполне определенные биологические реакции - от ощущения раздражения вплоть до поверхностных электрических разрядов. Эти реакции зависят от напряженности поля, условий окружающей среды и индивидуальной чувствительности. Порог непосредственного восприятия у 10% добровольцев находился в пределах от 2 до 20 кВ/м, в то время как у 5% было выявлено раздражающее действие, при напряженности поля 15–20 кВ/м . Искровые разряды от человека к земле воспринимали как болезненные 7% добровольцев, находившихся в поле с напряженностью в 5 кВ/м. Пороговое значение для разряда от заряженного предмета через заземленного человека зависит от габаритов этого предмета и поэтому требует конкретной оценки.

Поле высокой напряженности, быстро пульсирующие магнитные поля могут стимулировать ткани периферической или центральной нервной системы. Подобные явления могут возникать во время проведения магниторезонансной томографии и используются при транскраниальной магнитной стимуляции. Пороговое значение наведенного электрического поля для прямой стимуляции нерва может находиться на уровне всего лишь нескольких вольт на метр. Это пороговое значение, по-видимому, является постоянным в диапазоне частот от нескольких герц до нескольких килогерц. Лица, страдающие эпилепсией или предрасположенные к ней, по-видимому, являются

475

более чувствительными к индуцированным СНЧ электрическим полям в центральной нервной системе (ЦНС). Кроме того, чувствительность к электростимуляции ЦНС, по-видимому, обусловлена наличием в семье людей, страдающих эпилептическими припадками, а также использованием трициклических антидепрессантов, нейролептиков и других лекарств, понижающих эпилептический порог.

На функцию сетчатки, являющейся частью ЦНС, могут оказать влияние гораздо более слабые СНЧ магнитные поля , нежели те, которые вызывают прямую нервную стимуляцию. Ощущения вспышек света, именуемые «магнитными фосфенами» или «магнитофосфенами», возникают в результате взаимодействия индуцированного электрического поля с электрически возбудимыми клетками сетчатки. Пороговая напряженность наведенного электрического поля в околоклеточной жидкости сетчатки, согласно подсчетам, составляет от 10 до 100 мВ/м на частоте 20 Гц. Однако этим значениям присуща значительная неопределенность.

Менее ясными представляются данные в отношении других нейроповеденческих результатов, полученных в ходе исследований с участием добровольцев, такие как влияние на электрическую активность мозга, когнитивные функции, сон, сверхчувствительность и настроение. В целом подобные исследования проводились при уровнях воздействия ниже тех, которые необходимы для того, чтобы индуцировать вышеописанные явления. В результате были получены данные, в лучшем случае свидетельствующие о слабых и преходящих последствиях. Условия, необходимые для того, чтобы уяснить подобные реакции, в настоящее время определены недостаточно четко. Имеются данные, позволяющие предположить наличие обуславливаемого полем влияния на время реакции и снижение тщательности выполнения некоторых когнитивных задач, что подтверждается результатами исследований в отношении общей электрической активности мозга. Исследования в отношении того, оказывают ли магнитные поля влияние на качество сна, дают неоднородные результаты. Возможно, эта неоднородность частично объясняется различиями в постановке исследований.

Некоторые люди заявляют о своей повышенной чувствительности к электромагнитным полям в целом. Однако данные двойных слепых провокационных исследований позволяют предположить, что заявляемые симптомы не связаны с воздействием электромагнитных полей.

Имеются лишь разнородные и неубедительные данные о том, что воздействие электрических и магнитных полей СНЧ вызывает депрессивные симптомы или суициды. В силу этого данные считаются недостаточными.

Что касается животных, то возможность того, что воздействие полей СНЧ может влиять на нейроповеденческие функции, изучалась в ряде различных направлений при различных условиях воздействия. Неопровержимых результатов получено было немного. Имеются убедительные свидетельства того, что электрические поля промышленной частоты могут ощущаться животными скорее всего путем ощущения поверхностного заряда и могут вызывать кратковременное возбуждение или легкий стресс. Крысы чувствуют наличие поля в диапазоне интенсивностей от 3 до 13 кВ/м. Было обнаружено, что грызуны не переносят напряженность поля, превышающую 50 кВ/м. Другие возможные последствия, обусловленные воздействием поля, определены в значительно меньшей степени; лабораторные исследования свидетельствуют лишь о незначительных и кратковременных эффектах. Имеются данные о том, что воздействие магнитных полей может изменить действие опиоида и холинергических нейромедиаторных систем мозга. Это подтверждается результатами исследований, в которых изучалось воздействие полей на обезболивание, а также на пространственное запоминание и выполнение пространственных задач.

### 17.1.5 Нейроэндокринная система

Результаты исследований, проведенных с участием добровольцев, а также эпидемиологических исследований в местах проживания и в условиях производственных воздействий, позволяют предположить, что на нейроэндокринную систему не оказывает неблагоприятного влияния воздействие электрических или магнитных полей промышленной частоты. Это относится в особенности к уровням циркуляции специфических гормонов в нейроэндокринной системе, в том числе мелатонина, выделяемого шишковидной железой, а также ряда гормонов, участвующих в управлении обменом веществ и физиологическими процессами, которые выделяются гипофизом. Незначительные отличия наблюдались в отношении времени выделения мелатонина, что было обусловлено некоторыми особенностями воздействия, однако эти результаты не проявляются последовательно. Весьма трудно устранить возможное вмешательство различных экологических факторов и факторов образа жизни, которые могут также отражаться в уровнях гормонов. В большинстве лабораторных исследований по изучению эффектов воздействия полей СНЧ на уровни мелатонина у добровольцев в ночное время, после того, как были приняты меры, исключающие влияние мешающих факторов, никакого эффекта обнаружено не было.

Было проведено большое количество исследований на животных с целью изучения результатов воздействия электрических и магнитных полей промышленной частоты на уровни мелатонина в шишковидной железе и в сыворотке у крыс. В некоторых исследованиях отмечалось, что воздействие полей приводило к супрессии мелатонина в ночное время. Изменения в уровнях мелатонина, впервые наблюдавшиеся в ранних исследованиях при воздействии электрического поля до 100 кВ/м, повторно получать не

477

удалось. Результаты ряда более недавних исследований, в которых показывалось, что циркулярно поляризованные магнитные поля понижают уровень мелатонина в ночное время, слабо выглядят на фоне неподходящих сравнений с результатами, полученными для данных животных и более ранними результатами. Данные, полученные в результате других экспериментов с грызунами, в которых уровни интенсивности магнитного поля изменялись в диапазоне от нескольких микротесла до 5 мТл, носили двойственный характер в связи с тем, что в некоторых опытах происходило подавление мелатонина, а в других не отмечалось никаких изменений. У животных с сезонным циклом размножения результаты воздействия полей промышленной частоты на уровень мелатонина и обуславливаемый мелатонином репродуктивный статус, главным образом, отрицательные. Никаких убедительных свидетельств в отношении уровней мелатонина не было обнаружено в исследовании на человекообразных обезьянах, хронически подвергаемых воздействию полей промышленной частоты, хотя в более раннем исследовании с использованием двух животных отмечалась супрессия секреции мелатонина в результате нерегулярного и интермиттирующего воздействия полей.

Результаты воздействия СНЧ полей на продукцию и выделение мелатонина в изолированной шишковидной железе различались, хотя исследований in vitro проводилось немного. Данные о том, что воздействие полей СНЧ вмешивается в воздействие мелатонина на раковые клетки молочной железы, вызывают интерес. Однако недостатком этого является тот факт, что в клеточных линиях нередко наблюдается генотипическая и фенотипическая изменчивость в культуре, которая может препятствовать воспроизводству эксперимента в других лабораториях.

Никаких устойчивых результатов обнаружено не было в отношении обуславливающих стресс гормонов гипофизарно-адреналиновой оси у различных видов млекопитающих при одном возможном исключении возникновения кратковременного стрессового состояния, возникающего в связи с воздействием электрического поля СНЧ на достаточно заметном уровне. Аналогичным образом, несмотря на то, что было проведено небольшое количество исследований, наблюдались большей частью отрицательные или противоречивые результаты в отношении уровней гормона роста и гормонов, участвующих в регулировании метаболизма или связанных с контролем репродуктивного и сексуального развития.

В целом, эти данные не указывают на то, что электрические и/ или магнитные поля СНЧ оказывают влияние на нейроэндокринную систему таким образом, чтобы это производило неблагоприятное воздействие на здоровье человека, и поэтому эти данные считаются недостаточными.

### 17.1.6　Нейродегенеративные расстройства

Высказывалось предположение, что воздействие полей СНЧ обусловливает ряд нейродегенеративных заболеваний. В отношении болезни Паркинсона и множественного склероза количество исследований было незначительным, и доказательства взаимосвязи с этими заболеваниями отсутствуют. Что касается болезни Альцгеймера и бокового амиотрофического склероза, было опубликовано больше исследований. В ряде этих сообщений высказывается предположение, что лица, работающие в электроустановках, имеют больший риск бокового амиотрофического склероза. До сих пор не установлено никакого биологического механизма, который мог бы объяснить эту взаимосвязь, хотя это явление могло иметь место вследствие наличия неучтенных факторов, связанных с электрическими профессиями, как, например, удары электротоком. В целом, данные о взаимосвязи между воздействием полей СНЧ и боковым амиотрофическим склерозом считаются недостаточными.

Результаты нескольких исследований взаимосвязи между воздействием полей СНЧ и болезнью Альцгеймера противоречивы. Однако более качественные научные исследования, в которых основное внимание уделяется не смертности, а заболеваемости болезнью Альцгеймера, не указывают на какую-либо взаимосвязь. В целом, данные о взаимосвязи между воздействием полей СНЧ и болезнью Альцгеймера недостаточны.

### 17.1.7　Сердечно-сосудистые расстройства

Экспериментальные исследования как кратковременного, так и длительного воздействия указывают на то, что хотя электрошок является явной опасностью для здоровья, другие опасные последствия сердечно-сосудистого характера, связанные с полями СНЧ вряд ли могут возникнуть при уровнях воздействия, которые обычно имеют место в производственной и окружающей среде. Хотя в литературе сообщалось о различных сердечно-сосудистых изменениях, большинство последствий незначительны, и результаты, как в рамках самих исследований, так и при сравнении с другими исследованиями, противоречивы. За одним исключением: ни в одном из исследований по поводу заболеваемости и смертности, обусловленных сердечно-сосудистыми заболеваниями, не показана взаимосвязь с воздействием электрических или магнитных полей. Вопрос о том, существует ли взаимосвязь между воздействием полей и нарушением автономного контроля сердца, остается предметом догадок. В целом, данные не свидетельствуют о связи между воздействием полей СНЧ и сердечно-сосудистыми заболеваниями.

### 17.1.8　Иммунология и гематология

Данные о воздействии электрических или магнитных полей СНЧ на компоненты иммунной системы обычно противоречивы. На многие клеточные популяции и функциональные маркеры поля не оказывают никакого влияния. Однако в некоторых исследованиях с участием человека и с использованием полей от 10 мкТл до 2 мТл наблюдались изменения в естественных клетках-киллерах, число которых как уменьшалось, так и увеличивалось, а также в клетках белой крови, число которых оставалось без изменений или уменьшалось. В исследованиях на животных у самок мышей отмечалось уменьшение активности естественных клеток-киллеров, однако этого не наблюдалось у самцов мышей или у крыс обоего пола. Подсчет числа клеток белой крови также был противоречивым. В различных исследованиях сообщалось об уменьшении их числа или об отсутствии каких-либо изменений. В опытах на животных использовался еще более широкий диапазон - от 2 мкТл до 30 мТл. Трудность толкования потенциального влияния на здоровье при указанных данных объясняется значительными колебаниями в условиях воздействия полей и окружающих условий, сравнительно небольшим числом тестируемых субъектов и широким разнообразием конечных результатов.

Было проведено несколько исследований в отношении воздействия магнитных полей СНЧ на гематологическую систему. В ходе экспериментов по оценке дифференциации количества клеток красной крови дозы воздействия изменялись в диапазоне от 2 мкТл до 2 мТл. Никаких последовательных результатов острого воздействия магнитных полей СНЧ или сочетанного электрического и магнитного поля СНЧ не было обнаружено при проведении исследований с участием человека или животных.

В силу этого, в целом, данные в отношении последствий воздействия электрических или магнитных полей СНЧ на иммунную и гематологическую систему считаются недостаточными.

### 17.1.9 Воспроизводство и развитие

В целом, эпидемиологические исследования не указывают на какую-либо взаимосвязь нарушений репродуктивной функции человека в связи с воздействием полей СНЧ на мать или отца. Имеются некоторые данные об увеличении риска выкидыша, связанного с воздействием магнитного поля на будущую мать, однако эти данные являются недостаточными.

Воздействие электрических полей СНЧ с уровнями вплоть до 150 кВ/м изучалось на нескольких видах млекопитающих. Сюда относятся изучение крупных популяций и воздействие полей на протяжении нескольких поколений. Результаты исследований устойчиво указывают на отсутствие каких-либо отрицательных последствий для развития.

Воздействие магнитных полей СНЧ с уровнями до 20 мТл на млекопитающих не приводит к значительным нарушениям формирования внешних признаков, внутренних органов или скелета. В некоторых исследованиях указывается на увеличение частоты незначительных скелетных аномалий у крыс и мышей. Скелетные изменения являются сравнительно распространенным результатом тератологических исследований и нередко считаются биологически незначимыми . Однако нельзя исключать трудноуловимые влияния магнитных полей на развитие скелета. Исследований, в которых рассматриваются репродуктивные последствия, было опубликовано очень мало, и из них нельзя делать каких-либо выводов.

В нескольких исследованиях на экспериментальных моделях, не относящихся к классу млекопитающих (куриные эмбрионы, рыбы, морские ежи и насекомые), сообщается о результатах, которые указывают на то, что магнитные поля СНЧ в пределах микротеслы могут вносить нарушения в ранние этапы развития. Однако результаты изучения экспериментальных моделей, не относящихся к млекопитающим, имеют меньшую ценность при общей оценке токсичности в отношении развития, нежели исследования в этой области, касающиеся млекопитающих.

В целом, данные о последствиях для развития и репродуктивной системы являются недостаточными.

### 17.1.10 Онкологические заболевания

Классификация МАИР, относящая магнитные поля СНЧ к "возможно канцерогенным для человека" (IARC, 2002) основана на всех имеющихся данных до 2001 года включительно. Обзор литературы в данной монографии посвящен главным образом исследованиям, появившимся после обзора МАИР.

*Эпидемиология*

Классификация МАИР в значительной мере опирается на взаимосвязи, выявленные в ходе эпидемиологических исследований лейкозов у детей. Классификационная характеристика этих данных в качестве имеющих ограниченный характер не изменяется в связи с добавлением двух дополнительных исследований в области лейкозов у детей, опубликованных после 2002 года. Со времени публикации монографии МАИР данные в отношении других онкологических заболеваний у детей остаются недостаточными.

После публикации монографии МАИР появился ряд сообщений, касающихся риска рака молочной железы у взрослых, обусловленного воздействием магнитного поля СНЧ. Эти исследования шире, чем предыдущие и более беспристрастные, и в целом они дают отрицательный ответ. С наличием этих исследований данные о взаимосвязи между воздействием магнитного поля СНЧ и риском рака молочной железы, значительно ослабили свою позицию и не свидетельствуют о взаимосвязи подобного рода.

По поводу рака головного мозга и лейкозов у взрослых, новые исследования, опубликованные после монографии МАИР, не меняют вывод о том, что общий объем данных о взаимосвязи между магнитными полями СНЧ и риском этих заболеваний остается недостаточным.

Для всех других видов онкологических болезней, данные по-прежнему остаются недостаточными.

*Лабораторные исследования на животных*

В настоящее время подходящая животная модель для наиболее распространенной формы детского лейкоза, острого лимфобластного лейкоза, отсутствует. Три независимых крупномасштабных исследования, где были использованы крысы, не дали никаких данных в отношении взаимосвязи между воздействием магнитных полей СНЧ и заболеваемостью спонтанным раком молочной железы. В большинстве исследований сообщается об отсутствии связи воздействия магнитных полей СНЧ с лейкозом или лимфомой у грызунов. В нескольких крупномасштабных и продолжительных исследованиях с использованием грызунов не было выявлено какого-либо устойчивого увеличения заболеваемости каким-либо онкологическим заболеванием, в т.ч. заболеванием кроветворных органов, молочной железы, головного мозга и кожи.

В значительном числе исследований изучалось воздействие магнитных полей СНЧ на химически индуцированные опухоли молочной железы у крыс. Непоследовательность полученных результатов может объясняться в целом или частично различиями в проведении экспериментов, такими как использование специфических линий. Большинство исследований воздействия магнитного поля СНЧ на модели лейкоза/лимфомы, индуцированные химическим путем или радиацией, дают отрицательный ответ. В исследованиях повреждений печени, предшествующих новообразованиям, опухолей кожи, индуцированных химическим путем, и опухолей головного мозга сообщается главным образом об отрицательных результатах. В одном исследовании сообщается об активизации индуцированных ультрафиолетом опухолей кожи после воздействия магнитных полей СНЧ.

Две группы сообщают об увеличении числа разрывов цепочек ДНК в тканях головного мозга после воздействия in vivo магнитными полями СНЧ. Однако в других группах, использовавших различные модели генотоксичности у грызунов, данных о генотоксичности обнаружено не было. Результаты исследований, в которых изучалось не генотоксическое воздействие применительно к раку, неубедительны.

В целом, свидетельства о том, что воздействие магнитных полей СНЧ само по себе вызывает опухоли, отсутствуют. Данные о том, что воздействие магнитного поля СНЧ в сочетании с канцерогенами может активизировать развитие опухоли, недостаточны.

*Исследования in vitro*

Обычно в исследованиях воздействия поля СНЧ на клетки не выявляется генотоксичности при интенсивности поля менее 50 мТл. Заметным исключением являются данные недавнего исследования, в котором сообщается о повреждении ДНК при магнитной индукции всего лишь 35 мкТл. Однако эти исследования еще оцениваются, и, как мы понимаем, результаты являются неполными. Все больше появляется данных о том, что магнитные поля СНЧ могут взаимодействовать с агентами, наносящими повреждения ДНК.

Явные доказательства того, что активация при помощи магнитных полей СНЧ генов, участвующих в управлении клеточным циклом, отсутствуют. Однако систематические исследования с целью анализа реакции генома в целом еще необходимо провести.

Во многих других исследованиях на клеточном уровне, например в отношении клеточной пролиферации, апоптоза, кальциевой сигнализации и злокачественной трансформации, получены непоследовательные и неубедительные результаты.

*Общий вывод*

Опубликованные после монографии МАИР 2002 г. новые исследования на человеке, животных и in vitro не изменяют общую классификацию магнитных полей СНЧ как возможного канцерогена для человека.

### 17.1.11 Оценка риска для здоровья

В соответствии с Уставом ВОЗ здоровье является состоянием полного физического, душевного и социального благополучия, а не только отсутствием болезней и физических дефектов. Оценка риска представляет собой концептуальную схему структурированного изучения информации, имеющей отношение к медицинским или экологическим последствиям. Оценка риска для здоровья может использоваться в качестве вводного элемента процесса управления факторами риска, который охватывает все действия, которые необходимо произвести, чтобы решить, необходимо ли предпринимать какие-либо конкретные меры в отношении данной опасности, а также принятие этих мер.

При оценке риска для здоровья, достоверные данные в отношении здоровья человека, в тех случаях, когда они имеются, обычно более информативны, чем данные, полученные на животных. Исследования на животных и исследования in vitro могут подкреплять данные исследований о здоровье человека, заполнять пробелы в изучении здоровья человека или использоваться при принятии решений в опасных случаях, когда исследований с участием человека недостаточно или когда они отсутствуют.

Всякие исследования, имеющие как положительные, так и отрицательные результаты, необходимо подвергать оценке и обсуждать, исходя из их собственных достоинств, а затем рассматривать их все в совокупности, придерживаясь метода весомости доказательств. Важно определить, в какой степени какая-либо совокупность доказательств изменяет вероятность того, что определенное воздействие вызывает некий результат. Данные в отношении последствий обычно более убедительны, если результаты различных видов исследований (эпидемиологических и лабораторных) указывают на один и тот же вывод и/или когда многие исследования одного и того же типа приводят к одинаковому результату.

*Острые эффекты*

Острые биологические эффекты были установлены в связи с воздействием электрических и магнитных полей от крайне и сверхнизких до ОНЧ в диапазоне частот до 100 кГц. Это воздействие может иметь отрицательные последствия для здоровья. В силу этого необходимо устанавливать пределы воздействия. Существуют международные рекомендации по данному вопросу. Соблюдение этих рекомендаций обеспечивает надлежащую защиту от острых последствий.

*Хронические эффекты*

Научные данные, позволяющие предположить, что ежедневное хроническое низкоинтенсивное (более 0,3–0,4 мкТл) воздействие магнитного поля промышленной частоты представляет собой риск для здоровья, основаны на эпидемиологических исследованиях, свидетельствующих об устойчивой картине увеличения риска развития лейкоза у детей. Неопределенность оценки риска связана с тем, какое влияние может оказать неправильная классификация отклонений в контрольной и экспонированной выборках на наблюдаемую взаимосвязь между магнитными полями и лейкозами у детей. Кроме того, практически все лабораторные и механистические данные не свидетельствуют о взаимосвязи между слабыми магнитными полями СНЧ и нарушениями биологических функций или состоянием заболевания. Таким образом, в целом данные не являются достаточно убедительными, чтобы их можно было рассматривать в качестве причинных, однако они достаточно весомы, чтобы оставаться предметом озабоченности.

Несмотря на то, что причинная связь между воздействием магнитного поля и детскими лейкозами не установлена, возможное влияние его на здоровье населения должно было бы рассчитываться, допуская причинно-следственную связь, для того, чтобы включать это в политику как потенциально полезный элемент. Вместе с тем подобные расчеты в значительной степени зависят от распределения воздействия и других предположений и в силу этого являются неточными. Если исходить из того, что взаимосвязь является причинной, то количество случаев лейкозов у детей во всем мире, которые могли бы быть обусловлены воздействием магнитного поля, согласно расчету может составить от 100 до 2400 случаев в год. Однако это составляет 0,2 – 4,9% от общего числа случаев лейкозов, которое во всем мире в 2000 г. составляло 49 000. Таким образом, в глобальном плане влияние на здоровье населения, если таковое имеется, будет ограниченным и неопределенным. Был изучен ряд других заболеваний на предмет возможной обусловленности воздействием магнитного поля СНЧ. К ним относятся онкологические заболевания детей и взрослых, депрессия, самоубийства, репродуктивные дисфункции, нарушение развития, иммунологические модификации и неврологические болезни. Научные данные, подтверждающие взаимосвязь между магнитными полями СНЧ и каким-либо из заболеваний, гораздо слабее, чем в отношении лейкозов у детей, а в некоторых случаях (например, в том, что касается сердечно-сосудистых заболеваний или рака молочной железы) данные достаточны для того, чтобы была уверенность в том, что магнитные поля не являются причиной заболевания.

### 17.1.12 Мероприятия по защите

Для защиты против выявленных негативных последствий воздействия электрических и магнитных полей СНЧ необходимо устанавливать предельные уровни их воздействия. Эти нормативы должны быть определены на основе тщательного изучения всех необходимых научных данных.

Определенным образом были выявлены лишь эффекты острых воздействий, и для защиты от них разработаны две международные рекомендации, касающиеся предельно допустимых уровней воздействия (ICNIRP, 1998a; IEEE, 2002).

Наряду с определенно выявленными эффектами острых воздействий существуют неопределенности о наличии эффектов хронических воздействий в силу ограниченности данных о взаимосвязи между воздействием магнитных полей СНЧ и лейкозами у детей. Поэтому необходимо проявлять осторожный подход. Однако во имя предосторожности не рекомендуется занижать до какого-либо произвольного уровня нормативы предельных уровней воздействия, определенные в рекомендациях. Это подрывает научные основы, на которых построены эти нормативы, и, возможно, окажется дорогостоящим и необязательно эффективным способом защиты.

Осуществление других приемлемых мер предосторожности по снижению воздействия поля обоснованно и необходимо. Однако электроэнергия приносит несомненную пользу в здравоохранении, социальной и экономической областях, и меры предосторожности не должны ставить под угрозу эти преимущества. Кроме того, учитывая недостаточность данных о взаимосвязи между воздействием полей СНЧ и детскими лейкозами, а также ограниченное влияние на здоровье населения, если такая взаимосвязь имеется, преимущества мер по снижению воздействия полей на здоровье неясны. Таким образом, расходы на меры предосторожности должны быть весьма незначительными. Стоимость осуществления мер по снижению влияния полей в различных странах будет различна, что затрудняет разработку общей рекомендации в отношении уравновешивания расходов с потенциальной угрозой полей СНЧ.

Ввиду вышеизложенного, рекомендуется нижеследующее.

- Разработчикам политики необходимо устанавливать нормативы воздействия полей СНЧ, как для населения в целом, так и для условий профессиональных воздействий. Наилучшим руководством для определения обоих уровней воздействия и принципов научного пересмотра их являются международные рекомендации.

- Разработчикам политики необходимо организовать программы защиты от электрических и магнитных полей СНЧ, предусматривающие измерения полей от всех источников, с тем чтобы предельно допустимые уровни воздействия не превышались ни для населения в целом, ни для работающих.

- При условии того, что медицинские, социальные и экономические блага, предоставляемые электроэнергией, не поставлены под угрозу, оправдано и необходимо осуществление как можно более дешевых мер предосторожности по снижению воздействия полей.

- Разработчикам политики, плановикам и производителям необходимо предусматривать соблюдение дешевых мер защиты при строительстве новых сооружений и проектировнаии нового оборудования, включая электроприборы.

- Следует предусматривать внесение изменений в инженерную практику, направленных на снижение воздействия полей СНЧ, создаваемых оборудованием или приборами при условии, что при этом сохраняются другие дополнительные преимущества, такие как бóльшая безопасность и достигается это при незначительных или нулевых расходах.

- При переходе от одного типа оборудования к другому наряду с соображениями безопасности, надежности работы и экономичности необходимо учитывать проблему снижения интенсивности полей СНЧ, создаваемых этими приборами.

- Местным органам при строительстве новых установок или при замене старых, не упуская из внимания вопросы безопасности, необходимо регламентировать прокладку кабелей и проводов таким образом, чтобы это способствовало снижению непроизвольно возникающих токов в земле.

Активные меры по выявлению нарушений или существующих проблем в проложенных электрокабелях могут оказаться дорогостоящими и вряд ли будут оправданы.

- Национальным органам необходимо осуществлять эффективную и открытую стратегию коммуникаций, с тем чтобы все участники принимали информированные решения. Эта стратегия должна предусматривать информацию в отношении того, каким образом отдельные лица могут сами снизить воздействие полей.

- Местные органы должны улучшить планирование установок, являющихся источником СНЧ электромагнитных полей, предусматривая более активную консультацию с промышленностью, местным правительством и гражданами в процессе определения местоположения основных источников электромагнитных полей СНЧ.

- Правительство и промышленность должны содействовать проведению научно-исследовательских программ, направленных на понижение уровня неопределенности научных данных в отношении последствий воздействия полей СНЧ на человека.

## 17.2 Рекомендации для научных исследований

Выявление пробелов в знаниях, касающихся возможных последствий воздействия полей СНЧ для здоровья является главной составной частью оценки этого риска для здоровья. Нижеследующие рекомендации (обобщенные в Таблице 1) излагаются в отношении дальнейших научных исследований.

В качестве важнейшей необходимости требуется проведение дальнейших исследований в отношении промежуточных частот , под которыми обычно понимаются частоты от 300 Гц до 100 кГц, учитывая имеющийся пробел в этой области. Очень небольшой объем данных из необходимой базы знаний для оценки риска для здоровья был собран, и в большинстве существующих исследований результаты непоследовательны и нуждаются в дополнительном подтверждении. Общие требования формирования достаточной базы данных в отношении промежуточных частот с точки зрения оценки риска для здоровья состоят в оценке воздействия, эпидемиологических и лабораторных исследованиях с участием человека, а также в исследованиях на животных и на клеточном уровне (in vitro) (ICNIRP, 2003; ICNIRP, 2004; Litvak et al., 2002).

Для всех исследований с участием добровольцев настоятельно необходимо, чтобы исследования с участием человека проводились в полном согласии с этическими принципами, учитывая положения Хельсинской декларации (WMA, 2004).

Что касается лабораторных исследований, необходимо уделять приоритетное внимание опубликованным результатам, (i) в отношении которых имеются хотя бы скудные данные о воспроизведении или подтверждении, (ii) которые потенциально имеют отношение к канцерогенезу (например, генотоксичность), (iii) которые достаточно убедительны для использования механистического анализа и (iv) в которых присутствуют системы млекопитающих или человека.

### 17.2.1 Источники, измерения и воздействие на организм

Дальнейшая классификация жилья в различных странах, где имеет место высокий уровень воздействия полей СНЧ, с целью определения сравнительного воздействия внутренних и внешних источников полей, влияния порядка прокладки проводов и заземления, а также других характеристик жилья может помочь выявить соответствующие количественные характеристики воздействия, необходимые для эпидемиологической оценки. Важной частью этого является лучшее понимание воздействия полей СНЧ на плод в утробе матери и на детей, в особенности воздействие нагревательных электрокабелей в панелях пола жилых помещений и трансформаторов в многоквартирных зданиях.

Есть подозрение, что в некоторых случаях производственного воздействия СНЧ полей нынешние рекомендуемые нормативы экспозиции превышаются. Необходимо иметь больше информации в отношении воздействия полей (включая частоты, отличные от промышленной), связанных с условиями работы, например, работа по обслуживанию воздушных линий электропередачи под напряжением, работа внутри или вблизи створа магнита магнитно-резонансного томографа (и в силу этого воздействие полей СНЧ с переменным градиентом) и работа на транспортных системах. Аналогичным образом необходимо располагать дополнительными знаниями о подверженности воздействию населения, которое может оказаться близким к рекомендуемым нормативам, в том числе со стороны таких источников, как системы безопасности, библиотечные системы размагничивания, индукционное приготовление пищи и водонагревательные приборы.

Воздействие контактных токов предлагалось в качестве возможного объяснения взаимосвязи магнитных полей СНЧ с лейкозом у детей. Необходимы исследования в других странах, помимо США, для оценки возможности того, что порядок заземления электропроводки в жилых домах и прокладки водопроводов может способствовать возникновению контактных токов в жилье. Подобные исследования должны проводиться в приоритетном порядке в странах, в которых эпидемиологические данные в отношении полей СНЧ и лейкозов у детей вызывают озабоченность.

### 17.2.2 Дозиметрия

В прошлом большая часть лабораторных исследований основывалась на наведенных в организме электрических токах в качестве основного измеряемого параметра, и поэтому дозиметрические показатели определялись этим количественным фактором. Лишь недавно стали проводить работу по изучению взаимосвязи между воздействием внешнего поля и индуцированными электрическими полями. Чтобы лучше понимать биологические эффекты, необходимо иметь больше данных о внутренних электрических полях, возникающих при различных внешних воздействиях.

Необходимо произвести расчеты внутренних электрических полей, вызываемых совместным воздействием внешних электрических и магнитных полей в различных сочетаниях. Расчеты векторного сложения колебаний в различной фазе и воздействия электрических и магнитных полей в соответствии с их пространственным изменением необходимы для оценки основных вопросов, касающихся соблюдения нормативов.

До сих пор проводилось очень мало расчетов по перспективной модели беременной женщины и плода с учетом необходимого анатомического моделирования. Важное значение имеет расчет вероятного возрастания индукции электрических полей в плоде с точки зрения возможности возникновения лейкозов у детей. При этом большую роль играет производственное и внепроизводственное воздействие поля на материнский организм .

Имеется необходимость дополнительного усовершенствования микродозиметрических моделей, учитывающих клеточную архитектуру нейронных сетей и других сложных систем органов, которые более чувствительны к воздействию наведенных электрических полей. Этот процесс моделирования также должен принимать во внимание влияние на электрические потенциалы клеточной мембраны и на выделение нейромедиаторов.

### 17.2.3 Биофизические механизмы

Имеются три основных области, где довлеют очевидные ограничения для нынешнего понимания таких механизмов как механизма радикальных пар, магнитных частиц в организме и соотношений сигнал-шум в многоклеточных системах, таких как нейронные сети.

Механизм радикальных пар является одним из более вероятных механизмов низкоинтенсивного взаимодействия, однако еще надо доказать, что он способен вызывать значительные изменения в клеточном метаболизме и функциях. Особенно важно понять нижний предел воздействия, на котором он проявляется, с тем чтобы судить о том, может или не может этот механизм иметь отношение к канцерогенезу. Учитывая недавние исследования, при которых в иммунных клетках, подвергавшихся воздействию полей СНЧ, происходило усиление активных форм кислорода, рекомендуется использовать в качестве клеточных моделей для изучения возможностей механизма радикальных пар клетки иммунной системы, которые генерируют реактивные формы кислорода.

Хотя наличие магнитных частиц (магнетитовые кристаллы) в головном мозге человека согласно нынешним данным, не свидетельствует о какой-либо чувствительности к магнитным полям СНЧ в окружающей среде, в дальнейших теоретических и экспериментальных работах необходимо изучить, может ли при определенных условиях подобная чувствительность существовать. Кроме того, следует продолжить изучение всех влияний, которые может оказывать наличие магнетитов на вышеупомянутый механизм радикальных пар.

Необходимо проводить дальнейшее изучение того, в какой степени функционируют в мозгу многоклеточные механизмы в плане улучшения соотношения сигнал-шум, с тем, чтобы разработать теоретические принципы количественного исчисления этого явления или определения его предельных значений. Методом in vitro необходимо проводить дальнейшее изучение порога и частотной реакции нейронных сетей в гиппокампе и других частях мозга.

### 17.2.4   Нейроповедение

Рекомендуется проводить лабораторные исследования с привлечением добровольцев по вопросу о возможном влиянии полей на сон и на выполнение задач, требующих умственного напряжения, придерживаясь согласованной методологии,. Необходимо выявить зависимость реакции от интенсивности поля при более высоких значениях магнитной индукции, по сравнению с использовавшимися ранее, а также в широком диапазоне частот (т.е. в килогерцовом диапазоне).

Исследования с участием взрослых добровольцев и с использованием животных позволяют предположить, что при кратковременном воздействии интенсивных электрических или магнитных полей могут иметь место острые когнитивные последствия. Для разработки нормативов воздействия чрезвычайно важно представлять себе эти последствия, однако конкретные данные, касающиеся обусловленных полем результатов воздействия на организм детей, отсутствуют. Рекомендуется провести лабораторные исследования когнитивной функции и изменений в электроэнцефалограмме (ЭЭГ) у лиц, подвергшихся воздействию полей СНЧ, в том числе взрослых, регулярно подвергающихся производственным воздействиям, а также у детей.

Поведенческие исследования с использованием детенышей животных могут дать ценные данные для изучения возможных когнитивных последствий у детей. Следует изучить возможные последствия пре- и постнатального воздействия магнитных полей СНЧ на развитие нервной системы и когнитивные функции. Полезным дополнением к этим исследованиям может оказаться изучение последствий воздействия магнитных полей СНЧ и наведенных электрических полей на рост нервных клеток с использованием срезов головного мозга и нейронных культур.

Имеется необходимость дальнейшего изучения потенциальных последствий для здоровья, о которых позволяют предполагать экспериментальные данные об опиоидных и холинергических реакциях у животных. Следует расширить изучение модификации опиоидных и холинергических реакций у животных и определить параметры воздействия и биологическую основу подобных поведенческих реакций.

### 17.2.5 Нейроэндокринная система

Существующая база данных в отношении реакции нейроэндокринной системы не указывает на то, что воздействие полей СНЧ оказывает неблагоприятное влияние на здоровье человека. Поэтому в рекомендациях в отношении дополнительных исследований нет необходимости.

### 17.2.6 Нейродегенеративные расстройства

В ряде исследований наблюдалось увеличение риска бокового амиотрофического склероза у лиц, по роду занятий связанных с электричеством. Считается важным изучить эту взаимосвязь более подробно для того, чтобы выявить, участвуют ли магнитные поля СНЧ в возникновении этого редкого нейродегенеративного заболевания. Для этого требуется проведение крупномасштабных проспективных когортных исследований с информацией о воздействии магнитного поля СНЧ, о наличии ударов электрическим током, а также о воздействии других потенциальных факторов риска.

Остается сомнительным, являются ли магнитные поля СНЧ фактором риска в развитии болезни Альцгеймера. Имеющиеся в настоящее время данные недостаточны, и эту взаимосвязь необходимо изучить более подробно. Особое значение имеет использование данных о заболеваемости, а не о смертности.

### 17.2.7 Сердечно-сосудистые нарушения

Дополнительные исследования взаимосвязи между магнитными полями СНЧ и риском сердечно-сосудистых заболеваний приоритетными не считаются.

### 17.2.8 Иммунология и гематология

В изменениях, наблюдаемых в отношении иммунологических и гематологических параметров у взрослых, подвергшихся воздействию магнитных полей СНЧ, обнаруживается непоследовательность, а также в основном отсутствуют данные исследований в отношении детей. Поэтому рекомендация состоит в том, чтобы проводить исследования о последствиях воздействия полей СНЧ на развитие иммунной и кроветворной систем у животных раннего возраста.

### 17.2.9 Репродуктивные аспекты и развитие

Имеются определенные данные об увеличении риска выкидыша, обусловленного воздействием магнитного поля СНЧ. Принимая во внимание потенциально значимое влияние подобной взаимосвязи на здоровье населения, рекомендуется проведение дополнительных эпидемиологических исследований.

### 17.2.10 Онкологические заболевания

Наиболее приоритетным вопросом в этой области является разрешение противоречий между эпидемиологическими данными (которые указывают на взаимосвязь между воздействием магнитного поля СНЧ и увеличением риска лейкозов у детей) и экспериментальными и механистическими данными (которые на эту взаимосвязь не указывают). По этому вопросу рекомендуется проведение совместной работы эпидемиологов и ученых экспериментаторов. Чтобы новые эпидемиологические исследования оказались информативными, они должны быть сосредоточены на новых аспектах воздействия поля, на потенциальном взаимодействии с другими факторами или на группах лиц, подвергшихся высокоинтенсивному воздействию, или иным образом быть новаторскими в этой области исследований. Кроме того, также рекомендуется обновить существующие сводные данные путем дополнения данными недавних исследований и путем нового понимания результатов анализа.

Исследования в области рака головного мозга у детей дают неоднозначные результаты. Также как и в случае лейкозов у детей, сводный анализ исследований рака мозга у детей должен быть весьма информативным, и в силу этого таковой рекомендуется. Сводный анализ подобного рода может при небольшой стоимости дать более глубокое и более совершенное понимание существующих данных, включая возможность селекции ошибок при отборе, и, в том случае, если исследования достаточно однородны, может содействовать получению наиболее точной оценки риска.

Что касается рака молочной железы у взрослых, в самых последних исследованиях убедительно показано, что нет никакой взаимосвязи с воздействием магнитных полей СНЧ. Поэтому дополнительным исследованиям этой взаимосвязи следует придавать второстепенное значение.

В отношении лейкозов у взрослых и рака головного мозга рекомендация состоит в том, чтобы обновить информацию по существующим крупным когортам лиц, подвергающимся производственным воздействиям  Результаты исследований в области медицины труда, совокупных данных и мета-анализов по лейкозам и раку головного мозга неоднозначны и неубедительны.  Однако недавно были опубликованы новые данные, и их следует использовать для обновления вышеуказанных результатов.

Первоочередные действия состоят в том, чтобы изучить эпидемиологические данные путем реализации моделей in vitro и с использованием животных по исследованию реакций на низкоинтенсивные магнитные поля СНЧ, которые могли бы применяться в условиях различных лабораторий.

Следует разработать трансгенные модели грызунов для изучения лейкозов у детей, с тем чтобы имелись необходимые экспериментальные животные модели для изучения последствий воздействия магнитного поля СНЧ.  В противном случае, согласно имеющимся сегодня результатам исследований на животных, изолированно одни магнитные поля СНЧ не оказывают никакого канцерогенного действия.  Поэтому приоритетный характер следует придавать исследованиям in vitro и на животных, в которых магнитные поля СНЧ были бы тщательно изучены в качестве сопутствующих канцерогенным факторам.

Что касается других исследований in vitro, то эксперименты, в которых сообщается о генотоксичных эффектах интермиттирующего воздействия  магнитного поля СНЧ, должны быть повторены в других условиях.

### 17.2.11  Мероприятия по защите

Проведение исследований в области разработки политики охраны здоровья и осуществление этой политики в тех областях, где имеется научная неопределенность, рекомендуется, в особенности в отношении мер предосторожности, толкование мер предосторожности и оценки воздействия мер предосторожности с точки зрения магнитных полей СНЧ и других агентов, классифицируемых в качестве «возможных канцерогенов для человека». В тех случаях, когда имеется неуверенность в отношении потенциального  риска для здоровья, создаваемого каким-либо агентом, для общества, должны быть обеспечены  меры предосторожности, с тем чтобы создать необходимую защиту для населения и работающих.  По данному вопросу, касающемуся воздействия магнитных полей СНЧ, было проведено лишь ограниченное число исследований, и в силу важности этого вопроса необходимо заниматься более активными исследованиями.  Это может помочь странам сделать меры предосторожности частью своей политики в области охраны здоровья.

Рекомендуется проведение дополнительных исследований в отношении восприятия риска и коммуникации, которые конкретно затрагивают вопрос об электромагнитных полях.  Психологические и социологические факторы, которые влияют на восприятие риска в целом, были всесторонне изучены. Однако число исследований, направленных на анализ сравнительного значения этих факторов в случае электромагнитных полей или по выявлению других факторов, которые обусловлены электромагнитными полями, является ограниченным. Недавние исследования позволяют предположить, что меры предосторожности, некоторые несут в себе сообщения о риске, могут изменить восприятие риска, усиливая или сглаживая озабоченность этим вопросом. Поэтому необходимы более глубокие исследования в этой области.

Следует проводить исследования по разработке методов анализа издержки-преимущества/издержки-эффективность с точки зрения уменьшения воздействия магнитных полей СНЧ. Использование методов анализа издержки–преимущества и издержки–эффективность для оценки того, является ли данная политическая опция преимуществом для общества, было изучено во многих областях общественной политики. Необходима разработка схемы, которая установит параметры, необходимые для того, чтобы проводить такое изучение магнитных полей СНЧ. В силу неопределенности оценки необходимо предусматривать параметры, которые поддаются количественной оценке, и те, которые не поддаются такой оценке.

**Таблица 1. Рекомендации для дальнейших исследований**

| Источники, измерения и воздействия | Приоритетность |
| --- | --- |
| Дальнейшая характеристика жилых помещений с высоким воздействием магнитного поля СНЧ в различных странах | Средняя |
| Выявление пробелов в знаниях относительно воздействия полей СНЧ на рабочих местах, как например при магниторезонансной томографии | Высокая |
| Изучение возможности возникновения контактных токов у детей в связи с особенностями электропроводки в жилых помещениях вне США | Средняя |
| **Дозиметрия** | |
| Дополнительные дозиметрические расчеты, увязывающие внешние электрические и магнитные поля с внутренними электрическими полями, в особенности в том, что касается совокупного воздействия электрических и магнитных полей различной ориентации | Средняя |
| Расчет индуцированных электрических полей и токов у беременных женщин и в плоде | Средняя |
| Дальнейшее уточнение микродозиметрических моделей, учитывающих клеточную архитектуру нейронных сетей и другие сложные системы подорганов | Средняя |

## Биофизические механизмы

| | |
|---|---|
| Дальнейшие исследования механизмов радикальных пар в иммунных клетках, которые генерируют активные формы кислорода в процессе своей фенотипической функции | Средняя |
| Дальнейшие теоретические и экспериментальные исследования возможной роли магнетитов в чувствительности к магнитному полю СНЧ | Низкая |
| Определение пороговых реакций на внутренние электрические поля, индуцированные полями СНЧ, в многоклеточных системах, таких как нейронные сети, с использованием теоретических методов и методов in vitro | Высокая |

## Нейроповедение

| | |
|---|---|
| Когнитивные исследования, изучение сна и электроэнцефалограмм у добровольцев, в том числе у детей и лиц, подверженных воздействию полей по роду работы с применением широкого диапазона частот СНЧ при высоких плотностях потока | Средняя |
| Исследование влияния пре- и постнатального воздействия полей на последующее развитие когнитивной функции у животных | Средняя |
| Дальнейшее изучение опиоидных и холинергических реакций у животных | Низкая |

## Нейродегенеративные расстройства

| | |
|---|---|
| Дополнительное изучение риска бокового амиотрофического склероза у «лиц электрических профессий» в связи с экспозицией к СНЧ магнитному полю, а также болезни Альцгеймера в связи с воздействием магнитного поля СНЧ | Высокая |

## Иммунология и гематология

| | |
|---|---|
| Изучение последствий воздействия магнитного поля СНЧ на развитие иммунной и кроветворной систем у животных раннего возраста | Низкая |

## Репродуктивные аспекты и развитие

| | |
|---|---|
| Дополнительные исследования возможной связи между выкидышем и воздействием магнитного поля СНЧ | Низкая |

## Онкологические заболевания

| | |
|---|---|
| Обновление новой информацией существующих сводных результатов в отношении лейкозов у детей | Высокая |
| Совокупный анализ существующих исследований возникновения опухолей мозга у детей | Высокая |
| Обновление существующих мета-анализов, касающихся лейкозов у взрослых и опухолей мозга, а также когорт лиц, подверженных профессиональному воздействию полей по роду своих занятий | Средняя |

| | |
|---|---|
| Создание моделей детского лейкоза на базе трансгенных грызунов для использования в изучении полей СНЧ | Высокая |
| Оценка совместного канцерогенного действия путем исследований in vitro и на животных | Высокая |
| Попытка воспроизводства исследований в области генотоксичности, проводимых in vitro | Средняя |

### Защитные меры

| | |
|---|---|
| Исследования по разработке политики в области охраны здоровья и осуществление мер в тех областях, где имеется научная неопределенность | Средняя |
| Дальнейшие исследования в области восприятия риска и коммуникаций в отношении электромагнитных полей | Средняя |
| Разработка методов анализа издержки-преимущества / издержки-эффективность для смягчения результатов воздействия полей СНЧ | Средняя |

# 18 RESUMEN Y RECOMENDACIONES PARA ESTUDIOS POSTERIORES

En la presente monografía sobre Criterios de Salud Ambiental (EHC) se abordan los posibles efectos en la salud de la exposición a campos eléctricos y magnéticos de frecuencias extremadamente bajas (ELF). En ella se examinan las características físicas de los campos ELF, así como las fuentes de exposición y la medición. Sin embargo, sus principales objetivos son la revisión de la literatura científica sobre los efectos biológicos de la exposición a campos de ELF, a fin de evaluar cualquier riesgo para la salud proveniente de la exposición a dichos campos y utilizar esta evaluación de los riesgos de salud en la formulación de recomendaciones a las autoridades nacionales sobre los programas de protección de la salud.

Las frecuencias bajo consideración están comprendidas en el rango por encima de 0 Hz a 100 kHz. La inmensa mayoría de los estudios se han realizado sobre campos magnéticos en frecuencia de energía (50 ó 60 Hz) y muy pocos utilizando campos eléctricos en frecuencia de energía. Además, se han realizado varios estudios sobre campos de muy baja frecuencia (VLF, 3–30 kHz), campos magnéticos de gradientes invertidos utilizados en la imaginología de resonancia magnética y campos de VLF más débiles que emiten los monitores de visualización y los televisores.

En este capítulo se resumen las principales conclusiones y recomendaciones de cada sección, así como las conclusiones globales del proceso de evaluación de los riesgos de salud. Los términos utilizados en esta monografía para describir el peso de la evidencia para un resultado de salud determinado son los siguientes. Se dice que la evidencia es "limitada" cuando se reduce a un solo estudio o cuando hay cuestiones por resolver en relación con el diseño, la realización o la interpretación de varios estudios. La evidencia es "insuficiente" cuando no se puede interpretar que los estudios demuestran la presencia o la ausencia de un efecto debido a limitaciones cualitativas o cuantitativas importantes, o cuando no se dispone de datos.

También se encontraron brechas fundamentales en los conocimientos, y en la sección titulada "Recomendaciones para la investigación" se han resumido las investigaciones necesarias para llenar esas brechas.

## 18.1 Resumen

### 18.1.1 Fuentes, mediciones y exposiciones

Donde quiera que se genera, transmite o distribuye electricidad en tendidos o cables eléctricos o se utiliza en aparatos eléctricos existen campos eléctricos y magnéticos. Dado que el uso de la electricidad forma parte integrante de nuestro sistema de vida moderno, estos campos están omnipresentes en nuestro ambiente.

La unidad de intensidad de campo eléctrico es el voltio por metro ($V\ m^{-1}$) o el kilovoltio por metro ($kV\ m^{-1}$) y para los campos magnéticos la densidad de flujo se mide en teslas (T), o más habitualmente en mililteslas (mT) o en microteslas ($\mu T$).

La exposición residencial a campos magnéticos en frecuencia de energía no registra grandes variaciones en todo el mundo. La media geométrica del campo magnético en los hogares oscila entre 0,025 y 0,07 µT en Europa y entre 0,055 y 0,11 µT en los Estados Unidos. Los valores medios de los campos eléctricos entre el hogar son del orden de varias decenas de voltios por metro. En las proximidades de determinados aparatos eléctricos, los valores instantáneos del campo magnético pueden llegar a ser de unos pocos cientos de microteslas. Cerca de las líneas de energía, los campos magnéticos llegan a ser de alrededor de 20 µT y los campos eléctricos de varios miles de voltios por metro.

Son pocos los niños que tienen una exposición residencial promedio en el tiempo a campos magnéticos de 50 ó 60 Hz superior a los niveles asociados con un aumento de la incidencia de la leucemia infantil (ver la sección 18.1.10). Entre el 1% y el 4% tienen una exposición media superior a 0,3 µT y sólo del 1% al 2% tienen una exposición media que supera los 0,4 µT.

La exposición ocupacional, aunque predominantemente debido a los campos en frecuencia de energía, también puede incluir otras frecuencias. Se ha encontrado que el promedio de la exposición a campos magnéticos en el lugar de trabajo para las ocupaciones relacionadas con la electricidad es superior al de otros trabajos tales como el trabajo de oficina, con valores que oscilan entre 0.4–0.6 µT para los electricistas y los ingenieros eléctricos y alrededor de 1.0 µT en los trabajadores de líneas de energía, siendo máxima la exposición de los soldadores, los maquinistas de ferrocarril y los operadores de máquinas de coser (por encima de 3 µT). Las exposiciones máximas a campos magnéticos en el lugar de trabajo pueden llegar a ser de alrededor de 10 mT y están asociadas de manera invariable con la presencia de conductores portadores de corrientes altas. En la industria del suministro de energía eléctrica, los trabajadores pueden estar expuestos a campos eléctricos de hasta 30 kV m$^{-1}$.

### 18.1.2 Campos eléctricos y magnéticos dentro del cuerpo

La exposición a campos eléctricos y magnéticos externos de frecuencias extremadamente bajas induce campos eléctricos y corrientes dentro del cuerpo. La dosimetría describe la relación entre los campos externos y el campo eléctrico y la densidad de corriente inducidos en el cuerpo, u otros parámetros asociados con la exposición a estos campos. El campo eléctrico y la densidad de corriente inducidos localmente son de especial interés debido a que están relacionados con la estimulación de los tejidos excitables, tales como los nervios y los músculos.

Los cuerpos de las personas y animales perturban significativamente la distribución espacial de un campo eléctrico de ELF. En bajas frecuencias, el cuerpo es un buen conductor y las líneas del campo perturbado externas al cuerpo son casi perpendiculares a la superficie de éste. En la superficie del cuerpo expuesto se inducen cargas oscilantes, que a su vez inducen corrientes dentro del cuerpo. Las características fundamentales de la dosimetría para la exposición de las personas a campos eléctricos ELF son las siguientes:

- El campo eléctrico dentro del cuerpo suele ser de cinco a seis órdenes de magnitud inferior al campo eléctrico externo.

- Cuando la exposición es fundamentalmente al campo vertical, la dirección predominante de los campos inducidos también es vertical.

- Para un campo eléctrico externo determinado, los campos inducidos más fuertes corresponden al cuerpo humano en perfecto contacto con el suelo a través de los pies (eléctricamente aterrado) y los campos inducidos más débiles corresponden al cuerpo aislado del suelo (en "espacio libre").

- El flujo total de corriente en un cuerpo en perfecto contacto con el suelo esta determinado por el tamaño y la forma del cuerpo (incluida la postura) antes que la conductividad de los tejidos.

- La distribución de las corrientes inducidas a través de los diversos órganos y tejidos está determinada por la conductividad de dichos tejidos.

- La distribución de un campo eléctrico inducido también es afectada por la conductividad, pero menos que la corriente inducida.

- También hay un fenómeno independiente en el que la corriente se produce en el cuerpo por medio del contacto con un objeto conductor situado en un campo eléctrico.

Para los campos magnéticos, la permeabilidad de los tejidos es igual a la del aire, de manera que el campo en un tejido es igual al campo externo. Los cuerpos de las personas y de los animales no perturba significativamente el campo. La principal interacción de los campos magnéticos corresponde a la inducción de Faraday de campos eléctricos y las densidades de corriente asociadas en los tejidos conductores. Las características fundamentales de la dosimetría para la exposición de los seres humanos a campos magnéticos de ELF son las siguientes:

- El campo eléctrico y la corriente inducidos dependen de la orientación del campo externo. Los campos inducidos en el cuerpo considerado en conjunto son máximos cuando el campo está alineado de la parte anterior a la posterior del organismo, pero en algunos órganos concretos los valores máximos corresponden al campo alineado de un costado al otro.

- Los campos eléctricos más débiles son inducidos por un campo magnético orientado a lo largo del eje vertical del cuerpo.

- Para una intensidad y una orientación determinadas del campo magnético, se inducen campos eléctricos más altos en los cuerpos de mayor tamaño.

- La distribución del campo eléctrico inducido es afectada por la conductividad de los diversos órganos y tejidos. Éstos tienen un efecto limitado en la distribución de la densidad de corriente inducida.

### 18.1.3 Mecanismos biofísicos

Se examina la posibilidad de diversos mecanismos de interacción directa e indirecta propuestos para los campos eléctricos y magnéticos de ELF, en particular si una "señal" generada en un proceso biológico por la exposición a un campo se puede discriminar del ruido aleatorio inherente, y si el mecanismo desafía los principios científicos y los conocimientos científicos actuales. Muchos mecanismos se hacen posibles solamente en campos por encima de una intensidad determinada. No obstante, la ausencia de mecanismos posibles identificados no excluye la posibilidad de efectos en la salud incluso con niveles de campo muy bajos, siempre que se sigan los principios científicos básicos.

Entre los numerosos mecanismos propuestos para la interacción directa de los campos dentro del cuerpo humano, hay tres que destacan más que los otros por su potencial actuación a niveles más bajos del campo: los campos eléctricos inducidos en redes neurales, los pares de radicales y la magnetita.

Los campos eléctricos inducidos en los tejidos por la exposición a campos eléctricos o magnéticos de ELF estimulan directamente las fibras nerviosas mielinizadas aisladas de una forma posible desde el punto de vista biofísico cuando la intensidad del campo interno es superior a algunos voltios por metro. La transmisión sináptica en las redes neurales, en contraposición a las células aisladas, se puede ver afectada por campos mucho más débiles. Los organismos multicelulares suelen utilizar tal procesamiento de la señal por los sistemas nerviosos para detectar señales ambientales débiles. Para la discriminación en la red neural, se ha propuesto un límite inferior de 1 mV m$^{-1}$, pero de acuerdo con la evidencia actual parecen más probables valores umbral de alrededor de 10–100 mV m$^{-1}$.

El mecanismo par radical es una manera aceptada en que los campos magnéticos pueden influir en tipos específicos de reacciones químicas, por lo general aumentando las concentraciones de radicales libres reactivos en los campos bajos y reduciéndolas en los campos altos. Este aumento se ha visto en campos magnéticos de menos de 1 mT. Existe algunas evidencias que vinculan este mecanismo a la navegación de las aves durante la migración. Sobre una base teórica y debido a que los cambios producidos por los campos magnéticos de ELF y estáticos son similares, se sugiere que es poco probable que los campos en frecuencias de energía muy inferiores al campo geomagnético de unos 50 µT tenga mucha importancia biológica.

En los tejidos de los animales y seres humanos se encuentran cristales de magnetita, pequeños cristales ferromagnéticos de óxido de hierro de diversas formas, aunque en cantidades insignificantes. Al igual que los radicales libres, se han relacionado con la orientación y la navegación en los animales migratorios, aunque la presencia de cantidades insignificantes de magnetita en el cerebro humano no confiere la capacidad de detectar el débil campo geomagnético. Los cálculos basados en hipótesis extremas parecen indicar para los efectos de los campos de ELF en los cristales de magnetita un límite inferior de 5 µT.

Otras interacciones biofísicas directas de los campos, tales como la ruptura de enlaces químicos, las fuerzas sobre las partículas cargadas y los diversos mecanismos de "resonancia" de banda estrecha, no parecen explicar de manera verosímil las interacciones en los niveles de campo encontrados en los entornos público y ocupacional.

Con respecto a los efectos indirectos, la carga eléctrica superficial inducida por campos eléctricos puede se percibida y dar lugar a microchoques dolorosos al tocar un objeto conductor. Se pueden producir corrientes de contacto cuando, por ejemplo, los niños pequeños tocan un grifo en la bañera de algunos hogares. Esto produce en la médula ósea pequeños campos eléctricos, posiblemente por encima de los niveles de ruido de fondo. Sin embargo, se desconoce si representan un riesgo para la salud.

Las líneas de energía eléctrica de alto voltaje producen nubes de iones con carga eléctrica como consecuencia de la descarga de tipo corona. Se ha sugerido que podría aumentar la deposición sobre la piel y en las vías respiratorias dentro del cuerpo de los contaminantes del aire, posiblemente con efectos adversos en la salud. Sin embargo, parece probable que los iones del efecto corona tengan efectos escasos o nulos en los riesgos de salud a largo plazo, incluso en las personas más expuestas.

Ninguno de los tres mecanismos directos considerados anteriormente parece ser una causa posible del aumento de incidencia de enfermedades a los niveles de exposición que suele encontrar la población. De hecho, solamente comienzan a ser posibles a niveles varios órdenes de magnitud superiores, y los mecanismos indirectos todavía no se han investigado suficientemente. Esta ausencia de un mecanismo posible identificado no excluye la posibilidad de efectos adversos en la salud, pero hace necesaria la obtención de evidencias más sólidas a partir de la biología y la epidemiología.

### 18.1.4 Neurocomportamiento

La exposición a campos eléctricos en frecuencia de energía provoca respuestas biológicas bien definidas, que van desde la percepción hasta las molestias, por medio de los efectos de la carga eléctrica superficial. Estas respuestas dependen de la intensidad del campo, las condiciones ambientales y la sensibilidad individual. Los umbrales para la percepción directa por el 10% de un grupo de voluntarios fueron de 2 a 20 kV m$^{-1}$, mientras que el 5% encontraron molestias con 15–20 kV m$^{-1}$. Se observó que la descarga de chispas de la persona al suelo era dolorosa en el 7% de los voluntarios en un campo de 5 kV m$^{-1}$. Los umbrales para la descarga a partir de un objeto cargado a través de una persona aterrada eléctricamente dependen del tamaño del objeto, por lo que se requiere una evaluación específica.

Los campos magnéticos rápidamente pulsantes de intensidad elevada pueden estimular el tejido nervioso periférico o central; tales efectos se pueden presentar durante los procedimientos de imaginología por resonancia magnética (IRM) y se utilizan en la estimulación magnética transcraneal. Las intensidades umbrales de un campo eléctrico inducido para la estimulación directa de los nervios podrían ser de apenas unos voltios por metro. El umbral probablemente es constante dentro de un rango de frecuencias entre unos pocos hertzios y algunos kilohertzios. Es probable que las personas que sufren epilepsia o están predispuestas a ella sean más susceptibles a los campos eléctricos de ELF inducidos en el sistema nervioso central (SNC). Además, la sensibilidad del SNC al estímulo eléctrico está probablemente asociada con un historial familiar de convulsiones y el uso de antidepresivos tricíclicos, agentes neurolépticos y otros fármacos que reducen el umbral de convulsión.

La función de la retina, que forma parte del SNC, puede verse afectada por la exposición a campos magnéticos de ELF mucho más débiles que los causantes de una estimulación directa de los nervios. La interacción del campo eléctrico inducido con las células de la retina excitables eléctricamente da lugar a una sensación de destellos luminosos, denominados fosfenos magnéticos o magnetofosfenos. Las intensidades umbral de los campos eléctricos inducidos en el fluido extracelular de la retina se ha estimado que están comprendidas entre unos 10 y 100 mV m$^{-1}$ a 20 Hz. Sin embargo, existe una incertidumbre considerable la en relación con estos valores.

La evidencia de otros efectos neurocomportamentales en estudios con voluntarios, tales como los efectos en la actividad eléctrica del cerebro, la cognición, el sueño, la hipersensibilidad y el humor, son menos claras. En general, dichos estudios se han realizado con niveles de exposición por debajo de los necesarios para inducir los efectos descritos anteriormente, y en el mejor de los casos solamente se han obtenido evidencias de efectos sutiles y transitorios. Las condiciones necesarias para que se den tales respuestas no están bien definidas por el momento. Hay algunos indicios que parecen indicar la existencia de efectos dependientes del campo sobre el tiempo de reacción y sobre la precisión reducida en la realización de algunas funciones cognitivas, que están respaldados por los resultados de estudios sobre la actividad eléctrica general del cerebro. En los estudios en los que se investigó si los campos magnéticos afectaban a la calidad del sueño se han reportado resultados inconsistentes. Es posible que estas inconsistencias puedan atribuirse en parte a diferencias en el diseño de los estudios.

Algunas personas afirman que son hipersensibles a los CEM en general. Sin embargo, los resultados obtenidos en estudios doble ciego de provocación parecen indicar que los síntomas notificados no guardan relación con la exposición a dichos campos.

Las únicas evidencias que la exposición a campos eléctricos y magnéticos de ELF provoca síntomas depresivos o el suicidio son inconsistentes y no concluyentes. Por lo tanto, la evidencia es considerada inadecuada.

En animales, se ha estudiado desde varias perspectivas la posibilidad de que la exposición a campos de ELF afecte a las funciones neurocomportamentales, utilizando una serie de condiciones de exposición. Son pocos los efectos sólidamente establecidos. Existe evidencia convincente que los animales pueden detectar campos eléctricos en frecuencia de energía, muy probablemente como consecuencia de los efectos de la carga superficial, que pueden provocar agitación transitoria o un estrés ligero. En las ratas, la gama de detección está comprendida entre 3 y 13 kV m$^{-1}$. Se ha comprobado que los roedores muestran rechazo hacia las intensidades de campo superiores a 50 kV m$^{-1}$. Otros posibles cambios dependientes del campo no están bien definidos; los estudios de laboratorio solamente han proporcionado evidencias de efectos sutiles y transitorios. Existen algunas evidencias que la exposición a campos magnéticos puede modular las funciones de los sistemas de neurotransmisores opioides y colinérgicos en el cerebro, respaldadas por los resultados de estudios en los que se investigaron los efectos en la analgesia y en la adquisición y el desempeño de funciones de memoria espacial.

### 18.1.5  Sistema neuroendocrino

Los resultados de varios estudios en voluntarios, así como de estudios epidemiológicos residenciales y ocupacionales, sugieren que el sistema neuroendocrino no es afectado adversamente por la exposición a campos eléctricos o magnéticos en frecuencias de energía. Esto se aplica particularmente a los niveles circulantes de hormonas específicas del sistema neuroendocrino, como la melatonina, liberada por la glándula pineal (epífisis), y a varias hormonas liberadas por glándula pituitaria (hipófisis) que intervienen en el control del metabolismo y la fisiología del cuerpo. A veces se observaron ligeras diferencias en el tiempo de la liberación de la melatonina relacionadas con ciertas características de la exposición, pero estos resultados no fueron consistentes. Es muy difícil eliminar la posible confusión debida a diversos factores ambientales y al estilo de vida que también podrían influir en los niveles hormonales. En la mayor parte de los estudios de laboratorio sobre los efectos de la exposición a campos de ELF en los niveles nocturnos de melatonina en voluntarios no se encontró ningún efecto cuando se tuvo cuidado en el control de los posibles factores de confusión.

Del gran número de estudios en animales que investigan los efectos de los campos eléctricos y magnéticos en frecuencias de energía sobre los niveles de la melatonina pineal (en la epífisis) y en el suero, algunos reportaron que la exposición provocaba la supresión nocturna de la melatonina. Los cambios en los niveles de melatonina observados por primera vez en los estudios iniciales de exposición a campos eléctricos de hasta 100 kV m$^{-1}$ no pudieron reproducirse. Los resultados de una serie de estudios más recientes, que mostraban que los campos magnéticos polarizados circularmente suprimían los niveles nocturnos de melatonina, fueron debilitados por las comparaciones inapropiadas entre los animales expuestos y los controles históricos. Los datos de otros experimentos en roedores, que abarcaban niveles de intensidad comprendidos desde unos pocos microteslas a 5 mT, fueron equívocos, con algunos mostrando depresión de la melatonina, mientras que en otros no se observaron cambios. En animales de reproducción estacional, la evidencia de un efecto de la exposición a campos en frecuencia de energía sobre los niveles de la melatonina y en el estatus reproductivo dependiente de ésta son predominantemente negativas. En un estudio con primates no humanos sometidos a una exposición crónica a campos en frecuencia de energía no se detectó ningún efecto convincente en los niveles de melatonina, aunque en un estudio preliminar en el que se utilizaron dos animales se reporto la supresión de la melatonina en respuesta a una exposición irregular e intermitente.

Los efectos de la exposición a campos de ELF sobre la producción o liberación de melatonina en glándulas pineales aisladas fueron variables, aunque se han realizado relativamente pocos estudios in vitro. Las evidencias que la exposición a campos de ELF interfiere con la acción de la melatonina en las células de cáncer de mama in vitro son complicadas. Sin embargo, este sistema presenta el inconveniente que frecuentemente las líneas celulares muestran deriva genotípica y fenotípica en el cultivo que puede obstaculizar la transferibilidad posibilidad de transferencia entre laboratorios.

No se han observado efectos consistentes en las hormonas relacionadas con el estrés del eje hipófisis-glándulas suprarrenales en diversas especies de mamíferos, con la posible excepción de un estrés de corta duración tras el inicio de la exposición a campos eléctricos ELF de niveles suficientemente altos para poder percibirlos. Similarmente, si bien son pocos los estudios que se han realizado, en la mayoría se han observado efectos negativos o inconsistentes en los niveles de hormona del crecimiento y de las hormonas que intervienen en el control de la actividad metabólica o están asociadas con el control de la reproducción y el desarrollo sexual.

Considerados en conjunto, estos datos no indican que los campos eléctricos y/o magnéticos de ELF afecten al el sistema neuroendocrino de manera que se produzcan efectos adversos en la salud humana, por lo que las pruebas se consideran inadecuadas.

### 18.1.6 Trastornos neurodegenerativos

Se ha planteado la hipótesis que la exposición a campos de ELF puede estar asociada con varias enfermedades neurodegenerativas. En relación con la enfermedad de Parkinson y la esclerosis múltiple, el número de estudios ha sido pequeño y no hay evidencias de asociación con estas enfermedades. En el caso de la enfermedad de Alzheimer y la esclerosis lateral amiotrófica (ELA), se han publicado más estudios. Algunos de estos informes parecen indicar que las personas que trabajan en ocupaciones relacionadas con la electricidad podrían tener mayor riesgo de esclerosis lateral amiotrófica (ELA). Hasta ahora no se ha establecido ningún mecanismo biológico que pueda explicar esta asociación, aunque podría haber surgido debido a factores de confusión relacionados con las ocupaciones vinculadas a la electricidad, como los choques eléctricos. En conjunto, se considera que las pruebas de la asociación entre la exposición a campos de ELF y la esclerosis lateral amiotrófica son (inadecuadas) insuficientes.

Los pocos estudios en los que se ha investigado la asociación entre la exposición a campos ELF y la enfermedad de Alzheimer son contradictorios. Sin embargo, los estudios de mayor calidad que se concentraron en la morbilidad de la enfermedad de Alzheimer más que en la mortalidad no indicaron una asociación. En conjunto, las pruebas de una asociación entre la exposición a campos ELF y la enfermedad de Alzheimer son insuficientes.

### 18.1.7 Trastornos cardiovasculares

Los estudios experimentales de exposición tanto de corta como de larga duración indican que, si bien el choque eléctrico representa un peligro evidente para la salud, es improbable que se produzcan otros efectos cardiovasculares peligrosos asociados con los campos de ELF a los niveles de exposición ambiental u ocupacional comúnmente encontrados. Aunque se han reportado diversos cambios cardiovasculares en la literatura, la mayoría de los efectos son pequeños y los resultados no han sido consistentes en los estudios y entre ellos. Con una sola excepción, ninguno de los estudios de la morbilidad y mortalidad de las enfermedades cardiovasculares ha mostrado una asociación con la exposición. La posibilidad de que exista una asociación específica entre la exposición y el control autónomo alterado del corazón sigue siendo una mera especulación. En conjunto, las pruebas no respaldan una asociación entre la exposición a campos de ELF y las enfermedades cardiovasculares.

### 18.1.8 Inmunología y hematología

Las evidencias de los efectos de los campos eléctricos o magnéticos de ELF sobre los componentes del sistema inmunológico en general son inconsistentes. En muchos casos las poblaciones celulares y los marcadores funcionales no fueron afectados por la exposición. Sin embargo, en algunos estudios en seres humanos con campos desde 10 µT a 2 mT se observaron cambios en las células asesinas naturales (citolíticas) , que mostraron tanto un aumento como una disminución de su número, y en la cuenta total de células blancas (leucocitos), sin cambios o con una disminución del número. En estudios en animales, se observó una actividad reducida de las células citolíticas en ratones hembras, pero no en los machos ni en las ratas de ambos sexos. También en la cuenta de células blancas el recuento de leucocitos se obtuvieron resultados inconsistentes, con una disminución o ningún cambio en los distintos estudios. La gama de exposición de los animales fue aún más amplia, de 2 µT a 30 mT. La dificultad para interpretar el impacto potencial de estos datos en la salud radica en las grandes variaciones de las condiciones de exposición y ambientales, el número relativamente pequeño de individuos sometidos a prueba y la amplia variedad de efectos finales.

Son pocos los estudios realizados sobre los efectos de los campos magnéticos de ELF en el sistema hematológico. En los experimentos de evaluación de la cuenta diferencial de células blancas (leucocitos), las exposiciones fueron desde 2 μT a 2 mT. No se han encontrado efectos consistentes de la exposición aguda a campos magnéticos de ELF o a campos eléctricos y magnéticos de ELF combinados ni en los estudios con personas ni con animales.

Por consiguiente, de manera global las evidencias de los efectos de los campos eléctricos o magnéticos de ELF en los sistemas inmunológico y hematológico se consideran insuficientes.

### 18.1.9 Reproducción y desarrollo

En conjunto, los estudios epidemiológicos no han demostrado que haya una asociación entre resultados adversos en la reproducción humana con la exposición materna o paterna a campos de ELF. Hay algunas evidencias de un aumento del riesgo de aborto asociado con la exposición materna a campos magnéticos, pero son insuficientes.

Se han evaluado exposiciones a campos eléctricos de ELF de hasta 150 kV m$^{-1}$ en varias especies de mamíferos, incluidos estudios con grupos de gran tamaño y exposiciones durante varias generaciones. Los resultados, consistentemente, no mostraron ningún efecto adverso en el desarrollo.

La exposición de mamíferos a campos magnéticos de ELF de hasta 20 mT no da lugar a malformaciones externas, viscerales o esqueléticas graves. Algunos estudios muestran un aumento de pequeñas anomalías esqueléticas, tanto en ratas como en ratones. En estudios teratológicos son relativamente frecuentes las variaciones en el esqueleto, las cuales frecuentemente se consideran biológicamente insignificantes. Sin embargo, no se pueden excluir sutiles efectos de los campos magnéticos en el desarrollo del esqueleto. Se han publicado muy pocos estudios en los que se aborden los efectos en la reproducción, y de ellos no se puede extraer ninguna conclusión.

En varios estudios sobre modelos experimentales no mamíferos (embriones de pollo, peces, erizos de mar e insectos) se han reportado resultados mostrando que los campos magnéticos de ELF a niveles de microteslas pueden alterar el desarrollo inicial. Sin embargo, los resultados de los modelos experimentales no mamíferos en la evaluación global de la toxicidad en el desarrollo tienen un valor menor que los obtenidos en los estudios correspondientes con mamíferos.

En conjunto, las pruebas de efectos en el desarrollo y la reproducción son insuficientes.

### 18.1.10 Cáncer

La clasificación de la Agencia Internacional de Investigación del Cáncer (IARC) de los campos magnéticos de ELF como "posiblemente carcinogénicos para los seres humanos" (IARC, 2002) se basa en todos los datos disponibles hasta 2001 inclusive. El examen de la literatura en la presente monografía de los Criterios de Salud Ambiental se concentra principalmente en los estudios publicados después de la revisión de la IARC.

*Epidemiología*

En la clasificación de la IARC influyeron fuertemente las asociaciones observadas en los estudios epidemiológicos sobre la leucemia infantil. La clasificación de esta evidencia como limitada no cambia con la adición de dos estudios sobre leucemia infantil publicados después de 2002. Desde la publicación de la monografía de la IARC, las evidencias de otros casos de cáncer infantil siguen siendo insuficientes.

Con posterioridad a la monografía de la IARC se han publicado varios informes relativos al riesgo de cáncer de mama en mujeres adultas asociado con la exposición a campos magnéticos de ELF. Estos estudios son más amplios que los anteriores y menos susceptibles a sesgos, y en conjunto son negativos. Con estos resultados, la evidencia de una asociación entre la exposición a campos magnéticos de ELF y el riesgo de cáncer de mama en mujeres se debilitan considerablemente y no respaldan una asociación de este tipo.

En el caso del cáncer cerebral y la leucemia en adultos, los nuevos estudios publicados después de la monografía de la IARC no modifican la conclusión de que la evidencia global de una asociación entre los campos magnéticos de ELF y el riesgo de estas enfermedades siguen siendo insuficientes.

Para otras enfermedades y todos los demás tipos de cáncer, las pruebas permanecen insuficientes.

*Estudios en animales de laboratorio*

En la actualidad no hay ningún modelo animal adecuado para la forma más frecuente de leucemia infantil, la leucemia linfoblástica aguda. Tres estudios independientes de gran escala con ratas no proporcionaron ninguna evidencia de algún efecto de los campos magnéticos de ELF sobre la incidencia de tumores de mama espontáneos. La mayoría de los estudios no reportan ningún efecto de los campos magnéticos de ELF sobre la leucemia o los linfomas en modelos roedores. Varios estudios de gran escala de larga duración en roedores no han mostrado ningún aumento consistente de ningún tipo de cáncer, incluyendo tumores hematopoyéticos, de mama, cerebrales y de piel.

Un número sustancial de estudios examinaron los efectos de los campos magnéticos de ELF sobre tumores de mama inducidos por sustancias químicas en ratas. Se obtuvieron resultados inconsistentes, que pueden deberse totalmente o en parte a diferencias en los protocolos experimentales, tales como el uso de subrazas específicas. La mayoría de los estudios sobre los efectos de la exposición a campos magnéticos de ELF en modelos de leucemia/linfomas inducidos por sustancias químicas o por radiación fueron negativos. Los estudios de lesiones hepáticas preneoplásicas, tumores de piel inducidos por sustancias químicas y tumores cerebrales reportaron resultados predominantemente negativos. Un estudio reporto una aceleración de la tumorigenesís cutánea inducida por radiaciones ultravioleta (UV) tras la exposición a campos magnéticos de ELF.

Dos grupos han reportado un aumento de los niveles de ruptura de las cadenas de ADN en el tejido cerebral tras la exposición in vivo a campos magnéticos de ELF. Sin embargo, otros grupos, utilizando una variedad de diferentes modelos de genotoxicidad en roedores, no encontraron ninguna evidencia de efectos genotóxicos. Los resultados de los estudios de investigación sobre los efectos no genotóxicos pertinentes al cáncer no son concluyentes.

En conjunto no hay ninguna prueba que la exposición a campos magnéticos de ELF provoque por sí sola la aparición de tumores. La evidencia que la exposición a campos magnéticos de ELF puede potenciar el desarrollo de tumores en combinación con carcinógenos es inadecuada (insuficiente).

*Estudios in vitro*

En general, los estudios de los efectos de la exposición de células a campos de ELF no han mostrado ninguna inducción de genotoxicidad para campos por debajo de 50 mT. La notable excepción es la evidencia obtenida en estudios recientes en los que se han descrito daños en el ADN con campos de una intensidad de apenas 35 µT; sin embargo, estos estudios todavía están siendo evaluados y la comprensión de estos hallazgos todavía es incompleta. También existe evidencia creciente que los campos magnéticos de ELF pueden interactuar con agentes causantes de daños en el ADN.

No hay ninguna evidencia clara de la activación por campos magnéticos de ELF de genes asociados con el control del ciclo celular. Sin embargo, todavía no se han realizado estudios sistemáticos en los que se analice la respuesta del genoma completo.

Muchos otros estudios celulares, por ejemplo sobre proliferación celular, apoptosis, señalización del calcio y transformación maligna, han dado resultados inconsistentes o no concluyentes.

*Conclusión general*

Los nuevos estudios en seres humanos, en animales e in vitro, publicados desde la monografía de 2002 de la IARC, no modifican la clasificación global de los campos magnéticos de ELF como posibles carcinógenos para los seres humanos.

### 18.1.11 Evaluación de los riesgos de salud

Según la Constitución de la OMS, la salud es un estado de completo bienestar físico, mental y social, y no solamente la ausencia de afecciones o enfermedades. La evaluación de riesgo es un marco conceptual para una revisión estructurada de la información pertinente a la estimación de los resultados para la salud o el ambiente. La evaluación de riesgo de salud se puede utilizar como un aporte a la gestión del riesgo que acompaña a todas las actividades necesarias para adoptar decisiones sobre si una exposición requiere algunas acciones específicas y la aplicación de esas acciones.

En la evaluación de los riesgos para la salud humana, los datos válidos en seres humanos, siempre que se disponga de ellos, generalmente son más informativos que los obtenidos en animales. Los estudios en animales e in vitro pueden respaldar las pruebas procedentes de los estudios en seres humanos, llenar las brechas en la evidencia procedentes de los estudios en seres humanos o utilizarse para adoptar una decisión sobre los riesgos cuando los estudios en seres humanos son insuficientes o no existen.

Todos los estudios, ya sea con efectos positivos o negativos, necesitan ser evaluados juzgados por su propio valor, y luego en conjunto en un sistema basado en el peso de la evidencia. Es importante determinar en qué medida un conjunto de evidencias cambia la probabilidad de que la exposición dé lugar a un resultado. La evidencia de un efecto generalmente es reforzada si los resultados de distintos tipos de estudios (epidemiología y laboratorio) apuntan a la misma conclusión, o cuando estudios múltiples del mismo tipo dan el mismo resultado.

## Efectos agudos

Se han establecido los efectos biológicos agudos para la exposición a campos eléctricos y magnéticos de ELF en el rango de frecuencias de hasta 100 kHz que pueden tener consecuencias adversas para la salud. Por consiguiente, se necesitan límites de exposición. Existen recomendaciones internacionales en las que se ha abordado esta cuestión. La observancia de estas recomendaciones proporciona una protección adecuada frente a los efectos agudos.

## Efectos crónicos

La evidencia científica que sugiere que la exposición cotidiana crónica a campos magnéticos en frecuencia de energía de baja intensidad (por encima de 0,3–0,4 µT) representa un riesgo para la salud se basa en estudios epidemiológicos que demuestran que hay un patrón consistente de aumento del riesgo de leucemia infantil. Entre las incertidumbres que rodean la evaluación del peligro se incluyen el rol que que podrían desempeñar en la relación observada entre los campos magnéticos y la leucemia infantil el sesgo de selección de los controles y la clasificación errónea de la exposición. Además, virtualmente ninguna de las evidencias de laboratorio y mecanísticas respaldan una relación entre los campos magnéticos de ELF de bajo nivel y los cambios en la función biológica o el estado patológico. Por tanto, en el balance la evidencia no es lo suficientemente fuerte para considerar que hay una relación causal, pero sí para que se mantenga la preocupación.

Aunque no se ha establecido una relación causal entre la exposición a campos magnéticos y la leucemia infantil, se ha calculado el posible impacto en la salud pública suponiendo la existencia de causalidad, a fin de proporcionar un aporte potencialmente útil a las políticas. Sin embargo, estos cálculos dependen en gran medida de las distribuciones de la exposición y de otras hipótesis, por lo que son muy imprecisos. Suponiendo que la asociación sea causal, se puede estimar que el número de casos de leucemia infantil en todo el mundo que podrían atribuirse a la exposición es del orden de 100 a 2400 al año. Sin embargo, esto representa 0,2 a 4,9% de la incidencia anual total de casos de leucemia, estimados en 49 000 en todo el mundo en el año 2000. Por tanto, en un contexto mundial las repercusiones en la salud pública, si las hay, serían limitadas y dudosas.

Se ha investigado la posible asociación de otras enfermedades con la exposición a campos magnéticos de ELF. Entre ellas están el cáncer tanto en niños como en adultos, la depresión, el suicidio, la disfunción reproductiva, los trastornos del desarrollo, las modificaciones inmunológicas y las enfermedades neurológicas. La evidencia científica que respalda una vinculación entre los campos magnéticos de ELF y cualquiera de estas enfermedades es mucho más débil que para la leucemia infantil, y en algunos casos (por ejemplo en las enfermedades cardiovasculares o el cáncer de mama) la evidencia es suficiente para tener la confianza que los campos magnéticos no son causa de la enfermedad.

### 18.1.12 Medidas de protección

Es esencial que se apliquen límites de exposición, a fin de proteger contra los efectos adversos establecidos de la exposición a campos eléctricos y magnéticos de ELF. Estos límites de exposición deberían basarse en un examen exhaustivo de toda la evidencia científica relevante.

Solamente se han establecido los efectos agudos, y hay dos recomendaciones internacionales de límites de exposición (ICNIRP, 1998a; IEEE, 2002) destinadas a la protección frente a estos efectos.

Además de estos efectos agudos conocidos, hay incertidumbres acerca de la existencia de efectos crónicos, debido a que las pruebas de una vinculación entre la exposición a campos magnéticos de ELF y la leucemia infantil son limitadas. Por consiguiente, se justifica la utilización de enfoques de precaución. Sin embargo, no se recomienda la reducción de los valores límites de las recomendaciones sobre la exposición a algún nivel arbitrario en aras de la precaución. Dicha práctica socava el fundamento científico en el que se basan los límites y probablemente sea una manera costosa y no necesariamente eficaz de proporcionar protección.

La aplicación de otros procedimientos apropiados de precaución para reducir la exposición es razonable y se justifica. Sin embargo, la energía eléctrica aporta evidentes beneficios a la salud, sociales y económicos, y los enfoques de precaución no deberían comprometer esos beneficios. Además, teniendo en cuenta, por una parte la debilidad de la evidencia de una vinculación entre la exposición a campos magnéticos de ELF y la leucemia infantil y por otra parte el limitado impacto en la salud pública si existe una vinculación, no están claros los beneficios para la salud de una reducción de la exposición. Así pues, los costos de las medidas de precaución deberían ser muy bajos. Los costos de la aplicación de reducciones de la exposición variarán de un país a otro, por lo que resulta muy difícil formular una recomendación general para alcanzar un equilibrio entre los costos y los posibles riesgos derivados de los campos ELF.

En vista de lo expuesto, se recomienda lo siguiente.

- Los encargados de formular las políticas deberían establecer recomendaciones para la exposición a campos de ELF tanto del público en general como de los trabajadores. La mejor fuente de orientación para los niveles de exposición y los principios aplicables a la revisión científica son las recomendaciones internacionales.

- Los encargados de formular las políticas deberían establecer un programa de protección para los CEM ELF que incluya mediciones de los campos de todas las fuentes, a fin de asegurarse de que no se superen los límites de exposición del público en general o de los trabajadores.

- Siempre que no se pongan en peligro los beneficios para la salud, sociales y económicos de la energía eléctrica, es razonable y se justifica la aplicación de procedimientos de precaución de muy bajo costo para reducir la exposición.

- Los encargados de formular las políticas, los planificadores comunitarios y los fabricantes deberían aplicar medidas de muy bajo costo al construir nuevas instalaciones y diseñar nuevos equipos, incluyendo aparatos eléctricos.

- Se debe estudiar la introducción de cambios en las prácticas de ingeniería para reducir la exposición a campos de ELF procedentes de equipos o dispositivos, siempre que se obtengan otros beneficios adicionales, tales como mayor seguridad o un costo escaso o nulo.

- Cuando se planteen cambios en las fuentes existentes de campos ELF, se debería considerar los aspectos de seguridad, la fiabilidad y los aspectos económicos involucrados.

- Las autoridades locales deberían hacer cumplir las normas sobre las instalaciones eléctricas a fin de reducir corrientes a tierra accidentales cuando se construyan nuevos locales o cuando se renueven las instalaciones eléctricas ya existentes, manteniendo al mismo tiempo la seguridad. Las medidas preventivas para identificar infracciones o problemas existentes en las instalaciones eléctricas resultarían costosas y probablemente no estarían justificadas.

- Las autoridades nacionales deberían aplicar una estrategia eficaz y de comunicación abierta a fin de que todas las partes interesadas puedan adoptar decisiones fundamentadas; debe estar incluida la

511

información sobre la manera en que las personas pueden reducir su propia exposición.

- Las autoridades locales deben mejorar la planificación de las instalaciones emisoras de CEM ELF, incluyendo el mejoramiento de las consultas entre la industria, los gobiernos locales y los ciudadanos al establecer las principales fuentes de emisión de CEM ELF.

- Los gobiernos y la industria deberían promover programas de investigación para reducir la incertidumbre de la evidencia científica sobre los efectos de la exposición a campos ELF en la salud.

## 18.2    Recomendaciones para la investigación

La identificación de las brechas en los conocimientos relativos a los posibles efectos en la salud de la exposición a campos de ELF es una parte esencial de la presente evaluación de los riesgos de salud. Como consecuencia, se han formulado las siguientes recomendaciones para investigación adicional (resumidas en la Tabla 1).

Es primordial la necesidad de realizar nuevas investigaciones sobre las frecuencias intermedias (FI), usualmente comprendidas entre 300 Hz y 100 kHz, dada la presente falta de datos en esta área. Es muy escasa la base de conocimientos de la cual se dispone y que se necesita para la evaluación de los riesgos de salud, y en la mayoría de los estudios existentes se han obtenido resultados inconsistentes, que es necesario comprobar ulteriormente. Los requisitos generales para establecer una base de datos de FI que sea suficiente a la hora de evaluar los riesgos de salud incluye la evaluación de la exposición, estudios epidemiológicos, estudios humanos de laboratorio y estudios en animales y celulares (in vitro) (ICNIRP, 2003; ICNIRP, 2004; Litvak et al., 2002).

En los estudios de laboratorio se debe conceder prioridad a las respuestas reportadas (i) para las cuales exista por lo menos alguna evidencia de replicación o confirmación, (ii) que sean potencialmente pertinentes a la carcinogénesis (por ejemplo de genotoxicidad), (iii) que sean suficientemente sólidas para permitir un análisis mecanístico y (iv) que se produzcan en sistemas de mamíferos o seres humanos.

### 18.2.1    Fuentes, mediciones y exposiciones

La caracterización ulterior de los hogares con un exposición elevada a campos de ELF en los distintos países, a fin de identificar la contribución relativa de las fuentes internas y externas, la influencia de las prácticas de instalación del tendido eléctrico/aterramiento eléctrico y otras características del hogar, puede servir de ayuda para identificar un sistema de medición de la exposición pertinente a la evaluación epidemiológica. Un componente importante de esto es el mejor entendimiento de la exposición fetal e infantil a campos de ELF, especialmente los procedentes de la exposición residencial a la calefacción eléctrica debajo del piso en los domicilios y de los transformadores en los edificios de viviendas.

Se sospecha que en algunos casos de exposición ocupacional se superan los límites presentes de las recomendaciones sobre campos de ELF. Se necesita más información sobre la exposición (incluso a frecuencias que no son de energía) relacionada con el trabajo, por ejemplo, mantenimiento de líneas con tensión, el trabajo dentro o cerca del núcleo central de las magnetos de los aparatos de IRM (y en consecuencia con los campos de ELF de gradiente conmutada) y el trabajo en sistemas de transporte. Asimismo, se necesitan más conocimientos acerca de la exposición del público general que pueda acercarse a los límites de las recomendaciones, incluyendo fuentes tales como los sistemas de seguridad, los sistemas de desmagnetización de las bibliotecas, las cocinas de inducción y los calentadores de agua.

Se ha propuesto la exposición a corrientes de contacto como una posible explicación de la asociación de los campos magnéticos de ELF con la leucemia infantil. Es necesario realizar investigaciones en países distintos de los Estados Unidos para evaluar la posibilidad de que las prácticas de aterramiento eléctrico residenciales y la ductería de agua potable en las viviendas den lugar a corrientes de contacto. Dichos estudios tendrían prioridad en los países con resultados epidemiológicos importantes con respecto a los campos de ELF y la leucemia infantil.

### 18.2.2 Dosimetría

La mayor parte de las investigaciones de laboratorio realizadas en el pasado se basaban en corrientes eléctricas inducidas en el cuerpo como métrica básica, de manera que la dosimetría se concentraba en esta cantidad. Sólo en fechas recientes se ha comenzado a explorar la relación entre la exposición externa y los campos eléctricos inducidos. Para comprender mejor los efectos biológicos, se necesitan más datos sobre los campos eléctricos internos en distintas condiciones de exposición.

Se debe realizar un cálculo de los campos eléctricos internos, debido a la influencia combinada de los campos eléctricos y magnéticos externos en distintas configuraciones. Es necesaria la adición vectorial de las contribuciones fuera de fase y con variaciones espaciales de los campos eléctricos y magnéticos para evaluar el cumplimiento de las restricciones básicas.

Son muy pocos los cálculos que se han realizado sobre modelos avanzados de la mujer embarazada y el feto con modelos anatómicos apropiados. Es importante evaluar el posible aumento de la inducción de campos eléctricos en el feto en relación con el tema de la leucemia infantil. En este sentido son importantes la exposición ocupacional materna y residencial.

Existe la necesidad de seguir perfeccionando los modelos microdosimétricos, con el objetivo de tener en cuenta la estructura celular de las redes neurales y otros sistemas suborgánicos complejos identificados como más sensibles a los efectos de los campos eléctricos inducidos. En este proceso de modelamiento también se debe tener presente la influencia en los potenciales eléctricos de la membrana celular y en la liberación de neurotransmisores.

### 18.2.3 Mecanismos biofísicos

Existen tres áreas principales en los que son evidentes los límites del entendimiento actual de los mecanismos: el mecanismo par radical, las partículas magnéticas en el cuerpo y la relación señal a ruido en los sistemas multicelulares, tales como las redes neuronales.

El mecanismo par radical es uno de los mecanismos más verosímiles de interacción de bajo nivel, pero todavía no se ha demostrado que es capaz de mediar efectos significativos en el metabolismo y la función celular. Es particularmente importante entender el límite inferior de exposición al cual actúa, de manera que se pueda determinar si puede ser o no un mecanismo importante para la carcinogénesis. Teniendo en cuenta los estudios recientes en los que aumentaron las especies de oxígeno reactivo en células inmunitarias expuestas a campos de ELF, se recomienda el empleo de células del sistema inmunológico que generan especies de oxígeno reactivo como parte de su respuesta inmunitaria como modelos celulares para investigar el potencial del mecanismo par radical.

Aunque, de acuerdo con las evidencias actuales, la presencia de partículas magnéticas (cristales de magnetita) en el cerebro humano no parece conferir sensibilidad a los campos magnéticos de ELF del ambiente, se deberían explorar más enfoques teóricos y experimentales para estudiar si tal sensibilidad puede existir bajo determinadas condiciones. Además, se debería buscar cualquier modificación que pueda introducir la presencia de magnetita en el mecanismo par radical antes mencionado.

Se debe seguir investigando en qué medida actúan mecanismos multicelulares en el cerebro, de manera que mejoren las relaciones señal a ruido, a fin de desarrollar un marco teórico para su cuantificación o para determinar sus posibles límites. Se debe realizar investigación adicional del umbral y la respuesta de frecuencia de las redes neuronales en el hipocampo y en otras partes del cerebro utilizando métodos in vitro.

### 18.2.4 Neurocomportamiento

Se recomienda que los estudios de laboratorio basados en voluntarios sobre los posibles efectos en el sueño y en la realización de tareas que exijan un esfuerzo mental grande se lleven a cabo utilizando procedimientos metodológicos armonizados. Es necesario identificar las relaciones dosis-respuesta con densidades de flujo magnético superiores a las utilizadas anteriormente y con una gama amplia de frecuencias (es decir, en el rango de los kilohertz).

Los estudios realizados en voluntarios adultos y en animales sugieren que pueden producirse efectos cognitivos agudos con exposiciones de corto plazo a campos eléctricos o magnéticos intensos. La caracterización de tales efectos es muy importante para el desarrollo de orientación sobre la exposición, pero se carece de datos específicos concernientes a efectos dependientes del campo en niños. Se recomienda la realización de estudios de laboratorio en la cognición y los cambios en los electroencefalogramas (EEG) en personas expuestas a campos de ELF, incluyendo adultos sujetos habitualmente a exposición ocupacional y niños.

Los estudios de comportamiento con animales inmaduros proporcionan un indicador útil de los posibles efectos cognitivos en los niños. Se deben estudiar los posibles efectos de la exposición prenatal y postnatal a campos magnéticos de ELF en el desarrollo del sistema nervioso y la función cognitiva. Sería útil complementar estos estudios con investigaciones sobre los efectos de la exposición a campos magnéticos de ELF y campos eléctricos inducidos en el crecimiento de las células nerviosas, utilizando rebanadas de cerebro o neuronas cultivadas.

Es necesario seguir investigando las consecuencias potenciales en la salud sugeridas por los datos experimentales que muestran respuestas opioides y colinérgicas en animales. Se deberian ampliar los estudios en los que se examina la modulación de las respuestas opioides y colinérgicas en animales y se debería definir los parámetros de exposición y la base biológica de estas respuestas de comportamiento.

### 18.2.5 Sistema neuroendocrino

La base de datos existente sobre la respuesta neuroendocrina no indica que la exposición a campos de ELF tenga impactos adversos en la salud humana. Por consiguiente, no se formula ninguna recomendación para nuevas investigaciones.

### 18.2.6 Trastornos neurodegenerativos

En varios estudios se ha observado un aumento del riesgo de esclerosis lateral amiotrófica en las "ocupaciones eléctricas". Se considera importante realizar más investigación de esta asociación, a fin de descubrir si los campos magnéticos de ELF intervienen como causa de esta rara enfermedad neurodegenerativa. Esta investigación requiere estudios prospectivos de cohortes de gran envergadura con información sobre la exposición a campos magnéticos de ELF, a choques eléctricos así como exposición a otros posibles factores de riesgo.

Sigue siendo discutible si los campos magnéticos de ELF constituyen un factor de riesgo para la enfermedad de Alzheimer. Los datos disponibles en la actualidad no son suficientes, por lo que habría que estudiar más esta asociación. Tiene particular importancia el uso de datos sobre la morbilidad más que sobre la mortalidad.

### 18.2.7 Trastornos cardiovasculares

No se considera prioritaria la realización de investigaciones adicionales sobre la asociación entre los campos magnéticos de ELF y el riesgo de enfermedades cardiovasculares.

### 18.2.8　Inmunología y hematología

Los cambios observados en los parámetros inmunológicos y hematológicos en adultos expuestos a campos magnéticos de ELF mostraron inconsistencias, y esencialmente no se dispone de datos de investigación sobre niños. Por consiguiente, se recomienda la realización de estudios sobre los efectos de la exposición a campos de ELF en el desarrollo de los sistemas inmunológicos y hematopoyético en animales jóvenes.

### 18.2.9　Reproducción y desarrollo

Existen algunas evidencias de un aumento del riesgo de aborto asociado con la exposición a campos magnéticos de ELF. Teniendo en cuenta las repercusiones potencialmente elevadas de dicha asociación para la salud pública se recomienda la realización de nuevas investigaciones epidemiológicas.

### 18.2.10　Cáncer

La máxima prioridad de las investigaciones en esta área corresponde a la solución del conflicto entre los datos epidemiológicos (que muestran una asociación entre la exposición a campos magnéticos de ELF y un aumento del riesgo de leucemia infantil) y los datos experimentales y mecanísticos (que no respaldan esta asociación). Se recomienda la colaboración de epidemiólogos y científicos experimentales en este sentido. Para que los nuevos estudios epidemiológicos sean ilustrativos, se deben concentrar en nuevos aspectos de la exposición, en la interacción potencial con otros factores o en grupos muy expuestos, o bien introducir alguna otra innovación en esta esfera de investigación. Además, se recomienda también la actualización de los análisis combinados existentes, añadiendo datos de estudios recientes y aplicando nuevos conocimientos dentro del análisis.

En los estudios sobre el cáncer cerebral infantil se han obtenido resultados inconsistentes. Al igual con la leucemia infantil, el análisis de los estudios combinados sobre el cáncer cerebral infantil sería muy informativo, por lo que se recomienda. Un análisis de este tipo puede proporcionar sin grandes gastos mayor y mejor información sobre los datos existentes, incluyendo la posibilidad del sesgo de selección, y si los estudios son suficientemente homogéneos puede ofrecer la mejor estimación de riesgo.

En el caso del cáncer de mama en adultos, estudios más recientes han mostrado de manera convincente que no existe ninguna asociación con la exposición a campos magnéticos de ELF. Por consiguiente, la investigación adicional sobre esta asociación debe ser objeto de una prioridad muy baja.

En relación con la leucemia y el cáncer cerebral en adultos, se recomienda la actualización de las cohortes de gran envergadura existentes de personas expuestas ocupacionalmente. Los estudios ocupacionales, los análisis combinados y los metaanálisis para la leucemia y el cáncer cerebral han sido inconsistentes y no concluyentes. Sin embargo, posteriormente se han publicado nuevos datos que deberían utilizarse para actualizar estos análisis.

Se ha de conceder prioridad al abordar las evidencias epidemiológicas, mediante el establecimiento de modelos in vitro y animales apropiados para las respuestas a campos magnéticos de ELF de bajo nivel que sean ampliamente transferibles entre laboratorios.

Se deben desarrollar modelos de roedores transgénicos para la leucemia infantil, a fin de disponer de modelos de animales experimentales apropiados para estudiar los efectos de la exposición a campos magnéticos de ELF. De otra manera, para los estudios existentes en animales el peso de la evidencia es que no existen efectos carcinogénicos provenientes de los campos magnéticos de ELF actuando por sí solos. Por consiguiente, se debe conceder máxima prioridad a los estudios in vitro y en animales en los que se evalúen rigurosamente los campos magnéticos de ELF como cocarcinógenos.

Con respecto a otros estudios in vitro, se deben repetir los experimentos en los que se reportan los efectos genotóxicos de una exposición intermitente a campos magnéticos de ELF.

### 18.2.11 Medidas de protección

Se recomienda la realización de investigaciones sobre la formulación de políticas de protección de la salud y su aplicación en sectores con incertidumbre científica, en concreto sobre el uso del principio de precaución, su interpretación y la evaluación del impacto de las medidas de precaución para campos magnéticos de ELF y otros agentes clasificados como "posibles carcinógenos para los seres humanos". Cuando existen incertidumbres acerca del riesgo potencial para la salud que un agente plantea para la sociedad, medidas de precaución que pueden estar justificadas, a fin de asegurar la protección adecuada del público y los trabajadores. Son limitadas las investigaciones que se han realizado sobre este tema para campos magnéticos de ELF y, debido a su importancia, es necesario seguir investigando. Esto puede ayudar a los países a integrar el principio de precaución en sus políticas de protección de la salud.

Se aconsejan nuevas investigaciones sobre la percepción y comunicación del riesgo orientadas específicamente a los campos electromagnéticos. Se han investigado ampliamente los factores psicológicos y sociológicos que influyen en la percepción del riesgo en general. Sin embargo, han sido limitadas las investigaciones para analizar la importancia relativa de estos factores en el caso de los campos electromagnéticos o para identificar otros factores específicos de dichos campos. En estudios recientes se ha sugerido que las medidas de precaución que transmiten mensajes de riesgo implícitos pueden modificar la percepción del riesgo, aumentando o disminuyendo la preocupación. Por consiguiente, está justificada una investigación más profunda sobre este tema.

Se debe realizar la investigación sobre el desarrollo de un análisis de costo-beneficio / costo-efectividad para la mitigación de los campos magnéticos de ELF. El empleo del análisis de costo-beneficio y costo-efectividad para evaluar si una opción en materia de políticas es beneficiosa para la sociedad se ha investigado en muchos sectores de las políticas públicas. Es necesario formular un marco que permita identificar qué parámetros son necesarios a fin de realizar este análisis para campos magnéticos de ELF. Debido a las incertidumbres en la evaluación, se necesitará incorporar parámetros cuantificables y no cuantificables.

**Tabla 1. Recomendaciones para nuevas investigaciones**

| Fuentes, mediciones y exposiciones | Prioridad |
|---|---|
| Caracterización ulterior de los hogares con exposición elevada a campos magnéticos de ELF en distintos países | Media |
| Identificar las brechas en el conocimiento acerca de la exposición ocupacional a campos de ELF, tales como en las IRM | Alta |
| Evaluación de la capacidad de las instalaciones eléctricas residenciales fuera de los Estados Unidos para inducir corrientes de contacto en los niños | Media |
| **Dosimetría** | |
| Dosimetría computacional adicional de la relación de los campos eléctricos y magnéticos externos con los campos eléctricos internos, en particular con respecto a la exposición a campos eléctricos y magnéticos combinados en distintas orientaciones | Media |
| Cálculo de los campos eléctricos y las corrientes inducidos en las mujeres embarazadas y en el feto | Media |
| Mayor perfeccionamiento de los modelos microdosimétricos, teniendo en cuenta la estructura celular de las redes neurales y otros sistemas suborgánicos complejos | Media |
| **Mecanismos biofísicos** | |
| Mayor estudio de los mecanismos par radical en las células inmunitarias que generan especies de oxígeno reactivo como parte de su función fenotípica | Media |
| Nuevos estudios teóricos y experimentales de la posible función de la magnetita en la sensibilidad a campos magnéticos de ELF | Baja |
| Determinación de las respuestas umbral a campos eléctricos internos inducidos por campos de ELF en sistemas multicelulares, tales como las redes neurales, utilizando enfoques teóricos e in vitro | Alta |
| **Neurocomportamiento** | |
| Estudios de la función cognitiva, el sueño y el electroencefalograma (EEG) en voluntarios, con inclusión de niños y personas ocupacionalmente expuestas, utilizando un amplio rango de frecuencias de campos de ELF con densidades de flujo elevadas | Media |
| Estudios de la exposición prenatal y postnatal en la función cognitiva posterior en animales | Media |
| Nuevos estudios de las respuestas opioides y colinérgicas en animales | Baja |